Missing Data in Clinical Studies

Statistics in Practice

Advisory Editor

Stephen Senn
University of Glasgow, UK

Founding Editor

Vic Barnett
Nottingham Trent University, UK

Statistics in Practice is an important international series of texts which provide detailed coverage of statistical concepts, methods and worked case studies in specific fields of investigation and study.

With sound motivation and many worked practical examples, the books show in down-to-earth terms how to select and use an appropriate range of statistical techniques in a particular practical field within each title's special topic area.

The books provide statistical support for professionals and research workers across a range of employment fields and research environments. Subject areas covered include medicine and pharmaceutics; industry, finance and commerce; public services; the earth and environmental sciences, and so on.

The books also provide support to students studying statistical courses applied to the above areas. The demand for graduates to be equipped for the work environment has led to such courses becoming increasingly prevalent at universities and colleges.

It is our aim to present judiciously chosen and well-written workbooks to meet everyday practical needs. Feedback of views from readers will be most valuable to monitor the success of this aim.

A complete list of titles in this series appears at the end of the volume.

Missing Data in Clinical Studies

Geert Molenberghs
Center for Statistics
Hasselt University
Diepenbeek, Belgium

Michael G. Kenward
Medical Statistics Unit
London School of Hygiene and Tropical Medicine
London, UK

John Wiley & Sons, Ltd

Other Wiley Editorial Offices

John Wiley & Sons Inc., 111 River Street, Hoboken, NJ 07030, USA

Jossey-Bass, 989 Market Street, San Francisco, CA 94103-1741, USA

Wiley-VCH Verlag GmbH, Boschstr. 12, D-69469 Weinheim, Germany

John Wiley & Sons Australia Ltd, 42 McDougall Street, Milton, Queensland 4064, Australia

John Wiley & Sons (Asia) Pte Ltd, 2 Clementi Loop #02-01, Jin Xing Distripark, Singapore 129809

John Wiley & Sons Canada Ltd, 6045 Freemont Blvd, Mississauga, ONT, Canada L5R 4J3

Wiley also publishes its books in a variety of electronic formats. Some content that appears in print may not be available in electronic books.

Anniversary Logo Design: Richard J. Pacifico

British Library Cataloguing in Publication Data

A catalogue record for this book is available from the British Library

ISBN-13 978-0-470-84981-1 (HB)

Typeset in 10/12pt Galliard by Integra Software Services Pvt. Ltd, Pondicherry, India
Printed and bound in Great Britain by TJ International, Padstow, Cornwall
This book is printed on acid-free paper responsibly manufactured from sustainable forestry in which at least two trees are planted for each one used for paper production.

To Conny, An, and Jasper

To Pirkko

Contents

20   Sensitivity Happens   313

21   Regions of Ignorance and Uncertainty   329

22   Local and Global Influence Methods   353

23   The Nature of Local Influence   417

Preface

Three quarters of a century ago, Karl Pearson, Sir Ronald Fisher, Egon Pearson, and a good number of their contemporaries were concerned about the loss of balance that could arise if data collected from carefully designed experiments turned out to be incomplete. Their concern was wholly appropriate in the pre-automated computing era, when balance was an integral part of manageable statistical analyses. Following the Second World War there was a great increase in the development and practice of experimental and observational studies in human subjects. At the same time the regulation of such studies became – quite understandably, with the aberrations of the war fresh in mind – much more strict. Some decades later, the key paper of Rubin (1976) established *incomplete data* as a proper field of study in its own right within the domain of statistics. Subsequent major contributions in this field were the expectation–maximization algorithm (Dempster *et al.* 1977) and multiple imputation (Rubin 1987), to name but two. It can fairly be said that Little and Rubin's (1987) book, the first monograph encompassing the subject, marked the coming of age of the analysis of incomplete data as a field of research.

The intervening two decades have seen a tremendous amount of research output on the problem of missing data. It is possible to distinguish from this output several different strands. First, considerable attention has been paid to the accommodation of incompleteness in epidemiological and clinical studies in a practically accessible manner that provides due protection to the interests of both industry and the general public. This is particularly true for clinical trials within regulatory processes, with a variety of interested parties, including the regulatory authorities, the biopharmaceutical companies, and the clinical investigators, to name but a few, actively contributing to the debate. Second, methodological developments have continued apace, some of a highly sophisticated nature. We can usefully distinguish between a parametric school, essentially of a likelihood and Bayesian nature, with landmark contributions from Don Rubin, Rod Little, and many of their students and collaborators, and a semi-parametric school, built around Horvitz–Thompson and estimating equations ideas, with seminal contributions from Jamie Robins, Andrea Rotnitzky, and a variety of their students and co-workers.

There is noticeable divergence between the various lines of thinking. Ideally, there should be continuing dialogue, ranging from the very applied to the most theoretical researcher in the field, regardless of modelling and inferential preferences. At the same time, there is a broad consensus that no single modelling approach, no matter how sophisticated, can overcome the limitation of simply not having access to the missing data. All parties – academia, industry, and regulatory authorities – stress the need for, and importance of, sensitivity analysis. By this we mean, in a broad sense, the formal or informal assessment of the impact of incompleteness on key statistical inferences. Scientific research, standard operating procedures, and guidelines, such as International Conference on Harmonisation Guideline E9, all point in this same direction. There is considerably less agreement, however, as to how such sensitivity analyses should be conceived, conducted and presented in practice, and this is not surprising given both the early stage of, and feverish activity within, this particular area of missing data research.

A key prerequisite for a method to be embraced, no matter how important, is the availability of trustworthy and easy-to-use software, preferably in commercially or otherwise generally accessible *bona fide* packages. It is not an exaggeration to claim that the last decade has seen tremendous progress on this front. Such methods and techniques as direct likelihood and Bayesian analysis, multiple imputation, the expectation–maximization algorithm, and weighted estimating equations are appearing in SAS, Stata, S-Plus, R, and various other mainstream statistical packages.

These observations, developed through numerous lectures, shorter and longer courses, and through statistical consultancy with academic, biopharmaceutical, and governmental partners, led to the conception of this book. The opportunity to interact with audiences of various backgrounds and with a broad range of interests, across the globe, has been an invaluable educational experience for us. In turn, we hope the book will be of value to a wide audience, including applied statisticians and biomedical researchers, in particular in the biopharmaceutical industry, medical and public health research organizations, contract research organizations, and academic departments. We have chosen an explanatory rather than a research-oriented style of exposition, even though some chapters contain advanced material. A perspective is given in Chapter 1. We focus on practice rather than on mathematical rigour, and this is reflected in the large number of worked examples dotted throughout the text.

Many of the statistical analyses have been performed using such SAS procedures as MIXED, GENMOD, GLIMMIX, NLMIXED, MI, and MIANALYZE, with the addition of user-defined SAS macros, as well as functions in other packages, such as GAUSS, where the necessary facilities have not yet been implemented elsewhere. In spite of this, the methodological development and the analyses of the case studies alike are presented in a software-independent fashion. Illustrations on how to use SAS for a selected collection of model strategies are confined to a small number of chapters and sections, implying that the text can be read without problem if these software excursions are ignored. Selected programs, macros, output, and publicly available data sets can be found on Wiley's website, as well as on the authors' site (www.uhasselt.be/censtat).

Geert Molenberghs (Diepenbeek) and Michael G. Kenward (London)

Acknowledgements

This text has benefited tremendously from stimulating interaction and joint work with a number of colleagues. We are grateful to many for their kind permission to use their data. We gratefully acknowledge the support of: Marc Aerts (Universiteit Hasselt, Diepenbeek), Caroline Beunckens (Universiteit Hasselt, Diepenbeek), Luc Bijnens (Johnson & Johnson Pharmaceutical Research and Development, Beerse), Marc Buyse (International Drug Development Institute, Ottignies-Louvain-la-Neuve), James Carpenter (London School of Hygiene and Tropical Medicine), Raymond Carroll (Texas A&M University, College Station), Desmond Curran (Icon Clinical Research, Dublin), Stephen Evans (London School of Hygiene and Tropical Medicine), Garrett Fitzmaurice (Harvard School of Public Health, Boston), Els Goetghebeur (Universiteit Gent), Niel Hens (Universiteit Hasselt, Diepenbeek), Joseph Ibrahim (University of North Carolina, Chapell Hill), Ivy Jansen (Universiteit Hasselt, Diepenbeek), Emmanuel Lesaffre (Katholieke Universiteit Leuven), Stuart Lipsitz (Harvard School of Public Health, Boston), Rod Little (University of Michigan, Ann Arbor), Craig Mallinckrodt (Eli Lilly & Company, Indianapolis), Bart Michiels (Johnson & Johnson Pharmaceutical Research and Development, Beerse), James Roger (GlaxoSmithKline), Cristina Sotto (Universiteit Hasselt, Diepenbeek), Herbert Thijs (Universiteit Hasselt, Diepenbeek), Butch Tsiatis (North Carolina State University, Raleigh), Tony Vangeneugden (Tibotec, Mechelen), Stijn Vansteelandt (Universiteit Gent), Kristel Van Steen (Universiteit Gent), and Geert Verbeke (Katholieke Universiteit Leuven).

The feedback we received from our regular and short course audiences has been invaluable. We are grateful for such interactions in Argentina (Corrientes), Australia (Cairns, Coolangatta), Belgium (Beerse, Braine-l'Alleud, Brussels, Diepenbeek, Gent, Leuven, Wavre), Brazil (Londrina, Piracicaba), Canada (Toronto), Cuba (Havana, Varadero), Denmark (Copenhagen), Finland (Jokioinen, Tampere, Turku), France (Paris, Marseille, Toulouse, Vannes), Germany (Freiburg, Heidelberg), Greece (Athens), Ireland (Dublin), Korea (Seoul), the Netherlands (Rotterdam), New Zealand (Auckland, Christchurch, Hamilton), Spain (Barcelona, Pamplona, Santiago de Compostela), South Africa (Stellenbosch), Switzerland (Neuchâtel, Basle), the United Kingdom

(London, Manchester, Harlow, Sandwich, Stevenage, Sunningdale), and the United States of America (Ann Arbor, Arlington, Atlanta, Atlantic City, Minneapolis, New Jersey, New York City, Rockville, San Francisco, Seattle, Tampa, Washington, DC).

Several people have helped us with the computational side of the models presented. We mention in particular Caroline Beunckens, Ivy Jansen, Bart Michiels, Oliver Schabenberger (SAS Institute, Cary, North Carolina), Cristina Sotto, Herbert Thijs, and Kristel Van Steen.

We gratefully acknowledge support from Research Project Fonds voor We-tenschappelijk Onderzoek Vlaanderen G.0002.98, 'Sensitivity Analysis for Incomplete Data', NATO Collaborative Research Grant CRG 950648, 'Statistical Research for Environmental Risk Assessment', Belgian IUAP/PAI network 'Statistical Techniques and Modeling for Complex Substantive Questions with Complex Data', and US grants HL 69800, AHRQ 10871, HL 52329, HL 61769, GM 29745, MH 54693, CA 57030 and CA 70101 from the US National Institutes of Health, the Texas A&M Center for Environmental and Rural Health via a grant from the National Institute of Environmental Health Sciences (P3–ES09106), from the UK Economic and Social Research Council and National Health Service Research and Development Methodology Programme.

All along, it has been a fine experience working with our colleagues at John Wiley.

We are indebted to Conny, An, Jasper, and Pirkko, for their understanding and for time not spent with them while preparing this volume. Working on this book has been a period of close collaboration and stimulating exchange, which we will remember with affection for years to come.

Geert and Mike
Kessel-Lo, Belgium and Luton, England
September 2006

Part I
Preliminaries

1

Introduction

In this chapter we give a broad introduction to the problem of missing data. We provide a perspective on the topic, reviewing the main developments of the last century (Section 1.1), in the process paying special attention to the setting of clinical studies (Section 1.2). We examine the move towards more principled approaches, more elaborate modelling strategies and, most recently, the important role of sensitivity analysis (Section 1.3). Finally, we map out the developments and material that make up rest of the book (Section 1.4). In the next chapter we introduce the key sets of data that will be used throughout the book to illustrate the analyses.

1.1 FROM IMBALANCE TO THE FIELD OF MISSING DATA RESEARCH

It is very common for sets of quantitative data to be incomplete, in the sense that not all planned observations are actually made. This is especially true when studies are conducted on human subjects. Examples abound in epidemiologic studies (Piantadosi 1997; Clayton and Hills 1993; Green *et al.* 1997; Friedman *et al.* 1998), in clinical trials (Kahn and Sempos 1989; Lilienfeld and Stolley 1994; Selvin 1996), and in the social sciences, especially in sample surveys, psychometry, and econometrics (Fowler 1988, Schafer *et al.* 1993; Rubin 1987; Rubin *et al.* 1995), to name but a few areas.

Our focus in this book is on intervention-based clinical studies. We mean this in an inclusive sense, however, implying that the methodology presented may be appropriate outside this setting, for example in the context of epidemiological studies as well as experimental and observational data in non-human life sciences, including agricultural, biological, and environmental research.

Missing Data in Clinical Studies   G. Molenberghs and M.G. Kenward
© 2007 John Wiley & Sons, Ltd

Early work on the problem of missing data, especially during the 1920s and 1930s, was largely confined to algorithmic and computational solutions to the induced lack of balance or deviations from the intended study design. See, for example, the reviews by Afifi and Elashoff (1966) and Hartley and Hocking (1971). In the last quarter of the twentieth century, general algorithms, such as the expectation–maximization (EM: Dempster *et al.* 1977), and data imputation and augmentation procedures (Rubin 1987; Tanner and Wong 1987), combined with powerful computing resources, largely provided a solution to this aspect of the problem.

Rubin (1976) provided a formal framework for the field of incomplete data by introducing the important taxonomy of missing data mechanisms, consisting of *missing completely at random* (MCAR), *missing at random* (MAR), and *missing not at random* (MNAR). An MCAR mechanism potentially depends on observed covariates, but not on observed or unobserved outcomes. An MAR mechanism depends on the observed outcomes and perhaps also on the covariates, but not further on unobserved measurements. Finally, when an MNAR mechanism is operating, missingness does depend on unobserved measurements, perhaps in addition to dependencies on covariates and/or on observed outcomes. During the same era, the *selection model*, *pattern-mixture model*, and *shared-parameter model* frameworks were established. These are depicted schematically in Figure 1.1. In a selection model, the joint distribution of the ith subject's outcomes, denoted $\boldsymbol{Y}_i$, and vector of missingness indicators, written $\boldsymbol{R}_i$, is factored as the marginal outcome distribution and the conditional distribution of $\boldsymbol{R}_i$ given $\boldsymbol{Y}_i$. A pattern-mixture approach starts from the reverse factorization. In a shared-parameter model, a set of latent variables, latent classes, and/or random effects is assumed to drive both the $\boldsymbol{Y}_i$ and $\boldsymbol{R}_i$ processes. An important version of such a model further asserts that, conditional on the latent variables, $\boldsymbol{Y}_i$ and $\boldsymbol{R}_i$ exhibit no further dependence. Rubin (1976) contributed the concept of *ignorability*, stating that under precise conditions, the missing data mechanism can be ignored when interest lies in inferences about the measurement process. Combined with regularity conditions, ignorability applies to MCAR and MAR combined, when likelihood or Bayesian inference routes are chosen, but the stricter MCAR condition is required for frequentist inferences to be generally valid. A final distinction is made between missingness *patterns*. *Dropout* or *attrition* refers to the specific situation, arising in longitudinal studies, where subjects are observed without uninterruption from the beginning of the study until a given point in time, perhaps prior to the scheduled end of the study, when they drop out and do not return to the study. Given a rather strong focus in this book on longitudinal studies, dropout, an indicator of which is denoted by D_i, will occupy a prominent position. The general mechanism, where subjects can be observed and missing on any partition of the set of planned measurement occasions, is often called *non-monotone*

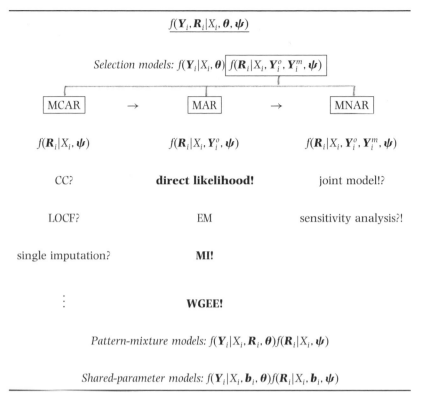

Figure 1.1 Schematic representation of the missing data frameworks and mechanisms, together with simple and more advanced methods, as well as sensitivity analysis. (MCAR, missing completely at random; MAR, missing at random; MNAR, missing not at random; CC, complete case analysis; LOCF, last observation carried forward; EM, expectation–maximization algorithm; MI, multiple imputation; WGEE, weighted generalized estimating equations.)

missingness. These and additional concepts are formalized and expanded upon in Chapter 3.

1.2 INCOMPLETE DATA IN CLINICAL STUDIES

In clinical trials, dropout is not only a common occurrence, there are also specific procedures for reporting and subsequently dealing with it. Patients who drop out of a clinical trial are usually listed on a separate withdrawal sheet of the case record form, with the reasons for withdrawal entered by the authorized investigator. Reasons frequently encountered are adverse events, illness not related to study medication, an uncooperative patient, protocol violation, and ineffective study medication. Further specifications may include so-called *loss to follow-up*. Based on this medically inspired typology, Gould (1980) proposed specific methods to handle this type of incompleteness.

Even though the primary focus of such trials is often on a specific time of measurement, usually the last, the outcome of interest is recorded in a longitudinal fashion, and dropout is a common occurrence. While dropout, in contrast to non-monotone missingness, may simplify model formulation and manipulation, the causes behind it can be more problematic. For example, dropout may derive from lack of efficacy, or from potentially serious and possible treatment-related side effects. In contrast, an intermittently missing endpoint value may be due more plausibly to the patient skipping a visit for practical or administrative reasons, to measurement equipment failure, and so on. In addition, one often sees that incomplete sequences in clinical trials are, for the vast majority, of a dropout type, with a relatively minor fraction of incompletely observed patients producing non-monotone sequences. For all of these reasons we will put major emphasis on the problem of dropout, although not entirely neglecting non-monotone missingness in the process.

In a strict sense the conventional justification for the analysis of data from a randomized trial is removed when data are missing for reasons outside the control of the investigator. Before one can address this problem, however, it is necessary to establish clearly the purpose of the study (Heyting *et al.* 1992). If one is working within a *pragmatic* setting, the event of dropout, for example, may well be a legitimate component of the response. It may make little sense to ask what response the subject would have shown had they remained on study, and the investigator may then require a description of the response *conditional* on a subject remaining in the trial. This, together with the pattern of missingness encountered, may then be the appropriate and valid summary of the outcome. We might call this a conditional description. Shih and Quan (1997) argue that such a description will be of more relevance in many clinical trials. On the other hand, from a more *explanatory* perspective, one might be interested in the behaviour of the responses that occurred irrespective of whether we were able to record them or not. This might be termed a *marginal* description of the response. For a further discussion of intention to treat and explanatory analyses in the context of dropout see Heyting *et al.* (1992) and Little and Yau (1996), as well as Section 4.5 of this volume. It is commonly suggested (Shih and Quan 1997) that such a marginal representation is not meaningful when the nature of dropout (e.g., death) means that the response cannot subsequently exist, irrespective of whether it is measured. While such dropout may in any particular setting imply that a marginal model is not helpful, it does not imply that it necessarily has no meaning. Provided that the underlying model does not attach a probability of one to dropout for a particular patient, then non-dropout and subsequent observations are an outcome consistent with the model and logically no different from any other event in a probability model. Such distinctions, particularly with respect to the conditional analysis, are complicated by the inevitable mixture of causes behind missing values. The conditional description is a mirror of what has been observed, and so its validity is less of an issue than its interpretation. In contrast, other methods of handling incompleteness make some correction or adjustment to what has been directly observed, and therefore address questions other than those corresponding to the conditional setting. In seeking to understand the validity of these analyses we need to compare their consequences with their aims.

Two simple, common approaches to analysis are (1) to discard subjects with incomplete sequences and (2) simple imputation. The first approach has the advantage of simplicity, although the wide availability of more sophisticated methods of analysis minimizes the significance of this. It is also an inefficient use of information. In a trivial sense it provides a description of the response conditional on a subject remaining in the trial. Whether this reflects a response of interest depends entirely on the mechanism(s) generating the missing values and the aims of the trial. It is not difficult to envisage situations where it can be very misleading, and examples of this exist in the literature (Kenward *et al.* 1994, Wang-Clow *et al.* 1995). Such imputation methods share the same drawbacks, although not all to the same degree. The data set that results will mimic a sample from the population of interest, itself determined by the aims of the analysis, only under particular and potentially unrealistic assumptions. Further, these assumptions depend critically on the missing value mechanism(s). For example, under certain dropout mechanisms the process of imputation may recover the actual marginal behaviour required while under other mechanisms it may be wildly misleading, and it is only under the simplest and most ignorable mechanisms that the relationship between imputation procedure and assumption is easily deduced. Little (1994a) gives two simple examples where the relationship is clear.

We therefore see that when there are missing values, simple methods of analysis do not necessarily imply simple, or even accessible, assumptions, and without understanding properly the assumptions being made in an analysis we are not in a position to judge its validity or value. It has been argued that while any particular *ad hoc* analysis may not represent the true picture behind the data, a collection of such analyses should provide a reasonable envelope within which the truth should lie. Even this claim is open to major criticisms, however, and we return to such ideas when sensitivity analyses are considered in Part III. In Chapter 4, after formally introducing of terminology and the necessary frameworks in Chapter 3, we provide a detailed examination of the advantages and drawbacks of simple methods, especially with a view to clinical trial practice.

As we explain in Chapter 4, it is unfortunate that so much emphasis has been given to methods such as *last observation carried forward* (LOCF), *complete case analysis* (CC), or simple forms of imputation. These are *ad hoc* methods defined *procedurally* in terms of manipulation of the data, rather than derived in a statistically principled way from the design of the trial and the aims of the analysis. As a consequence the relationship between their validity and underlying assumptions can be far from clear and, when the relevant assumptions *can* be identified, they are seen to be very strong and unrealistic. In the LOCF procedure the missing measurements are replaced by the last one available. In particular, even the strong MCAR assumption does not suffice to guarantee that an LOCF analysis is valid. On the other hand, under MAR, valid inferences can be obtained through a likelihood-based or Bayesian analysis, without the need for modelling the dropout process. As a consequence, one can simply use, for example, linear or generalized linear mixed models (Verbeke and Molenberghs 2000; Molenberghs and Verbeke 2005), without additional complication or effort. This does not imply that these particular analyses are appropriate for all questions that might be asked of trial data, but the clarity of the underlying assumptions means that appropriate modifications can be readily identified when non-MAR analyses are called for, for example with intention to treat (ITT) analyses when dropout is associated with termination of treatment.

We will argue in Chapter 4, through the cases studies in Chapters 5 and 6, and then further throughout Part III, that such MAR-based likelihood analyses not only enjoy much wider validity than the simple methods but, moreover, are simple to conduct, *without additional data manipulation*, using such tools as the SAS procedures MIXED, GLIMMIX, or NLMIXED. Thus, clinical trial practice should shift away from the *ad hoc* methods and focus on likelihood-based ignorable primary analyses instead. As will be argued further, the cost involved in having to specify a model will arguably be mild to moderate in realistic clinical trial settings. Thus, we promote the use of direct likelihood ignorable methods and demote the use of the LOCF and CC approaches. Mallinckrodt *et al.* (2003a, 2003b), Molenberghs *et al.* (2004), and Lavori *et al.* (1995) propose direct likelihood and multiple imputation methods, respectively, to deal with incomplete longitudinal data. Siddiqui and Ali (1998) compare direct likelihood and LOCF methods.

1.3   MAR, MNAR, AND SENSITIVITY ANALYSIS

From the previous section, it is clear that not only is it advisable to avoid simple *ad hoc* methods such as complete case analysis and last observation carried forward, but there exists more appropriate flexible, broadly valid and widely implemented methodology. Principled methods and techniques such as direct likelihood and Bayesian analyses, the EM algorithm, multiple imputation, and weighted generalized estimating equations are systematically reviewed in Part IV. All of these methods are valid under the relatively relaxed assumption of MAR.

At the same time, it is important to consider reasons for departures from MAR, and the possible consequences of this for the conclusions reached. One obvious example, mentioned above, concerns treatment termination among dropouts in an ITT analysis. More generally, the reasons for, and implications of, dropout are varied and it is therefore difficult, in fact usually impossible, to fully justify on a priori grounds the assumption of MAR. At first sight, this suggest a need for MNAR models. However, some careful considerations have to be made, the most important one of which is that no modelling approach, whether either MAR or MNAR, can recover the lack of information that occurs due to incompleteness of the data. These and related issues are given detailed treatment in Part IV.

An important feature of statistical modelling in the incomplete data setting is that the quality of the fit to the observed data need not reflect at all the appropriateness of the implied structure governing the unobserved data. This point is independent of the MNAR route taken, whether a parametric model of the type of Diggle and Kenward (1994) is chosen, or a semi-parametric approach such as in Robins *et al.* (1998). Hence in any incomplete data setting there cannot be anything that could be called a definitive analysis. Based on these considerations, it is advisable that, for primary analysis purposes, ignorable (MAR) likelihood-based methods be used. To explore the impact of deviations from the MAR assumption on the conclusions, one should then ideally conduct a sensitivity analysis, within which MNAR models can play a major role. The context of the trial and its aims can then be used to guide the choice of departures from MAR to explore in this sensitivity analysis.

The methods and strategies mentioned here have been added to Figure 1.1.

1.4   OUTLINE OF THE BOOK

In this book we place a strong emphasis on practical applications, and therefore we give more consideration to the explanation and illustration of concepts, and to proposing practicable modelling strategies, than to mathematical rigour. Excellent, rigorous accounts of missing data methodology can be found in Little and Rubin (1987, 2002), van der Laan and Robins (2003), and Tsiatis (2006). For these reasons, case studies feature prominently. In Chapter 2 we introduce a set of nine. The chapter also lists the places in the book where these sets of data are analysed so, if desired, their analyses can be followed in a step-by-step manner. In this chapter we also introduce eight additional examples which are used to further illustrate a range of points throughout the book.

In the final chapter of Part I we formalize the terminology, taxonomy, mechanisms, and frameworks introduced earlier in this chapter. This puts us in a position to provide a discussion of commonly used approaches in Part II and to provide a case for the need for a principled modelling approach (Chapter 4). The ideas laid down in this chapter are illustrated by means of two case studies, the orthodontic growth data (Chapter 5) and a series of depression trials (Chapter 6).

The MAR missingness mechanism, in particular in conjunction with ignorability, is the central idea in Part III. In Chapters 7, 8, and 9 we deal with the direct likelihood approach, the EM algorithm, and multiple imputation. All three have a likelihood (or Bayesian) basis. The semi-parametric weighted generalized estimating equations (WGEE) technique is discussed in Chapter 10. In spite of their different background, it is appealing to combine multiple imputation and WGEE ideas (Chapter 11). A tangential but nevertheless interesting caveat in the direct likelihood method, originating from the frequentist nature of some inferences surrounding the likelihood, is the subject of Chapter 12. This part of the book concludes with the analysis of a case study in ophthalmology (Chapter 13) and an overview of how the methods dealt with in earlier chapters can be implemented using the SAS software system (Chapter 14).

In Part IV we explore modelling strategies available under MNAR, organized by modelling framework: selection models in Chapter 15, pattern-mixture models in Chapter 16, and shared-parameter models in Chapter 17. The specialized topic of protective estimation, referring to mechanisms where missingness depends on unobserved but not on observed outcomes, is studied in Chapter 18.

In Part V we turn to the very important subject of sensitivity analysis. This can roughly be divided into two. First, in Chapters 19 and 20, we use a variety of arguments to illustrate the nature of sensitivity when data are incompletely observed, and provide some arguments as to why this is the case. Second, a number of sensitivity analysis tools are presented. In Chapter 21 we are concerned with the so-called *region of ignorance* and *region of uncertainty* concepts, while in Chapter 22 we develop in some detail methods based on local and global influence. The nature and behaviour of local influence are further scrutinized in Chapter 23. In Chapter 24 we bring together selection, pattern-mixture, and shared-parameter model concepts in what is called a latent-class mixture model.

The concluding chapters that make up Part VI report on two case studies. In Chapter 25 the opthalmology trial of Chapter 13 is revisited and subjected to a variety of analyses including assessment of sensitivity. In Chapter 26 we analyse quality-of-life data from a clinical trial with breast cancer patients.

We must emphasize that, in keeping with the theme of the book, our coverage should not in any sense be considered complete. The field of missing data is rapidly evolving, especially in the areas of more complex modelling strategies and sensitivity analysis. Therefore, we have settled for a wide range of instances of the various methods, selected because they make important points and/or can be used in practice. Throughout, we refer to key review papers, where the interested reader can often find more ample detail and further techniques not treated in this volume.

2

Key Examples

2.1 INTRODUCTION

In this chapter, nine key examples are introduced and explored to various degrees. Most, but not all, are clinical studies. Exceptions are the mastitis in dairy cattle data (Section 2.4) and the Slovenian public opinion survey case study (Section 2.10). The orthodontic growth data set, introduced in Section 2.3, while conducted in human subjects, is of more of an epidemiological nature. The others, the vorozole study (Section 2.2), the depression trials (Section 2.5), the fluvoxamine trial (Section 2.6), the toenail data (Section 2.7), the age-related macular degeneration trial (Section 2.8), and the analgesic trial (Section 2.9), are clinical studies. These examples have been selected for introduction in this chapter because they are either very illustrative for the kinds of data problems with which the book is concerned, and/or because they are analysed multiple times throughout the book.

Next to these nine key examples, a further set of eight examples can be found throughout the text. For ease of reference, we itemize them here. The Muscatine coronary risk factor study is analysed in Section 12.7. The Crépeau data, a halothane experiment in rats, are discussed in Section 12.8. A study in tinea pedis patients is reported in Section 15.4.3. In Chapter 18, two further analyses can be found: one related to the presence versus absence of colds (Section 18.3.6), the other the so-called six cities study (Section 18.4.3). Section 21.2 reports on the prevalence of HIV in Kenya. In Section 22.5, protein contents in dairy cattle are of interest. Finally, Sections 23.2 and 23.3 are devoted to the analysis of an anaesthesia study in rats.

In addition to the 17 real data sets listed, a number of points are made using various sets of artificial data. These can be found in Sections 8.7, 18.3.4, and 21.8.

Missing Data in Clinical Studies   G. Molenberghs and M.G. Kenward
© 2007 John Wiley & Sons, Ltd

2.2 THE VOROZOLE STUDY

This study was an open-label, multicentre, parallel group design conducted at 67 North American centres. Patients were randomized to either the new drug vorozole (2.5 mg taken once daily) or the standard drug megestrol acetate (40 mg four times daily). The patient population consisted of postmenopausal patients with histologically confirmed oestrogen-receptor positive metastatic breast carcinoma. All 452 randomized patients were followed until disease progression or death. The main objective was to compare the treatment groups with respect to response rate, whereas secondary objectives included a comparison relative to duration of response, time to progression, survival, safety, pain relief, performance status, and quality of life. Full details of this study are reported in Goss *et al.* (1999). In this book, we will focus on overall quality of life, measured by the total Functional Living Index: Cancer (FLIC: Schipper *et al.* 1984) – a higher FLIC score is the more desirable outcome. Even though this outcome is, strictly speaking, of the ordinal type, the total number of categories encountered exceeds 70, justifying the use of continuous outcome methods.

Patients underwent screening and, for those deemed eligible, a detailed examination at baseline (occasion 0) took place. Further measurement occasions were month 1, then from month 2 at bimonthly intervals until month 44.

Goss *et al.* (1999) analysed FLIC using a two-way analysis of variance (ANOVA) model with effects for treatment, disease status, as well as their interaction. No significant difference was found. Apart from treatment, important covariates are dominant site of the disease as well as clinical stage.

The data are analysed in Section 16.6 and in Chapter 26.

2.3 THE ORTHODONTIC GROWTH DATA

These data, introduced by Pothoff and Roy (1964), contain growth measurements for 11 girls and 16 boys. For each subject, the distance from the centre of the pituitary to the maxillary fissure was recorded at ages 8, 10, 12, and 14. The data were used by Jennrich and Schluchter (1986) to illustrate estimation methods for unbalanced data, where unbalancedness is now to be interpreted in the sense of an unequal number of boys and girls. Individual profiles and sex group by age means are plotted in Figure 2.1.

Little and Rubin (1987) deleted nine of the measurements at age 10, thereby producing nine incomplete subjects. They describe the mechanism to be such that subjects with a low value at age 8 are more likely to have a missing value at age 10. The data are presented in Table 2.1. The measurements that were deleted are marked with an asterisk.

Chapter 5 is devoted to the analysis of these data.

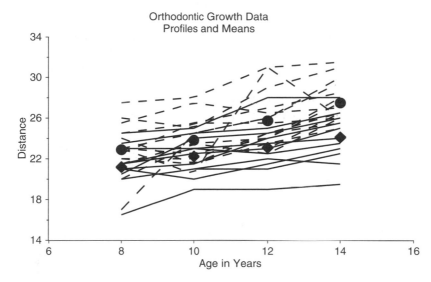

Figure 2.1 Orthodontic growth data. Observed profiles and group by age means. Solid lines and diamonds are for girls, dashed lines and bullets are for boys.

Table 2.1 Orthodontic growth data for 11 girls and 16 boys. Measurements marked * were deleted by Little and Rubin (1987).

	Age (in years)					Age (in years)			
Girl	8	10	12	14	Boy	8	10	12	14
1	21.0	20.0	21.5	23.0	1	26.0	25.0	29.0	31.0
2	21.0	21.5	24.0	25.5	2	21.5	22.5*	23.0	26.5
3	20.5	24.0*	24.5	26.0	3	23.0	22.5	24.0	27.5
4	23.5	24.5	25.0	26.5	4	25.5	27.5	26.5	27.0
5	21.5	23.0	22.5	23.5	5	20.0	23.5*	22.5	26.0
6	20.0	21.0*	21.0	22.5	6	24.5	25.5	27.0	28.5
7	21.5	22.5	23.0	25.0	7	22.0	22.0	24.5	26.5
8	23.0	23.0	23.5	24.0	8	24.0	21.5	24.5	25.5
9	20.0	21.0*	22.0	21.5	9	23.0	20.5	31.0	26.0
10	16.5	19.0*	19.0	19.5	10	27.5	28.0	31.0	31.5
11	24.5	25.0	28.0	28.0	11	23.0	23.0	23.5	25.0
					12	21.5	23.5*	24.0	28.0
					13	17.0	24.5*	26.0	29.5
					14	22.5	25.5	25.5	26.0
					15	23.0	24.5	26.0	30.0
					16	22.0	21.5*	23.5	25.0

Sources: Pothoff and Roy (1964) and Jennrich and Schluchter (1986).

2.4 MASTITIS IN DAIRY CATTLE

This example, concerning the occurrence of the infectious disease mastitis in dairy cows, was introduced in Diggle and Kenward (1994) and reanalysed in Kenward (1998). Data were available on the milk yields in thousands of litres of 107 dairy cows from a single herd in two consecutive years: Y_{ij} ($i = 1, \ldots, 107; j = 1, 2$). In the first year, all animals were supposedly free of mastitis; in the second year, 27 became infected. Mastitis typically reduces milk yield, and the question of scientific interest is whether the probability of occurrence of mastitis is related to the yield that would have been observed had mastitis not occurred. A graphical representation of the complete data is given in Figure 2.2. The data are analysed in Section 22.3.

2.5 THE DEPRESSION TRIALS

These data come from three clinical trials of antidepressants. The three trials contained 167, 342, and 713 patients with post-baseline data, respectively (Mallinckrodt *et al.* 2003b). The Hamilton Depression Rating Scale ($HAMD_{17}$) was used to measure the depression status of the patients. For each patient, a baseline assessment was available. Post-baseline visits differ by study (Table 2.2). Individual profiles of the change in $HAMD_{17}$ score from baseline for the first depression trial are shown in Figure 2.3.

For blinding purposes, therapies are recoded as A1 for primary dose of experimental drug, A2 for secondary dose of experimental drug, and B and C for non-experimental drugs. The treatment arms across the three studies are

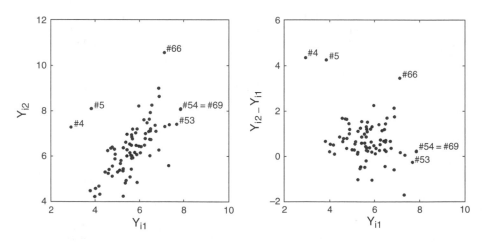

Figure 2.2 Mastitis in dairy cattle. Scatter plots of the second measurement versus the first measurement (left) and of the change versus the baseline measurement (right).

Table 2.2 Depression trials. Overview of number of patients and post-baseline visits per study.

	Number of patients	Numbering of post-baseline visits
Study 1	167	4–11
Study 2	342	4–8
Study 3	713	3–8

as follows: A1, B, and C for study 1; A1, A2, B, and C for study 2; A1 and B for study 3. The primary contrast is between A1 and C for studies 1 and 2, whereas in study 3 one is interested in A versus B.

In this case study, interest is in the difference between the treatment arms in mean change of the $HAMD_{17}$ score at the endpoint. However, as time evolves, more and more patients drop out, resulting in fewer observations for later visits. Indeed, a graphical representation of dropout, by study and by arm, is given in Figure 2.4. Due to this fact, observed mean profiles might be misleading if interpreted without acknowledging the diminishing basis of inference.

The data are analysed in Chapter 6 and then further in Sections 7.6, 10.5, 22.6, and 24.6.

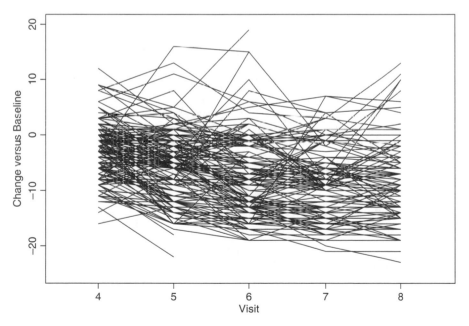

Figure 2.3 Depression trials. Individual profiles (top) and mean profiles by treatment arm (bottom) for the first study.

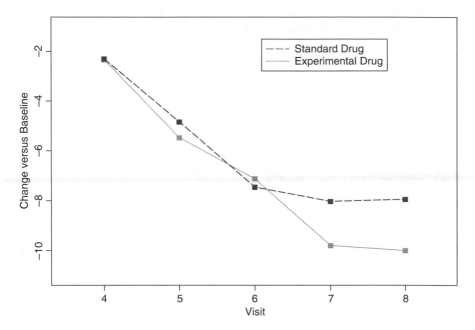

Figure 2.3 *Continued*

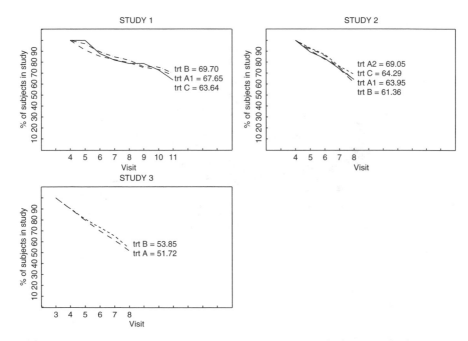

Figure 2.4 Depression trials. Evolution of dropout by study per treatment arm.

2.6   THE FLUVOXAMINE TRIAL

Accumulated experience with fluvoxamine, a serotonin reuptake inhibitor, in controlled clinical trials has shown it to be as effective as conventional antidepressant drugs and more effective than placebo in the treatment of depression (Burton 1991). However, many patients who suffer from depression have concomitant morbidity with conditions such as obsessive-compulsive disorder, anxiety disorders and, to some extent, panic disorders. In most trials, patients with comorbidity are excluded, and therefore, it is of interest to gather evidence as to the importance of such factors, with a view to improved diagnosis and treatment. The general aim of this study was to determine the profile of fluvoxamine in ambulatory clinical psychiatric practice.

A total of 315 patients were enrolled with one or more of the following diagnoses: depression, obsessive-compulsive disorder, and panic disorder. Several covariates were recorded, such as gender and initial severity on a five-point ordinal scale, where severity increases with category. After recruitment of each patient to the study, he or she was investigated at four occasions (weeks 2, 4, 8, and 12). On the basis of about 20 psychiatric symptoms, the therapeutic effect and the side effects were scored at each visit in an ordinal manner. Side effect is coded as: 1 = no; 2 = not interfering with functionality of patient; 3 = interfering significantly with functionality of patient; and 4 = the side effect surpasses the therapeutic effect. Similarly, the effect of therapy is recorded on a four-point ordinal scale: 1 = no improvement over baseline or worsening; 2 = minimal improvement (not changing functionality); 3 = moderate improvement (partial disappearance of symptoms); and 4 = important improvement (near complete disappearance of symptoms). Thus, a side effect occurs if new symptoms occur, while there is therapeutic effect if old symptoms disappear. These data were analysed by, among others, Molenberghs and Lesaffre (1994), Molenberghs *et al.* (1997), Lapp *et al.* (1998), Van Steen *et al.* (2001), and Jansen *et al.* (2003).

Table 2.3 gives the absolute and relative frequencies over the four categories of side effects and therapeutic effect for each of the four follow-up times. Because there are 315 subjects enrolled in the trial, it is clear that at these four times there are 16, 46, 72, and 89 subjects missing, respectively. The missing data patterns, common to both outcomes, are represented in Table 2.4. Note that a much larger fraction is fully observed than in, for example, the analgesic trial (Section 2.9). Among the incomplete sequences, dropout is much more common than intermittent missingness, the latter type confined to two sequences only. Observe that, unlike in Table 2.11, there are subjects, 14 in total, without any follow-up measurements. This group of subjects is still an integral part of the trial, as they contain baseline information, including covariate information and baseline assessment of severity of the mental illness.

The data are extensively analysed in Sections 15.4.2, 15.5.1, 16.8, 18.3.5, 20.4, 21.7, 22.8, and 22.10.

Table 2.3 Fluvoxamine trial. Absolute and relative frequencies of the four side effects and therapeutic effect categories for each of the four follow-up times.

	Week 2		Week 4		Week 8		Week 12	
Side effects								
0	128	42.8%	144	52.5%	156	64.2%	148	65.5%
1	128	42.8%	103	38.3%	79	32.5%	71	31.4%
2	28	9.4%	17	6.3%	6	2.5%	7	3.1%
3	15	5.2%	5	1.9%	2	0.8%	0	0.0%
Therapeutic effects								
0	19	6.4%	64	23.8%	110	45.3%	135	59.7%
1	95	31.8%	114	42.4%	93	38.3%	62	27.4%
2	102	34.1%	62	23.1%	30	12.4%	19	8.4%
3	83	27.8%	29	10.8%	10	4.1%	10	4.4%
Total	299		269		243		226	

Table 2.4 Fluvoxamine trial. Overview of missingness patterns and the frequencies with which they occur. (O, observed; M, missing.)

Measurement occasion					
Month 3	Month 6	Month 9	Month 12	Number	%
Completers					
O	O	O	O	224	71.11
Dropouts					
O	O	O	M	18	5.71
O	O	M	M	26	8.25
O	M	M	M	31	9.84
M	M	M	M	14	4.44
Non-monotone missingness					
M	O	O	O	1	0.32
M	M	M	O	1	0.32

2.7   THE TOENAIL DATA

The data introduced in this section were obtained from a randomized, double-blind, parallel group, multicentre study for the comparison of two oral treatments (in what follows coded as A and B) for toenail dermatophyte onychomycosis (TDO), described in full detail by De Backer *et al.* (1995). TDO is a common toenail infection, difficult to treat, affecting more than 2 out of every 100 persons (Roberts 1992). Antifungal compounds, classically used for treatment of TDO, need to be taken until the whole nail has grown out in a healthy manner. The development of new compounds, however, has reduced the treatment duration to 3 months. The aim of the present study was to compare the efficacy and safety of 12 weeks of continuous therapy with treatment A or with treatment B.

In total, 2×189 patients were randomized, distributed over 36 centres. Subjects were followed during 12 weeks (3 months) of treatment and then further, up to a total of 48 weeks (12 months). Measurements were taken at baseline, every month during treatment, and every 3 months afterwards, resulting in a maximum of seven measurements per subject. At the first occasion, the treating physician selects one of the affected toenails as the target nail, that is, the nail that will be followed over time. We will restrict our analyses to only those patients for whom the target nail was one of the two large toenails. This reduces our sample under consideration to 146 and 148 subjects, in group A and group B, respectively.

One of the responses of interest was the unaffected nail length, measured from the nail bed to the infected part of the nail, which is always at the free end of the nail, expressed in millimetres. This outcome has been studied extensively in Verbeke and Molenberghs (2000). Another important outcome in this study was the severity of the infection, coded as 0 (not severe) or 1 (severe). The question of interest was whether the percentage of severe infections decreased over time, and whether that evolution was different for the two treatment groups. A summary of the number of patients in the study at each time point and the number of patients with severe infections is given in Table 2.5. A graphical representation is given in Figure 2.5.

For a variety of reasons, the outcome was measured at all seven scheduled time points for only 224 (76%) of the 298 participants. Table 2.6 summarizes the number of available repeated measurements per subject for both treatment groups separately. We see that the occurrence of missingness is similar in both treatment groups.

The data are subjected to analysis in Section 7.4.

Table 2.5 Toenail data. Number and percentage of patients with severe toenail infection, for each treatment arm separately.

	Group A			Group B		
	No. severe	N	%	No. severe	N	%
Baseline	54	146	37.0	55	148	37.2
1 month	49	141	34.7	48	147	32.6
2 months	44	138	31.9	40	145	27.6
3 months	29	132	22.0	29	140	20.7
6 months	14	130	10.8	8	133	6.0
9 months	10	117	8.5	8	127	6.3
12 months	14	133	10.5	6	131	4.6

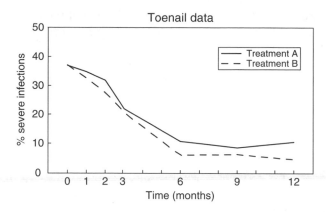

Figure 2.5 Toenail data. Evolution of the percentage of severe toenail infections in the two treatment groups separately.

Table 2.6 Toenail data. Number of available repeated measurements per subject, for each treatment arm separately.

No. of observations	Group A		Group B	
	N	%	N	%
1	4	2.74	1	0.68
2	2	1.37	1	0.68
3	4	2.74	3	2.03
4	2	1.37	4	2.70
5	2	1.37	8	5.41
6	25	17.12	14	9.46
7	107	73.29	117	79.05
Total:	146	100	148	100

2.8 AGE-RELATED MACULAR DEGENERATION TRIAL

These data arise from a randomized multicentre clinical trial comparing an experimental treatment (interferon-α) with a corresponding placebo in the treatment of patients with age-related macular degeneration. In this book we focus on the comparison between placebo and the highest dose (6 million units daily) of interferon-α (Z), but the full results of this trial have been reported elsewhere (Pharmacological Therapy for Macular Degeneration Study Group 1997). Patients with macular degeneration progressively lose vision. In the trial, visual acuity was assessed at different time points (4 weeks, 12 weeks, 24 weeks, and 52 weeks) through patients' ability to read lines of letters on standardized vision charts. These charts display lines of five letters of decreasing size, which the patient must read from top (largest letters) to bottom (smallest letters). The raw visual acuity is the total number of letters correctly read. In addition, one often refers to each line with at least four letters correctly read as a 'line of vision'. The primary endpoint of the trial was the loss of at least three lines of vision at 1 year, compared to baseline performance (a binary endpoint). The secondary endpoint of the trial was the visual acuity at 1 year (treated as a continuous endpoint). Buyse and Molenberghs (1998) examined whether the patient's performance at 6 months could be used as a surrogate for their performance at 1 year with respect to the effect of interferon-α. They looked at whether the loss of two lines of vision at 6 months could be used as a surrogate for the loss of at least three lines of vision at 1 year (Table 2.7). They also looked at whether visual acuity at 6 months could be used as a surrogate for visual acuity at 1 year.

Table 2.8 shows the visual acuity (mean and standard error) by treatment group at baseline, at 6 months, and at 1 year. Visual acuity can be measured in several ways. First, one can record the number of letters read. Alternatively, dichotomized versions (less than 3 lines of vision lost, or at least 3 lines of vision lost) can be used as well. Therefore, these data will be useful to illustrate methods for the joint modelling of continuous and binary outcomes, with or without taking the longitudinal nature into account. In addition, though there are 190 subjects with both month 6 and month 12 measurements available,

Table 2.7 Age-related macular degeneration trial. Loss of at least three lines of vision at 1 year by loss of at least two lines of vision at 6 months and by randomized treatment group (placebo versus *interferon-α*).

| | **12 months** | | | |
| | **Placebo** | | **Active** | |
6 months	**0**	**1**	**0**	**1**
No event (0)	56	9	31	9
Event (1)	8	30	9	38

Table 2.8 Age-related macular degeneration trial. Mean (standard error) of visual acuity at baseline, at 6 months and at 1 year by randomized treatment group (*placebo* versus *interferon-α*).

Time point	Placebo	Active	Total
Baseline	55.3 (1.4)	54.6 (1.3)	55.0 (1.0)
6 months	49.3 (1.8)	45.5 (1.8)	47.5 (1.3)
1 year	44.4 (1.8)	39.1 (1.9)	42.0 (1.3)

Table 2.9 Age-related macular degeneration trial. Overview of missingness patterns and the frequencies with which they occur. (O observed, M, missing.)

4 wks	12 wks	24 wks	52 wks	Number	%
Measurement occasion					
Completers					
O	O	O	O	188	78.33
Dropouts					
O	O	O	M	24	10.00
O	O	M	M	8	3.33
O	M	M	M	6	2.50
M	M	M	M	6	2.50
Non-monotone missingness					
O	O	M	O	4	1.67
O	M	M	O	1	0.42
M	O	O	O	2	0.83
M	O	M	M	1	0.42

the total number of longitudinal profiles is 240, but for only 188 of these have the four follow-up measurements been made.

Fifty incomplete subjects could therefore be considered for analysis as well. Both intermittent missingness as well as dropout occurs. An overview is given in Table 2.9.

Thus, 78.33% of the profiles are complete, while 18.33% exhibit monotone missingness. Out of the latter group, 2.5% or 6 subjects have no follow-up measurements. The remaining 3.33%, representing 8 subjects, have intermittent missing values. Thus, as in many of the examples seen already, dropout dominates intermediate patterns as the source of missing data.

The data are analysed in Chapters 13 and 25.

2.9   THE ANALGESIC TRIAL

These data come from a single-arm clinical trial involving 395 patients who are given analgesic treatment for pain caused by chronic non-malignant disease. Treatment was to be administered for 12 months and assessed by means of a five-point 'Global Satisfaction Assessment' (GSA) scale,

$$
\text{GSA} = \begin{cases} 1 & \text{very good,} \\ 2 & \text{good,} \\ 3 & \text{indifferent,} \\ 4 & \text{bad,} \\ 5 & \text{very bad.} \end{cases}
$$

Some analyses were done on a dichotomized version:

$$\text{GSABIN} = \begin{cases} 1 & \text{if GSA} \leq 3, \\ 0 & \text{otherwise.} \end{cases}$$

Apart from the outcome of interest, a number of covariates are available, such as age, sex, weight, duration of pain in years prior to the start of the study, type of pain, physical functioning, psychiatric condition, respiratory problems, etc.

GSA was rated by each person four times during the trial, at months 3, 6, 9, and 12. An overview of the frequencies by follow-up time is given in Table 2.10. Inspection of Table 2.10 reveals that the total in each column is variable. This

Table 2.10 Analgesic trial. Absolute and relative frequencies of the five GSA categories for each of the four follow-up times.

GSA	Month 3		Month 6		Month 9		Month 12	
1	55	14.3%	38	12.6%	40	17.6%	30	13.5%
2	112	29.1%	84	27.8%	67	29.5%	66	29.6%
3	151	39.2%	115	38.1%	76	33.5%	97	43.5%
4	52	13.5%	51	16.9%	33	14.5%	27	12.1%
5	15	3.9%	14	4.6%	11	4.9%	3	1.4%
Total	385		302		227		223	

Table 2.11 Analgesic trial. Overview of missingness patterns and the frequencies with which they occur. (O, observed; M, missing.)

	Measurement occasion				
Month 3	Month 6	Month 9	Month 12	Number	%
Completers					
O	O	O	O	163	41.2
Dropouts					
O	O	O	M	51	12.91
O	O	M	M	51	12.91
O	M	M	M	63	15.95
Non-monotone missingness					
O	O	M	O	30	7.59
O	M	O	O	7	1.77
O	M	O	M	2	0.51
O	M	M	O	18	4.56
M	O	O	O	2	0.51
M	O	O	M	1	0.25
M	O	M	O	1	0.25
M	O	M	M	3	0.76

is due to missingness. At 3 months, 10 subjects lack a measure, with these numbers being 93, 168, and 172 at subsequent times.

An overview of the extent of missingness is shown in Table 2.11. Note that only around 40% of the subjects have complete data. Both dropout and intermittent patterns of missingness occur, the former amounting to roughly 40%, with close to 20% for the latter. This example underscores that a satisfactory longitudinal analysis will often have to address the missing data problem. These data are analysed in Sections 7.7 and 10.6.

2.10 THE SLOVENIAN PUBLIC OPINION SURVEY

In 1991 Slovenians voted for independence from the former Yugoslavia in a plebiscite. To prepare for this result, the Slovenian government collected data in the Slovenian public opinion survey, a month before the plebiscite. Rubin *et al.* (1995) studied the three fundamental questions added to the survey and, in comparing it to the plebiscite's outcome, drew conclusions about the missing data process.

The three questions added were: (1) Are you in favour of Slovenian independence? (2) Are you in favour of Slovenia's secession from Yugoslavia? (3) Will you attend the plebiscite? In spite of their apparent equivalence, questions (1) and (2) are different since independence would have been possible in confederal form as well and therefore the secession question is added. Question (3) is highly relevant since the political decision was taken that not attending was treated as an effective no to question (1). Thus, the primary estimand is the proportion θ of people who will be considered as voting yes, which is the fraction of people answering yes to both the attendance and independence question. The raw data are presented in Table 2.12. We will return to this question in Sections 19.4 and 21.9.

Table 2.12 Slovenian public opinion survey. The don't know category is indicated by *.

		Independence		
Secession	**Attendance**	**Yes**	**No**	*
Yes	Yes	1191	8	21
	No	8	0	4
	*	107	3	9
No	Yes	158	68	29
	No	7	14	3
	*	18	43	31
*	Yes	90	2	109
	No	1	2	25
	*	19	8	96

The data were introduced into the statistical literature by Rubin *et al.* Vehovar (1995) and used by Molenberghs *et al.* (2001a) to illustrate their sensitivity analysis tool, the interval of ignorance. Thus, while not a clinical study, we have chosen to maintain these data as a key set, enabling us to illustrate a number of points.

Analyses are presented in Sections 19.4 and 21.9.

Terminology and Framework

3.1 MODELLING INCOMPLETENESS

To incorporate incompleteness into the modelling process, we need to reflect on the nature of the missing value mechanism and its implications for statistical inference. Rubin (1976) and Little and Rubin (2002, Chapter 6) distinguish between different missing value processes. A process is termed *missing completely at random* (MCAR) if missingness is independent of both unobserved and observed outcomes, and *missing at random* (MAR) if, conditional on the observed data, missingness is independent of the unobserved outcomes; otherwise, the process is termed *missing not at random* (MNAR). A more formal definition of these concepts is given in Section 3.4.

Given MAR, a valid analysis can be obtained through a likelihood-based analysis that ignores the missing value mechanism, provided the parameters describing the measurement process are functionally independent of the parameters describing the missingness process, the so-called parameter distinctness condition. This situation is termed ignorable by Rubin (1976) and Little and Rubin (2002) and leads to considerable simplification in the analysis (Diggle 1989; Verbeke and Molenberghs 2000); see also Section 3.5 below.

In practice, the reasons for missingness are likely to be many and varied, and it is therefore difficult to justify solely on a priori grounds the assumption of missingness at random. Arguably, under MNAR, a wholly satisfactory analysis of the data is not feasible, and it should be noted that the data alone cannot distinguish between MAR and MNAR mechanisms.

In the light of this, one approach could be to estimate from the available data the parameters of a model representing a MNAR mechanism. It is typically difficult to justify the particular choice of missingness model, and it does not

Missing Data in Clinical Studies   G. Molenberghs and M.G. Kenward
© 2007 John Wiley & Sons, Ltd

necessarily follow that the data contain information on the parameters of the particular model chosen. These points have been studied in Jansen *et al.* (2006b) and are discussed in Chapter 20. Where such information exists (and as we emphasize below this is normally derived from untestable modelling assumptions), the fitted model can be seen as providing some insight into the fit of the MAR model to the observed data. Only through external assumptions can we use this subsequently to make inferences about the missing value process. Consequently the approach is potentially useful for assessing the sensitivity of the conclusions to assumptions about the missing value process, but not for making definitive statements about it. Several authors have used MNAR models that explicitly model the dropout process, and attempted from these to draw conclusions about the missing value mechanism. These include Diggle and Kenward (1994) in the context of continuous longitudinal data and Molenberghs *et al.* (1997) for ordinal outcomes. Overviews of and extensive discussion on this topic can be found in Little (1995), Diggle *et al.* (2002), Verbeke and Molenberghs (2000) and Molenberghs and Verbeke (2005). Further early approaches for continuous data were proposed by Laird *et al.* (1987), Wu and Bailey (1988, 1989), Wu and Carroll (1988), and Greenlees *et al.* (1982). Proposals for categorical data were made by Baker and Laird (1988), Stasny (1986), Baker *et al.* (1992), Conaway (1992, 1993), and Park and Brown (1994).

A feature common to all complex (MNAR) modelling approaches is that they rely on untestable assumptions about the relationship between the measurement and missing value processes. An obvious consequence of this is that one should therefore avoid missing data as much as possible and, when the problem arises, ensure that all practicable efforts are made to collect information on the reasons for this. As an example, consider a clinical trial where outcome and missingness are both strongly related to a specific covariate X and where, conditionally on X, the response Y and the missing data process R are independent. In the selection framework (Sections 1.2 and 3.4), we then have that $f(Y, R|X) = f(Y|X)f(R|X)$, implying MCAR, whereas omission of X from the model may imply MAR or even MNAR, which has important consequences for selecting valid statistical methods.

Different MNAR models may fit the observed data equally well, but have quite different implications for the unobserved measurements, and hence for the conclusions to be drawn from the respective analyses. Without additional information we can only distinguish between such models using their fit to the observed data, and so goodness-of-fit tools typically do not provide a relevant means of choosing between such models. It follows that there is an important role for sensitivity analysis in assessing inferences from incomplete data. Sensitivity analysis is introduced, and various informal and formal methods discussed, in Part V.

In Section 3.2 we set the scene by introducing terminology that will be used throughout the remainder of the book. In Section 3.3 we sketch the broad frameworks for incomplete data modelling. Missing data patterns, informally introduced in the previous section and in Section 1.2, are formalized in Section 3.4. Ignorability is the subject of Section 3.5. Section 3.6 sketches a general pattern-mixture model framework.

3.2 TERMINOLOGY

The following terminology is based on the standard framework of Rubin (1976) and Little and Rubin (2002). It allows us to place formal conditions on the missing value mechanism which determine how the mechanism may influence subsequent inferences. Assume that for each independent unit $i = 1, \ldots, N$ in the study, it is planned to collect a set of measurements Y_{ij} ($j = 1, \ldots, n_i$). In a longitudinal study, i indicates the subject and j the measurement occasion. For multivariate studies, j refers to the particular outcome variable. In a hierarchical data setting, with more than two levels, j can be taken to refer generically to all sub-levels, in which case it would become a vector-valued indicator. The index i is always reserved for units (blocks) of independent replication.

We group the outcomes into a vector $\boldsymbol{Y}_i = (Y_{i1}, \ldots, Y_{in_i})'$. In addition, for each occasion j we define

$$R_{ij} = \begin{cases} 1 & \text{if } Y_{ij} \text{ is observed,} \\ 0 & \text{otherwise.} \end{cases}$$

These *missing data indicators* R_{ij} are organized into a vector $\boldsymbol{R}_i$ of parallel structure to $\boldsymbol{Y}_i$.

We then partition $\boldsymbol{Y}_i$ into two subvectors such that $\boldsymbol{Y}_i^o$ is the vector containing those Y_{ij} for which $R_{ij} = 1$, and $\boldsymbol{Y}_i^m$ contains the remaining components. These subvectors are referred to as the *observed* and *missing* components, respectively. The following terminology is adopted. *Complete data* refers to the vector $\boldsymbol{Y}_i$ of planned measurements. This is the outcome vector that would have been recorded if no data had been missing. The vector $\boldsymbol{R}_i$ and the process generating $\boldsymbol{R}_i$ are referred to as the *missing data process*. The *full data* $(\boldsymbol{Y}_i, \boldsymbol{R}_i)$ consist of the complete data, together with the missing data indicators. Note that, unless all components of $\boldsymbol{R}_i$ equal one, the full data components are never jointly observed but rather one observes the measurements $\boldsymbol{Y}_i^o$ together with the dropout indicators $\boldsymbol{R}_i$, which we refer to as the *observed data*.

When missingness is restricted to dropout or attrition, we can replace the vector $\boldsymbol{R}_i$ by a scalar variable D_i, the *dropout indicator*. In this case, each vector $\boldsymbol{R}_i$ is of the form $(1, \ldots, 1, 0, \ldots, 0)$ and we can define the scalar dropout indicator

$$D_i = 1 + \sum_{j=1}^{n_i} R_{ij}. \tag{3.1}$$

For an incomplete sequence, D_i denotes the occasion at which dropout occurs. For a complete sequence, $D_i = n_i + 1$. In both cases, D_i is equal to one plus the length of the measurement sequence, whether complete or incomplete. Sometimes it is convenient to define an alternative dropout indicator, $T_i = D_i - 1$, that indicates the number of measurements actually taken, rather than the first occasion at which the planned measurement has not been taken.

Dropout, or attrition, is an example of a *monotone* pattern of missingness. Missingness is termed monotone when there exists a permutation of the measurement occasions such that a measurement earlier in the permuted sequence is observed for at least those subjects who are observed at later measurements. Note that, for this definition to be meaningful, we need to have a balanced design in the sense of a common set of designed measurement occasions. Other patterns are called *non-monotone*.

3.3   MISSING DATA FRAMEWORKS

We now consider in turn the so-called *selection, pattern-mixture,* and *shared-parameter* modelling frameworks.

When data are incomplete due to the operation of a random (missing value) mechanism the appropriate starting point for a model is the full data density

$$f(\boldsymbol{y}_i, \boldsymbol{r}_i | X_i, W_i, \boldsymbol{\theta}, \boldsymbol{\psi}), \tag{3.2}$$

where X_i and W_i denote design matrices for the measurement and missingness mechanism, respectively. The corresponding parameter vectors are $\boldsymbol{\theta}$ and $\boldsymbol{\psi}$, respectively.

The *selection model* factorization is based on

$$f(\boldsymbol{y}_i, \boldsymbol{r}_i | X_i, W_i, \boldsymbol{\theta}, \boldsymbol{\psi}) = f(\boldsymbol{y}_i | X_i, \boldsymbol{\theta}) f(\boldsymbol{r}_i | \boldsymbol{y}_i, W_i, \boldsymbol{\psi}), \tag{3.3}$$

where the first factor is the marginal density of the measurement process and the second one is the density of the missingness process, conditional on the outcomes. The name is chosen because $f(\boldsymbol{r}_i | \boldsymbol{y}_i, W_i, \boldsymbol{\psi})$ can be seen as describing a unit's self-selection mechanism to either continue or leave the study. The term originates from the econometric literature (Heckman 1976) and it can be thought of in terms of a subject's missing values being 'selected' through the probability model, given their measurements, whether observed or not.

An alternative family is based on so-called *pattern-mixture models* (Little 1993, 1994a, 1995). These are based on the factorization

$$f(\boldsymbol{y}_i, \boldsymbol{r}_i | X_i, W_i, \boldsymbol{\theta}, \boldsymbol{\psi}) = f(\boldsymbol{y}_i | \boldsymbol{r}_i, X_i, \boldsymbol{\theta}) f(\boldsymbol{r}_i | W_i, \boldsymbol{\psi}). \tag{3.4}$$

The pattern-mixture model allows for a different response model for each pattern of missing values, the observed data being a mixture of these weighted by the probability of each missing value or dropout pattern.

The third family is referred to as *shared-parameter models*:

$$f(\boldsymbol{y}_i, \boldsymbol{r}_i | X_i, W_i, \boldsymbol{\theta}, \boldsymbol{\psi}, \boldsymbol{b}_i) = f(\boldsymbol{y}_i | \boldsymbol{r}_i, X_i, \boldsymbol{\theta}, \boldsymbol{b}_i) f(\boldsymbol{r}_i | W_i, \boldsymbol{\psi}, \boldsymbol{b}_i), \qquad (3.5)$$

where we explicitly include a vector of unit-specific latent (or random) effects $\boldsymbol{b}_i$ of which one or more components are shared between both factors in the joint distribution. Early references to such models are Wu and Carroll (1988) and Wu and Bailey (1988, 1989). A sensible assumption is that Y_i and R_i are conditionally independent, given the random effects $\boldsymbol{b}_i$. The random effects $\boldsymbol{b}_i$ can be used to define an appropriate hierarchical model. The same vector can then be used to describe the missing data process. The shared parameter $\boldsymbol{b}_i$ can be thought of as referring to a latent trait driving both the measurement and missingness processes.

The natural parameters of selection models, pattern-mixture models, and shared-parameter models have different interpretations, and transforming one statistical model from one of the frameworks to another is generally not straightforward.

3.4 MISSING DATA MECHANISMS

Rubin's taxonomy of missing value processes (Rubin 1976; Little and Rubin 2002), informally introduced in Section 1.2 and mentioned in Section 3.1, is fundamental to the modelling of incomplete data. It is perhaps most naturally expressed within the selection modelling framework for which it is based on the second factor of (3.3):

$$f(\boldsymbol{r}_i | \boldsymbol{y}_i, W_i, \boldsymbol{\psi}) = f(\boldsymbol{r}_i | \boldsymbol{y}_i^o, \boldsymbol{y}_i^m, W_i, \boldsymbol{\psi}). \qquad (3.6)$$

Under an *MCAR* mechanism, the probability of an observation being missing is independent of the responses,

$$f(\boldsymbol{r}_i | \boldsymbol{y}_i, W_i, \boldsymbol{\psi}) = f(\boldsymbol{r}_i | W_i, \boldsymbol{\psi}), \qquad (3.7)$$

and therefore (3.3) simplifies to

$$f(\boldsymbol{y}_i, \boldsymbol{r}_i | X_i, W_i, \boldsymbol{\theta}, \boldsymbol{\psi}) = f(\boldsymbol{y}_i | X_i, \boldsymbol{\theta}) f(\boldsymbol{r}_i | W_i, \boldsymbol{\psi}), \qquad (3.8)$$

implying that both components are independent. The implication is that the joint distribution of $\boldsymbol{y}_i^o$ and $\boldsymbol{r}_i$ becomes

$$f(\boldsymbol{y}_i^o, \boldsymbol{r}_i | X_i, W_i, \boldsymbol{\theta}, \boldsymbol{\psi}) = f(\boldsymbol{y}_i^o | X_i, \boldsymbol{\theta}) f(\boldsymbol{r}_i | W_i, \boldsymbol{\psi}). \qquad (3.9)$$

Under MCAR, the observed data can be analysed as though the pattern of missing values was predetermined. In whatever way the data are analysed, whether using a frequentist, likelihood, or Bayesian procedure, the process(es) generating the missing values can be ignored. For example, in this situation simple averages of the observed data at different occasions provide unbiased estimates of the corresponding population averages. The observed data can be regarded as a random sample of the complete data.

Note that this definition and the ones to follow are made conditionally on the covariates. When the covariates, assembled into X_i and W_i, are removed, the nature of a mechanism may change. In defining these mechanisms some authors distinguish between those made conditionally or not on the covariates.

Under an *MAR* mechanism, the probability of an observation being missing is *conditionally* independent of the unobserved outcome(s), given the values of the observed outcome(s):

$$f(\boldsymbol{r}_i|\boldsymbol{y}_i, W_i, \boldsymbol{\psi}) = f(\boldsymbol{r}_i|\boldsymbol{y}_i^o, W_i, \boldsymbol{\psi}). \tag{3.10}$$

Again the joint distribution of the observed data can be partitioned,

$$f(\boldsymbol{y}_i, \boldsymbol{r}_i|X_i, W_i, \boldsymbol{\theta}, \boldsymbol{\psi}) = f(\boldsymbol{y}_i|X_i, \boldsymbol{\theta})f(\boldsymbol{r}_i|\boldsymbol{y}_i^o, W_i, \boldsymbol{\psi}), \tag{3.11}$$

and hence at the observed data level,

$$f(\boldsymbol{y}_i^o, \boldsymbol{r}_i|X_i, W_i, \boldsymbol{\theta}, \boldsymbol{\psi}) = f(\boldsymbol{y}_i^o|X_i, \boldsymbol{\theta})f(\boldsymbol{r}_i|\boldsymbol{y}_i^o, W_i, \boldsymbol{\psi}). \tag{3.12}$$

Given the simplicity of (3.12), handling MAR processes is typically easier than handling MNAR.

Although the MAR assumption is particularly convenient in that it leads to considerable simplification in the issues surrounding the analysis of incomplete longitudinal data, an investigator is rarely able to justify its adoption, and so in many situations the final class of missing value mechanisms cannot be ruled out. Part III of this book is devoted to the MAR setting.

In the *MNAR* case, neither MCAR nor MAR holds. Under MNAR, the probability of a measurement being missing depends on unobserved outcome(s). No simplification of the joint distribution is possible and the joint distribution of the observed measurements and the missingness process has to be written as

$$f(\boldsymbol{y}_i^o, \boldsymbol{r}_i|X_i, W_i, \boldsymbol{\theta}, \boldsymbol{\psi}) = \int f(\boldsymbol{y}_i|X_i, \boldsymbol{\theta})f(\boldsymbol{r}_i|\boldsymbol{y}_i, W_i, \boldsymbol{\psi})d\boldsymbol{y}_i^m. \tag{3.13}$$

Inferences can only be made by making further assumptions, about which the observed data alone carry no information. Ideally, if such models are to be used, the choice of such assumptions should be guided by external information, but the degree to which this is possible varies greatly across application areas and applications. Such models can be formulated within each of the three main families: selection, pattern-mixture, and shared-parameter models. The differences between the families are especially important in the MNAR case, and lead to quite different, but complementary, views of the missing value problem. Little (1995), Hogan and Laird (1997), and Kenward and Molenberghs (1999) provide detailed reviews. See also Verbeke and Molenberghs (2000) and Molenberghs and Verbeke (2005).

It has been shown, for dropout in longitudinal studies, how Rubin's classification can be applied in the pattern-mixture framework as well (Molenberghs *et al.* 1998b; Kenward *et al.* 2003). We will discuss these points in Section 3.6.

The MCAR–MAR–MNAR terminology is independent of the inferential framework chosen. This is different for the concept of *ignorability*, which depends crucially on this framework (Rubin 1976). We will turn to this issue in the next section.

3.5   IGNORABILITY

In this section we focus on likelihood-based estimation. The full data likelihood contribution for unit *i* takes the form

$$L^*(\boldsymbol{\theta}, \boldsymbol{\psi}|X_i, W_i, \boldsymbol{y}_i, \boldsymbol{r}_i) \propto f(\boldsymbol{y}_i, \boldsymbol{r}_i|X_i, W_i, \boldsymbol{\theta}, \boldsymbol{\psi}).$$

Because inference has to be based on what is observed, the full data likelihood L^* needs to be replaced by the observed data likelihood L:

$$L(\boldsymbol{\theta}, \boldsymbol{\psi}|X_i, W_i, \boldsymbol{y}_i^o, \boldsymbol{r}_i) \propto f(\boldsymbol{y}_i^o, \boldsymbol{r}_i|X_i, W_i, \boldsymbol{\theta}, \boldsymbol{\psi}) \tag{3.14}$$

with

$$f(\boldsymbol{y}_i^o, \boldsymbol{r}_i|\boldsymbol{\theta}, \boldsymbol{\psi}) = \int f(\boldsymbol{y}_i, \boldsymbol{r}_i|X_i, W_i, \boldsymbol{\theta}, \boldsymbol{\psi}) d\boldsymbol{y}_i^m$$

$$= \int f(\boldsymbol{y}_i^o, \boldsymbol{y}_i^m|X_i, \boldsymbol{\theta}) f(\boldsymbol{r}_i|\boldsymbol{y}_i^o, \boldsymbol{y}_i^m, W_i, \boldsymbol{\psi}) d\boldsymbol{y}_i^m. \tag{3.15}$$

Under an MAR process, we obtain

$$f(\boldsymbol{y}_i^o, \boldsymbol{r}_i|\boldsymbol{\theta}, \boldsymbol{\psi}) = \int f(\boldsymbol{y}_i^o, \boldsymbol{y}_i^m|X_i, W_i, \boldsymbol{\theta}) f(\boldsymbol{r}_i|\boldsymbol{y}_i^o, W_i, \boldsymbol{\psi}) d\boldsymbol{y}_i^m$$

$$= f(\boldsymbol{y}_i^o|X_i, W_i, \boldsymbol{\theta}) f(\boldsymbol{r}_i|\boldsymbol{y}_i^o, W_i, \boldsymbol{\psi}). \tag{3.16}$$

Thus, the likelihood factors into two components of the same functional form as the general factorization (21.1) of the complete data. If, further, $\boldsymbol{\theta}$ and $\boldsymbol{\psi}$ are disjoint in the sense that the parameter space of the full vector $(\boldsymbol{\theta}', \boldsymbol{\psi}')'$ is the product of the parameter spaces of $\boldsymbol{\theta}$ and $\boldsymbol{\psi}$, then inference can be based solely on the marginal observed data density. This technical requirement is referred to as the separability condition. However, some caution should still be used when constructing precision estimators. This point is discussed in detail in Chapter 12.

In conclusion, when the separability condition is satisfied, *within the likelihood framework*, ignorability is equivalent to the union of MAR and MCAR. A formal derivation is given in Rubin (1976), where it is also shown that the same requirements hold for Bayesian inference, but that for frequentist inference to be ignorable, MCAR is the corresponding sufficient condition. Of course, it is possible that at least part of the scientific interest is directed towards the missing data process. Then ignorability is still useful since the measurement model and missingness model questions can be addressed through separate models, rather than jointly.

Classical examples of the more stringent condition with frequentist methods are ordinary least squares (see Chapter 7) and the generalized estimating equations approach of Liang and Zeger (1986). The latter produce unbiased estimators in general only under MCAR. Robins *et al.* (1995) and Rotnitzky and Robins (1995) have established that some progress can be made under MAR and that, even under MNAR processes, these methods can be applied (Rotnitzky and Robins 1997; Robins *et al.* 1998). Their method, discussed in Chapter 10, is based on including weights that depend on the missingness probability, proving the point that at least some information on the missingness mechanism should be included and, thus, that ignorability does not hold outside the likelihood framework.

3.6 PATTERN-MIXTURE MODELS

Pattern-mixture models (PMMs) were introduced in Section 3.3 as one of the three major frameworks within which missing data models can be developed. Little (1993, 1994a, 1995) originally proposed the use of PMMs as a viable alternative to selection models, and we will return to the topic at length in Chapter 16.

An important issue is that PMMs are by construction underidentified, that is, overspecified. Little (1993, 1994a) solves this problem through the use of identifying restrictions: inestimable parameters of the incomplete patterns are set equal to (functions of) the parameters describing the distribution of the completers. Identifying restrictions are not the only way to overcome underidentification, and we will discuss alternative approaches in Chapter 16. Although some authors perceive this underidentification as a drawback, it can be viewed as an asset because it forces one to reflect on the assumptions being made, and the assumptions are necessarily transparent. This can serve as a useful starting point for sensitivity analysis.

Little (1993, 1994a) advocated the use of identifying restrictions and presented a number of examples. One of these, *available case missing values* (ACMV), is the natural counterpart of MAR in the PMM framework, as was established by Molenberghs *et al.* (1998b). Specific counterparts to MNAR selection models were studied by Kenward *et al.* (2003). These will be discussed in what follows.

In line with Molenberghs *et al.* (1998b), we restrict attention to monotone patterns, dropping the unit index i from the notation, for simplicity. In general, let us assume that there are $t = 1, \ldots, n = T$ dropout patterns, where the dropout indicator, introduced in (3.1), is $d = t+1$. The indices j for measurement occasions and t for dropout patterns assume the same values, but using both simplifies notation.

For pattern t, the complete data density is given by

$$f_t(y_1, \ldots, y_T) = f_t(y_1, \ldots, y_t) f_t(y_{t+1}, \ldots, y_T | y_1, \ldots, y_t). \qquad (3.17)$$

The first factor is clearly identified from the observed data, while the second factor is not. It is assumed that the first factor is known or, more realistically, modelled using the observed data. Then identifying restrictions are applied in order to identify the second component.

Although, in principle, completely arbitrary restrictions can be used by means of any valid density function over the appropriate support, strategies that imply links back to the observed data are likely to have more practical relevance. One can base identification on all patterns for which a given component, y_s say, is identified. A general expression for this is

$$f_t(y_s | y_1, \ldots, y_{s-1}) = \sum_{j=s}^{T} \omega_{sj} f_j(y_s | y_1, \ldots, y_{s-1}), \quad s = t+1, \ldots, T. \qquad (3.18)$$

Let $\boldsymbol{\omega}_s$ denote the set of ω_{sj}s used, the components of which are typically positive. Every $\boldsymbol{\omega}_s$ that sums to one provides a valid identification scheme.

Let us incorporate (3.18) into (3.17):

$$f_t(y_1, \ldots, y_T) = f_t(y_1, \ldots, y_t) \prod_{s=0}^{T-t-1} \left[\sum_{j=T-s}^{T} \omega_{T-s,j} f_j(y_{T-s} | y_1, \ldots, y_{T-s-1}) \right]. \qquad (3.19)$$

We will consider three special but important cases, associated with such choices of $\boldsymbol{\omega}_s$ in (3.18). Little (1993) proposes *complete case missing values* (CCMV), which uses the following identification:

$$f_t(y_s | y_1, \ldots, y_{s-1}) = f_T(y_s | y_1, \ldots, y_{s-1}), \quad s = t+1, \ldots, T, \qquad (3.20)$$

corresponding to $\omega_{sT} = 1$ and all others zero. In other words, information which is unavailable is always borrowed from the completers. Alternatively, the nearest identified pattern can be used:

$$f_t(y_s | y_1, \ldots, y_{s-1}) = f_s(y_s | y_1, \ldots, y_{s-1}), \quad s = t+1, \ldots, T, \qquad (3.21)$$

corresponding to $\omega_{ss} = 1$ and all others zero. We will refer to these restrictions as *neighbouring case missing values* (NCMV).

The third special case of (3.18) is ACMV. ACMV is reserved for the counterpart of MAR in the PMM context. The corresponding ω_s vectors can be shown (Molenberghs *et al.* 1998b) to have components:

$$\omega_{sj} = \frac{\alpha_j f_j(y_1,\ldots,y_{s-1})}{\sum_{\ell=s}^{T} \alpha_\ell f_\ell(y_1,\ldots,y_{s-1})} \tag{3.22}$$

$(j = s,\ldots,T)$, where α_j is the fraction of observations in pattern j (Molenberghs *et al.* 1998b).

This MAR–ACMV link connects the selection and pattern-mixture families. It is of further interest to consider specific sub-families of the MNAR family. In the context of selection models for longitudinal data, one typically restricts attention to a class of mechanisms where dropout may depend on the current, possibly unobserved, measurement, but not on future measurements. The entire class of such models will be termed *missing non-future dependent* (MNFD). Although they are natural and easy to consider in a selection model situation, there exist important examples of mechanisms that do not satisfy MNFD, such as shared-parameter models (Wu and Bailey 1989; Little 1995).

Kenward *et al.* (2003) have shown there is a counterpart to MNFD in the pattern-mixture context. The conditional probability of pattern t in the MNFD selection models obviously satisfies

$$f(r = t|y_1,\ldots,y_T) = f(r = t|y_1, \ldots,y_{t+1}). \tag{3.23}$$

Within the PMM framework, we define *non-future dependent missing value* (NFMV) restrictions as follows: for all $t \geq 2$, for all $j < t-1$,

$$f(y_t|y_1,\ldots,y_{t-1},r = j) = f(y_t|y_1,\ldots,y_{t-1},r \geq t-1). \tag{3.24}$$

NFMV is not a single set of restrictions, but rather leaves one conditional distribution per incomplete pattern unidentified:

$$f(y_{t+1}|y_1,\ldots,y_t,r = t). \tag{3.25}$$

In other words, the distribution of the 'current' unobserved measurement, given the previous ones, is unconstrained. Note that (3.24) excludes such mechanisms as CCMV and NCMV. Kenward *et al.* (2003) have shown that, for longitudinal data with dropouts, MNFD and NFMV are equivalent.

For pattern t, the complete data density is given by

$$f_t(y_1,\ldots,y_T) = f_t(y_1,\ldots,y_t)f_t(y_{t+1}|y_1,\ldots,y_t)$$
$$\times f_t(y_{t+2},\ldots,y_T|y_1,\ldots,y_{t+1}). \tag{3.26}$$

```
SEM  :  MCAR  ⊂  MAR   ⊂  MNFD  ⊂  general MNAR
          ↕          ↕          ↕              ↕
PMM  :  MCAR  ⊂  ACMV  ⊂  NFMV  ⊂  general MNAR
                           ⊂    ≠    ∪
                              interior
```

Figure 3.1 Relationship between nested families within the selection model (SEM) and pattern-mixture model (PMM) families. (MCAR, missing completely at random; MAR, missing at random; MNAR, missing not at random; MNFD, missing non-future dependence; ACMV, available case missing values; NFMV, non-future missing values; interior, restrictions based on a combination of the information available for other patterns. The ⊂ symbol here indicates 'is a special case of'. The ↕ symbol indicates correspondence between a class of SEM models and a class of PMM models.)

It is assumed that the first factor is known or, more realistically, modelled using the observed data. Then identifying restrictions are applied to identify the second and third components. First, from the data, estimate $f_t(y_1, \ldots, y_t)$. Second, the user has full freedom to choose

$$f_t(y_{t+1} | y_1, \ldots, y_t). \tag{3.27}$$

Substantive considerations could be used to identify this density. Alternatively, a family of densities might be considered by way of sensitivity analysis. Third, using (3.24), the densities $f_t(y_j | y_1, \ldots, y_{j-1}), j \geq t + 2$, are identified. This identification involves not only the patterns for which y_j is observed, but also the pattern for which y_j is the current and hence the first unobserved measurement. An overview of the connection between selection and pattern-mixture models is given in Figure 3.1.

Two obvious mechanisms, within the MNFD family but outside MAR, are NFD1 (NFD standing for 'non-future dependent') – choose (3.27) according to CCMV – and NFD2 – choose (3.27) according to NCMV. NFD1 and NFD2 are strictly different from CCMV and NCMV.

Part II
Classical Techniques and the Need for Modelling

4

A Perspective on Simple Methods

4.1 INTRODUCTION

As stated earlier, incomplete data issues complicate the analysis of clinical and other studies in humans. In this chapter, a number of simple methods will be discussed, with emphasis on complete case (CC) analysis and last observation carried forward (LOCF). It will then be shown how a direct likelihood analysis, using the ignorability results of Section 3.5, is a more attractive, flexible, broadly valid, and, most importantly, principled alternative. In the following two chapters, these points will be underscored using case studies. Part III will then expand upon and broaden the scope of ignorability.

Before starting, however, it is useful to reflect on the precise nature of the research question that needs answering. This is directly connected to the measurement model, and to the method for dealing with incompleteness. We will briefly introduce each of these in turn.

4.1.1 Measurement model

When measurements are collected repeatedly, a choice has to be made regarding the modelling approach to the measurement sequence. Several views are possible.

View 1 refers to a choice to analyse the entire longitudinal sequence, because the research question is phrased in terms of at least one longitudinal aspect, such as the difference in slope between groups. Then there is little or no alternative other than to formulate a longitudinal model.

Missing Data in Clinical Studies   G. Molenberghs and M.G. Kenward
© 2007 John Wiley & Sons, Ltd

View 2 refers to the situation where interest is focused on a well-defined point in time. Very often this will be the last occasion; without loss of generality, let us assume this to be the case. There are two important sub-cases to be considered.

Under *View 2a* we understand that the research question is in terms of the *last planned occasion*. Such an analysis is complicated by the missingness since typically a number of response sequences will terminate before the planned end of the study. It is primarily for this situation that a number of simple methods have been devised, such as a CC analysis or LOCF. We will show in this and subsequent chapters that, with the aid of a longitudinal model, together with likelihood or equivalent machinery, the need for deletion or single imputation can be avoided.

With *View 2b* we cover the situation where interest genuinely focuses on the *last observed measurement*. Since this is, by definition, the time at which dropout occurs, it can sensibly be considered of interest in its own right. For example, outcomes and covariate information collected at or just before the moment of dropout can shed light on the dropout mechanisms, help to diversify between patient groups, etc.

While Views 1 and 2a necessitate reflection on the missing data mechanism, View 2b, in a sense, avoids the missing data problem because the question is couched completely in terms of observed measurements. Of course, an investigator should reflect very carefully on whether View 2b represents a relevant and meaningful scientific question (Shih and Quan 1997), and View 2b also implies that the time to the last observation made should be of direct interest.

4.1.2 Method for handling missingness

In principle, a choice has to be made regarding the modelling approach for the missingness process. Note that, under certain assumptions, however, this process can be ignored. The best known situation is a likelihood-based or Bayesian ignorable analysis (Section 3.5). Apart from that, the simple methods – such as CC, LOCF, and other simple imputation methods – typically do not explicitly address the missingness process either.

4.2   SIMPLE METHODS

4.2.1   Complete case analysis

A complete case analysis includes in the analysis only those cases for which all measurements were recorded. This method has obvious advantages. It is very simple to describe and, since the data structure is as planned, standard statistical tools can be used. Arguably, the restoration of a rectangular data structure was historically the most compelling reason to apply this method, but modern computational facilities have moved the problem far beyond this consideration. Further, because estimation is based solely on the same subset of completers, there is a common basis for inference, whichever analysis is employed.

Unfortunately, the method suffers from severe drawbacks. First, there is nearly always a substantial loss of information, leading to inefficient estimators. For example, suppose there are 20 measurements, with 10% of missing data on each measurement. Suppose, further, somewhat unrealistically, that missingness on the different measurements is independent; then the estimated percentage of incomplete observations is as high as 87%. The impact on precision and power is dramatic. Even though the reduction of the number of complete cases will be less dramatic in realistic settings where the missingness indicators are correlated, the effect just sketched will often undermine a CC analysis. In addition, and very important, severe bias can result when the missingness mechanism is MAR but not MCAR. Indeed, should an estimator be consistent in the complete data problem, then the derived CC analysis is consistent only if the missingness process is MCAR.

4.2.2 Imputation methods

An alternative way to obtain a data set to which complete data methods can be applied is based on completion rather than deletion. Commonly, the observed values are used as a basis to impute values for the missing observations. As with CC, imputation methods had the historical advantage of restoring a rectangular data matrix and, in addition, preserving balance in the sense that the same number of subjects per treatment arm or per experimental condition was preserved. However valid these may have been in the pre-automated computation era, such considerations are no longer relevant.

There are several ways in which the observed information can be used. Before discussing some of these, we will point to some common pitfalls. Little and Rubin (1987, 2002) were among the first to provide a comprehensive treatment. Great care has to be taken with imputation strategies. Dempster and Rubin (1983) write:

> The idea of imputation is both seductive and dangerous. It is seductive because it can lull the user into the pleasurable state of believing that the data are complete after all, and it is dangerous because it lumps together situations where the problem is sufficiently minor that it can be legitimately handled in this way and situations where standard estimators applied to the real and imputed data have substantial biases.

For the large family of now standard modelling tools for large and complex data sets, imputation is almost always detrimental to the inferences made.

Thus, the user of imputation strategies faces several dangers. First, the imputation model could be wrong and, hence, the point estimates would be biased. Second, even for a correct imputation model, the uncertainty resulting from missingness is masked. Even when one is reasonably sure about the mean value the unknown observation *would have had*, the actual stochastic realization, depending on both the mean and error structures, is still unknown. In addition, most methods require the MCAR assumption to hold, while some, such as LOCF, even require additional and often unrealistically strong assumptions.

LOCF will be treated separately in Section 4.2.3 since it can, although it need not, be seen as an imputation strategy. Here, we will briefly describe two other imputation methods. The idea behind *unconditional mean imputation* (Little and Rubin 2002) is to replace a missing value with the average of the observed values on the same variable over the other subjects. Thus, the term *unconditional* refers to the fact that one does not use (i.e., condition on) information on the subject for which an imputation is generated. Since imputed values are unrelated to a subject's other measurements, it is not unlikely for most if not all aspects of a longitudinal or otherwise hierarchical model to be distorted (Verbeke and Molenberghs 2000). In this sense, unconditional mean imputation can be equally as damaging as LOCF.

What is traditionally called *Buck's method*, or *conditional mean imputation* (Buck 1960; Little and Rubin 2002) is technically hardly more complex than mean imputation. Let us describe it for a single multivariate normal sample. The first step is to estimate the mean vector $\boldsymbol{\mu}$ and the covariance matrix Σ from the complete cases, assuming that $\boldsymbol{Y}_i \sim N(\boldsymbol{\mu}, \Sigma)$. For a subject with missing components, the regression of the missing components $\boldsymbol{Y}_i^m$ on the observed ones $\boldsymbol{y}_i^o$ is

$$\boldsymbol{Y}_i^m | \boldsymbol{y}_i^o \sim N(\boldsymbol{\mu}^m + \Sigma^{mo}(\Sigma^{oo})^{-1}(\boldsymbol{y}_i^o - \boldsymbol{\mu}_i^o), \Sigma^{mm} - \Sigma^{mo}(\Sigma^{oo})^{-1}\Sigma^{om}). \tag{4.1}$$

In the second step the conditional mean from the regression of the missing components on the observed ones is calculated and substituted for the missing values. Buck (1960) showed that, under mild conditions, the method is valid for MCAR mechanisms. Little and Rubin (2002) added that the method is valid under certain types of MAR mechanism, at least regarding point estimation. Even though the distribution of the observed components is allowed to differ between complete and incomplete observations, it is very important that the regression of the missing components on the observed ones *is* constant across missingness patterns. Again, this method shares with other single imputation strategies the problem that, although point estimation may be consistent, the precision will be overestimated. There is a connection between the *concept* of conditional mean imputation, a likelihood-based ignorable analysis (Section 4.6), and multiple imputation (Chapter 9), in the sense that the latter two methods produce expectations for the missing observations that are formally equal to those obtained under a conditional mean imputation.

The imputation methods reviewed here are clearly not the only ones. Little and Rubin (2002) mention several others. Methods such as hot deck imputation are based on filling in missing values from 'matching' subjects, where an appropriate matching criterion is used.

Almost all imputation techniques suffer from the following limitations:

1. The performance of imputation techniques is unreliable. Situations where they do work are difficult to distinguish from situations were they prove misleading.
2. Imputation often requires *ad hoc* adjustments to obtain satisfactory point estimates.
3. The methods fail to provide simple, correct estimators of precision.

In addition, most methods require the MCAR assumption to hold and some even go beyond MCAR in their requirements.

The main advantage, shared with CC analysis, is that complete data software can be used. While a CC analysis is even simpler since one does not need to address the imputation task, the imputation family uses all, and in fact too much, of the available information. With the availability of flexible commercial software tools for the analysis of longitudinal data, most of which can deal with unbalanced data, it is no longer necessary to restrict oneself to complete data methods.

4.2.3   Last observation carried forward

In this approach every missing value is replaced by the last observed value from the same subject. Whenever a value is missing, the last observed value is substituted. The technique can be applied to both monotone and non-monotone missing data. It is typically applied to settings where incompleteness is due to attrition.

Very strong and often unrealistic assumptions have to be made to ensure the validity of this method. First, one has to believe that a subject's measurements stay at the same level from the moment of dropout onwards (or during the period they are unobserved, in the case of intermittent missingness). In a clinical trial setting, one might believe that the response profile *changes* as soon as a patient goes off treatment and even that it would flatten. However, the constant profile assumption is even stronger. Further, this method shares with other single imputation methods the problem that it overestimates the precision by treating imputed and actually observed values on equal footing.

LOCF can, but need not, be viewed as an imputation strategy, depending on which of the Views 1, 2a, or 2b of Section 4.1 are taken. When View 1 or 2a is adopted, the aforementioned problems apply, certainly with View 2a, but even more so with View 1. Verbeke and Molenberghs (1997, Chapter 5) have shown that all features of a linear mixed model (group difference, evolution over time, variance structure, correlation structure, random-effects structure, etc.) can be severely affected by application of this technique.

When View 2b is adopted, the scientific question is in terms of the last observed measurement. This situation is often considered to be a genuine motivation for LOCF. However, there still are two fundamental objections. First, several questions so defined have a very unrealistic and *ad hoc* flavour. Clearly, measurements at (self-selected) dropout times are lumped together with measurements made at the (investigator-defined) end of the study. Second and very importantly, it is noteworthy that LOCF should be seen as logically different from View 2b. Indeed, whichever imputation method is chosen, or even, when no imputation at all takes place, this analysis would always be the same. The only condition is that no measurements are deleted (as in the CC analysis). Thus, when View 2b is considered plausible, the problem of missingness is avoided and hence cannot provide any evidence about the relative performance of methods to deal with missingness.

There is a considerable literature pointing out these, and other, problems with LOCF as an analysis technique. Publications include Gibbons *et al.* (1993), Verbeke and Molenberghs (2000), Lavori *et al.* (1995), Siddiqui *et al.* (1998), Heyting *et al.* (1992), Mallinckrodt *et al.* (2001a, 2001b, 2003a, 2003b), Molenberghs *et al.* (2004), Molenberghs and Verbeke (2005), Carpenter *et al.* (2004), and Beunckens *et al.* (2005).

Despite these shortcomings, LOCF has, in many areas, been the long-standing method of choice for the primary analysis in clinical trials because of its simplicity, ease of implementation, and belief that the potential bias from carrying observations forward leads to a 'conservative' analysis. We will return to these points in the next section.

The following example, using the hypothetical data in Table 4.1, illustrates the handling of missing data via LOCF. For patient 3, the last observed value, 19, is used to compute the mean change to endpoint for treatment group 1; and, for patient 6, the last observed value, 20, is used to compute the mean change to endpoint for treatment group 2. The imputed data are considered to

Table 4.1 Artificial incomplete data.

			Week					
Patient	Treatment	Baseline	1	2	3	4	5	6
1	1	22	20	18	16	14	12	10
2	1	22	21	18	15	12	9	6
3	1	22	22	21	20	19	*	*
4	2	20	20	20	20	21	21	22
5	2	21	22	22	23	24	25	26
6	2	18	19	20	*	*	*	*

be as informative as the actual data because the analysis does not distinguish between the actually observed data and the imputed data.

The assertion that LOCF yields conservative results does not appear to have arisen from formal proofs or rigorous empirical study. In the next section, it will be clear that LOCF can exaggerate the magnitude of treatment effects and inflate Type I error, that is, falsely conclude a difference exists when in fact the difference is zero.

Furthermore, mean change from baseline to endpoint is only a snapshot view of the response profile of a treatment. Gibbons *et al.* (1993) stated that endpoint analyses are insufficient because the evolution of response over time must be assessed to completely understand a treatment's efficacy profile. By its very design, LOCF change to endpoint cannot assess response profiles over time. Furthermore, advances in statistical theory and in computer hardware and software have made many alternative methods simple and easy to implement.

4.3 PROBLEMS WITH COMPLETE CASE ANALYSIS AND LAST OBSERVATION CARRIED FORWARD

Using the simple but insightful setting of two repeated follow-up measures, the first of which is always observed while the second can be missing, we establish some properties of the LOCF and CC estimation procedures under different missing data mechanisms. In this way, we are able to bring LOCF and CC within a general framework that makes clear their relationships with more formal modelling approaches and so provide a foundation for a coherent comparison among them. The use of a moderate amount of algebra will enable us to reach a number of interesting conclusions.

Let us assume that each subject i is to be measured on two occasions $t_i = 0, 1$. Subjects are randomized to one of two treatment arms: $T_i = 0$ for the standard arm and 1 for the experimental arm. The probability of a measurement being observed on the second occasion ($D_i = 2$) is p_0 and p_1 for treatment groups 0 and 1, respectively. We can write the means of the observations in the two dropout groups as follows:

$$\text{dropouts, } D_i = 1, \quad \beta_0 + \beta_1 T_i + \beta_2 t_i + \beta_3 T_i t_i, \tag{4.2}$$

$$\text{completers, } D_i = 2, \quad \gamma_0 + \gamma_1 T_i + \gamma_2 t_i + \gamma_3 T_i t_i. \tag{4.3}$$

The true underlying population treatment difference at time $t_i = 1$, as determined from (4.2)–(4.3), is equal to

$$\Delta_{\text{true}} = p_1(\gamma_0 + \gamma_1 + \gamma_2 + \gamma_3) + (1 - p_1)(\beta_0 + \beta_1 + \beta_2 + \beta_3)$$

$$- [p_0(\gamma_0 + \gamma_2) + (1 - p_0)(\beta_0 + \beta_2)]. \tag{4.4}$$

If we use LOCF as the estimation procedure, the expectation of the corresponding estimator equals

$$\Delta_{\text{LOCF}} = p_1(\gamma_0 + \gamma_1 + \gamma_2 + \gamma_3) + (1 - p_1)(\beta_0 + \beta_1)$$
$$- [p_0(\gamma_0 + \gamma_2) + (1 - p_0)\beta_0]. \tag{4.5}$$

Alternatively, if we use CC, the above expression changes to

$$\Delta_{\text{CC}} = \gamma_1 + \gamma_3. \tag{4.6}$$

Clearly these are, in general, both biased estimators.

We will now consider the special but important cases where the true missing data mechanisms are MCAR and MAR, respectively. Each of these will impose particular constraints on the β and γ parameters in model (4.2)–(4.3). Under MCAR, the β parameters are equal to their γ counterparts and (4.4) simplifies to

$$\Delta_{\text{MCAR,true}} = \beta_1 + \beta_3. \tag{4.7}$$

Suppose we apply the LOCF procedure in this setting. The expectation of the resulting estimator then simplifies to

$$\Delta_{\text{MCAR,LOCF}} = \beta_1 + (p_1 - p_0)\beta_2 + p_1\beta_3. \tag{4.8}$$

The bias is given by the difference between (4.7) and (4.8):

$$B_{\text{MCAR,LOCF}} = (p_1 - p_0)\beta_2 - (1 - p_1)\beta_3. \tag{4.9}$$

While of a simple form, we can learn several things from this expression by focusing on each of the terms in turn. First, suppose $\beta_3 = 0$ and $\beta_2 \neq 0$, implying that there is no differential treatment effect between the two measurement occasions but there is an overall time trend. Then the bias can go in both directions depending on the sign of $p_1 - p_0$ and the sign of β_2. Note that $p_1 = p_0$ only in the very special case the dropout rate is the same in both treatment arms. Whether or not this is the case has no impact on the status of the dropout mechanism (it is MCAR in either case, even though in the second case dropout is treatment-arm dependent), but is potentially very important for the bias implied by LOCF. Second, suppose $\beta_3 \neq 0$ and $\beta_2 = 0$. Then, again, the bias can go in both directions depending on the sign of β_3, that is, depending on whether the treatment effect at the second occasion is larger or smaller than the treatment effect at the first occasion. In conclusion, even under the unrealistically strong assumption of MCAR, we see that the bias in the LOCF estimator typically does not vanish and, even more importantly, the bias can be positive or negative, and can even induce an apparent treatment effect when there is none.

In contrast, as can be seen from (4.6) and (4.7), the CC analysis is clearly unbiased.

Let us now turn to the MAR case. In this setting, the constraint implied by the MAR structure of the dropout mechanism is that the conditional distribution of the second observation given the first is the same in both dropout groups (Molenberghs *et al.* 1998b). Based on this result, the expectation of the second observation in the standard arm of the dropout group is

$$E(Y_{i2}|D_i = 1, T_i = 0) = \gamma_0 + \gamma_2 + \sigma(\beta_0 - \gamma_0) \tag{4.10}$$

where $\sigma = \sigma_{12}\sigma_{11}^{-1}$, in which σ_{11} is the variance of the first observation in the fully observed group and σ_{12} is the corresponding covariance between the pair of observations. Similarly, in the experimental group, we obtain

$$E(Y_{i2}|D_i = 1, T_i = 1) = \gamma_0 + \gamma_1 + \gamma_2 + \gamma_3 + \sigma(\beta_0 + \beta_1 - \gamma_0 - \gamma_1). \tag{4.11}$$

The true underlying population treatment difference (4.4) then becomes

$$\Delta_{\text{MAR,true}} = \gamma_1 + \gamma_3 + \sigma[(1 - p_1)(\beta_0 + \beta_1 - \gamma_0 - \gamma_1) - (1 - p_0)(\beta_0 - \gamma_0)]. \tag{4.12}$$

In this case, the bias in the LOCF estimator can be written as:

$$\begin{aligned} B_{\text{MAR,LOCF}} =& p_1(\gamma_0 + \gamma_1 + \gamma_2 + \gamma_3) + (1 - p_1)(\beta_0 + \beta_1) \\ &- p_0(\gamma_0 + \gamma_2) - (1 - p_0)\beta_0 - \gamma_1 - \gamma_3 \\ &- \sigma[(1 - p_1)(\beta_0 + \beta_1 - \gamma_0 - \gamma_1) \\ &- (1 - p_0)(\beta_0 - \gamma_0)]. \end{aligned} \tag{4.13}$$

Again, although involving more complicated relationships, it is clear that the bias can go in either direction, thus contradicting the claim often put forward that the LOCF procedure, even though biased, is a conservative one. Further, it is far from clear what conditions need to be imposed in this setting for the corresponding estimator to be either unbiased or conservative.

The bias in the CC estimator case takes the form

$$B_{\text{MAR,CC}} = -\sigma[(1 - p_1)(\beta_0 + \beta_1 - \gamma_0 - \gamma_1) - (1 - p_0)(\beta_0 - \gamma_0)]. \tag{4.14}$$

Even though this expression is simpler than in the LOCF case, it is still true that the bias can operate in both directions.

Thus, in all cases, LOCF typically produces bias whose direction and magnitude depend on the true but unknown treatment effects. This implies that great caution is needed when using this method. In contrast, an ignorable likelihood based analysis, as outlined in Sections 4.4 and 4.6, and using results from Section 3.5, provides a consistent estimator of the true treatment difference at the second occasion under both MCAR and MAR, provided the regression model of the second measurement on the first one is of a linear form. While this is an assumption, it is rather a mild one in contrast to the very stringent conditions required to justify the LOCF method, even when the qualitative features of the bias are considered more important than the quantitative ones. It is worth observing that the LOCF method does not even work under the strong MCAR conditions, whereas the CC approach does.

4.4   USING THE AVAILABLE CASES: A FREQUENTIST VERSUS A LIKELIHOOD PERSPECTIVE

In Section 3.5 it was shown, using results from Rubin (1976), that a likelihood analysis is valid when applied to an incomplete set of data, provided the missing data are MAR and under some mild regularity conditions. This implies that likelihood-based and Bayesian analyses are viable candidates for the routine primary analysis of clinical trial data. This result has some interesting implications for standard results, such as the equivalence of least-squares regression and normal distribution based regression. While they produce the same point estimator and asymptotically the same precision estimator *for balanced and complete data*, this is no longer true in the incomplete data setting. The former method is frequentist in nature, the second one likelihood-based. We will illustrate this result for a simple, bivariate normal population with missingness in Section 4.4.1. An analogous result for an incomplete contingency table will be derived in Section 4.4.2.

4.4.1   A bivariate normal population

Consider a bivariate normal population,

$$\begin{pmatrix} Y_{i1} \\ Y_{i2} \end{pmatrix} \sim N\left(\begin{pmatrix} \mu_1 \\ \mu_2 \end{pmatrix}, \begin{pmatrix} \sigma_{11} & \sigma_{12} \\ & \sigma_{22} \end{pmatrix} \right), \tag{4.15}$$

out of which $i = 1, \ldots, N$ subjects are sampled, each of which is supposed to provide $j = 1, 2$ measurements. Assume further that d subjects complete the study and $N - d$ drop out after the first measurement occasion.

In a frequentist available case method each of the parameters in (4.15) is estimated using the available information (Little and Rubin 2002; Verbeke and Molenberghs 2000). This implies μ_1 and σ_{11} would be estimated using all N subjects, whereas only the remaining d contribute to the other three parameters. For the mean parameters, this produces

$$\widehat{\mu_1} = \frac{1}{N} \sum_{i=1}^{N} y_{i1}, \tag{4.16}$$

$$\widetilde{\mu}_2 = \frac{1}{d}\sum_{i=1}^{d} y_{i2}; \tag{4.17}$$

maximum likelihood estimators are indicated by hats, while tildes are used for frequentist, least-squares type estimators. This method is valid only under MCAR. An added disadvantage is that, since different information is used for different parameters, and when samples are small, it is possible to produce, for example, non-positive definite covariance matrices, even though consistency under MCAR is not jeopardized. Further, application of the method to more complex designs is less than straightforward. Fortunately, there is no need to apply the method since the likelihood approach is more broadly valid and, at the same time, computationally easier.

To obtain an explicit expression for the likelihood-based estimators, along the lines of Little and Rubin (2002), observe that the conditional density of the second outcome given the first one, based on (4.15), can be written as

$$Y_{i2}|y_{i1} \sim N(\beta_0 + \beta_1 y_{i1}, \sigma^2_{2|1}), \tag{4.18}$$

where

$$\beta_1 = \rho\frac{\sigma_2}{\sigma_1},$$

$$\beta_0 = \mu_2 - \beta_1\mu_1 = \mu_2 - \rho\frac{\sigma_2}{\sigma_1}\mu_1,$$

$$\sigma^2_{2|1} = \sigma^2_2(1-\rho^2).$$

Now the maximum likelihood estimator for the first mean coincides with (4.16), underscoring the fact that ordinary least squares and maximum likelihood provide the same point estimators, when the data are complete. For the second mean, however, we now obtain:

$$\widehat{\mu}_2 = \frac{1}{N}\left\{\sum_{i=1}^{d} y_{i2} + \sum_{i=d+1}^{N}\left[\bar{y}_2 + \widehat{\beta}_1(y_{i1} - \bar{y}_1)\right]\right\} \tag{4.19}$$

Here, $\bar{y}_1$ is the mean of the measurements at the first occasion among the completers. Several observations can be made. First, under MCAR, the completers and dropouts have equal distributions at the first occasion, and hence the correction term has expectation zero, again rendering the frequentist and likelihood methods equivalent, *even though they do not produce exactly the same point estimator*. Second, when there is no correlation between the first and second measurements, the regression coefficient $\beta_1 = 0$, and hence there is no correction either.

Note that, in practice, the estimators do not have to be derived explicitly. While they are insightful, standard likelihood-based analyses, for example using standard software, will automatically ensure that corrections of the type (4.19) are used. Thus, for example, it would be sufficient to estimate the parameters in (4.15) using the SAS procedure MIXED, as long as complete and incomplete sequences are passed on to the procedure.

Further, the coefficient β_1 depends on the variance components σ_{11}, σ_{12}, and σ_{22}. This implies that a misspecified variance structure may lead to bias in $\widehat{\mu_2}$. Thus, the well-known independence between the distributions of the estimators for μ and Σ in multivariate normal population holds, once again, only when the data are balanced and complete.

4.4.2   An incomplete contingency table

Analogous to the incomplete bivariate normal sample of the previous section, it is insightful to consider an incomplete 2×2 contingency table:

$$
\begin{array}{|c|c|}\hline Y_{1,11} & Y_{1,12} \\ \hline Y_{1,21} & Y_{1,22} \\ \hline\end{array}
\begin{array}{|c|}\hline Y_{0,} \\ \hline Y_{1,} \\ \hline\end{array},
\tag{4.20}
$$

where $Y_{r,jk}$ refers to the number of subjects in the completer ($r = 1$) and dropout ($r = 0$) groups, respectively, with response profile (j, k). Since for the dropouts only the first outcome is observed, only summaries $Y_{r=0,j}$ are observable. Using all available data, the probability of success at the first time is estimated as

$$
\widehat{\pi}_1 = \frac{Y_{1,1+} + Y_{0,1+}}{N},
\tag{4.21}
$$

where $+$ instead of a subscript refers to summing over the corresponding subscript. When the available cases only are used, the estimator for the success probability at the second time is

$$
\widetilde{\pi}_2 = \frac{Y_{1,+1}}{d}.
\tag{4.22}
$$

Once again, information from the incomplete subjects is not used. It is easy to show that the maximum likelihood estimator under MAR, that is, ignorability, equals

$$
\widehat{\pi}_2 = \frac{Y_{1,+1} + Y_{0,1} \cdot \frac{Y_{1,11}}{Y_{1,1+}} + Y_{0,2} \cdot \frac{Y_{1,21}}{Y_{1,2+}}}{N}.
\tag{4.23}
$$

The second and third terms in (4.23) result from splitting the partially classified counts according to the corresponding conditional distributions in the first table.

4.5 INTENTION TO TREAT

A related and, for the regulatory clinical trial context, very important set of assertions is the following:

1. An ignorable likelihood analysis can be specified a priori in a protocol without any difficulty.
2. An ignorable likelihood analysis is consistent with the intention to treat (ITT) principle, even when only the measurement at the last occasion is of interest (provided that the treatment compliance of those who drop out is assumed to be the same as those who remain).
3. The difference between an LOCF and an ignorable likelihood analysis can be both liberal and conservative.

The first is easy to see since, given ignorability, formulating a linear mixed model or another likelihood-based approach for either complete or incomplete data involves exactly the same steps.

Let us expand on the second issue. It is often believed that when the last measurement is of interest a test for the treatment effect at the last occasion neglects sequences with dropout, even when such sequences contain post-randomization outcomes. As a result, it is often asserted that to be consistent with ITT some form of imputation, based on an incomplete patient's data, for example using LOCF, is necessary. However, as shown in Section 4.4.1, likelihood-based estimation of means in an incomplete multivariate setting involves adjustment in terms of the conditional expectation of the unobserved measurements given the observed ones. Thus, a likelihood-based ignorable analysis should be seen as a proper way to accommodate information on a patient with post-randomization outcomes, even when such a patient's profile is incomplete. This fact, in conjunction with the use of treatment allocation as randomized rather than as received, shows that direct likelihood is fully consistent with ITT.

Regarding the third issue, consider a situation where the treatment difference increases over time, reaches a maximum around the middle of the study period, with a decline thereafter until complete disappearance at the end of the study. Suppose, further, that the bulk of dropout occurs around the middle of the study. Then an endpoint analysis based on MAR will produce the correct nominal level, whereas LOCF might reject the null hypothesis too often. When considering LOCF, we often have in mind examples in which the disease shows progressive improvement over time. However, when the goal of a treatment is maintenance of condition in a progressively worsening disease state, LOCF can exaggerate the treatment benefit. For example, in Alzheimer's disease the goal is to prevent the patient from worsening. Thus, in a one-year trial where a patient on active treatment drops out after one week, carrying the last value forward implicitly assumes no further worsening. This is obviously not conservative.

4.6   CONCLUDING REMARKS

We have noted that in many settings the MAR assumption is more reasonable than the MCAR assumption or the set of assumptions that has to be made for an LOCF analysis. Likelihood-based and Bayesian methodology offers a general framework from which to develop valid analyses under the MAR assumption. Flexible longitudinal methods such as the linear mixed model (Verbeke and Molenberghs 2000) and the generalized linear mixed model (Molenberghs and Verbeke 2005) can be used in a routine fashion under MAR. In many settings, a saturated group by time model for the mean, combined with an unstructured covariance matrix, can be considered. When outcomes are continuous, this leads to a classical, general multivariate normal model. In the next chapter, we will show that such analyses do not have to be seen as making more assumptions than, say, a multivariate analysis of variance (MANOVA), an ANOVA for each time point, or a simple t test. The method easily extends towards more elaborate covariance structures, often thought to derive from random effects and/or serial correlation. Most importantly, all of them are valid under MAR, provided the model is correctly specified. Specific choices for such a model in the continuous data case were termed *mixed-effects model repeated measures* analysis by Mallinckrodt *et al.* (2001a, 2001b, 2003a, 2003b).

Molenberghs *et al.* (2004) discussed the sense in which likelihood-based MAR methods are consistent with the ITT principle, and in fact are an improvement over LOCF in this regard, via appropriate use of all available data on all patients.

5

Analysis of the Orthodontic Growth Data

5.1 INTRODUCTION AND MODELS

Jennrich and Schluchter (1986), Little and Rubin (2002), and Verbeke and Molenberghs (1997, 2000) each fitted the same eight models to the orthodontic growth data introduced in Section 2.3. The models can be expressed within the general linear mixed models family (Verbeke and Molenberghs 2000):

$$Y_i = X_i\boldsymbol{\beta} + Z_i\boldsymbol{b}_i + \boldsymbol{\varepsilon}_i, \tag{5.1}$$

where

$$\boldsymbol{b}_i \sim N(\mathbf{0}, D),$$

$$\boldsymbol{\varepsilon}_i \sim N(\mathbf{0}, \Sigma_i),$$

and $\boldsymbol{b}_i$ and $\boldsymbol{\varepsilon}_i$ are statistically independent. Here, Y_i is the (4×1) response vector, X_i is a $(4 \times p)$ design matrix for the fixed effects, $\boldsymbol{\beta}$ is a vector of unknown fixed regression coefficients, Z_i is a $(4 \times q)$ design matrix for the random effects, $\boldsymbol{b}_i$ is a $(q \times 1)$ vector of normally distributed random parameters, with covariance matrix D, and $\boldsymbol{\varepsilon}_i$ is a normally distributed (4×1) random error vector, with covariance matrix Σ. Since every subject contributes exactly four measurements at exactly the same time points, it is possible to drop the subscript i from the error covariance matrix Σ_i unless, for example, sex is thought to influence the residual covariance structure. The random error $\boldsymbol{\varepsilon}_i$ encompasses both cross-sectional (as in a cross-sectional study) and serial correlation. The design will be a function of age, sex, and/or the interaction between both. Let us indicate

Missing Data in Clinical Studies   G. Molenberghs and M.G. Kenward
© 2007 John Wiley & Sons, Ltd

boys (girls) with $x_i = 0$ ($x_i = 1$). Time, expressed as age of the child, takes four values: $t_{ij} \equiv t_j = 8, 10, 12, 14$.

In Section 5.2 the original, complete set of data is analysed, with direct likelihood methodology applied to the incomplete version of the data in Section 5.3. These analyses are compared with the simple ones in Section 5.4. A perspective on how to implement the methodology in SAS is given in Section 5.5. Finally, implications for power are discussed in Section 5.6.

5.2   THE ORIGINAL, COMPLETE DATA

Table 5.1 summarizes model fitting and comparison for the eight models originally considered by Jennrich and Schluchter (1987). The initial model 1 assumes an unstructured group by time model, producing eight mean parameters. In addition, the variance–covariance matrix is left unstructured, yielding an additional 10 parameters. First the mean structure is simplified, followed by the covariance structure. Models 2 and 3 consider the mean profiles to be non-parallel and parallel straight lines, respectively. While the second model fits adequately, the third one does not, based on conventional likelihood ratio tests. Thus, the crossing lines will be retained. Models 4 and 5 assume the variance–covariance structure to be of a banded (Toeplitz) and first-order autoregressive (AR(1)) type, respectively. Model 6 assumes the covariance structure to arise from correlated random intercepts and random slopes. In model 7, a compound symmetry (CS) structure is assumed, which can be seen as the marginalization of a random-intercepts model. Finally, model 8 assumes

Table 5.1 Growth data: complete data set. Model fit summary. (Par., number of model parameters; -2ℓ, minus twice the log-likelihood; Ref., reference model for likelihood ratio test; G^2, likelihood ratio test statistic value; d.f., corresponding number of degrees of freedom; RI, random intercepts; RS, random slopes; CS, compound symmetry.)

	Mean	Covariance	Par.	-2ℓ	Ref.	G^2	d.f.	p-value
1	unstructured	unstructured	18	416.509				
2	$\neq$ slopes	unstructured	14	419.477	1	2.968	4	0.5632
3	$=$ slopes	unstructured	13	426.153	2	6.676	1	0.0098
4	$\neq$ slopes	Toeplitz	8	424.643	2	5.166	6	0.5227
5	$\neq$ slopes	AR(1)	6	440.681	2	21.204	8	0.0066
					4	16.038	2	0.0003
6	$\neq$ slopes	RI+RS	8	427.806	2	8.329	6	0.2150
7	$\neq$ slopes	CS (RI)	6	428.639	2	9.162	8	0.3288
					4	3.996	2	0.1356
					6	0.833	2	0.6594
					6	0.833	1:2	0.5104
8	$\neq$ slopes	simple	5	478.242	7	49.603	1	< 0.0001
					7	49.603	0:1	< 0.0001

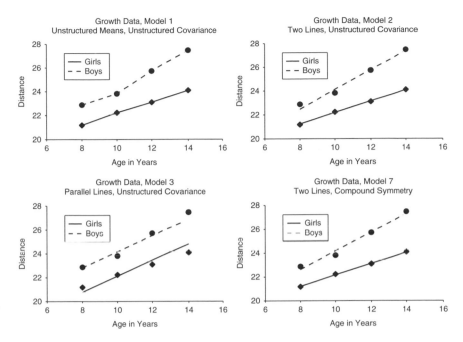

Figure 5.1 Growth data. Profiles for the complete data, for a selected set of models.

uncorrelated measurements. Of these, models 4, 6, and 7 are well fitting. Model 7, being the most parsimonious one, will be retained.

5.3 DIRECT LIKELIHOOD

Let us now fit the same eight models to the trimmed version of the data set, as presented by Little and Rubin (2002), using direct likelihood methods. This implies the same models are fitted with the same software tools, but now to a reduced set of data. Molenberghs and Verbeke (1997) presented CC and LOCF analyses for the same eight models. In the next section, we will compare the analyses of the original, non-trimmed data, to CC, LOCF, and direct likelihood analyses. Figure 5.1 shows the observed and fitted mean structures for models 1, 2, 3, and 7. Note that observed and fitted means coincide for model 1. This is in line with general theory, since the model saturates the group by time mean structure *and*, in addition, the data are balanced. The same will not be true in the next section, where direct likelihood is applied to the trimmed set of data.

Table 5.2 presents the counterpart to Table 5.1 for the incomplete data and using direct likelihood. Note that the same model 7 is selected. Were simple methods to be used, quite a different picture would emerge, as is clear from Table 5.3.

Table 5.2 Growth data. Direct likelihood analysis. Model fit summary. (Par., number of model parameters; -2ℓ, minus twice the log-likelihood; Ref., reference model for likelihood ratio test; G^2, likelihood ratio test statistic value; d.f., corresponding number of degrees of freedom; CS, compound symmetry.)

	Mean	Covariance	Par.	-2ℓ	Ref.	G^2	d.f.	p
1	unstructured	unstructured	18	386.957				
2	≠ slopes	unstructured	14	393.288	1	6.331	4	0.1758
3	= slopes	unstructured	13	397.400	2	4.112	1	0.0426
4	≠ slopes	banded	8	398.030	2	4.742	6	0.5773
5	≠ slopes	AR(1)	6	409.523	2	16.235	8	0.0391
6	≠ slopes	random	8	400.452	2	7.164	6	0.3059
7	≠ slopes	CS	6	401.313	6	0.861	2	0.6502
					6	0.861	1:2	0.5018
8	≠ slopes	simple	5	441.583	7	40.270	1	<0.0001
					7	40.270	0:1	<0.0001

Table 5.3 Growth data. Finally selected model under a number of simple missing data handling mechanisms. (Par., number of parameters; CS, compound symmetry; a suffix 'a' on a model number refers to a variation on one of the models in Tables 5.1 and 5.2.)

Method	Model	Mean	Covariance	Par.
Complete case	7a	= slopes	CS	5
LOCF	2a	quadratic	unstructured	16
Unconditional mean	7a	= slopes	CS	5
Conditional mean	1	unstructured	unstructured	18

Let us return to the results of the direct likelihood analysis. Figure 5.2 displays the fit of models 1, 2, 3, and 7. In contrast to Figure 5.1, observed and expected means now do not coincide under model 1, even though it saturates the group by age mean structure. This is entirely in line with the developments given in Section 4.4. The likelihood takes into account the expectation of the missing measurements, given the observed ones. In our case, this only occurs at the age of 10. Comparing the small (all children) with the large (remaining children) bullets and diamonds, it is clear that those remaining in the study have larger measurements than those removed. The direct likelihood correction has produced estimates at the age of 10 that are situated below the observed means. Obviously, the likelihood tends to overcorrect in this case. The reason for this is that the estimated correlation between ages 8 and 10 is substantially larger than the correlation between ages 10 and 12. Such variability is not unexpected in relatively small samples. Hence, careful reflection on the variance–covariance structure is much more important here than when data are complete and balanced. We return to these points in the next section.

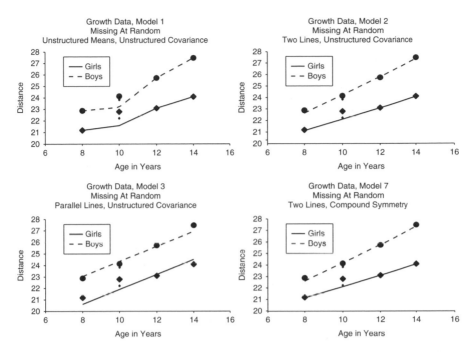

Figure 5.2 Profiles for the growth data set, from a selected set of models. MAR analysis. (The small symbols at age 10 are the observed group means for the complete data set.)

5.4 COMPARISON OF ANALYSES

In the previous section we illustrated the points made in the previous chapter, namely that such simple methods as CC and LOCF, as well as other simple imputation methods, can be quite distorting, whereas direct likelihood retains its validity under MAR. One might argue that the price to pay is the need to fit a model to the entire longitudinal sequence, even in circumstances where scientific interest focuses on the last planned measurement occasion. For continuous data, an obvious choice for such a full longitudinal model is the linear mixed model, as exemplified in Section 5.1.

However, for balanced longitudinal data, where the number of subjects is sufficiently large compared with the number of measurement occasions (a rough rule of thumb $N \geq 10n$ is suggested later in Section 5.6), a full multivariate normal can often be considered. An example is model 1 fitted to the growth data. Such a model does not make assumptions beyond those made by, say, a MANOVA, an ANOVA for each time point or, equivalently, a t test per time point. This is illustrated in Table 5.4, using model 1 fitted to the complete and trimmed growth data. Means for boys at ages 8 and 10 are displayed. Whenever the data are balanced, the means are the same regardless of which estimation method is used. Standard errors are asymptotically the same and even in a small

Table 5.4 Growth data. Likelihood, MANOVA, and ANOVA analyses for the original data and the trimmed data (observed, CC, and LOCF). Means for boys at ages 8 and 10 are displayed. (ML, maximum likelihood; REML, restricted maximum likelihood.)

Principle	Method	Boys at age 8	Boys at age 10
Original	ML	22.88 (0.56)	23.81 (0.49)
	REML ≡ MANOVA	22.88 (0.58)	23.81 (0.51)
	ANOVA per time	22.88 (0.61)	23.81 (0.53)
Observed	ML	22.88 (0.56)	23.17 (0.68)
	REML	22.88 (0.58)	23.17 (0.71)
	MANOVA	24.00 (0.48)	24.14 (0.66)
	ANOVA per time	22.88 (0.61)	24.14 (0.74)
CC	ML	24.00 (0.45)	24.14 (0.62)
	REML ≡ MANOVA	24.00 (0.48)	24.14 (0.66)
	ANOVA per time	24.00 (0.51)	24.14 (0.74)
LOCF	ML	22.88 (0.56)	22.97 (0.65)
	REML ≡ MANOVA	22.88 (0.58)	22.97 (0.68)
	ANOVA per time	22.88 (0.61)	22.97 (0.72)

sample like the one considered here, differences are negligible. Note that CC overestimates the means since the subjects removed from analysis have lower means than average, and LOCF underestimates the mean at age 10, since the age 8 measurement is carried forward.

When the observed data are analysed, it is clear that the results from the direct likelihood analyses (maximum likelihood and restricted maximum likelihood), valid under MAR, diverge from the frequentist MANOVA and ANOVA analyses, which are valid only under MCAR. MANOVA effectively reduces to CC, due to its inability to take incomplete sequences into account. ANOVA produces a frequentist available case analysis, with correct inferences only at measurement occasions with complete data.

Once again, we observe that direct likelihood overcorrects, leading to mean estimates that are slightly too small. This is not due to bias, but rather to small-sample variability. It underscores the necessity to correctly specify the variance–covariance structure, and to ensure that its constituent parameters are estimated sufficiently accurately. Otherwise, the likelihood corrections outlined in Section 4.4 do not perform well.

Let us consider Table 5.5 to gain further insight into the need for an adequate specification of the covariance structure. We retain an unstructured group by age mean structure, and pair it with three covariance structures. Apart from an unstructured residual covariance matrix (model 1), we also consider a CS structure (model 7b) and an independence structure (model 8b).

When the data are complete, the choice of covariance structure is immaterial for the point estimates, whereas the choice is crucial when data are incomplete. Next to the overcorrection of model 1 at age 10, model 7b exhibits quite acceptable behaviour, but model 8b coincides with and hence is as bad as CC

Table 5.5 Growth data. Comparison of mean estimates for boys at ages 8 and 10, complete and incomplete data, using direct likelihood, an unstructured mean model, and various covariance models.

Data	Mean	Covariance	Boys at age 8	Boys at age 10
Complete	unstructured	unstructured	22.88	23.81
	unstructured	CS	22.88	23.81
	unstructured	simple	22.88	23.81
Incomplete	unstructured	unstructured	22.88	23.17
	unstructured	CS	22.88	23.52
	unstructured	simple	22.88	24.14

at age 10. The adequate performance of model 7b is due to the fact that the expected mean of a missing age 10 measurement gives equal weight to all surrounding measurements, rather than overweighting the age 8 measurement due to an accidentally high correlation. The zero correlations in model 8b do not allow for such a correction and hence the information that the ages 8, 12, and 14 measurements for the incomplete profiles are relatively low is wasted.

Figure 5.3 presents the mean fit associated with all three models, for both sexes. Whereas the models, fitted to the complete data, would all simply pass through the large bullets and diamonds, the differences clearly emerge from the line profiles when the models are fitted to the incomplete data. Once more,

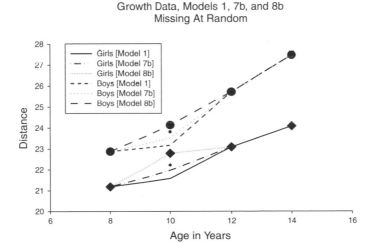

Figure 5.3 Growth data. Fitted mean profiles to the incomplete data, using maximum likelihood, an unstructured mean model and unstructured (model 1), CS (model 7b), and independence (model 8b) covariance structure.

the best fit is obtained with model 7b (CS), which treats all 'neighbouring' measurements equally when predicting a missing observation at the age of 10, from the measurements taken at the ages 8, 12, and 14.

5.5   EXAMPLE SAS CODE FOR MULTIVARIATE LINEAR MODELS

When fitting model 1 to the complete growth data set, the following code can be used:

```
proc mixed data = help method = ml;
title 'Model 1';
class sex idnr age;
model measure = age*sex / noint solution;
repeated / type = un subject = idnr r rcorr;
run;
```

A small precaution is needed when fitting the code to the incomplete data. When the nine lines, corresponding to the nine missing measurements, are removed from the data set, it is implicitly assumed that the remaining measurements, actually corresponding to ages 8, 12, and 14, would correspond to ages 8, 10, and 12. To avoid problems, therefore, it is best to rewrite the REPEATED statement as

```
repeated age / type = un subject = idnr r rcorr;
```

This form of the code would always be valid, and therefore it is good defensive programming practice always to include the variable specifying the time ordering in the REPEATED statement.

For models where age is also used as a continuous – and not merely as a class – variable, a second copy is needed, so that age can be used as a continuous and a class variable at the same time:

```
data help;
set growthav;
agec = age;
run;
proc mixed data = help method = ml;
title 'Model 2';
class sex idnr agec;
model measure = sex age*sex / solution;
repeated agec / type = un subject = idnr r rcorr;
run;
```

5.6 COMPARATIVE POWER UNDER DIFFERENT COVARIANCE STRUCTURES

In advocating the use of the unstructured covariance matrix for analysing repeated measurements data we need to be sure that this is not an excessively inefficient procedure. Here we examine the effect on power for (1) treatment-by-time interaction and (2) final time point comparison, with two treatment groups, when moving from a structured to an unstructured covariance matrix. Such a comparison can only be made meaningfully for tests with the correct nominal size, and to ensure this we need each test to be valid under a given *true* covariance matrix. This implies that all structures compared directly must be nested, with the true matrix the most parsimonious. We consider here three sets of such nested structures. The number of parameters are expressed in terms of the maximum number of follow-up times (n):

1. The first-order autoregressive (AR) series:

   AR(1)   first-order autoregressive, 2 parameters;
   ARH(1)   heterogeneous first-order autoregressive, $n+1$ parameters;
   AD(1)   first-order ante-dependence structure, $2n-1$ parameters;
   UN   unstructured, $n(n+1)/2$ parameters.

2. The first-order moving-average (MA) series:

   TOEP(2)   order 2 Toeplitz, 2 parameters;
   TOEPH(2) heterogeneous order 2 Toeplitz, $n+1$ parameters;
   UN(2)   order 2 banded unstructured, $2n-1$ parameters;
   UN   unstructured, $n(n+1)/2$ parameters.

3. The compound symmetric (CS) series:

   CS   compound symmetry, 2 parameters;
   CSH   heterogeneous compound symmetry, $n+1$ parameters;
   UN   unstructured, $n(n+1)/2$ parameters.

For each set it is assumed that the data actually follow the most parsimonious structure (AR(1), TOEP(2), CS) with a correlation of 0.5. To compare the power of the relevant tests (interaction or final time point) under the different structures we consider the set of alternative hypotheses which generate a power of 80% under the most parsimonious structure. The other structures must necessarily have less power than this (under the same alternatives): we are interested in the size of the differences. The power has been calculated using the Kenward and Roger small-sample adjustment to the Wald statistic and its degrees of freedom (Kenward and Roger 1997).

Two values of n are considered, 5 and 10; and four sample sizes (N): 12, 24, 48, and 96. We are assuming that one-third of subjects drop out in the patterns given in Table 5.6 (in sets of 12; 'M' implies missing) with dropout distributed evenly between the two groups.

Table 5.6 Power calculations. Dropout pattern in the two treatment groups. (O, observed; M, missing.)

n = 5

1	2	3	4	5	Replication
		Time			
O	O	O	O	O	8
O	O	O	O	M	1
O	O	O	M	M	1
O	O	M	M	M	1
O	M	M	M	M	1

n = 10

1	2	3	4	5	6	7	8	9	10	Replication
				Time						
O	O	O	O	O	O	O	O	O	O	8
O	O	O	O	O	O	O	O	O	M	1
O	O	O	O	O	O	O	M	M	M	1
O	O	O	O	O	M	M	M	M	M	1
O	O	O	M	M	M	M	M	M	M	1

Table 5.7 contains the powers as a percentage, for the three sets under all combinations of structure, number of times, and number of subjects for the treatment-by-time interaction (on $n - 1$ d.f.) and the final time point comparison (on 1 d.f.), respectively.

We first note that very similar patterns of power apply to each of the three series of structures, so no distinction will be made among these in the following. The impact of a particular covariance structure on power depends both on how well it is estimated, and on the role of the structure in the estimate of the relevant effects and in their estimated precision. We expect this impact to be much higher in the interaction test, and this is shown clearly in the results in Table 5.7. With smaller sample sizes the unstructured covariance matrix leads to great loss of power, an extreme result occurring with 10 time points and only 12 subjects, for which the power appears hardly greater than the size of the test. In fact for such tiny sample sizes the approximation on which these calculations are made breaks down, and entirely different approaches to analysis are recommended in such extreme cases. Such settings are not common, however, and as the sample sizes increase to about $10n$ the power of the unstructured test is about 65% compared to 80% for the most parsimonious structure, and about 77% for the heterogeneous structures. Note that the most parsimonious structures are rarely adequate in real problems, so this comparison provides an exaggerated

Table 5.7 Power calculations. Power, as a percentage, under all combinations of structure, number of times, and number of subjects.

n	Series AR	N 12	24	48	96	Series MA	N 12	24	48	96	Series CS	N 12	24	48	96
Treatment-by-time interaction															
5	AR(1)	80	80	80	80	TOEP(2)	80	80	80	80	CS	80	80	80	80
	ARH(1)	47	66	73	77	TOEPH(2)	54	68	76	77	CSH	47	65	73	77
	AD(1)	38	60	71	73	UN(2)	36	59	71	75					
	UN	26	52	66	68	UN	26	52	67	68	UN	26	52	66	68
10	AR(1)	80	80	80	80	TOEP(2)	80	80	80	80	CS	80	80	80	80
	ARH(1)	30	53	66	73	TOEPH(2)	46	61	71	76	CSH	36	57	69	74
	AD(1)	20	45	62	71	UN(2)	19	43	61	71					
	UN	5	21	50	64	UN	5	21	47	64	UN	5	21	48	65
Final time point comparison															
5	AR(1)	80	80	80	80	TOEP(2)	80	80	80	80	CS	80	80	80	80
	ARH(1)	69	76	78	79	TOEPII(2)	75	78	79	80	CSH	72	77	79	79
	AD(1)	68	76	78	79	UN(2)	68	76	78	79					
	UN	68	76	78	79	UN	68	75	78	79	UN	69	76	78	79
10	AR(1)	80	80	80	80	TOEP(2)	80	80	80	80	CS	80	80	80	80
	ARH(1)	68	76	78	79	TOEPH(2)	77	78	79	80	CSH	72	77	79	79
	AD(1)	67	75	78	79	UN(2)	67	75	78	79					
	UN	67	75	78	79	UN	67	75	78	79	UN	68	75	78	79

view of the loss of power under the unstructured matrix. For practical purposes the loss of power is not serious (for the interaction test) with sample sizes greater than $10n$.

The covariance structure plays a much smaller role in the final time point test, and again this is reflected very clearly in the results in the table. Apart from the very small sample size ($N = 12$), the loss of power under the unstructured matrix is negligible and its use should be considered in all but the very smallest problems; and, as remarked above, in such very small problems alternative analysis strategies are probably advisable anyway.

5.7   CONCLUDING REMARKS

We have shown, using a simple but illustrative example, that for balanced, complete data, a sufficiently general longitudinal model, such as a multivariate normal or general linear mixed model, will have similar or identical behaviour to ANOVA or simple t tests. However, when fitted to incomplete data, the likelihood-based methods are more broadly valid since they only require the missing data mechanism to be missing at random, rather than missing completely at random.

We have also shown that there is an increase in sensitivity of the estimation of mean model with respect to the fitted covariance model. Too simple a covariance structure may lead to bias in certain mean model parameters. We therefore wish to avoid putting unnecessary constraints on this structure, but this must be balanced against the loss of power which arises from the estimation of the covariance parameters. An unstructured matrix should therefore be the first choice unless the trial size is small enough to imply that this would lead to a non-trivial loss in power. The results shown above in Section 5.6 suggest that for final time point comparisons this loss will be minimal in all but the very smallest trials. For full comparison of treatment profiles over time the impact on power is greater and the rule of thumb $N \geq 10n$ is suggested for sample sizes large enough to justify the automatic use of an unstructured covariance matrix. Otherwise careful reflection is needed on the choice of a more parsimonious structure. A compromise between flexibility and parsimony is needed, and intermediate structures such as those with unconstrained variances across time (so-called heterogeneous and ante-dependence structures, for example) are potentially useful for this.

6

Analysis of the Depression Trials

We now analyse the three clinical trials introduced in Section 2.5. The primary null hypothesis (zero difference between the treatment and placebo in mean change of the $HAMD_{17}$ total score at the endpoint) is tested using a model of the type (5.1). The model includes the fixed categorical effects of treatment, investigator, time, and treatment-by-time interaction, as well as the continuous, fixed covariates of baseline score and baseline score-by-time interaction. In line with the protocol design, we use the heterogeneous compound symmetric covariance structure. The Kenward–Roger (Kenward and Roger 1997) procedure will be used to calculate standard errors, Wald tests, and reference denominator degrees of freedom. The significance of differences in least-squares means is based on Type III tests. These examine the significance of each partial effect, that is, the significance of an effect with all the other effects in the model. Analyses are implemented using the SAS procedure MIXED.

Given this description, the effect of simple approaches, such as LOCF and CC, versus MAR, can be studied in terms of their impact on various linear mixed model aspects (fixed effects, variance structure, correlation structure). It will be shown that the impact of the simplifications can be noticeable. This is the subject of Section 6.1, dedicated to View 1 of Section 4.1.1. Section 6.2 focuses on Views 2a and 2b, where the last planned occasion and the last measurement obtained are of interest, respectively. In addition, we consider the issues arising when switching from a two-treatment arm to an all-treatment arm comparison.

Missing Data in Clinical Studies   G. Molenberghs and M.G. Kenward
© 2007 John Wiley & Sons, Ltd

6.1   VIEW 1: LONGITUDINAL ANALYSIS

For each study in this longitudinal analysis, we will only consider the treatments that are of direct interest. This means we estimate the main difference between these treatments (treatment main effect) as well as the difference between both over time (treatment-by-time interaction). Treatment main effect estimates and standard errors, *p*-values for treatment main effect and treatment-by-time interaction, and estimates for the within-patient correlation are reported in Table 6.1. When comparing LOCF, CC, and MAR, there is little difference between the three methods, in either the treatment main effect or the treatment-by-time interaction. Nevertheless, some important differences will be established between the strategies in terms of other model aspects. These will be seen to be in line with the reports in Verbeke and Molenberghs (1997, 2000).

Two specific features of the mean structure are the time trends and the treatment effects (over time). We discuss these in turn. The placebo time trends and the treatment effects (*i.e.*, differences between the active arms and the placebo arms) are displayed in Figures 6.1 and 6.2, respectively. Both LOCF and CC are different from MAR, with a larger difference for CC. The effect is strongest in the third study. It is striking that different studies lead to different conclusions in terms of relative differences between the approaches. While there is a relatively small difference between the three methods in study 2 and a mild one for study 1, for study 3 there is a strong separation between LOCF and CC on the one hand, and MAR on the other hand. Importantly, the *average* effect is smaller for MAR than for LOCF and CC. This result is in agreement with the results in Section 4.3, which showed that the direction of the bias on LOCF is in fact hard to anticipate, and should not be taken for granted.

Table 6.1   Depression trials. View 1. Treatment effects (standard errors: s.e.), *p*-values for treatment main effect and for treatment by time interaction, and within-patient correlation coefficients.

Study	Method	Treatment effect (s.e.)	p-value Effect	p-value Interaction	Within-patient correlation
1	LOCF	−1.60 (1.40)	0.421	0.565	0.65
	CC	−1.96 (1.38)	0.322	0.684	0.57
	MAR	−1.81 (1.24)	0.288	0.510	0.53
2	LOCF	−1.61 (1.05)	0.406	0.231	0.54
	CC	−1.97 (1.16)	0.254	0.399	0.37
	MAR	−2.00 (1.12)	0.191	0.138	0.39
3	LOCF	1.12 (0.71)	0.964	<0.001	0.74
	CC	1.75 (0.77)	0.918	<0.001	0.57
	MAR	2.10 (0.69)	0.476	<0.001	0.60

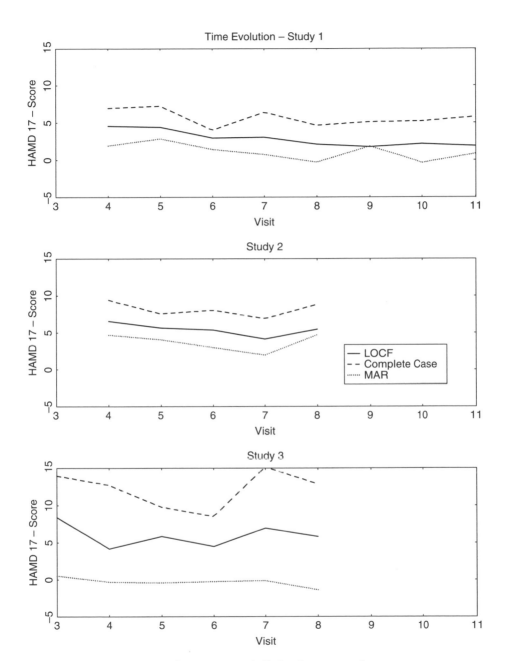

Figure 6.1 Depression trials. Summary of all placebo time evolutions.

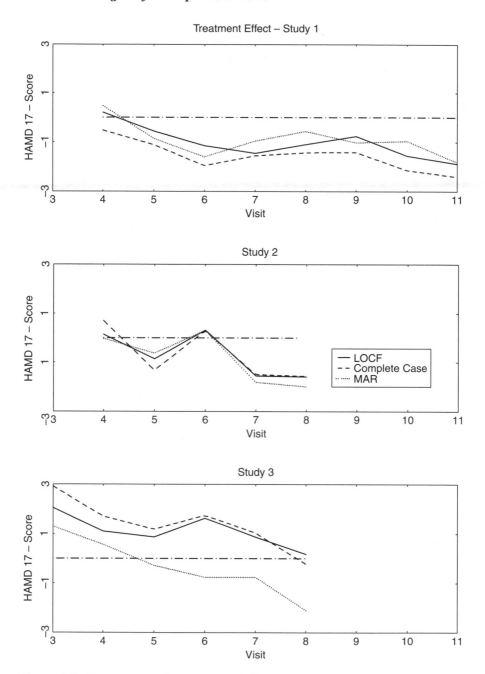

Figure 6.2 Depression trials. Summary of all treatment effects.

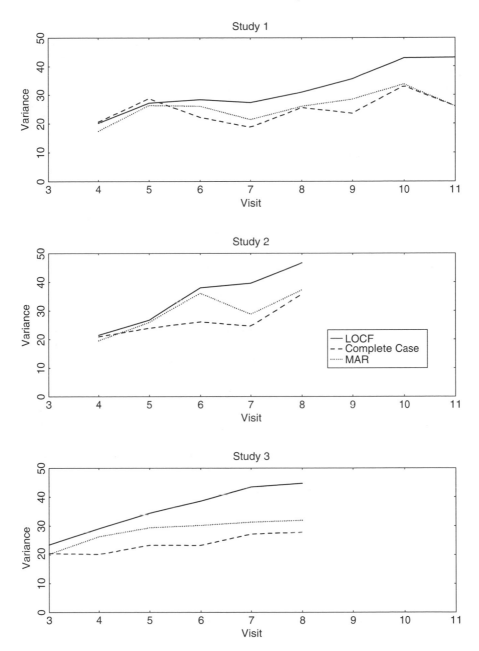

Figure 6.3 Depression trials. Variance functions by study and by method.

The variance–covariance structure employed is heterogeneous compound symmetry variance structure (CSH), with a common correlation and a variance specific to each measurement occasion. The latter feature allows us to plot the fitted variance function over time. This is done in Figure 6.3. It is very noticeable that MAR and CC produce a relatively similar variance structure, which tends to rise only mildly. LOCF, on the other hand, deviates from both and points towards a (linear) increase in variance. If further modelling is done, MAR and CC produce homogeneous or classical compound symmetry (CS) and hence a random-intercept structure. LOCF, on the other hand, suggests a random-slope model. The reason for this discrepancy is that an incomplete profile is completed by means of a flat profile. Within a pool of linearly increasing or decreasing profiles, this leads to a progressively wider spread as study time elapses. Noting that the fitted variance function has implications for the computation of mean model standard errors, the potential for misleading inferences is clear.

The fitted correlations are given in Table 6.1. Clearly, CC and MAR produce virtually the same correlation. However, the correlation coefficient estimated under LOCF is much stronger. This is entirely due to the fact that, after dropout, a constant value is imputed for the remainder of the study period, thereby increasing the correlation between the repeated measurements. Of course, the problem is even more severe than is shown by this analysis since, under LOCF, a constant correlation structure can be changed into one which progressively strengthens as time elapses. It should be noted that the correlation structure has an impact on all longitudinal aspects of the mean structure. For example, estimates and standard errors of time trends and estimated interactions of time with covariates can all be affected. In particular, if the estimated correlation is too high, the time trend can be ascribed a precision which is too high, implying the potential for a *liberal* error.

In conclusion, all aspects of the multivariate linear mixed model (mean structure and covariance structure) may be influenced by the method of analysis. This is in line with results reported in Verbeke and Molenberghs (1997, 2000). It is important to note that, generally, the direction of the errors (conservative or liberal) is not clear a priori, since different distortions (in mean, variance, or correlation structure) may counteract each other. We will now study a number of additional analyses that are highly relevant from a clinical trial point of view.

6.2 VIEWS 2A AND 2B AND ALL VERSUS TWO TREATMENT ARMS

When emphasis is on the last measurement occasion, LOCF and CC are straightforward to use. When the last observed measurement is of interest, the corresponding analysis is not different from that obtained under LOCF. In these cases, a *t* test will be used. Note that it is still possible to obtain inferences from a full linear mixed-effects model in this context. While this seems less sensible, since one obviously would get distorted estimates of longitudinal characteristics such as time evolution, we nevertheless add these for the sake of comparison. Note that the *t*-test analysis is more in line with clinical trial practice.

For MAR, by its very nature, one is drawn to consider the incomplete profiles, to use the information contained in these for the correct estimation of effects at later times, where there may be some missingness. Thus, one has to consider the full linear mixed model, in line with suggestions made in Chapter 4.

An additional issue that occurs whenever there are more than two treatment arms is whether one uses all treatments or only the two of interest. This choice has an effect on the *p*-value in the linear mixed model case. Consider, for example, the covariance structure. Model-based smoothing of the covariance structure takes place either on two arms or on all arms. Hence, due to correlations between model parameters, the estimated treatment effects and also the resulting *p*-values might change. Generally, one might argue that efficiency can be gained by using all treatment arms, but this comes at the cost of an increased risk of misspecification. This risk can be avoided by assuming a treatment-arm-specific covariance matrix in conjunction with a treatment-arm-specific mean evolution. For the *t* tests, however, there is no change. Of course, one might entertain the possibility of correcting for multiple comparisons when more than two arms are involved, but this is not our current focus of interest, and does not substantially affect our conclusions.

Table 6.2 summarizes results in terms of *p*-values. In study 3, which has a relatively large sample size, all *p*-values indicate a significant difference with the sole exception, very importantly, of the *t* tests under LOCF. This re-emphasizes the problems with the LOCF method as discussed in Section 6.1. In studies 1 and 2, more subtle differences are observed.

For study 1, we have the following conclusions. All mixed models lead to borderline differences: LOCF and CC are not significant, MAR is borderline

Table 6.2 Depression trials. Views 2a and 2b: *p*-values ('mixed' refers to the assessment of treatment at the last visit based on a linear mixed model).

Method	Model	Data used	Study 1	Study 2	Study 3
CC	Mixed	All treatments	0.076	0.055	0.001
		Two treatments	0.070	0.088	0.001
CC	*t* test	All treatments	0.092	0.156	0.017
		Two treatments	0.092	0.156	0.017
LOCF	Mixed	All treatments	0.053	0.052	0.001
		Two treatments	0.056	0.082	0.001
	t test	All treatments	0.246	0.172	0.120
		Two treatments	0.246	0.172	0.120
MAR	Mixed	All treatments	0.052	0.048	0.001
		Two treatments	0.047	0.077	0.001

(depending on the number of treatments included). An endpoint analysis (i.e., using the last available measurement) leads to a completely different picture, with results that are clearly far from significance. For study 2, the mixed models lead to small differences, with a noticeable shift towards borderline significance for MAR with all treatments. An endpoint analysis shows, again, results that are notably different (non-significant) from the mixed models.

If the t tests under LOCF and CC are compared with the mixed analysis of MAR, studies 1 and 2 show dramatic differences. Such a comparison is not contrived since the t tests for LOCF and CC are well in line with common data-analytic practice and under MAR only the mixed analysis makes sense.

These results, in conjunction with those of Section 6.1, underscore the limitations of LOCF and CC. By selecting a subset (CC), a different type of patient might be retained in the treated versus the untreated arm. This can be explained by a difference in therapeutic effect, a difference in side effects or a combination thereof. As with CC, the difference of complete versus incomplete observations can cause distortions within an LOCF analysis. In addition to differences in sets to which the techniques are applied, there are further distortions which take place in the mean structure, the variance structure and the correlation structure. These effects may counteract and/or strengthen each other, depending on the situation.

In conclusion, use of likelihood-based ignorable methods is more justifiable than LOCF and CC.

Part III
Missing at Random and Ignorability

7

The Direct Likelihood Method

7.1 INTRODUCTION

In Chapter 4 we provided a general perspective on the relative position of simple methods, such as complete case analysis and last observation carried forward, in comparison with the more principled approach of direct likelihood analysis, that is, the likelihood-based way of using the available cases. This method was presented as the preferred one among those considered thus far, based on the ignorability theory laid out in Section 3.5. The various methods were there illustrated and juxtaposed using two case studies: the orthodontic growth data in Chapter 5 and the depression trials in Chapter 6.

In this chapter, we expand upon the direct likelihood method. In Section 7.2 this is placed in a broader perspective, including a number of alternative methods to be described in later chapters, such as multiple imputation (Chapter 9), the expectation–maximization algorithm (Chapter 8) and weighted generalized estimating equations (Chapter 10). We then focus on the direct likelihood method in the two important cases of continuous and discrete repeatedly measured outcomes. In Section 7.3 we present a version of the linear mixed model as a key modelling framework which can usefully be combined with the concept of ignorability. This generalizes the earlier use of the model, as encountered in Chapter 5. In Section 7.4 we illustrate the method using the toenail data. In Section 7.5 we sketch the generalized linear mixed model framework, which is useful for analysing longitudinal data of a non-Gaussian type. In Sections 7.6 and 7.7 we report on two case studies, the data for which were introduced in Sections 2.5 and 2.9, respectively. In the first we consider a binary version of the continuous outcome studied in Chapter 6 from a series of trials on depression. In the second we model a longitudinally measured score

Missing Data in Clinical Studies   G. Molenberghs and M.G. Kenward
© 2007 John Wiley & Sons, Ltd

from a trial on chronic pain. A further case study, of age-related macular degeneration, is presented in Chapter 13.

In addition to the subsequent chapters already mentioned, this part of the book contains a comparative study of weighted and multiple imputation based generalized estimating equations (Chapter 11). The precise scope of the likelihood framework used in, for example, the current chapter is studied in Chapter 12. Finally, the extent to which the SAS system can be used for these analyses is the subject of Chapter 14.

7.2   IGNORABLE ANALYSES IN PRACTICE

The key message from Section 3.5 is that, under the assumption of MAR and the mild separability condition, likelihood-based and Bayesian analyses are valid, provided all available data are analysed. This means, for example for the growth data set analysed in Chapter 5, that a direct likelihood analysis will be based on 18 children with four measurements and 9 children with three measurements, as was illustrated in Section 5.3. In Section 5.5 we emphasized that little or no additional (SAS) code is needed to undertake such an analysis. In other words, virtually the same code, used to analyse the original, complete data, can be used here as well. One might then wonder why it has taken so long for this flexible and simple paradigm to enter the mainstream of analysis. Arguably, the main reason is the availability of convenient commercial software tools. In the past many packages featured some multivariate analysis tools, such as the GLM procedure in SAS. However, these tended to delete all units that were not fully complete. This forced the user into a complete case analysis. Only during the past one-and-a-half decades has software development seen the advent of so-called longitudinal, or repeated measures, analysis tools. For example, as exemplified in Section 5.5, the SAS procedure MIXED can be used to analyse continuous repeated measurements, with the SAS procedures GENMOD, GLIMMIX, and NLMIXED applicable for the general, typically non-Gaussian, situation. Similar procedures and functions exist in other packages, such as R, S-Plus, and Stata. Thus, generally, any module with likelihood estimation facilities which can handle incompletely observed subjects in the way described above, will provide the correct likelihood and lead to valid estimates, likelihood ratios, and so on, under the MAR assumption.

A few remarks apply. First, it has been shown that it is better to use the observed information matrix, rather than the expected (Kenward and Molenberghs 1998), when data are MAR. This point is elaborated in Chapter 12. Second, ignoring the missing data mechanism assumes there is no scientific interest in the said mechanism. When this is untrue, the analyst can, without any problem, fit appropriate models to the missing data indicators, much as is done in Section 10.4. Third, regardless of the elegance and beauty of the direct likelihood analysis, MNAR can almost never be ruled out as a mechanism, and therefore one ought to consider the possible impact of such mechanisms as well. This point will be taken up in Parts IV and V. Fourth, a commonly used analysis tool for incomplete non-Gaussian data is generalized estimating equations (GEE: Liang and Zeger 1986). Due to its non-likelihood, and hence frequentist, nature, an MAR mechanism is not ignorable when GEE is the mode of analysis. Specific solutions have been proposed for this situation, as can be found in Chapter 10.

While direct likelihood is an appealing mode of analysis in a wide variety of situations, there are a number of alternative methods of practical relevance. In Chapter 9, multiple imputation (Rubin 1987) will be presented. Broadly, the method consists of replacing missing values multiple times, using an appropriate Bayesian predictive distribution. The data sets thus completed allow for the same analysis as one would undertake had the data been complete. A straightforward final step combines the multiple estimates into a single one, and provides an estimate of precision that accommodates the incompleteness of the data. In certain settings multiple imputation approximates a Bayesian analysis and so may provide results that are very similar indeed to those derived from a direct likelihood approach. In other settings the two may diverge, and we explore this in the chapter. In most examples, a direct likelihood analysis requires numerical maximization of the likelihood. This can be done in many ways, and some specific examples of this for non-Gaussian outcomes are described in Section 7.5. An important and very general algorithm for maximizing the likelihood of incomplete data is the so-called expectation–maximization (EM) algorithm (Dempster *et al.* 1977). It has been, and is, useful in a number of data-augmentation settings including, apart from incomplete data, random-effects models, latent classes, and mixture distributions. We consider this in Chapter 8.

7.3   THE LINEAR MIXED MODEL

While, by definition, direct likelihood ideas can be used with a variety of likelihoods, the linear mixed model (Laird and Ware 1982; Verbeke and Molenberghs 2000) is a useful and sensible choice. As illustrated in Sections 5.2–5.4, it encompasses the general multivariate normal model. Therefore, it generalizes and coincides with commonly used methods applied to complete data sets, such as (multivariate) analysis of variance and a *t* test at a given time point. But whereas, for example, ANOVA is valid only under MCAR, the linear mixed model formulation, by virtue of its likelihood basis, allows for a valid analysis under MAR. It also allows one to incorporate a variety of features, such as individual and/or population-averaged longitudinal profiles of specific parametric shapes, hierarchies resulting from a multi-centre or multi-country nature of a trial, and meta-analysis. Therefore, we will introduce this model, already applied in the specific situation of the orthodontic growth data in Chapter 5, in full generality here. Detailed accounts can be found, for example, in Verbeke and Molenberghs (2000), Fitzmaurice *et al.* (2004), and Molenberghs and Verbeke (2005).

Let Y_{ij} be the jth measurement for the ith subject or cluster ($i = 1, \ldots, N$; $j = 1, \ldots, n_i$). Further, $\boldsymbol{Y}_i = (Y_{i1}, \ldots, Y_{in_i})'$ is the n_i-dimensional vector grouping all observations available for subject i. Assuming, for example, an average trend for Y as a function of time t_{ij}, group x_i, and their interaction, a multivariate regression model would be obtained:

$$Y_{ij} = \beta_0 + \beta_1 t_{ij} + \beta_2 x_i + \beta_3 t_{ij} x_i + \varepsilon_{ij}, \qquad (7.1)$$

with the assumption that the error components ε_{ij} are normally distributed with mean zero. In vector notation, we obtain $\boldsymbol{Y}_i = X_i \boldsymbol{\beta} + \boldsymbol{\varepsilon}_i$ for an appropriate design matrix X_i, with $\boldsymbol{\beta} = (\beta_0, \beta_1, \beta_2, \beta_3)'$ and with $\boldsymbol{\varepsilon}_i = (\varepsilon_{i1}, \varepsilon_{i2}, \ldots, \varepsilon_{in_i})'$. The model is completed by specifying an appropriate covariance matrix V_i for $\boldsymbol{\varepsilon}_i$, leading to the multivariate model

$$\boldsymbol{Y}_i \sim N(X_i \boldsymbol{\beta}, V_i). \qquad (7.2)$$

General designs, using a variety of covariates, their transformations and interactions, can be employed to construct the design matrix X_i.

Assuming that $V_i = \sigma^2 I_{n_i}$, with I_{n_i} the identity matrix of dimension n_i, corresponds to assuming that the repeated measurements Y_{ij} on a given subject are independent, a very unrealistic assumption in most longitudinal settings. In the case of balanced data, that is, when a fixed number $n \equiv n_i$ of measurements is taken for all subjects, and when measurements are taken at fixed time points $t_{ij} \equiv t_j$, for all i and j, a useful covariance model is $V_i = V$, where V is a general (unstructured) $n \times n$ positive definite covariance matrix. This yields the classical multivariate regression model (Seber 1984, Chapter 8).

Depending on the context and the actual data at hand, other choices may be appropriate. For example, a first-order autoregressive model assumes that the covariance between two measurements Y_{ij} and Y_{ik} from the same subject i is of the form $\sigma^2 \rho^{|t_{ij} - t_{ik}|}$ for unknown parameters σ^2 and ρ. Another example is compound symmetry, which assumes the covariance to be of the form $\sigma^2 + \gamma \delta_{jk}$ for unknown parameters σ^2 and γ and where δ_{jk} equals one for $j = k$ and zero otherwise. These are examples of homogeneous covariance structures since they assume the variance of all Y_{ij} to be equal. Heterogeneous versions can be formulated as well (Verbeke and Molenberghs 2000). Examples of such heterogeneous structures have been given and studied in Section 5.6.

Apart from a, perhaps structured, multivariate model formulation, the so-called random-effects approach toward extending the univariate linear regression model to longitudinal settings can be followed. It is based on the assumption that, for every subject, the response can be modelled by a linear regression model, but with subject-specific regression coefficients. A specific instance was given in Section 5.3. For example, starting from (7.1), but explicitly allowing for subject-specific intercepts and slopes, one obtains

$$Y_{ij} = (\beta_0 + b_{i0}) + (\beta_1 + b_{i1})t_{ij} + \beta_2 x_i + \beta_3 t_{ij} x_i + \varepsilon_{ij}. \tag{7.3}$$

As before, $\boldsymbol{\varepsilon}_i = (\varepsilon_{i1}, \varepsilon_{i2}, \ldots, \varepsilon_{in_i})'$ is assumed to be normally distributed with mean vector zero, and some covariance matrix which we now denote by Σ_i. Because subjects are randomly sampled from a population of subjects, it is natural to assume that the subject-specific regression coefficients $\boldsymbol{b}_i = (b_{i0}, b_{i1})'$ are normally distributed with mean zero and covariance G.

The above model is a special case of the general linear mixed model which assumes that the vector $\boldsymbol{Y}_i$ of repeated measurements for the ith subject satisfies

$$\boldsymbol{Y}_i | \boldsymbol{b}_i \sim N(X_i \boldsymbol{\beta} + Z_i \boldsymbol{b}_i, \Sigma_i), \tag{7.4}$$

$$\boldsymbol{b}_i \sim N(\boldsymbol{0}, G), \tag{7.5}$$

for $n_i \times p$ and $n_i \times q$ known design matrices X_i and Z_i, for a p-dimensional vector $\boldsymbol{\beta}$ of unknown regression coefficients, for a q-dimensional vector $\boldsymbol{b}_i$ of subject-specific regression coefficients assumed to be sampled from the q-dimensional normal distribution with mean zero and covariance G, and with Σ_i a covariance matrix parameterized through a set of unknown parameters. The components in $\boldsymbol{\beta}$ are called 'fixed effects', the components in $\boldsymbol{b}_i$ are called 'random effects'. The fact that the model contains fixed as well as random effects motivates the term 'mixed models'.

The fitting of a linear mixed model is usually based on the marginal model that, for subject i, is multivariate normal with mean $X_i \boldsymbol{\beta}$ and covariance $V_i(\boldsymbol{\alpha}) = Z_i G Z_i' + \Sigma_i$, where we make explicit the dependence of V_i on the vector $\boldsymbol{\alpha}$ of parameters in the covariance matrices G and Σ_i. The parameters in $\boldsymbol{\alpha}$ are usually called 'variance components'. The classical approach to estimation and inference is based on maximum likelihood (ML). Assuming independence across subjects, the likelihood takes the form

$$L_{\mathrm{ML}}(\boldsymbol{\theta}) = \prod_{i=1}^{N} \left\{ (2\pi)^{-n_i/2} |V_i(\boldsymbol{\alpha})|^{-\frac{1}{2}} \right.$$

$$\left. \times \exp\left[-\frac{1}{2} (\boldsymbol{Y}_i - X_i \boldsymbol{\beta})' V_i^{-1}(\boldsymbol{\alpha}) (\boldsymbol{Y}_i - X_i \boldsymbol{\beta}) \right] \right\}. \tag{7.6}$$

Estimation of $\boldsymbol{\theta}' = (\boldsymbol{\beta}', \boldsymbol{\alpha}')$ requires joint maximization of (7.6) with respect to all elements in $\boldsymbol{\theta}$. In general, no analytic solutions are available, calling for numerical optimization routines. In practice a modification of (7.6) is used called restricted maximum likelihood (REML) estimation (Harville 1974), which leads to smaller bias in the variance component estimators than full maximum likelihood. Verbeke and Molenberghs (2000) provide a full account of ML and REML in this context.

When inferences on the fixed effects $\boldsymbol{\beta}$ are of interest, it is customary to use t or F distributions, with the denominator degrees of freedom estimated from the data. This is often based on so-called Satterthwaite-type approximations (Satterthwaite 1941; Kenward and Roger 1997), and is only fully developed for the case of linear mixed models. The method of Kenward and Roger (1997) works very well in both large and small samples, and is generally considered the optimal choice.

When interest is also in inference for some of the variance components in $\boldsymbol{\alpha}$, classical asymptotic Wald, likelihood ratio, and score tests can be used. However, due to restrictions on the parameter spaces, some hypotheses of interest may be on the boundary of the parameter space, implying that classical testing procedures are no longer valid. In some special but important cases, analytic results are available on how to correctly test such hypotheses. We therefore refer to Stram and Lee (1994, 1995) for results on the likelihood ratio test, to Verbeke and Molenberghs (2003) for results on the score test, and to Molenberghs and Verbeke (2006) for some general considerations. A detailed discussion on inference for the marginal linear mixed model can be found in Verbeke and Molenberghs (2000, Chapter 6). See also Molenberghs and Verbeke (2005).

When there is scientific interest in the random effects as well, so-called empirical Bayes estimation methods can be used (Laird and Ware 1982). Accounts are given in Verbeke and Molenberghs (2000), Fitzmaurice *et al.* (2004), and Molenberghs and Verbeke (2005).

7.4   ANALYSIS OF THE TOENAIL DATA

We now analyse the toenail data, introduced in Section 2.7, first under the assumption of an MCAR process, then considering an MAR process.

An exploratory graphical tool for studying average evolutions over time is to plot the sample average at each occasion versus time, thereby including all patients still available at that occasion. For the toenail example, this is shown in Figure 7.1(a). The graph suggests that there is very little difference between both groups, with marginal superiority of treatment A.

Note that the sample averages at a specific occasion are unbiased estimators of the mean responses of those subjects still in the study at that occasion. Hence, the average profiles in Figure 7.1(a) only reflect the marginal average evolutions if, at each occasion, the mean response of those still in the study equals the mean response of those who have dropped out. Thus, we have to assume that the mean of the response, conditional on dropout status, is independent of the dropout status.

Similar assumptions for variances, correlations, and so on are needed for drawing valid inferences, based on sample statistics of the observed data. This

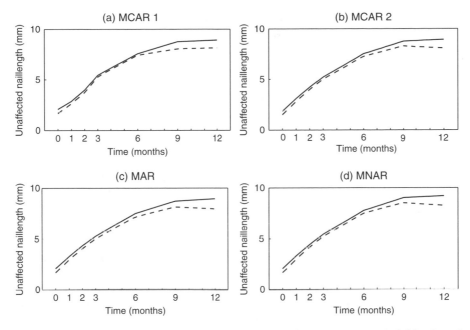

Figure 7.1 Toenail data. Estimated mean profile under treatment A (solid line) and treatment B (dashed line), obtained under different assumptions for the measurement model and the dropout model. (a) Completely random dropout, without parametric model for the average evolution in both groups. (b) Completely random dropout, assuming quadratic average evolution for both groups. (c) Random dropout, assuming quadratic average evolution for both groups. (d) Non-random dropout, assuming quadratic average evolution for both groups.

means assuming the response Y and the dropout time D to be independent, that is, MCAR.

Under the assumption of MCAR, a complete case or available case analysis would be valid, though inefficient, as indicated in Section 4.2. Note that the vector of all 14 sample averages plotted in Figure 7.1(a) can be interpreted as the ordinary least-squares estimate obtained from fitting a two-way ANOVA model to all available measurements, thereby ignoring the dependence between repeated measures within subjects. Under MCAR, this provides an unbiased estimator for the marginal average evolution in the population. Further, it follows from the theory on generalized estimating equations (Liang and Zeger 1986) that this ordinary least-squares estimator is asymptotically normally distributed, and valid standard errors are obtained from the sandwich estimator (see Section 10.3.2). Hence, Wald-type statistics are readily available for testing hypotheses or for the calculation of approximate confidence intervals.

For these data, we have used the sample averages displayed in Figure 7.1(a) to test for any differences between the two treatment groups. The resulting Wald statistic equals $\chi^2 = 4.704$ on 7 degrees of freedom, from which we conclude that there is no evidence in the data for any difference between both groups ($p = 0.696$). Note that the above methodology also applies if we assume the outcome to satisfy a general linear regression model, where the average evolution in both groups may be assumed to be of a specific parametric form. We compared both treatments assuming that the average evolution is quadratic over time, with regression parameters possibly depending on treatment. The resulting ordinary least-squares profiles are shown in Figure 7.1(b). The main difference with the profiles obtained from a model with unstructured mean evolutions (Figure 7.1(a)) is seen during the treatment period (first 3 months). The Wald test statistic, employed for testing treatment differences, now equals $\chi^2 = 2.982$ on 3 degrees of freedom ($p = 0.394$), yielding the same conclusion as before.

In practice, patients often leave the study prematurely for reasons related to the outcome of interest, rendering MCAR less plausible as a mechanism and suggesting that MAR, or perhaps even MNAR, ought to be explored. We will now turn to MAR-based analyses.

To this effect, a selection model will be formulated. A formal discussion of selection models is deferred to Part IV. We will use the functional form of $f(d_i|\mathbf{y}_i)$ to discriminate between different types of dropout processes. Recall from Section 3.5 that under MCAR or MAR, the joint density of observed measurements and dropout indicator factors is

$$f(\mathbf{y}_i^o, d_i) = \begin{cases} f(\mathbf{y}_i^o)f(d_i) & \text{under MCAR,} \\ f(\mathbf{y}_i^o)f(d_i|\mathbf{y}_i^o) & \text{under MAR,} \end{cases}$$

from which it follows that a marginal model for the observed data $\mathbf{y}_i^o$ only is required. Moreover, the measurement model $f(\mathbf{y}_i^o)$ and the dropout model $f(d_i)$ or $f(d_i|\mathbf{y}_i^o)$ can be fitted separately, provided that the parameters in both models are functionally independent of each other (separability).

We will now fit a selection model to the toenail data, assuming random dropout. Our primary goal is to test for any treatment differences; hence, we do not need to explicitly consider a dropout model. Rather, it is sufficient to specify a marginal model for the observed outcomes $\mathbf{Y}_i^o$. The measurement model we consider here assumes a quadratic evolution for each subject, possibly with subject-specific intercepts, and we allow the stochastic error components to be correlated within subjects. More formally, we assume that $\mathbf{Y}_i^o$ satisfies the following linear mixed-effects model:

$$Y_{ij}^o = \begin{cases} (\beta_{A0} + b_i) + \beta_{A1}t_{ij} + \beta_{A2}t_{ij}^2 + \varepsilon_{(1)ij} + \varepsilon_{(2)ij} & \text{group A,} \\ (\beta_{B0} + b_i) + \beta_{B1}t_{ij} + \beta_{B2}t_{ij}^2 + \varepsilon_{(1)ij} + \varepsilon_{(2)ij} & \text{group B.} \end{cases} \quad (7.7)$$

All random components have zero mean. The random-intercept variance is d_{11}. The variance of the measurement error $\varepsilon_{(1)i}$ is $\sigma^2 I_{n_i}$, whereas the variance of the serial process $\varepsilon_{(2)i}$ is $\tau^2 H_i$, where H_i follows from the particular serial process considered. The unknown parameters β_{A0}, β_{A1}, β_{A2}, β_{B0}, β_{B1}, and β_{B2} describe the average quadratic evolution of Y_i^o over time.

Let us first assume that $\varepsilon_{(1)ij}$ is absent from the model. The estimated average profiles obtained from fitting model (7.7) to the toenail data are shown in Figure 7.1(c). Note that there is very little difference from the ordinary least-squares average profiles shown in Figure 7.1(b) and obtained under the MCAR assumption. The observed likelihood ratio statistic for testing for treatment differences equals $2 \ln \lambda = 4.626$ on 3 degrees of freedom. Hence, under model (7.7) and under the assumption of random dropout, there is little evidence for any average difference between the treatments A and B ($p = 0.201$).

7.5   THE GENERALIZED LINEAR MIXED MODEL

When outcomes are of a non-Gaussian type, a variety of full likelihood-based models can be considered. Molenberghs and Verbeke (2005) distinguish between marginal, conditional, and random-effects models. We will return to marginal models in Chapter 10 and focus here on random-effects models, the most commonly encountered one being the generalized linear mixed model, which combines generalized linear model concepts with ideas from linear mixed models. This likelihood-based framework also easily extends to fully non-linear models for Gaussian and non-Gaussian outcomes.

As before, Y_{ij}, is the jth outcome measured for subject i, $i = 1, \ldots, N, j = 1, \ldots, n_i$, and Y_i is the n_i-dimensional vector of all measurements available for cluster i. It is assumed that, conditionally on q-dimensional random effects b_i, assumed to be drawn independently from $N(0, G)$, the outcomes Y_{ij} are independent with densities of the exponential-family form

$$f_i(y_{ij}|b_i, \beta, \phi) = \exp\left\{\phi^{-1}[y_{ij}\theta_{ij} - \psi(\theta_{ij})] + c(y_{ij}, \phi)\right\},$$

with $\eta(\mu_{ij}) = \eta(E(Y_{ij}|b_i)) = x'_{ij}\beta + z'_{ij}b_i$ for a known link function $\eta(\cdot)$, where x_{ij} and z_{ij} are p-dimensional and q-dimensional vectors of known covariate values, with β a p-dimensional vector of unknown fixed regression coefficients, with ϕ a scale parameter, and with θ_{ij} the natural (or canonical) parameter. Further, let $f(b_i|G)$ be the density of the $N(0, G)$ distribution for the random effects b_i.

Due to the above independence assumption, this model is often referred to as a *conditional independence* model. This assumption is the basis of the implementation in the NLMIXED procedure. Just as in the linear mixed model case, the model can be extended with residual correlation, in addition to the one induced by the random effects. Such an extended model has been implemented in the SAS procedure GLIMMIX, and its predecessor the GLIMMIX macro. This advantage is counterbalanced by bias induced by the optimization routine employed by GLIMMIX. It is important to realize that GLIMMIX can be used without random effects as well, thus effectively producing a marginal model, with estimates and standard errors similar to those obtained with GEE, as discussed in Section 10.3.3.

As for the linear mixed model case, inference is conventionally based on the marginal model for $\boldsymbol{Y}_i$ which is obtained from integrating out the random effects. The likelihood contribution of subject i then becomes

$$f_i(\boldsymbol{y}_i|\boldsymbol{\beta}, G, \phi) = \int \prod_{j=1}^{n_i} f_{ij}(y_{ij}|\boldsymbol{b}_i, \boldsymbol{\beta}, \phi)\, f(\boldsymbol{b}_i|G)\, d\boldsymbol{b}_i,$$

from which the likelihood for $\boldsymbol{\beta}, G$, and ϕ is derived as

$$
\begin{aligned}
L(\boldsymbol{\beta}, G, \phi) &= \prod_{i=1}^{N} f_i(\boldsymbol{y}_i|\boldsymbol{\beta}, G, \phi) \\
&= \prod_{i=1}^{N} \int \prod_{j=1}^{n_i} f_{ij}(y_{ij}|\boldsymbol{b}_i, \boldsymbol{\beta}, \phi)\, f(\boldsymbol{b}_i|G)\, d\boldsymbol{b}_i.
\end{aligned}
\tag{7.8}
$$

The key problem in maximizing the resulting likelihood is the presence of N integrals over the q-dimensional random effects. In some special cases, these integrals can be solved analytically. However, since no analytic expressions are available for these integrals, numerical approximation is needed. Here, we will focus on the most frequently used approaches to this. In general, the numerical approximations can be subdivided into those that are based on the approximation of: first, the integrand; second, the data; and third, the integral itself. Extensive overviews of currently available approximations can be found in Pinheiro and Bates (2000), Tuerlinckx *et al.* (2004), Skrondal and Rabe-Hesketh (2004), and Molenberghs and Verbeke (2005).

When integrands are approximated, the goal is to obtain a tractable integral such that closed-form expressions can be found, making the numerical maximization of the approximated likelihood feasible. Several methods have been proposed, but basically all come down to Laplace-type approximations of the function to be integrated (Tierney and Kadane 1986).

A second class of approaches is based on a decomposition of the data into the mean and an appropriate error term, with a Taylor series expansion of the mean which is a non-linear function of the linear predictor. All methods in this class differ in the order of the Taylor approximation and/or the point around which the approximation is expanded. More specifically, one considers the decomposition

$$Y_{ij} = \mu_{ij} + \varepsilon_{ij} = h(\boldsymbol{x}'_{ij}\boldsymbol{\beta} + \boldsymbol{z}'_{ij}\boldsymbol{b}_i) + \varepsilon_{ij}, \tag{7.9}$$

in which $h(\cdot)$ equals the inverse link function $\eta^{-1}(\cdot)$, and where the error terms have the appropriate distribution with variance equal to $\mathrm{var}(Y_{ij}|\boldsymbol{b}_i) = \phi v(\mu_{ij})$

for $v(\cdot)$ the usual variance function in the exponential family. Note that, with the natural link function,

$$v(\mu_{ij}) = \frac{\partial h}{\partial \eta}(\boldsymbol{x}'_{ij}\boldsymbol{\beta} + \boldsymbol{z}'_{ij}\boldsymbol{b}_i).$$

Several approximations of the mean μ_{ij} in (7.9) can be considered. One possibility is to consider a linear Taylor expansion of (7.9) around current estimates $\widehat{\boldsymbol{\beta}}$ and $\widehat{\boldsymbol{b}}_i$ of the fixed effects and random effects, respectively. This will result in the expression

$$\boldsymbol{Y}^*_i \;\;\equiv\;\; \widehat{W}^{-1}_i(\boldsymbol{Y}_i - \widehat{\boldsymbol{\mu}}_i) + X_i\widehat{\boldsymbol{\beta}} + Z_i\widehat{\boldsymbol{b}}_i \;\approx\; X_i\boldsymbol{\beta} + Z_i\boldsymbol{b}_i + \boldsymbol{\varepsilon}^*_i, \qquad (7.10)$$

with $\widehat{W}_i$ equal to the diagonal matrix with diagonal entries equal to $v(\widehat{\mu}_{ij})$, and for $\boldsymbol{\varepsilon}^*_i$ equal to $\widehat{W}^{-1}_i\boldsymbol{\varepsilon}_i$, which still has mean zero. Note that (7.10) can be viewed as a linear mixed model for the pseudo-data $\boldsymbol{Y}^*_i$, with fixed effects $\boldsymbol{\beta}$, random effects $\boldsymbol{b}_i$, and error terms $\boldsymbol{\varepsilon}^*_i$.

This immediately yields an algorithm for fitting the original generalized linear mixed model. Given starting values for the parameters $\boldsymbol{\beta}$, G and ϕ in the marginal likelihood, empirical Bayes estimates are calculated for $\boldsymbol{b}_i$, and pseudo-data $\boldsymbol{Y}^*_i$ are computed. Then the approximate linear mixed model (7.10) is fitted, yielding updated estimates for $\boldsymbol{\beta}$, G, and ϕ. These are then used to update the pseudo-data, and this whole scheme is iterated until convergence is reached.

The resulting estimates are called *penalized quasi-likelihood* (PQL) estimates in the literature (Molenberghs and Verbeke 2005), or *pseudo-quasi-likelihood* in the documentation of the GLIMMIX procedure (http://support.sas.com/rnd/app/da/glimmix.html) because they can be obtained by optimizing a quasi-likelihood function which only involves first- and second-order conditional moments, augmented with a penalty term on the random effects. The pseudo-likelihood terminology derives from the fact that the estimates are obtained by (restricted) maximum likelihood of the pseudo-response or working variable.

An alternative approximation is very similar to the PQL method, but is based on a linear Taylor expansion of the mean μ_{ij} in (7.9) around the current estimates $\widehat{\boldsymbol{\beta}}$ for the fixed effects and around $\boldsymbol{b}_i = \boldsymbol{0}$ for the random effects. The resulting estimates are called *marginal quasi-likelihood* (MQL) estimates. We refer to Breslow and Clayton (1993) and Wolfinger and O'Connell (1993) for more details. Since the linearizations in the PQL and the MQL methods lead to linear mixed models, the implementation of these procedures is often based on feeding updated pseudo-data into software for the fitting of linear mixed models. However, it should be emphasized that intermediate results from these procedures should be interpreted with great care. For example, reported (log-)likelihood values correspond to the assumed normal model for the pseudo-data and should not be confused with the (log-)likelihood for the generalized linear mixed model for the actual data under analysis. Further, fitting of linear mixed models can be based on ML as well as REML estimation. Hence, within the PQL and MQL frameworks, both methods can be used for the fitting of the linear model to the pseudo-data, yielding (slightly) different results. Finally, the quasi-likelihood methods discussed here are very similar to the method of linearization that will be discussed in Section 10.3.3 for fitting generalized estimating equations. The difference is that here, the correlation between repeated measurements is modelled through the inclusion of random effects, conditionally on which repeated measures are assumed independent, while in the GEE approach this association is modelled through a marginal working correlation matrix.

Note that, when there are no random effects, both this method and GEE reduce to a marginal model, the difference being in the way the correlation parameters are estimated. In both cases, it is possible to allow for misspecification of the association structure by resorting to empirically corrected standard errors. When this is done, the methods are valid under MCAR. If one has confidence in the specified correlation structure, purely model-based inference can be conducted and hence the methods are valid when missing data are MAR.

A third method of numerical approximation is based on the approximation of the integral itself, and is particularly useful where the above two approximation are inadequate. Of course, a wide selection of numerical integration tools, available from the optimization literature, can be applied. Several of these have been implemented in various software tools for generalized linear mixed models. A general class of quadrature rules selects a set of abscissae and constructs a weighted sum of function evaluations over those. In the particular context of random-effects models, so-called *adaptive* quadrature rules can be used (Pinheiro and Bates 1995, 2000), were the numerical integration is centred around the empirical Bayes estimates of the random effects, and the number of quadrature points is then selected in terms of the desired accuracy.

To illustrate the main ideas, we consider Gaussian and adaptive Gaussian quadrature, designed for the approximation of integrals of the form

$$\int f(z)\phi(z)dz,$$

for a known function $f(z)$ and for $\phi(z)$ the density of the (multivariate) standard normal distribution. We will first standardize the random effects such that they get the identity covariance matrix. Let $\boldsymbol{\delta}_i$ be equal to $\boldsymbol{\delta}_i = G^{-1/2}\mathbf{b}_i$. We then have that $\boldsymbol{\delta}_i$ is normally distributed with mean $\mathbf{0}$ and covariance I. The linear predictor then becomes $\theta_{ij} = \mathbf{x}'_{ij}\boldsymbol{\beta} + \mathbf{z}'_{ij}G^{1/2}\boldsymbol{\delta}_i$, so the variance components in G have been moved to the linear predictor. The likelihood contribution for subject i then equals

$$f_i(\boldsymbol{y}_i|\boldsymbol{\beta}, G, \phi) = \int \prod_{j=1}^{n_i} f_{ij}(y_{ij}|\mathbf{b}_i, \boldsymbol{\beta}, \phi) \, f(\mathbf{b}_i|G) \, d\mathbf{b}_i. \tag{7.11}$$

Obviously, (7.11) is of the form $\int f(z)\phi(z)dz$ as required to apply (adaptive) Gaussian quadrature.

In Gaussian quadrature, $\int f(z)\phi(z)dz$ is approximated by the weighted sum

$$\int f(z)\phi(z)dz \approx \sum_{q=1}^{Q} w_q \, f(z_q).$$

Q is the order of the approximation. The higher Q the more accurate the approximation will be. Further, the so-called nodes (or quadrature points) z_q are solutions to the Qth-order Hermite polynomial, while the w_q are well-chosen weights. The nodes z_q and weights w_q are reported in tables. Alternatively, an algorithm is available for calculating all z_q and w_q for any value Q (Press *et al.* 1992). In the case of univariate integration, the approximation consists of subdividing the integration region into intervals, and approximating the surface under the integrand by the sum of surfaces of the so-obtained approximating rectangles. An example is given in the left-hand panel of Figure 7.2, for the case of $Q = 10$ quadrature points. A similar interpretation is possible for the approximation of multivariate integrals. Note that the figure immediately highlights one of the main disadvantages of (non-adaptive) Gaussian quadrature: the fact that the quadrature points z_q are chosen based on $\phi(z)$, independent of the function $f(z)$ in the integrand. Depending on the support of $f(z)$, the z_q will or will not lie in the region of interest. Indeed, the

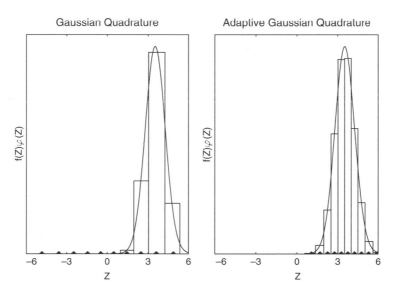

Figure 7.2 Graphical illustration of Gaussian (left) and adaptive Gaussian (right) quadrature of order $Q = 10$. The black triangles indicate the position of the quadrature points, while the rectangles indicate the contribution of each point to the integral.

quadrature points are selected to perform well when $f(z)\phi(z)$ approximately behaves like $\phi(z)$, that is, like a standard normal density function. This will be the case, for example, if $f(z)$ is a polynomial of a sufficiently low order. In our applications, however, the function $f(z)$ will take the form of a density from the exponential family, hence an exponential function. It may then be helpful to rescale and shift the quadrature points such that more quadrature points lie in the region of interest. This is shown in the right-hand panel of Figure 7.2, and is called adaptive Gaussian quadrature.

In general, the higher the order Q, the better the approximation will be of the N integrals in the likelihood. Typically, adaptive Gaussian quadrature needs (much) less quadrature points than classical Gaussian quadrature. On the other hand, adaptive Gaussian quadrature requires for each unit the numerical maximization of a function of the form $\ln(f(z)\phi(z))$ for the calculation of $\hat{z}$. This implies that adaptive Gaussian quadrature is much more time-consuming.

Since fitting of generalized linear mixed models is based on ML principles, inferences for the parameters are readily obtained from classical ML theory.

7.6   THE DEPRESSION TRIALS

We now fit generalized linear mixed models to the depression trials introduced in Section 2.5 and analysed previously in Chapter 6. Marginal models, based on weighted generalized estimating equations, will be considered in Section 10.5. While the continuous outcome was the focus of Chapter 6, we will now consider an analysis of the binary outcome defined as 1 if the $HAMD_{17}$ score is larger than 7, and 0 otherwise. These analyses are in line with Jansen *et al.* (2006a), Dmitrienko *et al.* (2005, Chapter 5), Molenberghs and Verbeke (2005, Chapter 27), and Molenberghs *et al.* (2005).

The likelihood-based nature of the generalized linear mixed model enables us to invoke the standard ignorability theory of Section 3.5, similar to the earlier applications for continuous outcomes, as in Chapters 5 and 6 and Section 7.4.

The model considered takes the form

$$\text{logit}[P(Y_{ij} = 1 | x_i, T_i, t_j, b_i)] = \beta_0 + b_i + \beta_{14}I(t_j = 4) + \beta_{15}I(t_j = 5)$$

$$+ \beta_{16}I(t_j = 6) + \beta_{17}I(t_j = 7) + \beta_2 x_i + \beta_3 T_i, \tag{7.12}$$

where $b_i \sim N(0, \tau^2)$ is a random intercept for subject i, x_i is the baseline value, T_i is the treatment indicator, and t_j is the time at which measurement j is taken. Since the follow up times range from 4 to 8, $t_j = j + 3$ for $j = 1, \ldots, 5$. Finally, $I(\cdot)$ is an indicator function.

Dmitrienko *et al.* (2005, Chapter 5) and Molenberghs *et al.* (2005) have indicated that here too the choice between adaptive and non-adaptive quadrature, the number of quadrature points, and the choice between quasi-Newton and

Table 7.1 Depression trials. Results of fitting random-effects model (7.12). Parameter estimates (standard errors) for generalized linear mixed model with adaptive Gaussian quadrature (Num. int.) and penalized-quasi likelihood methods (PQL). Interaction terms are not shown.

Effect	Parameter	PQL	Num. int.
Intercept	β_0	$-1.70\,(1.06)$	$-2.31\,(1.34)$
Visit 4	β_{14}	$0.66\,(1.48)$	$0.64\,(1.75)$
Visit 5	β_{15}	$-0.44\,(1.29)$	$-0.78\,(1.51)$
Visit 6	β_{16}	$0.17\,(1.22)$	$0.19\,(1.41)$
Visit 7	β_{17}	$-0.23\,(1.25)$	$-0.27\,(1.43)$
Baseline	β_2	$0.10\,(0.06)$	$0.15\,(0.07)$
Treatment	β_3	$-0.84\,(0.55)$	$-1.20\,(0.72)$
Random-intercept variance	τ^2	$2.53\,(0.53)$	$5.71\,(1.53)$

Newton–Raphson have a noticeable impact on the results, where adaptive quadrature and Newton–Raphson iteration produce the most reliable results, with no difference in the parameter estimates and standard errors observed, whether 10, 20, or 50 quadrature points are used. The latter results are contrasted with PQL based estimates in Table 7.1.

Once again, there are considerable differences between both approaches, and the PQL estimates are rather close to the GEE estimates. This indicates that, though the method is in principle likelihood-based, the inadequacy of the approximation undermines its validity under MAR to a greater extent than when data are complete; hence, where practicable, numerical integration is to be preferred. Turning to the treatment effect at endpoint, this is not significant in either of the analyses, but the difference in p-values is noticeable: $p = 0.0954$ for numerical integration and $p = 0.1286$ with PQL.

7.7 THE ANALGESIC TRIAL

We now turn to the trial on chronic pain, introduced in Section 2.9. We begin by considering the following model for the binary outcome:

$$Y_{ij}|b_i \sim \text{Bernoulli}(\pi_{ij}),$$
$$\text{logit}(\pi_{ij}) = \beta_0 + b_i + \beta_1 t_{ij} + \beta_2 t_{ij}^2 + \beta_3 x_i, \tag{7.13}$$

where

$$\pi_{ij} = \text{logit}[P(Y_{ij} = 1|b_i, t_{ij}, x_i)],$$

t_{ij} is the time of measurement, x_i is pain control assessment at baseline, and b_i is the random intercept for patient i, assumed to follow $b_i \sim N(0, \tau^2)$. Molenberghs

Table 7.2 Analgesic trial. Parameter estimates (standard errors) for generalized linear mixed models (7.13) and (7.14), obtained by means of adaptive Gaussian quadrature with 20 quadrature points.

Effect	Parameter	Estimate (s.e.) binary	Estimate (s.e.) ordinal
Intercept	β_1	4.05 (0.71)	
Intercept 1	α_1		$-1.56\,(0.55)$
Intercept 2	α_2		1.03 (0.54)
Intercept 3	α_3		3.89 (0.56)
Intercept 4	α_4		6.21 (0.60)
Time	β_2	$-1.16\,(0.47)$	$-0.54\,(0.31)$
Time^2	β_3	0.24 (0.09)	0.11 (0.06)
Baseline PCA	β_4	$-0.30\,(0.14)$	$-0.32\,(0.14)$
Random-intercept variance	τ^2	2.53 (0.68)	4.44 (0.60)

and Verbeke (2005, Chapter 17), fitted model (7.13) using a variety of methods (MQL, PQL, numerical integration) and software tools (the SAS procedures GLIMMIX and NLMIXED, MLwiN, and MIXOR). We restrict attention to adaptive Gaussian quadrature, with 20 quadrature points, using the SAS procedure NLMIXED. Results are presented in Table 7.2.

Let us now switch to the original, five-point ordinal outcome, the GSA scale defined in Section 2.9. The ordinal marginal equivalent to (7.13) is

$$\text{logit}[P(Y_{ij} \leq k | t_{ij}, x_i, b_i)] = \alpha_k + b_i + \beta_2 t_{ij} + \beta_3 t_{ij}^2 + \beta_4 x_i \qquad (7.14)$$

$(k = 1, \ldots, 4)$. The sole difference is that the single intercept term β_0 has been replaced by a set of four intercepts, one less than the number of categories. Since all other effects are independent of the cut-off category k, the model is said to be of the *proportional odds* type. Results are presented in Table 7.2. We note that there is similarity between the binary and ordinal analyses, in line with expectations. Furthermore, these analyses underscore the ease with which incomplete longitudinal data can be analysed by way of direct likelihood.

8

The Expectation–Maximization Algorithm

8.1 INTRODUCTION

In Part II and Chapter 7 we proposed direct likelihood as the preferred approach for analysing incomplete (longitudinal) data, when the MAR assumption is deemed plausible. In some settings the appropriate likelihood is comparatively easy to construct and maximize. However, this is not always the case, and in this chapter and the next we consider methods that exploit comparatively simple complete data calculations to simplify the problem of dealing with less amenable incomplete data problems. In the next chapter we consider multiple imputation, a method that extends to analyses well beyond the MAR-based likelihood methods. In the present chapter we consider the expectation–maximization (EM) algorithm, a convenient and widely applicable computational technique that can be used when the observed data likelihood is awkward and/or difficult to compute, in contrast to the methods for Gaussian and non-Gaussian longitudinal data proposed in Chapter 7.

The EM algorithm is a general-purpose iterative algorithm for calculating maximum likelihood estimates in parametric models for incomplete data. Within each iteration of the EM algorithm there are two steps, called the expectation step, or E step, and the maximization step, or M step. The name EM algorithm was coined by Dempster *et al.* (1977), who provided a general and unified formulation of the algorithm, its basic properties, and many examples and applications of it. The books by Little and Rubin (1987), Schafer (1997), and McLachlan and Krishnan (1997) provide detailed descriptions and applications of the algorithm.

Missing Data in Clinical Studies   G. Molenberghs and M.G. Kenward
© 2007 John Wiley & Sons, Ltd

The fundamental idea behind the EM algorithm is to associate with the given incomplete data problem, a complete data problem for which maximum likelihood estimation is computationally more tractable. Starting from suitable initial parameter values, the E and M steps are repeated until convergence. Given a set of parameter estimates, such as the mean vector and covariance matrix for a multivariate normal setting, the E step calculates the conditional expectation of the complete data log-likelihood given the observed data and the parameter estimates. This step often reduces to calculating simple sufficient statistics. Given the complete data log-likelihood, the M step then finds the parameter estimates to maximize the complete data log-likelihood from the E step.

An initial criticism of the method was that the algorithm did not produce estimates of the covariance matrix of the maximum likelihood estimators. However, a number of developments have provided methods for such obtaining these (Louis 1982). Another issue is the slow convergence that can happen in certain settings. This has resulted in the development of modified versions of the algorithm as well as many Monte Carlo based methods and other extensions (McLachlan and Krishnan 1997). In turns out that estimation of precision and speed of convergence are intimately linked, as both are based upon the matrix of second derivatives of the observed data likelihood, that is, the Hessian matrix or, similarly, the information matrix.

The condition for the EM algorithm to be valid, in its basic form, is ignorability and hence MAR. The use of EM in the MNAR context is touched upon in Section 15.4.

The principles of the EM algorithm and its sub-tasks are introduced in Section 8.2. The concept of observed and missing information is formalized in Section 8.3 and applied to the rate of convergence (Section 8.4), speeding up of the algorithm (Section 8.5), and precision estimation (Section 8.6). A simple but illustrative example is presented in Section 8.7.

8.2   THE ALGORITHM

We now present each of the three steps of the EM algorithm: the initial step, the expectation or E step, and the maximization or M step.

8.2.1   The initial step

Let $\theta^{(0)}$ be an initial parameter vector, which can be found from, for example, a complete case analysis, an available case analysis, or a simple method of imputation. Such an estimate is needed for the algorithm to start. Note that the initial estimate is allowed to be biased and/or inefficient. While it will, under broad conditions, not affect the event of reaching a maximum, a poor initial estimate can slow the iterative process considerably.

8.2.2 The E step

Given current values $\boldsymbol{\theta}^{(t)}$ for the parameters, the E step computes the objective function, which, in the case of the missing data problem, is equal to the expected value of the observed data log-likelihood, given the observed data and the current parameters

$$Q(\boldsymbol{\theta}|\boldsymbol{\theta}^{(t)}) = \int \ell(\boldsymbol{\theta}|\,\boldsymbol{Y})f(\boldsymbol{Y}^m|\boldsymbol{Y}^o,\boldsymbol{\theta}^{(t)})d\boldsymbol{Y}^m = E\left[\ell(\boldsymbol{\theta}|\boldsymbol{Y})|\boldsymbol{Y}^o,\boldsymbol{\theta}^{(t)}\right], \qquad (8.1)$$

that is, substituting the expected value of $\boldsymbol{Y}^m$, given $\boldsymbol{Y}^o$ and $\boldsymbol{\theta}^{(t)}$. In some cases, this substitution can take place directly at the level of the data, but often it is sufficient to substitute only the function of $\boldsymbol{Y}^m$ appearing in the complete data log-likelihood. For exponential families, the E step reduces to the computation of complete data sufficient statistics.

8.2.3 The M step

In the M step $\boldsymbol{\theta}^{(t+1)}$ is calculated, the parameter vector that maximizes the log-likelihood of the imputed data (or the imputed log-likelihood). Formally, $\boldsymbol{\theta}^{(t+1)}$ satisfies

$$Q(\boldsymbol{\theta}^{(t+1)}|\boldsymbol{\theta}^{(t)}) \geq Q(\boldsymbol{\theta}|\boldsymbol{\theta}^{(t)}), \qquad \text{for all } \boldsymbol{\theta}.$$

One can show that the observed data likelihood increases at every step. Because the log-likelihood is bounded from above, eventual convergence follows.

The fact that the EM algorithm is guaranteed to converge to a, possibly local, maximum is a great advantage. However, a disadvantage is that this convergence is slow (linear or superlinear), and that precision estimates are not automatically provided.

8.3 MISSING INFORMATION

To provide a framework for the examination of convergence monitoring, acceleration, and precision estimation, we now turn our attention to the principle of *missing information*. We use obvious notation for the observed and expected information matrices for the complete and observed data. Let

$$I(\boldsymbol{\theta}, Y^o) = \frac{\partial^2 \ln \ell(\boldsymbol{\theta})}{\partial\boldsymbol{\theta}\partial\boldsymbol{\theta}'}$$

be the matrix of the negative of the second-order partial derivatives of the (incomplete data) log-likelihood function with respect to the elements of $\boldsymbol{\theta}$, that is, the observed information matrix for the observed data model. The expected information matrix for the observed data model is termed $\mathcal{J}(\boldsymbol{\theta},\ \boldsymbol{Y}^o)$. By analogy with the complete data $\boldsymbol{Y} = (\boldsymbol{Y}^o, \boldsymbol{Y}^m)$, we let $I_c(\boldsymbol{\theta}, \boldsymbol{Y})$ and $\mathcal{J}_c(\boldsymbol{\theta}, \boldsymbol{Y})$, be the observed and expected information matrices for the complete data model, respectively. Now, both likelihoods are connected by the relation

$$\ell(\boldsymbol{\theta}) = \ell_c(\boldsymbol{\theta}) - \ln\frac{f_c(\boldsymbol{y}^0, \boldsymbol{y}^m | \boldsymbol{\theta})}{f_c(\boldsymbol{y}^0 | \boldsymbol{\theta})} = \ell_c(\boldsymbol{\theta}) - \ln f(\boldsymbol{y}^m | \boldsymbol{y}^o, \boldsymbol{\theta}).$$

This equality carries over to the information matrices in the sense that

$$I(\boldsymbol{\theta}, \boldsymbol{Y}^o) = I_c(\boldsymbol{\theta}, \boldsymbol{Y}) + \frac{\partial^2 \ln f(\boldsymbol{y}^m | \boldsymbol{y}^o, \boldsymbol{\theta})}{\partial \boldsymbol{\theta} \partial \boldsymbol{\theta}'}.$$

Taking expectations over $\boldsymbol{Y}|\boldsymbol{Y}^o = \boldsymbol{y}^o$ leads to

$$I(\boldsymbol{\theta}, \boldsymbol{y}^o) = \mathcal{J}_c(\boldsymbol{\theta}, \boldsymbol{y}^o) - \mathcal{J}_m(\boldsymbol{\theta}, \boldsymbol{y}^o),$$

where $\mathcal{J}_m(\boldsymbol{\theta}, \boldsymbol{y}^o)$ is the expected information matrix for $\boldsymbol{\theta}$ based on $\boldsymbol{Y}^m$ when conditioned on $\boldsymbol{Y}^o$. This information can be viewed as the 'missing information', resulting from observing $\boldsymbol{Y}^o$ only and not also $\boldsymbol{Y}^m$. This leads to the *missing information principle*,

$$\mathcal{J}_c(\boldsymbol{\theta}, \boldsymbol{y}) = I(\boldsymbol{\theta}, \boldsymbol{y}) + \mathcal{J}_m(\boldsymbol{\theta}, \boldsymbol{y}),$$

which has the following interpretation: the (conditionally expected) complete information equals the observed information plus the missing information.

8.4 RATE OF CONVERGENCE

The notion that the rate at which the EM algorithm converges depends upon the amount of missing information in the incomplete data compared to the hypothetical complete data, will be made explicit by deriving results regarding the rate of convergence in terms of information matrices (McLachlan and Krishnan 1997).

Under regularity conditions, the EM algorithm will converge linearly. By using a Taylor series expansion, we can write

$$\boldsymbol{\theta}^{(t+1)} - \boldsymbol{\theta}^* \simeq J(\boldsymbol{\theta}^*)[\boldsymbol{\theta}^{(t)} - \boldsymbol{\theta}^*],$$

where $\boldsymbol{\theta}^*$ is the parameter vector value for which the likelihood attains its maximum. Thus, in a neighbourhood of $\boldsymbol{\theta}^*$, the EM algorithm is essentially a linear iteration with rate matrix $J(\boldsymbol{\theta}^*)$, as $J(\boldsymbol{\theta}^*)$ is typically non-zero. For this reason, $J(\boldsymbol{\theta}^*)$ is often referred to as the matrix rate of convergence, or simply the rate of convergence. For vector $\boldsymbol{\theta}^*$, a measure of the actual observed convergence rate is the global rate of convergence, which can be assessed by

$$r = \lim_{t \to \infty} \frac{||\boldsymbol{\theta}^{(t+1)} - \boldsymbol{\theta}^*||}{||\boldsymbol{\theta}^{(t)} - \boldsymbol{\theta}^*||},$$

where $||\cdot||$ is any norm on d-dimensional Euclidean space $\mathbb{R}^d$, and d is the number of missing values. In practice, during the process of convergence, r is typically assessed as

$$r = \lim_{t \to \infty} \frac{||\boldsymbol{\theta}^{(t+1)} - \boldsymbol{\theta}^{(t)}||}{||\boldsymbol{\theta}^{(t)} - \boldsymbol{\theta}^{(t-1)}||}.$$

Under regularity conditions, it can be shown that r is the largest eigenvalue of the $d \times d$ rate matrix $J(\boldsymbol{\theta}^*)$.

Now $J(\boldsymbol{\theta}^*)$ can be expressed in terms of the observed and missing information:

$$J(\boldsymbol{\theta}^*) = I_d - I_c(\boldsymbol{\theta}^*, \mathbf{Y}^o)^{-1} I(\boldsymbol{\theta}^*, \mathbf{Y}^o) = \mathcal{I}_c(\boldsymbol{\theta}^*, \mathbf{Y}^o)^{-1} \mathcal{I}_m(\boldsymbol{\theta}^*, \mathbf{Y}^o).$$

This means that the rate of convergence of the EM algorithm is given by the largest eigenvalue of the information ratio matrix $\mathcal{I}_c(\boldsymbol{\theta}, \mathbf{Y}^o)^{-1} \mathcal{I}_m(\boldsymbol{\theta}, \mathbf{Y}^o)$, which measures the proportion of information about $\boldsymbol{\theta}$ that is missing by not observing $\mathbf{Y}^m$ in addition to $\mathbf{Y}^o$. The greater the proportion of missing information, the slower the rate of convergence. The fraction of information loss may vary across different components of $\boldsymbol{\theta}$, suggesting that certain components of $\boldsymbol{\theta}$ may approach $\boldsymbol{\theta}^*$ rapidly using the EM algorithm, while other components may require a large number of iterations. Further, exceptions to the convergence of the EM algorithm to a local maximum of the likelihood function occur if $J(\boldsymbol{\theta}^*)$ has eigenvalues exceeding unity.

8.5 EM ACCELERATION

Using the concept of the rate matrix,

$$\boldsymbol{\theta}^{(t+1)} - \boldsymbol{\theta}^* \simeq J(\boldsymbol{\theta}^*)[\boldsymbol{\theta}^{(t)} - \boldsymbol{\theta}^*],$$

we can solve this approximate equality for $\boldsymbol{\theta}^*$ to yield

$$\widetilde{\boldsymbol{\theta}}^* = (I_d - J)^{-1}(\boldsymbol{\theta}^{(t+1)} - J\boldsymbol{\theta}^{(t)}).$$

The J matrix can be determined empirically, using a sequence of subsequent iterates. It also follows from the observed and complete (or, equivalently) missing information:

$$J = I_d - \mathcal{I}_c(\boldsymbol{\theta}^*, \mathbf{Y})^{-1} I(\boldsymbol{\theta}^*, \mathbf{Y}).$$

Here, $\widetilde{\boldsymbol{\theta}}^*$ can then be seen as an accelerated iterate.

8.6   CALCULATION OF PRECISION ESTIMATES

Although the observed information matrix is not directly accessible, it has been shown by Louis (1982) that

$$I_m(\boldsymbol{\theta}, \boldsymbol{Y}^o) = E[\boldsymbol{S}_c(\boldsymbol{\theta}, \boldsymbol{Y})\boldsymbol{S}_c(\boldsymbol{\theta Y})' | \boldsymbol{y}^o] - \boldsymbol{S}(\boldsymbol{\theta}, \boldsymbol{Y}^o)\boldsymbol{S}(\boldsymbol{\theta}, \boldsymbol{Y}^o)',$$

for appropriate score vectors $\boldsymbol{S}$, $\boldsymbol{S}_c$. This leads to an expression for the observed information matrix in terms of complete data quantities that are available (McLachlan and Krishnan 1997):

$$I(\boldsymbol{\theta}, \boldsymbol{Y}^o) = I_m(\boldsymbol{\theta}, \boldsymbol{Y}^o) - E[\boldsymbol{S}_c(\boldsymbol{\theta}, \boldsymbol{Y})\boldsymbol{S}_c(\boldsymbol{\theta}, \boldsymbol{Y})' | \boldsymbol{y}^o] + \boldsymbol{S}(\boldsymbol{\theta}, \boldsymbol{Y}^o)\boldsymbol{S}(\boldsymbol{\theta}, \boldsymbol{Y}^o)'.$$

From this equation, the observed information matrix can be estimated as

$$I(\widehat{\boldsymbol{\theta}}, \boldsymbol{Y}^o) = I_m(\widehat{\boldsymbol{\theta}}, \boldsymbol{Y}^o) - E[\boldsymbol{S}_c(\widehat{\boldsymbol{\theta}}, \boldsymbol{Y})\boldsymbol{S}_c(\widehat{\boldsymbol{\theta}}, \boldsymbol{Y})' | \boldsymbol{y}^o],$$

where $\widehat{\boldsymbol{\theta}}$ is the maximum likelihood estimator.

8.7   A SIMPLE ILLUSTRATION

We will illustrate the principle of the EM algorithm using a simple, artificial, multinomial setting, considered by Dempster *et al.* (1977) in their original paper on the EM algorithm and also in Little and Rubin (2002).

The data and the complete and incomplete data models are presented in Figure 8.1. The key feature, which turns this problem into an incomplete data problem, is the fact that the counts Y_{11} and Y_{12} are not separately observed, but their total Y_i^o is.

Complete data:	Y_{11}	Y_{12}	Y_2	Y_3	Y_4
Complete data model:	$\frac{1}{2}$	$\frac{1}{4}\theta$	$\frac{1}{4}(1-\theta)$	$\frac{1}{4}(1-\theta)$	$\frac{1}{4}\theta$

Observed data:	Y_1^o		Y_2^o	Y_3^o	Y_4^o
Observed data model:	$\frac{1}{2}+\frac{1}{4}\theta$		$\frac{1}{4}(1-\theta)$	$\frac{1}{4}(1-\theta)$	$\frac{1}{4}\theta$
Observed counts:	125		18	20	34

Figure 8.1   Multinomial example. Complete and observed data and model.

The data can be analysed in at least three obvious ways: (1) by means of direct likelihood, using a non-iterative solution; (2) also by direct likelihood, but using an iterative solution; and (3) using the EM algorithm.

The log-likelihood for the (hypothetical) complete data is

$$\ell_c(\theta) = \sum_{j=1}^{5} \ln[\pi_j(\theta)]$$

$$= Y_{11}(125; \theta) \ln\left(\frac{1}{2}\right) + Y_{12}(125; \theta) \ln\left(\frac{1}{4}\theta\right) + 18 \ln\left(\frac{1}{4}(1-\theta)\right)$$

$$+ 20 \ln\left(\frac{1}{4}(1-\theta)\right) + 34 \ln\left(\frac{1}{4}\theta\right), \tag{8.2}$$

and its counterpart for the observed data is

$$\ell(\theta) = \sum_{j=1}^{4} \ln[\pi_j^o(\theta)]$$

$$= 125 \ln\left(\frac{1}{2} + \frac{1}{4}\theta\right) + 18 \ln\left\{\frac{1}{4}(1-\theta)\right\}$$

$$+ 20 \ln\left\{\frac{1}{4}(1-\theta)\right\} + 34 \ln\left(\frac{1}{4}\theta\right). \tag{8.3}$$

A non-iterative solution starts from the first-order derivative $S(\theta)$ of the observed data log-likelihood (8.3):

$$4S(\theta) = \frac{y_1}{2+\theta} - \frac{y_2}{1-\theta} - \frac{y_3}{1-\theta} + \frac{y_4}{\theta} = 0. \tag{8.4}$$

Rewriting (8.4) produces a quadratic equation:

$$-197\theta^2 + 150\theta + 68 = 0,$$

with two solutions $\theta_1 = 0.6268$ and $\theta_2 = -0.5507$, of which the proper solution obviously is: $\widehat{\theta} = 0.626821497871$. The unusually large number of decimal places is given to monitor the convergence of the iterative procedures in what follows.

Turning to an iterative solution of the observed data likelihood, we first define the matrix that connects the observed to the complete data:

$$C = \begin{pmatrix} 1 & 1 & 0 & 0 & 0 \\ 0 & 0 & 1 & 0 & 0 \\ 0 & 0 & 0 & 1 & 0 \\ 0 & 0 & 0 & 0 & 1 \end{pmatrix}. \tag{8.5}$$

This matrix is called a *coarsening matrix* by Molenberghs and Goetghebeur (1997). Using (8.5), $\pi^o(\theta) = C\pi(\theta)$. Writing

$$\pi(\theta) = \begin{pmatrix} 0.50 \\ 0 \\ 0.25 \\ 0.25 \\ 0 \end{pmatrix} + \begin{pmatrix} 0 \\ 0.25 \\ -0.25 \\ -0.25 \\ 0.25 \end{pmatrix} \theta = X_0 + X_1\theta,$$

the score function (8.4) can be written as

$$S(\theta) = X_1' C'\{C\mathrm{cov}(Y)C'\}^-(Y^o - nC\pi),$$

and the second derivative is

$$H(\theta) = nX_1' C'\{C\mathrm{cov}(Y)C'\}^- CX_1,$$

from which the updating algorithm follows:

$$\theta^{(t+1)} = \theta^{(t)} + \frac{S(\theta^{(t)})}{H(\theta^{(t)})}.$$

As always, at maximum, $W(\theta)$ can be used to estimate standard errors.

Before applying the direct likelihood iterative solution, we first turn to the EM algorithm. Likelihood (8.2) for the complete data gives rise to the objective function

$$Q(\theta|\theta^{(t)}) = Y_{11}(125; \theta^{(t)})\ln\left(\frac{1}{2}\right) + Y_{12}(125; \theta^{(t)})\ln\left(\frac{1}{4}\theta\right)$$

$$+ 18\ln\left\{\frac{1}{4}(1-\theta)\right\} + 20\ln\left\{\frac{1}{4}(1-\theta)\right\}$$

$$+ 34\ln\left(\frac{1}{4}\theta\right). \tag{8.6}$$

The E step requires the calculation of $Y_{11}(125; \theta^{(t)})$ and $Y_{12}(125; \theta^{(t)})$:

$$Y_{11}(125; \theta^{(t)}) = 125 \cdot \frac{2}{2 + \theta^{(t)}},$$

$$Y_{12}(125; \theta^{(t)}) = 125 \cdot \frac{\theta^{(t)}}{2 + \theta^{(t)}}.$$

For the M step, observe first that the complete data objective function is

$$4 \cdot S_c(\theta) = \frac{Y_{12}^{(t)}}{\theta} - \frac{Y_2}{1-\theta} - \frac{Y_3}{1-\theta} + \frac{Y_4}{\theta} = 0,$$

which, upon rewriting, is seen to produce a linear equation,

$$Y_{12}^{(t)} + Y_4 = \theta(Y_{12}^{(t)} + Y_2 + Y_3 + Y_4),$$

leading to the solution

$$\theta^{(t+1)} = \frac{Y_{12}^{(t)} + Y_4}{Y_{12}^{(t)} + Y_2 + Y_3 + Y_4} = \frac{Y_{12}^{(t)} + 34}{Y_{12}^{(t)} + 18 + 20 + 34}.$$

The iteration history for both iterative methods is given in Table 8.1. The iteration history of the sufficient statistics $Y_{11}^{(t)}$ and $Y_{12}^{(t)}$ is given in Table 8.2.

Note that the convergence of the EM algorithm is considerably slower than the Newton–Raphson based convergence. In addition, note that convergence is faster if the convergence rate is smaller, as the rate describes the contraction of the difference between subsequent parameter values and the maximum.

Table 8.1 Multinomial example. Iteration history for direct likelihood maximization using Newton–Raphson and for the EM algorithm.

	Newton–Raphson		EM	
t	$\theta^{(t)}$	Rate	$\theta^{(t)}$	Rate
1	0.500000000000	0.0506	0.500000000000	0.1464
2	0.633248730964	0.0447	0.608247422680	0.1346
3	0.626534069270	0.0449	0.624321050369	0.1330
4	0.626834428416	0.0449	0.626488879080	0.1328
5	0.626820916320	0.0449	0.626777322347	0.1327
6	0.626821524027	0.0449	0.626815632110	0.1327
7	0.626821496695	0.0449	0.626820719019	0.1327
8	0.626821497924	0.0453	0.626821394456	0.1327

Table 8.2 Multinomial example. Iteration history of the sufficient statistics $Y_{11}^{(t)}$ and $Y_{12}^{(t)}$ with the EM algorithm.

t	$Y_{11}^{(t)}$	$Y_{12}^{(t)}$
1	100.000	25.0000
2	95.8498	29.1502
3	95.2627	29.7373
4	95.1841	29.8159
5	95.1737	29.8263
6	95.1723	29.8277
7	95.1721	29.8279
8	95.1721	29.8279

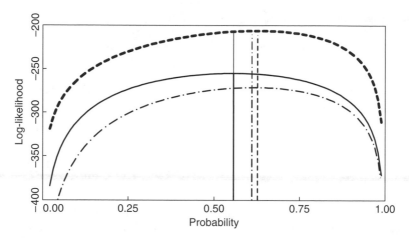

Figure 8.2 Multinomial example. Observed data log-likelihood (dashed curve) and two subsequent complete data log-likelihoods (1, solid curve; 2, dot-dashed curve).

The observed data log-likelihood and its complete data counterpart for two subsequent iterations are given in Figure 8.2. When considering the log-likelihood values at maximum *of the complete data log-likelihoods*, they seemingly decrease between subsequent cycles. However, they cannot be compared directly, as the function itself changes at every cycle. The complete data log-likelihood is merely a device for optimization and cannot be used directly for likelihood ratio tests or precision estimation. As stated in Sections 8.5 and 8.6, asymptotic covariance matrices and thus standard errors do not follow immediately, and additional work is required.

Regarding the estimation of precision, it is easy enough to use direct likelihood methods, that is, to use the information matrix derived from the observed data likelihood,

$$I(\theta) = \frac{y_1}{(2+\theta)^2} + \frac{(y_2+y_3)}{(1-\theta)^2} + \frac{y_4}{\theta^2},$$

which, evaluated in the maximum likelihood estimator $\widehat{\theta} = 0.6268$, yields $\widehat{\mathcal{I}} = 377.516$. The asymptotic standard error is the inverse square root of this quantity, that is 0.051.

Now the complete data score is

$$S_c(\theta, \boldsymbol{Y}) = \frac{Y_{12}+y_4}{\theta} - \frac{y_2+y_3}{1-\theta},$$

and the complete data information is

$$I_c(\theta, \boldsymbol{Y}) = \frac{Y_{12}+y_4}{\theta^2} + \frac{y_2+y_3}{(1-\theta)^2},$$

with expectation

$$\mathcal{I}_c(\theta, \boldsymbol{y}^o) = \frac{E[Y_{12}|y_1] + y_4}{\theta^2} + \frac{y_2 + y_3}{(1-\theta)^2},$$

and

$$E(Y_{12}|y_1) = y_1 \cdot \frac{\frac{1}{4}\theta}{\frac{1}{2} + \frac{1}{4}\theta}.$$

The missing information is

$$\mathcal{I}_m(\theta, \boldsymbol{y}^o) = \text{var}[S_c(\theta, \boldsymbol{Y})|\boldsymbol{y}^o)]$$

$$= \text{var}\left[\left(\frac{Y_{12} + y_4}{\theta} - \frac{y_2 + y_3}{1-\theta}\right)\bigg| y\right]$$

$$= \frac{1}{\theta^2}\text{var}(Y_{12}|y)$$

$$= \frac{1}{\theta^2} \cdot y_1 \cdot \frac{\frac{1}{4}\theta}{\frac{1}{2} + \frac{1}{4}\theta} \cdot \frac{\frac{1}{2}}{\frac{1}{2} + \frac{1}{4}\theta}$$

$$= \frac{1}{\theta^2} \cdot y_1 \cdot \frac{\frac{1}{8}\theta}{(\frac{1}{2} + \frac{1}{4}\theta)^2}.$$

Substituting the observed data values and the maximum likelihood estimate for θ yields $\mathcal{I}_c(\widehat{\theta}, \boldsymbol{y}^o) = 435.318$, $\mathcal{I}_m(\widehat{\theta}, \boldsymbol{y}^o) = 57.801$ and hence $I(\widehat{\theta}, \boldsymbol{y}^o) = 435.318 - 57.801 = 377.516$, in perfect agreement with the direct likelihood derivation.

To conclude, note that the ratio

$$J(\widehat{\theta}) = \frac{\mathcal{I}_m(\widehat{\theta}, y)}{\mathcal{I}_c(\widehat{\theta}, y)} = \frac{57.801}{435.318} - 0.1328,$$

in agreement with the convergence rate observed earlier.

8.8   CONCLUDING REMARKS

The expectation–maximization algorithm has been presented as an important tool for maximizing less amenable (log-)likelihoods that is valid under MAR and with existing extensions under MNAR (see Section 15.4). The EM algorithm can be used not only when data are incomplete, but in many settings where the observed data are a subset of the data considered in the model. Examples include grouped data, censored data, partially classified data, as well as latent class, latent variable, and random-effects models. In many practical situations arising in clinical studies, direct likelihood and multiple imputation will be sufficiently versatile to obviate the need for using the EM algorithm, but it does have important roles in some settings as a general-purpose optimization tool, and is used to provide initial parameter estimates in some implementations of multiple imputation.

9

Multiple Imputation

9.1 INTRODUCTION

Since its introduction nearly 30 years ago (Rubin 1978) multiple imputation has become an important and influential approach for dealing with the statistical analysis of incomplete data. It now has a very large bibliography, including several reviews and texts (Rubin 1987, 1996; Rubin and Schenker 1986; Schafer 1997, 1999; Horton and Lipsitz 2001). Its domain of application has spread steadily from sample surveys to include many diverse areas such as the analysis of observational data from public health research and clinical trials. In parallel with these developments, tools for multiple imputation have been incorporated into several mainstream statistical packages. In this chapter we provide an introduction to the multiple imputation procedure and indicate some of the roles it may have to play in the current setting.

The overall approach is sketched out in Section 9.2 and an outline theoretical justification is presented in Section 9.3. We consider the inferential part of the procedure in Section 9.4, its relative efficiency in Section 9.5, and discuss how imputations may be made in Section 9.6. Some possible roles for multiple imputation in the current setting are discussed in Section 9.7

An illustration, using the age-related macular degeneration study introduced in Section 2.8, is deferred to Chapter 13.

9.2 THE BASIC PROCEDURE

The key idea of the multiple imputation (MI) procedure is to replace each missing value with a set of M plausible values. Each value is a *Bayesian* draw from the conditional distribution of the missing observation given the

Missing Data in Clinical Studies   G. Molenberghs and M.G. Kenward
© 2007 John Wiley & Sons, Ltd

observed data, made in such a way that the set of imputations properly represents the information about the missing value that is contained in the observed data for the chosen model. The imputations produce M 'completed' data sets, each of which is analysed using the method that would have been appropriate had the data been complete. The model for the latter analysis is called the *substantive* model, while that used to produce the imputations is called the *imputation* model. One great strength of the MI procedure is that, to a certain extent, these two models can be considered separately. MI is most straightforward to use under MAR, and most software implementations make this assumption. However, it is quite possible to apply it in MNAR settings, and this is particularly convenient when certain classes of pattern-mixture model are used to construct the imputation model. Two examples are Little and Yau (1996) and Thijs *et al.* (2002). There are many developments and extensions of the basic MI concept; for example, Aerts *et al.* (2002) develop a local MI method and Lipsitz *et al.* (1998) propose a semi-parametric MI approach.

Multiple imputation involves three distinct phases or, using Rubin's (1987) terminology, tasks:

1. The missing values are filled in M times to generate M complete data sets.
2. The M complete data sets are analysed by using standard procedures.
3. The results from the M analyses are combined into a single inference.

It is worth noting that the first and third tasks can be conducted by the SAS procedures MI and MIANALYZE, respectively, at least for particular imputation models. The second task is performed using one of the standard data-analytic procedures.

The actual procedure is as follows. Suppose that we are interested in making inferences about the $k \times 1$ parameter vector $\boldsymbol{\beta}$ from the substantive model and that we are able to make appropriate Bayesian posterior draws from the imputation model. We return later to see how this might be done in practice. Replacing the missing data by their corresponding imputation samples, M completed data sets are constructed. Denote by $\hat{\boldsymbol{\beta}}^{m}$ and V^m respectively the estimate of $\boldsymbol{\beta}$ and its covariance matrix from the mth completed data set $(m = 1, \ldots, M)$. The MI estimate of $\boldsymbol{\beta}$ is the simple average of the estimates,

$$\hat{\boldsymbol{\beta}}^{*} = \frac{1}{M} \sum_{m=1}^{M} \hat{\boldsymbol{\beta}}^{m}.$$

We also need a measure of precision for $\hat{\boldsymbol{\beta}}^{*}$ that properly reflects the uncertainty in the imputations. One great practical advantage of MI is the existence of a simple expression for the covariance matrix of $\hat{\boldsymbol{\beta}}^{*}$ that can be applied very generally and uses only complete data quantities. This is known as Rubin's variance formula (Rubin 1987) and combines within- and between-imputation variability in an intuitively appealing way. Define

$$W = \frac{1}{M} \sum_{m=1}^{M} V^m$$

to be the average within-imputation covariance matrix, and

$$B = \frac{1}{M-1} \sum_{m=1}^{M} (\hat{\boldsymbol{\beta}}^m - \hat{\boldsymbol{\beta}}^*)(\hat{\boldsymbol{\beta}}^m - \hat{\boldsymbol{\beta}}^*)'$$

to be the between-imputation covariance matrix of $\hat{\boldsymbol{\beta}}^m$. Then an estimate of the covariance matrix of $\hat{\boldsymbol{\beta}}^*$ is given by

$$V = W + \left(\frac{M+1}{M}\right) B.$$

Apart from an adjustment to accommodate the finite number of imputations used, this is a very straightforward combination of between- and within-imputation variability.

9.3   THEORETICAL JUSTIFICATION

At the heart of the MI method is a Bayesian argument. Suppose we have a problem with two parameters γ_1, γ_2 and data y. In a Bayesian analysis these have a joint posterior distribution

$$f(\gamma_1, \gamma_2 \mid y).$$

Now suppose that our focus is on γ_2, with γ_1 being regarded as a nuisance. Because the posterior can be partitioned as

$$f(\gamma_1, \gamma_2 \mid y) = f(\gamma_1 \mid y)f(\gamma_2 \mid \gamma_1, y),$$

it can be seen that the marginal posterior for γ_2 can be expressed as

$$f(\gamma_2 \mid y) = E_{\gamma_1}\{f(\gamma_2 \mid \gamma_1, y)\}.$$

In particular, the posterior mean and variance for γ_2 can be expressed

$$E(\gamma_2 \mid y) = E_{\gamma_1}\{E_{\gamma_2}(\gamma_2 \mid \gamma_1, y)\},$$
$$\text{var}(\gamma_2 \mid y) = E_{\gamma_1}\{\text{var}_{\gamma_2}(\gamma_2 \mid \gamma_1, y)\} + \text{var}_{\gamma_1}\{E_{\gamma_2}(\gamma_2 \mid \gamma_1, y)\}.$$

These can be approximated using empirical moments. Let γ_1^m, $m = 1, \ldots, M$, be draws from the marginal posterior distribution of γ_1. Then, approximately,

$$E(\gamma_2 \mid y) \simeq \frac{1}{M} \sum_{m=1}^{m} \{E_{\gamma_2}(\gamma_2 \mid \gamma_1^m, y)\} = \tilde{\gamma}_2$$

say, and

$$\operatorname{var}(\gamma_2 \mid y) = \frac{1}{M} \sum_{m=1}^{m} \operatorname{var}_{\gamma_2}(\gamma_2 \mid \gamma_1^m, y) + \frac{1}{M-1} \sum_{m=1}^{m} \{E_{\gamma_2}(\gamma_2 \mid \gamma_1^m, y) - \tilde{\gamma}_2\}^2.$$

These formulae can be generalized in an obvious way for vector-valued parameters.

The final link between these expressions and the MI procedure is then to use γ_2 to represent the parameters of the substantive model and γ_1 to represent the missing data.

It is assumed that in sufficiently large samples the conditional posterior moments for γ_2 can be approximated by maximum likelihood, or equivalent efficient, estimators from the completed data sets. This makes it clear why we need to use imputation (conditional predictive) draws from a proper Bayesian posterior. In this way we can see that the MI estimates of the parameters of interest and their variance approximate the first two moments of the posterior distribution in a fully Bayesian analysis. The large-sample approximation of the posterior also suggests that MI should be applied to a parameter on the scale for which the posterior is better approximated by the normal distribution, for example using log odds ratios when the parameter of interest is an odds ratio.

9.4   INFERENCE UNDER MULTIPLE IMPUTATION

From a Bayesian perspective the foregoing is a relatively straightforward approximate procedure, provided we are able to make the appropriate posterior draws for the imputations. However, in practice the final step of MI is a frequentist one. Tests and confidence intervals are based on the approximate pivot

$$P = (\hat{\boldsymbol{\beta}}^* - \boldsymbol{\beta})' V^{-1} (\hat{\boldsymbol{\beta}}^* - \boldsymbol{\beta}).$$

In a conventional, regular, problem this would have an asymptotic χ_k^2 distribution. However, in the MI setting, the asymptotic results and hence the χ^2 reference distributions do not solely depend on the sample size N, but also on the number of imputations M. Therefore, Li *et al.* (1991) propose the use of an $F_{k,w}$ reference distribution for the scaled statistic

$$F = \frac{P}{k(1+r)}$$

with

$$w = 4 + (\tau - 4)\left[1 + \frac{(1 - 2\tau^{-1})}{r}\right]^2,$$

$$r = \frac{1}{k}\left(1 + \frac{1}{M}\right)\text{tr}(BW^{-1}),$$

$$\tau = k(M - 1).$$

Here, r is the average relative increase in variance due to missingness across the components of $\boldsymbol{\beta}$. The limiting distribution of F, as $M \to \infty$, is the χ_k^2 distribution. This procedure is applicable for any vector of parameters from the substantive model, or any linear combination of these.

9.5   EFFICIENCY

Multiple imputation is attractive because it can be highly efficient even for small values of M. In many applications, as few as 3–5 imputations are sufficient to obtain excellent results. Rubin (1987, p. 114) shows that the efficiency of an estimate based on M imputations is approximately

$$\left(1 + \frac{\gamma}{M}\right)^{-1},$$

where γ is the fraction of missing information for the quantity being estimated. The fraction γ quantifies how much more precise the estimate might have been if no data had been missing. The efficiencies achieved for various values of M and rates of missing information are shown in Table 9.1. This table shows that gains rapidly diminish after the first few imputations. In many situations there simply is little advantage in producing and analysing more than a few imputed data sets. There are exceptions to this rule, however, and in some of the clinical trial examples considered by Carpenter *et al.* (2006) substantially more imputations are needed to stabilize the results. Increasing the number of imputations also improves the precision of the between-imputation covariance matrix B and, when k is not small, may be necessary to provide a non-singular estimate of this.

Table 9.1 Relative efficiency (per cent) of MI estimation by number of imputations M and fraction of missing information γ.

			γ		
m	0.1	0.3	0.5	0.7	0.9
2	95	87	80	74	69
3	97	91	86	81	77
5	98	94	91	88	85
10	99	97	95	93	92
20	100	99	98	97	96

9.6 MAKING PROPER IMPUTATIONS

Unsurprisingly, many of the practical issues with MI concern the choice of, and Bayesian draws from, the imputation model. Schafer (1997, pp. 109–110) summarizes the formal requirements for an MI to be valid. For the simplest settings it is possible to check formally that these conditions hold. For more realistic problems such a justification is difficult to construct, and broader guidelines are needed. Rubin (1987, pp. 126–127) provides the following:

- Draw imputations following the Bayesian paradigm as repetitions from a Bayesian posterior distribution of the missing values under the chosen models for non-response and data, or an approximation to this posterior distribution that incorporates appropriate between-imputation variability.
- Choose models of non-response appropriate for the posited response mechanism.
- Choose models for the data that are appropriate for the complete data statistics likely to be used – if the model for the data is correct, then the model is appropriate for all complete data statistics.

In general, the imputation model should contain variables known to be predictive of missingness and accommodate structure – for example interactions – in the substantive model. In particular, for imputing covariates, the outcome variable must be included as an explanatory variable in the model. Failure to accommodate the structure appropriately can cause bias in the resulting analysis (Fay 1992). It has been suggested that inferences are fairly robust to the choice of imputation distribution itself. Clearly this depends very much on the setting, in particular on the substantive model and the nature, pattern and quantity of the missing data.

Suppose in a given problem that a unit provides (potentially) p variables $z = (z_1, \ldots, z_p)'$. Divide these into those observed and those (potentially) missing: z_o and z_m. Each of these may be an outcome or an explanatory variable in the substantive model, or may be in the imputation model only (as an explanatory variable). In its most general form the imputation model provides a, typically multivariate, regression of z_m on z_o with conditional distribution

$$g(z_m \mid z_o, r)$$

where r, a vector of indicator variables, is the observed pattern of missingness for this particular unit. If the missing data mechanism is assumed to be ignorable then r can be dropped from this to give

$$g(z_m \mid z_o),$$

which provides considerable simplification. In particular, for simpler modelling structures the required imputation model can be estimated from the completers only, that is, those units without missing data.

Care needs to be taken in conceptualizing ignorability when the missingness pattern is non-monotone (Robins and Gill 1997; see also Chapter 19 below). If different units have different non-monotone patterns of missingness then it is difficult to conceive of plausible missing value mechanisms that maintain the ignorability assumption. One route is to assume that different mechanisms apply to different units, but this can appear rather contrived. In practice, to keep the problem manageable, this issue is usually put to one side, and r is simply omitted from the imputation model.

The main problem is then to construct and fit an appropriate imputation model $g(z_m \mid z_o)$, and make posterior Bayesian draws from it. This means, among other things, that uncertainty about the parameters of this model must be properly incorporated. Such draws can be made in many different ways, often involving some form of approximation. Particular methods may be better suited to particular settings, so we will concentrate below on those that are especially relevant in the clinical trial context. First, we consider some general approaches to the problem. In most settings, for example with missing longitudinal outcomes or missing covariates in observational studies, the missing data will be potentially *multivariate*. The imputation model will need to reflect this, so all methods of drawing imputations that are practically relevant need to handle multivariate data. In some contexts the missing variables will of different types, for example measured, discrete, binary or ordinal. Joint modelling of such disparate variables in a flexible and convenient way is itself an important statistical problem. Broadly two approaches to this have emerged in the MI setting.

First, for all but nominal variables, a joint multivariate normal distribution is assumed. This requires considerable approximation for highly non-normal variables, such as binary, but some authors have justified the use of such approximations; see, for example, Schafer (1997, Chapters 4 and 5). Some success has even been reported using a normal regression model for the extreme case of missing binary data (*e.g.*, Schafer 1997, Section 5.1), although predictably issues arise when probabilities are extreme (Schafer and Schenker 2000). Various methods can then be used to fit and make Bayesian draws from the joint distribution.

In many settings simpler approximate imputation draws can be used. A range of such methods for generating proper imputations is given in Little and Rubin (2002, Section 10.2.3). In sufficiently large samples we can often do acceptably well by approximating the posterior predictive distribution using a multivariate normal distribution with mean and covariance matrix taken from the maximum likelihood estimates. Under MAR it is, in principle, possible to obtain these from the completers only, which leads to considerable simplification and may be acceptably precise when the proportion of missing data is not great.

We illustrate this approach using a simple normal regression imputation model, from which values of x_i are to be imputed given the observed values of y_i:

$$x_i \mid y_i \sim N(\xi + \eta y_i, \tau^2). \tag{9.1}$$

Under MAR we can use maximum likelihood to get consistent estimators, $\widehat{\gamma}$ and $\widehat{\tau}^2$ say, of $\gamma = (\xi, \eta)'$ and τ^2, from the complete pairs. In this particular setting, of course, maximum likelihood is equivalent to simple least squares.

Approximate draws from a Bayesian posterior for the parameters of the imputation model (9.1) can be made as follows:

$$\tilde{\tau}^2 = (m-2)\widehat{\tau}^2/X \text{ for } X \sim \chi^2_{m-2},$$

$$\tilde{\gamma} \sim N(\widehat{\gamma}, \tilde{\tau}^2(F'F)^{-1}),$$

where m is the number of completers, and F is the $m \times 2$ matrix with rows consisting of $(1, y_i)$ from the completers.

Finally, the missing x_i are drawn from

$$x_i \sim N((1, y_i)\tilde{\gamma}, \tilde{\tau}^2).$$

This method is simple to extend for longitudinal data with attrition (dropout), where at each time point previously imputed values are used in the imputation model as predictors. More generally, such approaches can be applied with maximum likelihood estimators from other classes of regression model where it is assumed that the large-sample posterior can be approximated by the maximum likelihood estimator and its large-sample covariance matrix. These need not be confined to the use of the data from the completers only.

For general missing data patterns with a multivariate normal imputation model, small-sample draws can be constructed comparatively simply using Markov chain Monte Carlo (MCMC) methods; Schafer (1997, Section 5.4) gives details. Broadly, in statistical applications, MCMC is used to generate pseudo-random draws from multidimensional and otherwise intractable probability distributions via Markov chains. A Markov chain is a sequence of random variables in which the distribution of each element depends on the value of the previous one(s). In the MCMC method, one constructs a Markov chain long enough for the distribution of the elements to stabilize to a common distribution. This stationary distribution is the one of interest. By repeatedly simulating steps of the chain, draws from the distribution of interest are generated.

More precisely, the MCMC method works as follows in the multivariate normal setting. In the first step, starting values need to be chosen. This can be done by computing a vector of means and a covariance matrix from the complete data. These are used to estimate the parameters of the prior distributions for means and variances of the multivariate normal distribution with an informative prior. The next step is then the imputation step: values for missing data items are simulated by randomly selecting a value from the available distribution of values, that is, the predictive distribution of missing values given the observed values. In the posterior step, the posterior distribution of the mean and covariance parameters is updated, by updating the parameters governing their distribution (e.g., the inverted Wishart distribution for the variance–covariance matrix and the normal distribution for the means). This is then followed by sampling from the posterior distribution of mean and covariance parameters, based on the updated parameters. The imputation and the posterior steps are then iterated until the distribution is stationary. This implies that the mean vector and covariance matrix are unchanged throughout the iterative process. Finally, we use the imputations from the final iteration to yield a data set that has no missing values.

With monotone missingness it is expected that the MCMC approach and approximate regression method should lead to very similar answers. The difference is due largely to the different prior distributions used. Both methods are available in the SAS procedure MI. Multivariate nominal discrete data can be handled using a log-linear model (Schafer 1997, Section 8), and again facilities are available for this in the SAS procedure MI.

The second broad approach is different from that just described in that it does not start with the construction of well-defined *joint* distribution for the variables to be imputed. Rather, it starts with a collection of univariate conditionals which, it is hoped, correspond to a genuine joint distribution. Draws are made from these using a sequential procedure which is analogous to a Gibbs sampler, such as the one underlying the MCMC approach described above. However, it can be demonstrated formally that the resulting draws converge to samples from a well-defined multivariate posterior distribution only in the case of multivariate normal data with monotone missingness.

The main idea in this approach is that a univariate conditional model is constructed for each potentially missing variable which is appropriate to the type, such as a logistic regression for a binary variable. The other potentially missing variables are then used as explanatory variables in each univariate imputation model. This is attractive in that it avoids the inevitable concerns about approximations that accompany the use of the multivariate normal based approach described above. Using the previous notation this model, for the kth missing variable (of q), would be for the conditional distribution

$$[z_k \mid z_1, \dots, z_{k-1}, z_{k+1}, \dots, z_q, \mathbf{z}_o], \ k = 1, \dots, q.$$

Cycling through all q models in turn, univariate posterior draws are then made, given current values of the other variables. The whole cycle is then repeated, usually a small number of times, typically 10–20. One set of MIs is taken from the final cycle. The whole process is then repeated M times. Most implementations use approximate large-sample draws from the univariate models. The great advantage of this approach is that each type of variable is modelled appropriately. The disadvantage is that, in general, there is no guarantee that the distribution of the draws converges to a valid joint posterior distribution. Some limited simulation studies do seem to suggest that the method can perform quite well in certain settings. The overall approach was developed independently by Taylor *et al.* (2002) who called it the the *sequential regression imputation method*, and van Buuren *et al.* (1999) who used the term *multiple chained equations*. These methods are particularly attractive with sets of observational data when many different covariates may be incomplete.

A third approach, which is less relevant in the current setting, uses non-parametric methods through Bayesian versions of hot-deck imputation. Herzog and Rubin (1983) and Heitjan and Rubin (1991) are comparatively early examples. The appropriate role of these is, however, with large surveys, which takes us away from the present concerns. A related approach that avoids an explicit parametric imputation model uses the so-called *propensity score*. This was originally defined as the conditional probability of assignment to a particular treatment given a vector of observed covariates (Rosenbaum and Rubin 1983). In the missing data setting a propensity score is generated for each variable with missing values to indicate the probability of observations being missing. The observations are then grouped based on these propensity scores, and an approximate Bayesian bootstrap imputation (Rubin 1987) is applied to each group. The propensity score method uses only the covariate information associated with whether the imputed variable values are missing. It does not use the associations among variables. As a consequence, while it can be effective for inferences about the distributions of individual imputed variables, it is not appropriate for analyses involving relationships among variables.

In the current setting we are mainly (although not wholly) dealing with sets of longitudinal data, in which sequences are incomplete. For such problems the most appropriate approach is the one first described above, in particular as implemented in the SAS procedure MI.

9.7   SOME ROLES FOR MULTIPLE IMPUTATION

Suppose that we use a multivariate normal model for continuous repeated responses as set out in Chapter 7 and then, rather than using a direct likelihood analysis, instead use MI for the missing responses employing a multivariate normal imputation model that is wholly consistent with the chosen substantive model. How would we expect the results to differ from the likelihood analysis? In practice, we would expect very similar results; indeed, as the number of imputations (M) increases, the results from the two analyses should converge (apart from small differences due to the asymptotic approximations involved). With finite M the maximum likelihood estimators are actually more efficient, although the difference may be very small.

To illustrate this point this we consider model 1 from Sections 5.2 and 5.3, consisting of separate unstructured profiles for boys and girls, and a fully unstructured 4×4 variance–covariance matrix. We focus on the mean for boys at the incompletely observed age 10 measurement. We use MI with a full multivariate normal imputation model for the missing data and $M = 5$ imputations. The mean, obtained from the original data, is 23.81 (standard error 0.51). The estimate obtained from direct likelihood was 23.17 (s.e. 0.68 with ML and 0.71 using REML). Based on the MI analysis, the estimate equals 22.69 (s.e. 0.81). Thus, in this simple and small example, MI performs similarly, as expected, even though it somewhat extends the slight overcorrection already seen with direct likelihood.

This raises the question as to when MI offers advantages over direct likelihood analyses. When covariates are missing, it offers an intuitively attractive and very manageable method for dealing with potentially very complex problems, for which likelihood analyses may be impracticable or, at least, very awkward. When responses only are missing, and likelihood analyses are relatively simple to do, as in the above example, it offers little. However, we have only considered the use of an imputation model which is 'consistent' with the substantive model in the sense that the two models (substantive and imputation) can both be derived from an overall model for the complete data. As Meng (1994) shows, it is one of the great strengths of MI that these two models do not have to be consistent in this sense. Meng introduces the term 'uncongenial' for an imputation model which is not consistent with the substantive model, and it is with these that MI has much to offer in the current setting. Here are three examples of situations in which such uncongenial imputation models might be of value.

Estimating equation methods. For some problems, such as fitting population-averaged models to repeated binary outcomes, non-likelihood methods of analysis might have advantages, especially when a full likelihood analysis is complicated and/or very demanding computationally. In particular, generalized estimating equations (Zeger and Liang 1986) are commonly used in such settings. Such methods are valid under MCAR but not MAR. In the next chapter we see how validity under MAR can be realized using appropriate weighting of the estimating equations. An alternative to this is to use MI in which the imputation model is consistent with the MAR assumption, but not necessarily congenial with the chosen substantive model. The population-averaged (or marginal) substantive model does not specify the entire joint distribution of the repeated outcomes (in particular, the dependence structure is left unspecified), and so cannot be used as a basis for constructing the imputation model. Several alternatives are possible. One could 'complete' the specification of the model by introducing dependence structure and impute from this. But such models are not convenient imputation models for the same reason they are not convenient substantive models and, if this route is pursued, one may as well anyway use a direct likelihood analysis in the first place. An alternative is to use a convenient and sufficiently rich joint model for the imputations, but one which is not parameterized in a population-averaged way, and so is uncongenial. Two possible types of such imputation model are (1) a generalized linear mixed model in which the dependence is induced through subject random effects, and (2) a log-linear model. The latter is a relatively simple choice for which imputation procedures are already implemented in widely available software. We return to this in Chapter 11.

The introduction of additional predictors. It may be that there are variables that are predictive of missingness on which we do *not* wish to condition, so they are not to be included in the substantive model. This can be done by *jointly* modelling the outcome and additional predictor variables, but this can lead to considerable additional complications and, further, removes the intuitive appeal of keeping the substantive model that would have been used had the data been complete. A straightforward alternative that does keep the original substantive model is to use MI in which these extra variables are included in the in the (now uncongenial) imputation model.

   An example of this would be if there were a measure of non-compliance which was strongly associated with dropout, where subjects who drop out are likely to be non-compliers. For an intention-to-treat analysis it is important that the imputation model for such subjects reflects their degree of compliance. In such a case non-compliance must be included in the imputation model to allow such distinctions to be made, but, as a post-randomization outcome, they must certainly not be in the substantive model.

Sensitivity analysis and MNAR imputations. We stress in Part V the importance of assessing the sensitivity to the underlying assumptions, especially MAR, of primary direct likelihood analyses. Multiple imputation provides a particularly convenient method for this. The same primary likelihood analysis can be kept for the substantive model, but the imputation model can be modified to allow for non-random imputations. This is particularly convenient when MNAR pattern-mixture models are used for the imputation model whose components can be constructed out of the fitted MAR model. The approach is very flexible, and many alternative forms of MNAR model can be considered in this way. Two very different examples of this are given by Little and Yau (1996) and Kenward *et al.* (2003). We explore this approach, with some examples, in much more detail in Part V.

9.8   CONCLUDING REMARKS

In this chapter we have outlined the main Bayesian principles behind multiple imputation and shown how it is carried out in a generic way; in particular, the stages of imputation, combination and inference have been described. We have discussed alternative methods for making proper imputations. Finally, we have distinguished those settings in the current clinical trial context in which multiple imputation provides real advantages over direct likelihood methods. Principally, these are those situations in which covariates are missing, and in which we wish to use uncongenial imputation models, especially as part of a sensitivity analysis. A case study using multiple imputation is presented in Chapter 13.

10

Weighted Estimating Equations

10.1 INTRODUCTION

The principled methods that we have met so far in this book for accommodating missing data mechanisms that are not MCAR have all involved, directly or indirectly, integration (or averaging) over the distribution of the missing data. For example, this is done directly in constructing the likelihood for the observed data (Chapter 7) and indirectly when using multiple imputation (Chapter 9). All such methods require assumptions to be made about this distribution, often in the form of its conditional distribution given the observed data and, as we emphasize in Part V, the resulting conclusions can be very sensitive to these. An alternative method for correcting for missing value mechanisms that are not strictly MCAR uses instead information about the missingness probabilities themselves. The idea, called inverse probability weighting (IPW), has its roots in survey analysis (Horvitz and Thompson 1952). We provide a very intuitive introduction to the idea in the next section. In its basic form the method has the advantage of robustness, in that it does not depend on knowledge of the distribution of the unobserved data. However, the price that is paid for this is inefficiency; see Clayton *et al.* (1998), for example. The reason for this is that the method in its basic form uses only the data from completers. Empirical evidence does suggest, however, that this can be less of an issue in some settings with missing binary data. Problems can also arise due to the fact that the resulting estimates may be unstable because certain subsets of the population have small missingness probabilities (Little and Rubin 2002, p. 49).

In this chapter we are mainly concerned with applying the ideas of IPW to settings where other approaches, such as direct likelihood, are not so convenient. We are principally concerned with the most common example of

---

Missing Data in Clinical Studies   G. Molenberghs and M.G. Kenward
© 2007 John Wiley & Sons, Ltd

this: the problem of fitting marginal models to non-normal outcomes, a setting in which generalized estimating equations are commonly used. In Section 10.3 we outline the basic ideas involved in the marginal modelling of non-normal data, and the use of generalized estimating equations. We show in Section 10.4 how IPW can be integrated quite conveniently into this set-up when we are faced with longitudinal data with dropout. In Sections 10.5 and 10.6 we describe applications of the approach using two of our illustrative examples.

In Section 10.7 we return to the problem of the inefficiency of IPW. In a series of papers over the last decade (principally Robins and Rotnitzky 1995; Robins *et al.* 1995; and Scharfstein *et al.* 1999), Robins and colleagues have proposed improved IPW estimates which are theoretically more efficient under the MAR assumption. A further development, the so-called doubly robust, or doubly protected, estimators, introduced in the discussion rejoinder in Scharfstein *et al.* (1999) and in the contribution to the discussion of Bickel and Kwon (2001) by Robins and Rotnitzky, are robust under certain conditions to misspecification of the model for the probability of response. We give an introduction to the ideas behind this form of double robustness that is based on the development in Carpenter *et al.* (2006). As yet the technical nature of these methods and the lack of available generally applicable software have restricted their accessibility and uptake by the wider research community. This is likely to change, however, in the future.

10.2   INVERSE PROBABILITY WEIGHTING

We introduce the idea of inverse probability weighting by giving a very intuitive view of the way in which it can correct the bias associated with missing data that are not MCAR. Consider a binary (0/1) outcome. Suppose that we wish to estimate the proportion of 1s in a population represented by a random sample of 12 subjects. Suppose further that all 1s are observed, but only half of subjects with a 0 are actually observed. This is an MNAR missingness mechanism. We might have the following data:

Subject	1	2	3	4	5	6	7	8	9	10	11	12
Actual outcome	1	0	0	0	1	0	1	0	0	0	1	0
Observed outcome	1	?	?	0	1	?	1	0	0	1	1	?

An unbiased estimator of the true population proportion is given by the actual proportion of successes, in this case equal to $4/12 = 1/3$. Of course, if some data are missing we do not have this estimate available to us. The proportion of successes among the *observed* data, on the other hand (the completers), is $4/8 = 1/2$. This is biased, and will remain so however large the sample becomes under this MNAR scheme. In this artificial setting we know that (on average) half of the zero outcomes are unobserved so, to compensate, double weight can be given to each of these, leading to the IPW estimate

$$\frac{4}{4+2\times 4} = \frac{1}{3},$$

equal in this case to the unbiased estimate. The exact equality here is a little contrived, and is a consequence of choosing to have exactly half of the zero outcomes missing in the sample. In practice this will only happen on average. Nevertheless, the IPW estimator is consistent under the conditions of the example. This is the essence of the approach developed by Horvitz and Thompson (1952).

We now move to a more realistic, but still very simple, example: linear regression. Suppose that we have n independent pairs $\{Y_i, x_i\}$ such that

$$E(Y_i) = \beta_0 + \beta_1 x_i = x_i'\boldsymbol{\beta}, \quad i = 1, \ldots, n,$$

and

$$Y_i \sim N(0, \sigma^2), \quad \text{independently.}$$

The ordinary least-squares regression line (in this case maximum likelihood) is obtained by solving the normal equations for $\boldsymbol{\beta}$:

$$\sum_{i=1}^{n} x_i'(y_i - x_i'\widehat{\boldsymbol{\beta}}) = \mathbf{0}.$$

Suppose now that some outcome (Y_i) observations are missing, and let R_i be the binary missing value indicator ($R_i = 0$ implies that Y_i is missing). It is easily checked that the following normal equations remain unbiased (hence consistent for $\boldsymbol{\beta}$):

$$\sum_{\text{observed}} x_i(y_i - x_i'\widehat{\boldsymbol{\beta}}) + \sum_{\text{missing}} x_i(y_i^* - x_i'\widehat{\boldsymbol{\beta}}) = 0, \tag{10.1}$$

where

$$y_i^* = E_{Y_i|r_i}(Y_i).$$

If R_i is independent of Y_i (everything assumed conditional on x_i), then

$$y_i^* = E_{Y_i|r_i}(Y_i) = E_{Y_i}(Y_i) = x_i'\widehat{\boldsymbol{\beta}}$$

and

$$\sum_{\text{observed}} x_i(y_i - x_i'\widehat{\boldsymbol{\beta}});$$

that is, use the completers only. The assumption above is equivalent to MCAR, and in this setting, without imposing a distribution on the x_i, there is no relevant additional information in the incomplete pairs.

Suppose now that R_i and Y_i are *not* independent. If the conditional distribution of $Y_i \mid r_i$ were *known* we could still use (10.1), and this is, for example, the basis of tobit regression. But, suppose that we do not know this distribution, but instead know, or can estimate, the missingness probabilities

$$\pi_i = P(R_i = 1 \mid \boldsymbol{y}_i, x_i).$$

Then it is easily seen that the IPW normal equations are unbiased (for known π_i),

$$\sum_{\text{observed}} \frac{\boldsymbol{x}_i(y_i - \boldsymbol{x}_i'\widehat{\boldsymbol{\beta}})}{\pi_i} = 0,$$

and hence consistent for $\boldsymbol{\beta}$. When consistent estimates of π_i are available, then, given suitable regularity conditions, consistency for $\boldsymbol{\beta}$ is maintained. There are fairly obvious caveats about these probabilities not becoming too small, and, in particular, not equalling zero.

We can now apply this to a fairly general setting where we have an unbiased estimating equation for some parameter vector $\boldsymbol{\beta}$ and vector of observations (outcome and/or explanatory) $\boldsymbol{z}_i$:

$$\boldsymbol{S}(\boldsymbol{\beta}) = \sum_{i=1}^{n} \boldsymbol{S}_i(\boldsymbol{z}_i, \widehat{\boldsymbol{\beta}}) = \boldsymbol{0}.$$

If $R_i = 1$ is now the event of observing a complete set $\boldsymbol{z}_i$ then the following IPW estimating equation is still unbiased:

$$\sum_{\text{observed}} \frac{\boldsymbol{S}_i(\boldsymbol{z}_i, \widehat{\boldsymbol{\beta}})}{P(R_i = 1)} = 0. \tag{10.2}$$

Again, to use this in practice we would need suitable estimates of the probabilities, using, for example logistic regression. The method is most obviously applicable under MAR, for then there is a direct route to obtaining the estimate of these. We return in Section 10.4 to a practical implementation of this in the context of dropout when a marginal model is to be fitted using generalized estimating equations. First we recall the basic ideas behind conventional generalized estimating equations.

10.3 GENERALIZED ESTIMATING EQUATIONS FOR MARGINAL MODELS

10.3.1 Marginal models for non-normal data

Marginal models describe the measurements within a repeated or multivariate sequence Y_i, conditional on covariates, but not on other measurements, nor on unobserved (latent) structures. While full likelihood approaches exist for such models (Molenberghs and Verbeke 2005), outside the multivariate normal linear model setting they can be very demanding in computational terms, and this explains the popularity of so-called generalized estimating equations (GEE: Liang and Zeger 1986), on which we focus here. In their basic form, these produce consistent estimators and valid inferences under MCAR, but not under MAR. Hence our interest in using IPW in this setting.

In SAS, the GENMOD procedure provides facilities for using GEE, using the basic approach outlined in Section 10.3.2. The GLIMMIX procedure provides an alternative so-called linearization-based approach for this, and this is described in Section 10.3.3. A number of additional extensions of and modifications to GEE exist, as well as alternative non-likelihood-based methods, such as empirically generalized least-squares and pseudo-likelihood methods. They are not considered here, and we refer the interested reader to Molenberghs and Verbeke (2005).

10.3.2 Generalized estimating equations

Generalized estimating equations (Liang and Zeger 1986) are useful when scientific interest focuses on the first moments of the outcome vector. Examples include time evolutions in the response probability, treatment effect, their interaction, and the effect of (baseline) covariates on these probabilities. GEE will allow the researcher to use a 'fix' for the correlations between measurements, present in the second moments, and to ignore the higher-order moments, whilst still obtaining valid inferences, with reasonable efficiency.

The GEE methodology is based on solving the equations

$$S(\boldsymbol{\beta}) = \sum_{i=1}^{N} \frac{\partial \boldsymbol{\mu}_i}{\partial \boldsymbol{\beta}'} (\phi A_i^{1/2} R_i A_i^{1/2})^{-1} (\boldsymbol{y}_i - \boldsymbol{\mu}_i) = \boldsymbol{0}, \tag{10.3}$$

in which the marginal covariance matrix V_i has been decomposed into $\phi A_i^{1/2} R_i A_i^{1/2}$, with A_i the matrix with the marginal variances on the main diagonal and zeros elsewhere, $R_i = R_i(\boldsymbol{\alpha})$ the marginal correlation matrix, often referred to as the *working* correlation matrix, and ϕ an overdispersion parameter.

Usually, the marginal covariance matrix contains a vector $\boldsymbol{\alpha}$ of unknown parameters which is replaced for practical purposes by a consistent estimator.

Assuming that the marginal mean $\boldsymbol{\mu}_i$ has been correctly specified as $h(\boldsymbol{\mu}_i) = X_i\boldsymbol{\beta}$, it can be shown that, under mild regularity conditions, the estimator $\widehat{\boldsymbol{\beta}}$ obtained from solving (10.3) is asymptotically normally distributed with mean $\boldsymbol{\beta}$ and covariance matrix

$$I_0^{-1}I_1I_0^{-1}, \tag{10.4}$$

where

$$I_0 = \left(\sum_{i=1}^{N} \frac{\partial \boldsymbol{\mu}_i'}{\partial \boldsymbol{\beta}} V_i^{-1} \frac{\partial \boldsymbol{\mu}_i}{\partial \boldsymbol{\beta}'} \right),$$

$$I_1 = \left(\sum_{i=1}^{N} \frac{\partial \boldsymbol{\mu}_i'}{\partial \boldsymbol{\beta}} V_i^{-1} \mathrm{var}(\boldsymbol{y}_i) V_i^{-1} \frac{\partial \boldsymbol{\mu}_i}{\partial \boldsymbol{\beta}'} \right).$$

In practice, $\mathrm{var}(\boldsymbol{y}_i)$ in (10.4) is replaced by $(\boldsymbol{y}_i - \boldsymbol{\mu}_i)(\boldsymbol{y}_i - \boldsymbol{\mu}_i)'$, which is unbiased on the sole condition that the mean was correctly specified.

Note that valid inferences can now be obtained for the mean structure, assuming only that the model assumptions with respect to the first-order moments are correct.

Liang and Zeger (1986) proposed moment-based estimates for the working correlation. For this, they first define deviations

$$e_{ij} = \frac{y_{ij} - \mu_{ij}}{\sqrt{v(\mu_{ij})}} \tag{10.5}$$

and then estimate overdispersion and correlation parameters in terms of cross-products and squares of (10.5), respectively. For example, under exchangeable working correlation assumptions, a moment-based estimator for the single α parameter is

$$\widehat{\alpha} = \frac{1}{N} \sum_{i=1}^{N} \frac{1}{n_i(n_i - 1)} \sum_{j \neq k} e_{ij}e_{ik},$$

with the corresponding estimator for the dispersion parameter given by

$$\widehat{\phi} = \frac{1}{N} \sum_{i=1}^{N} \frac{1}{n_i} \sum_{j=1}^{n_i} e_{ij}^2.$$

10.3.3   A method based on linearization

In can be seen that conventional GEE is derived from the score equations of the corresponding likelihood models. In a sense, GEE is obtained from considering only a subvector of the full vector of scores, corresponding to the first moments only (the outcomes themselves). On the other hand, they can also be seen as an extension of quasi-likelihood ideas, in which appropriate modifications are made to the scores to make these sufficiently flexible and to 'work' at the same time.

An alternative approach consists of linearizing the outcome, in the sense of Nelder and Wedderburn (1972), to construct a working variate, to which then weighted least squares is applied. In other words, iteratively reweighted least squares can be used (McCullagh and Nelder 1989). Within each step, the approximation produces all elements typically encountered in a multivariate normal model, and hence corresponding software tools can be used.

We write the outcome vector in a classical (multivariate) generalized linear models fashion:

$$\boldsymbol{y}_i = \boldsymbol{\mu}_i + \boldsymbol{\varepsilon}_i, \tag{10.6}$$

where, as usual, $\boldsymbol{\mu}_i = E(\boldsymbol{y}_i)$ is the systematic component and $\boldsymbol{\varepsilon}_i$ is the random component, typically following from a multinomial distribution. We assume that $\text{var}(\boldsymbol{y}_i) = \text{var}(\boldsymbol{\varepsilon}_i) = \Sigma_i$. The model is further specified by assuming

$$\boldsymbol{\eta}_i = g(\boldsymbol{\mu}_i),$$

$$\boldsymbol{\eta}_i = X_i \boldsymbol{\beta},$$

where $\boldsymbol{\eta}_i$ is the usual set of linear predictors, $g(\cdot)$ is a vector link function, typically made up of logit components, X_i is a design matrix and $\boldsymbol{\beta}$ are the regression parameters.

Estimation proceeds by solving iteratively the equation

$$\sum_{i=1}^{N} X_i' W_i X_i \boldsymbol{\beta} = \sum_{i=1}^{N} W_i \boldsymbol{y}_i^*, \tag{10.7}$$

where a working variate $\boldsymbol{y}_i^*$ has been defined, following from a first-order Taylor series expansion of $\boldsymbol{\eta}_i$ around $\boldsymbol{\mu}_i$:

$$\boldsymbol{y}_i^* = \widehat{\boldsymbol{\eta}}_i + (\boldsymbol{y}_i - \widehat{\boldsymbol{\mu}}_i) \widetilde{F}_i^{-1},$$

$$\widetilde{F}_i = \left. \frac{\partial \boldsymbol{\mu}_i}{\partial \boldsymbol{\eta}_i} \right|_{\beta = \widetilde{\beta}}. \tag{10.8}$$

The weights in (10.7) are specified as

$$W_i = F_i' \widetilde{\Sigma}_i^{-1} F_i. \tag{10.9}$$

In these equations $\widetilde{\beta}$ and $\widetilde{\Sigma}$ are evaluated at the current iteration step. Note that in the specific case of an identity link, $\boldsymbol{\eta}_i = \boldsymbol{\mu}_i$, $F_i = I_{n_i}$, and $\boldsymbol{y}_i = \boldsymbol{y}_i^*$, from which a standard multivariate regression follows.

The linearization-based method can be implemented using the SAS macro GLIMMIX and the SAS procedure GLIMMIX, by ensuring no random effects are included. Empirically corrected standard errors can be obtained by including the 'empirical' option.

10.4 WEIGHTED GENERALIZED ESTIMATING EQUATIONS

We now see how IPW can be incorporated into the conventional GEE set-up. The basic principle follows that described in Section 10.2 but, following the development in Robins *et al.* (1995), we now adapt this to the specific setting of GEE applied to longitudinal measurements with dropout. The basic idea is to use (10.2), where the weight is now obtained from the inverse probability of a subject dropping out at that particular measurement occasion, that is, of providing the actual set of measurements observed:

$$\nu_{ij} = P(D_i = j)$$

$$= \begin{cases} P(D_i = j | D_i \geq j) & j = 2, \\ P(D_i = j | D_i \geq j) \prod_{k=2}^{j-1} [1 - P(D_i = k | D_i \geq k)] & j = 3, \ldots, n_i, \\ \prod_{k=2}^{n_i} [1 - P(D_i = k | D_i \geq k)] & j = n_i + 1. \end{cases}$$

The estimating functions from (10.2), $S_i(z_i, \boldsymbol{\beta})$, then take the specific GEE form, to give

$$S(\boldsymbol{\beta}) = \sum_{i=1}^{N} \frac{1}{\nu_i} \frac{\partial \boldsymbol{\mu}_i}{\partial \boldsymbol{\beta}'} (\phi A_i^{1/2} R_i A_i^{1/2})^{-1} (\boldsymbol{y}_i - \boldsymbol{\mu}_i) = \boldsymbol{0},$$

or

$$S(\boldsymbol{\beta}) = \sum_{i=1}^{N} \sum_{d=2}^{n+1} \frac{I(D_i = d)}{\nu_{id}} \frac{\partial \boldsymbol{\mu}_i(d)}{\partial \boldsymbol{\beta}'} (\phi A_i^{1/2} R_i A_i^{1/2})^{-1} (d) (\boldsymbol{y}_i(d) - \boldsymbol{\mu}_i(d)) = \boldsymbol{0},$$

where $\boldsymbol{y}_i(d)$ and $\boldsymbol{\mu}_i(d)$ are the first $d - 1$ elements of $\boldsymbol{y}_i$ and $\boldsymbol{\mu}_i$ respectively. We define $\frac{\partial \boldsymbol{\mu}_i}{\partial \boldsymbol{\beta}'}(d)$ and $(\phi A_i^{1/2} R_i A_i^{1/2})^{-1}(d)$ analogously, in line with the definition in Robins *et al.* (1995).

10.5 THE DEPRESSION TRIALS

We illustrate the GEE and weighted GEE (WGEE) concepts using the depression trials introduced in Section 2.5, analysed in continuous form in Chapter 6, and in binary form in Section 7.6, using a generalized linear mixed model.

Using the same notation as in Section 7.6, the marginal mean function is specified as

$$\text{logit}[P(Y_{ij} = 1|x_i, T_i, t_j)]$$
$$= \beta_0 + \beta_{14}I(t_j = 4) + \beta_{15}I(t_j = 5)$$
$$+ \beta_{16}I(t_j = 6) + \beta_{17}I(t_j = 7) + \beta_2 x_i + \beta_3 T_i, \qquad (10.10)$$

where x_i is the baseline value, T_i is the treatment indicator, and t_j is the time at which measurement j is taken. Since the follow-up times range from 4 to 8, $t_j = j + 3$ for $j = 1, \ldots, 5$. Finally, $I(\cdot)$ is an indicator function.

Given the incomplete nature of the data, and in the absence of strong reasons for assuming MCAR, it is worthwhile considering the use of IPW. For this we need to construct appropriate weights, based on the probability of dropping out at a given time, given (1) that the patient is still in the study, (2) past response measurements, and (3) covariate values. We restrict attention to just the previous outcome and treatment indicator:

$$\text{logit}[P(D_i = j|D_i \geq j)] = \psi_0 + \psi_1 y_{i,j-1} + \gamma T_i, \qquad (10.11)$$

where $y_{i,j-1}$ clearly is the binary indicator at the previous occasion. The resulting model is of a standard logistic regression or probit regression type, and can be easily fitted using standard logistic regression software, such as the SAS procedures GENMOD and LOGISTIC. The result of fitting this logistic regression did not reveal strong evidence for a dependence on the previous outcome (estimate -0.097, s.e. 0.351), or on the treatment allocation (estimate 0.065, s.e. 0.314).

Results of fitting the standard GEE as well as weighted GEE, combined with the results of the linearization-based method, are presented in Table 10.1. Apart from treatment allocation, the effect of baseline value and indicators for time

Table 10.1 Depression trials. Results of marginal models: parameter estimates (model-based standard errors; empirically corrected standard errors) for standard unweighted and weighted GEE (denoted GEE and WGEE, respectively) and the linearization-based method. Interaction terms are not shown.

Effect	GEE	WGEE	Linearization
Intercept	-1.22 (0.77; 0.79)	-0.56 (0.63; 0.91)	-1.23 (0.75; 0.79)
Treatment	-0.71 (0.38; 0.38)	-0.91 (0.32; 0.41)	-0.67 (0.37; 0.38)
Visit 4	0.43 (1.05; 1.22)	-0.15 (0.85; 1.90)	0.45 (1.05; 1.22)
Visit 5	-0.45 (0.91; 1.23)	-0.23 (0.68; 1.54)	-0.47 (0.92; 1.23)
Visit 6	0.06 (0.86; 1.03)	0.15 (0.69; 1.13)	0.05 (0.86; 1.03)
Visit 7	-0.25 (0.89; 0.91)	-0.27 (0.78; 0.89)	-0.25 (0.89; 0.91)
Baseline	0.08 (0.04; 0.04)	0.06 (0.03; 0.05)	0.08 (0.04; 0.04)

at visits 4, 5, 6, and 7 were included in the model. Further, the interactions between treatment and visit and between baseline and visit were included in the model.

Although GEE and its linearization-based version produce very similar results, in line with earlier observations, there are differences with the weighted version, in parameter estimates as well as standard errors. For all but one parameter, the effect associated with the last visit, WGEE has notably less precision. Although it is to be expected that WGEE will be less efficient than a corresponding likelihood-based analysis, it is not obvious that it will be more or less precise that unweighted GEE. The comparison is complicated by the potential invalidity of the unweighted analysis under MAR. With both estimates and standard errors differing between the methods, the resulting inferences can be different. For example, the treatment effect parameter is non-significant with GEE ($p = 0.0633$ with standard GEE and $p = 0.1184$ with the linearized version), while a significant difference is found under the correct WGEE analysis ($p = 0.0268$). Also, the difference is marked for treatment effect at endpoint: $p = 0.0658$ with standard GEE and $p = 0.0631$ with the linearized version, while a significant difference is found under the correct WGEE analysis ($p = 0.0289$).

Thus, one may fail to detect such important effects as treatment differences when GEE is used rather than the admittedly somewhat more laborious, and typically less precise WGEE.

10.6 THE ANALGESIC TRIAL

We now return to the analgesic trial introduced in Section 2.9 and analysed by means of a generalized linear mixed model in Section 7.7. We will consider both a GEE as well as a WGEE analysis of the binary version of the global satisfaction assessment outcome, based on the marginal logit:

$$\text{logit}[P(Y_{ij} = 1 | t_j, \text{PCA0}_i)] = \beta_0 + \beta_1 t_j + \beta_2 t_j^2 + \beta_3 \text{PCA0}_i,$$

with x_i baseline pain control assessment and t_j the time at which measurement j is taken. A logistic regression is built for the dropout indicator in terms of the previous outcome (for which the ordinal version is used by means of four dummies), pain control assessment at baseline, physical functioning at baseline, and genetic disorder measured at baseline:

$$\text{logit}[P(D_i = j | D_i \geq j, \cdot)]$$
$$= \psi_0 + \psi_{11} I(\text{GSA}_{i,j-1} = 1) + \psi_{12} I(\text{GSA}_{i,j-1} = 2)$$
$$+ \psi_{13} I(\text{GSA}_{i,j-1} = 3) + \psi_{14} I(\text{GSA}_{i,j-1} = 4)$$
$$+ \psi_2 \text{PCA0}_i + \psi_3 \text{PF}_i + \psi_4 \text{GD}_i,$$

where $GSA_{i,j-1}$ is the five-point outcome at the previous time, $I(\cdot)$ an indicator function, $PCA0_i$ pain control assessment at baseline, PF_i physical functioning at baseline, and GD_i genetic disorder at baseline.

All of these effects are significant, with parameter estimates and standard errors given in Table 10.2, implying that there is evidence against MCAR in favour of MAR. This result is in contrast with that obtained in Section 10.5 for the depression trials. Parameter estimates and standard errors for standard GEE and weighted GEE are presented in Table 10.3. Although the evidence against MCAR is strong, the effect of the method chosen is noticeable but not large. As seen with the depression example, WGEE again tends to produce larger standard errors. Correction for the missingness mechanism has the effect of reducing the magnitude of the parameter estimates. In both cases, unstructured working assumptions were used. There is a noticeable effect on the working correlation matrix as well. With GEE, we obtain

$$R_{UN,GEE} = \begin{pmatrix} 1 & 0.173 & 0.246 & 0.201 \\ & 1 & 0.177 & 0.113 \\ & & 1 & 0.456 \\ & & & 1 \end{pmatrix},$$

whereas the WGEE version is

$$R_{UN,GEE} = \begin{pmatrix} 1 & 0.215 & 0.253 & 0.167 \\ & 1 & 0.196 & 0.113 \\ & & 1 & 0.409 \\ & & & 1 \end{pmatrix}.$$

Of course, in line with general warnings issued in Section 10.3.2, care should be taken with interpreting the working correlation structure. In principle, it is a set of nuisance parameters, merely included to obtain reasonably efficient GEE estimates.

Table 10.2 Analgesic trial. Parameter estimates (standard errors) for a logistic regression model to describe dropout.

Effect	Parameter	Estimate (s.e.)
Intercept	ψ_0	$-1.80(0.49)$
Previous GSA=1	ψ_{11}	$-1.02\ (0.41)$
Previous GSA=2	ψ_{12}	$-1.04\ (0.38)$
Previous GSA=3	ψ_{13}	$-1.34\ (0.37)$
Previous GSA=4	ψ_{14}	$-0.26\ (0.38)$
Baseline PCA	ψ_2	$0.25\ (0.10)$
Physical functioning	ψ_3	$0.009\ (0.004)$
Genetic dysfunctioning	ψ_4	$0.59\ (0.24)$

Table 10.3 Analgesic trial. Parameter estimates (empirically corrected standard errors) for standard GEE and weighted GEE (WGEE) fitted to the monotone sequences.

Effect	Parameter	GEE	WGEE
Intercept	β_1	2.95 (0.47)	2.17 (0.69)
Time	β_2	−0.84 (0.33)	−0.44 (0.44)
Time^2	β_3	0.18 (0.07)	0.12 (0.09)
Baseline PCA	β_4	−0.24 (0.10)	−0.16 (0.13)

10.7 DOUBLE ROBUSTNESS

We complete this chapter by considering more recent developments by Robins and colleagues that are designed to improve the efficiency of IPW, and we introduce in a fairly elementary way the idea of double robustness. This section is based on the development in Carpenter *et al.* (2006). Following these authors, we use the simple regression setting for this with three covariates $x_i = \{x_{i1}, x_{i2}, x_{i3}\}$, in which x_{i1} is observed with probability

$$\pi_i = P(R_i = 1 \mid y_i, x_{i2}, x_{i3}).$$

For this set-up we can write the simple weighted estimating equation (10.2) as

$$\sum_{i=1}^{n} \frac{R_i}{\pi_i} x_i (Y_i - x_i' \beta) = 0. \tag{10.12}$$

This includes only those subjects who were fully observed, and this is where the information is lost relative to likelihood-based methods, which include information on partially observed subjects (see, for example, Schafer 1997, p. 25). Now we note that any term with expectation zero can be added to (10.12) without changing its property of unbiasedness, and so the resulting parameter estimators will still be consistent. A plausible proposal is therefore to modify (10.12) to give

$$\sum_{i=1}^{n} \left[\frac{R_i}{\pi_i} x_i (Y_i - x_i' \beta) - \left(\frac{R_i}{\pi_i} - 1 \right) \phi (Y_i, x_{i2}, x_{i3}) \right]. \tag{10.13}$$

Here $\phi(\cdot)$ is some function of the data $(Y_i, x_{2,i}, x_{3,i})$. Thus, through this term, information from subjects who are missing x_{i1} contributes to the estimation. Further, applying a conditional expectation argument to (10.13), we see that the expectation is again zero, because the expectation of $R_i \mid y_i, x_i = \pi_i$, so the expectation of $\{R_i/\pi_i - 1\}$ is 0 and the additional term vanishes from (10.13). Thus the parameter estimators remain consistent.

To use (10.13) in practice, we have to choose the function ϕ. In order to motivate the choice of ϕ, an analogy from the geometry of regression may be helpful. In regression, we calculate the orthogonal projection of the space spanned by the response Y onto that spanned by the covariates X. The residual of this projection, $Y - X(X'X)^{-1}X'Y$ then has no greater variance than Y.

Likewise here, the residual of the orthogonal projection of the function of the data

$$\frac{R_i}{\pi_i}x_i(Y_i - \beta'x_i)$$

onto the space of mean-zero functions

$$\Lambda = \left[\left(\frac{R_i}{\pi_i} - 1\right)\phi(Y_i, x_{i2}, x_{i3}) : \phi \text{ arbitrary}\right]$$

has no greater variance. However, as we saw following (10.13), this projection remains an unbiased estimating equation.

The calculation of this projection follows certain rules, which are described in Robins and Rotnitzky (1995). Roughly speaking, they are derived by formulating the regression problem in Hilbert spaces formed of functions with mean zero, where the inner product is the covariance. The efficiency of estimators is then improved by making them orthogonal to the tangent space for the (possibly infinite-dimensional parameter indexing the) MAR missingness model (i.e., the general non-parametric MAR model for π, which might have, for example, a particular logistic form in our example), denoted by Λ. Applying these rules gives that

$$\phi_{\text{opt}}(Y_i, x_{i2}, x_{i3}) = E[x_i(Y_i - x_i'\beta)|Y_i, x_{i2}, x_{i3}]. \tag{10.14}$$

where the conditional expectations are taken over the true conditional distribution. Of course, in practice, the parameters of this distribution are not known, so will have to be estimated from the data. We return to this point in the discussion below.

Substituting (10.14) into (10.13), more efficient estimates of β are obtained by solving

$$\sum_{i=1}^{n}\left[\frac{R_i}{\pi_i}x_i(Y_i - x_i'\beta) - \left(\frac{R_i}{\pi_i} - 1\right)E\{x_i(Y_i - x_i'\beta)|Y_i, x_{i2}, x_{i3}\}\right] = 0. \tag{10.15}$$

The estimators obtained by solving (10.15) are known as *semi-parametric* estimators, because they do not model the entire distribution. For this reason, they are generally not as efficient as the maximum likelihood estimate obtained using the correct model. However, the efficiency of estimators solving (10.15) can be improved to achieve the minimum variance possible among all consistent asymptotically normal estimators under the given semi-parametric model. This minimum will usually coincide with the semi-parametric variance bound (defined as the supremum of the Cramér–Rao bounds under all parametric models that satisfy the semi-parametric model and contain the truth), although in certain situations it may be greater or ill defined (Newey 1990). The advantage, of course, of semi-parametric estimators is they can remain consistent where maximum likelihood estimators from a misspecified parametric model are inconsistent.

The steps necessary to *improve* the efficiency of (10.15) are most accessibly discussed in Rotnitzky and Robins (1997). Specifically, in our set-up, the term $x_i(Y_i - x_i'\beta)$ in (10.15) is replaced by $d(x_i)(Y_i - x_i'\beta)$. The function $d(x_i)$ is found iteratively. In practice, this procedure is difficult, even in our relatively simple situation. There do not appear to be any published analyses in real settings where this has been used.

The estimators obtained by solving (10.15) are regular and asymptotically linear (rejoinder to Scharfstein *et al.* 1999) so they are asymptotically normally distributed, and their variance can be estimated using a sandwich estimator as follows. Suppose we write the estimating equation for β as $\sum_{i=1}^{n} S_i(\beta) = 0$ (a 4×1 vector, including the constant), and the estimating equation for the logistic regression of the probability of observing x_{i1}, parameterized by α, as $\sum_{i=1}^{n} V_i(\alpha) = 0$ (again a 4×1 vector in the current example, including the constant). Let $w_i(\beta, \alpha) = (S', V')'$. Further, let

$$A = \sum_{i=1}^{n} \begin{pmatrix} \dfrac{\partial}{\partial \beta} S_i & \dfrac{\partial}{\partial \alpha} S_i \\ 0 & \dfrac{\partial}{\partial \alpha} V_i \end{pmatrix}_{\widehat{\beta}, \widehat{\alpha}}.$$

Then the sandwich estimator of the variance of $\widehat{\beta}$ is the upper 4×4 block of

$$A^{-1} \left[\sum_{i=1}^{n} w_i(\widehat{\beta}, \widehat{\alpha}) w_i'(\widehat{\beta}, \widehat{\alpha}) \right] (A^{-1})'.$$

In practice, it is more laborious to estimate the off-diagonal term in A, as we cannot use standard software. Further, as shown by van der Laan and Robins (2003, p. 135, Theorem 2.3) and more intuitively in Section 6.1 of Robins *et al.* (1994), setting them to zero results, under MAR, in overestimation of the variance, and conservative inferences.

Clearly, obtaining fully efficient parameter estimates through IPW is going to be difficult in general. However, in practical situations (10.15) may be efficient enough. Further, as with fully efficient estimators, the solutions to (10.15) have the intriguing additional property of *double robustness*.

Before we describe double robustness, recall that efficient IPW estimators require three models.

1. The substantive model which relates the outcome to explanatory variables/covariates of interest.

2. A model for the probability of observing the data. This is usually a logistic model of some form. If, as in our linear regression example, only a single variable is missing, it is a logistic model: in this case for observing x_{1i}. More generally, it will be built from a series of logistic regressions using a conditional argument as we have used above in Sections 10.4–10.6.
3. A model for the joint distribution of the partially and fully observed data, which is compatible with the substantive model in (1). In our regression set-up, the joint model would be multivariate normal. While, in principle, a correctly specified model for

$$\{x_i (Y_i - x_i'\beta) \,|\, Y_i, x_{2i}, x_{3i}\}$$

is sufficient, without specifying a joint model for the partially and fully observed data, it is usually difficult to choose it to be compatible with model (1).

Now, in common with statistical methods for complete data, if model (1) is wrong, for example because a key confounder is omitted, then estimates of all parameters will typically be inconsistent.

The intriguing property of (10.15) is that if *either* model (2) or model (3) is wrong, but not both, the estimators in model (1) are still consistent. This is because in either case, the expectation of the estimating equation is still zero at $\beta = \beta_{\text{true}}$. In the case where model (3) is wrong, but (2) is correct, this follows from the discussion following (10.15) as ϕ can be arbitrary. In the case where model (2) is wrong, but (3) is correct, this follows because we can change the order of conditional expectations. We first take expectations conditional on $(Y_i, R_i, x_{2i}, x_{3i})$ so, as we assume MAR, terms involving R_i cancel. We then change the order of conditional expectations on what remains, so that the expectation of $Y_i|x_i$ is first. As $\beta = \beta_{\text{true}}$, this means the remaining term is zero. This robustness to two possible sources of error is known as *double robustness* (sometimes *double protection*). If the protection afforded by this is apparent in practice, it is a potentially significant advantage of (10.15) in the analysis of complex data sets.

10.8 CONCLUDING REMARKS

Inverse probability weighting offers the attractive possibility of correcting for MAR missingness without needing to make assumptions about the conditional distribution of the unobserved data given the observed. Instead, only a model for the missingness process is required. In a general sense the price of this advantage is decreased efficiency. In its basic form IPW uses only information from completers, although this can be modified when dealing with dropout from longitudinal studies. IPW also provides a potentially attractive route when direct likelihood and related methods depend on computationally awkward joint models, as, for example, with marginal models for multivariate binary data. Non-likelihood methods of estimation, such as GEE, are not valid under MAR, but IPW can be used to adjust for MAR missingness in such settings. The resulting analyses, as described in Section 10.4 and illustrated in Sections 10.5 and 10.6, are not especially complicated.

In the last ten years the theory of IPW estimators has been greatly developed, in particular to include sensitivity analysis when data are missing and in terms of the interesting concept of double robustness. Comprehensive accounts are provided by van der Laan and Robins (2003) and Tsiatis (2006). At the moment the technically advanced nature of much of the material and the lack of widely available and generally applicable software has meant that the more sophisticated versions of the method are not yet in widespread use. However, developments on both fronts continue and it is very likely that these techniques will move into more mainstream use in the future.

11

Combining GEE and MI

11.1 INTRODUCTION

In Chapter 10 GEE, a special case of inverse probability weighting, was introduced as a useful device for the analysis of incomplete sequences, under the assumption of MAR. In Chapter 9 multiple imputation (MI) was described, and this suggests an alternative approach to handling MAR missingness when using GEE: use MAR-based MI together with a final GEE analysis for the substantive model. This is an example of using an *uncongenial* imputation model (see Section 9.7), and emphasizes the valuable flexibility that this facility brings to MI. We refer to this combination of MI and GEE as 'MI-GEE'. In the previous chapter we looked at inverse probability weighting.

In this chapter, we will compare both approaches, inverse probability weighting and MI-based, through the use of a so-called asymptotic simulation study, where all possible outcome combinations are considered, weighted by the probability associated with them by the data-generating mechanism. The behaviour of both methods in terms of mean squared error (MSE) and bias will be studied, under correctly specified and misspecified models. In this way, robustness of both methods under misspecification of either the dropout model, the imputation model, or the substantive model can be explored.

The data generation, imputation, and substantive models are considered in Section 11.2. In Section 11.3, a distinction is made between GEE on the one hand and a transition model on the other hand, as candidate substantive models for the MI analysis. Section 11.4 is devoted to a simulation study, with the design outlined in Section 11.4.1 and the results discussed in Section 11.4.2.

Missing Data in Clinical Studies   G. Molenberghs and M.G. Kenward
© 2007 John Wiley & Sons, Ltd

11.2   DATA GENERATION AND FITTING

While each of the two methods, WGEE and MI-GEE, depends on a GEE analysis, for which no full measurement model specification is necessary, we need to generate data from a fully specified model for the measurement and dropout mechanisms. In MI-GEE, in addition, an imputation model must be constructed. Molenberghs and Verbeke (2005) distinguish between three model families: marginal models, conditional models, and random-effects models. GEE (Chapter 10) is typically associated with first family, and the generalized linear mixed model (Section 7.5) belongs to the third. For data-generating purposes we will use the marginally based Bahadur model and a conditionally oriented transition model. Each of these will be described in turn.

11.2.1   The Bahadur model

Bahadur (1961) proposed a marginal model for binary outcomes, accounting for the association via marginal correlations. Define the marginal probability $\pi_{ij} = E(Y_{ij}) = P(Y_{ij} = 1)$, and define standardized deviations

$$\varepsilon_{ij} = \frac{Y_{ij} - \pi_{ij}}{\sqrt{\pi_{ij}(1 - \pi_{ij})}} \text{ and } e_{ij} = \frac{y_{ij} - \pi_{ij}}{\sqrt{\pi_{ij}(1 - \pi_{ij})}}, \qquad (11.1)$$

where y_{ij} is an actual value of the binary response variable Y_{ij}. Further, let $\rho_{ij_1j_2} = E(\varepsilon_{ij_1}\varepsilon_{ij_2}), \rho_{ij_1j_2j_3} = E(\varepsilon_{ij_1}\varepsilon_{ij_2}\varepsilon_{ij_3}), \ldots, \rho_{i12\ldots n_i} = E(\varepsilon_{i1}\varepsilon_{i2}\ldots\varepsilon_{in_i})$; then the general Bahadur model can be represented by the expression

$$f(\boldsymbol{y}_i) = f_1(\boldsymbol{y}_i)c(\boldsymbol{y}_i), \qquad (11.2)$$

where

$$f_1(\boldsymbol{y}_i) = \prod_{j=1}^{n_i} \pi_{ij}^{y_{ij}}(1 - \pi_{ij})^{1-y_{ij}}$$

and

$$c(\boldsymbol{y}_i) = 1 + \sum_{j_1 < j_2} \rho_{ij_1j_2}e_{ij_1}e_{ij_2} + \sum_{j_1 < j_2 < j_3} \rho_{ij_1j_2j_3}e_{ij_1}e_{ij_2}e_{ij_3}$$
$$+ \ldots + \rho_{i12\ldots n_i}e_{i1}e_{i2}\ldots e_{in_i}.$$

Thus, the probability mass function is the product of the independence model $f_1(\boldsymbol{y}_i)$ and the correction factor $c(\boldsymbol{y}_i)$. One possible viewpoint is to consider the factor $c(\boldsymbol{y}_i)$ as a model for overdispersion. Molenberghs and Verbeke (2005) provide an overview of marginal models.

11.2.2   A transition model

In a conditional model the parameters describe a feature (e.g., probability, odds, logit) of (a set of) outcomes, given values for the other outcomes (Cox 1972). The best-known example is undoubtedly the log-linear model.

In a transition model, a measurement Y_{ij} in a longitudinal sequence is described as a function of previous outcomes, or history, $\boldsymbol{h}_{ij} = (Y_{i1}, \ldots, Y_{i,j-1})$. One can write a regression model for the outcome Y_{ij} in terms of $\boldsymbol{h}_{ij}$, or alternatively the error term ε_{ij} can be written in terms of previous error terms. The order of a transition model is the number of previous measurements that is still considered to influence the current one. A model is called stationary if the functional form of the dependence is the same regardless of the actual time at which it occurs.

A particular version of a transition model is a stationary first-order autoregressive model for binary longitudinal outcomes, which is the following logistic regression type model:

$$\text{logit}[P(Y_{ij} = 1 | \boldsymbol{x}_{ij}, Y_{i,j-1} = y_{i,j-1}, \boldsymbol{\beta}, \alpha)] = \boldsymbol{x}'_{ij}\boldsymbol{\beta} + \alpha y_{i,j-1}. \qquad (11.3)$$

Extension to the second or higher orders is obvious.

11.3   MI-GEE AND MI-TRANSITION

Multiple imputation was formally introduced in Chapter 9. We now use the transition model above as the imputation model for the MI analysis. The number of imputations will be set equal to $M = 5$. We consider two possible substantive models: (1) a marginal model fitted using GEE and (2) a transition model fitted using maximum likelihood.

In WGEE all subjects are given weights, calculated using the hypothesized dropout model, so any misspecification of this dropout model will affect all subjects, and thus the final results. On the other hand, when considering MI together with GEE or a transition model (in what follows, we refer to these as MI-GEE and MI-transition, respectively), a misspecification made in the imputation step will only affect the unobserved (i.e., imputed) but not the observed part of the data. Meng's (1994) results show that, as long as such an uncongenial imputation model is not grossly misspecified, this approach will perform well. The relative impact of misspecification on the various methods will be studied next, by way of an asymptotic simulation study.

11.4   AN ASYMPTOTIC SIMULATION STUDY

In this section, we will quantify the bias induced by misspecification in WGEE, MI-GEE, and MI-transition, for a variety of settings. Given that the outcomes and the missing data process take a discrete form, quantification of this bias under specific assumptions about the non-response process can be done via a method first proposed by Rotnitzky and Wypij (1994). In this, a data set is constructed that contains all possible outcomes, weighted by their probability of occurrence under the true model. This implies the sum of the weights equals one. A model is then fitted to this artificial set of data with appropriate probability weighting. The resulting inferences are asymptotic and it is then straightforward to derive, for example, the asymptotic bias of the estimators.

11.4.1 Design

In the asymptotic simulation study, we distinguish between two stages: (1) the data-generating stage and (2) the analysis stage. At the first stage, a data-generating model is defined. Under the selection model framework, this generating model consists of a measurement model on the one hand, and a dropout model, given the measurement model, on the other hand. For the simulation study, a binary outcome at three time points was first simulated using either of two measurement models: a Bahadur model or a second-order autoregressive (AR(2)) transition model. Then, for the dropout model, an MAR mechanism was considered. This results in two data-generating models, which will be called respectively GM I (Bahadur measurement model and MAR dropout model) and GM II (AR(2) measurement model and MAR dropout model).

In addition, the measurement model incorporates a dichotomous covariate, such as a treatment *versus* placebo classification. Then, assuming that dropout can only occur after the first time point, there are three possible dropout patterns: (1) dropout at the second time point, (2) dropout at the third time point, or (3) no dropout. From this set-up, a total of 48 possible observed outcome sequences arise, because for each of the two covariate levels there are $2^3 = 8$ possible outcome vectors, each having three dropout possibilities.

The second step consists of the analysis. For the WGEE approach, this stage requires the specification of a marginal measurement model and a dropout model. For MI-transition, a conditional mean model is needed instead. For the MI-GEE and MI-transition approaches, the dropout process is accommodated in the imputation model.

In specifying the dropout model for WGEE, or imputation model for MI-GEE and MI-transition, both an MAR and an MCAR process have been considered. More specifically, for WGEE and MAR dropout, predictors include the two-level covariate and the previous outcome, while for the MCAR case, only the two-level covariate was used as predictor. On the other hand, for the multiple imputation approaches and for an MAR imputation model, missing values at the second time point are imputed using a logistic regression with measurements at the first time point, as well as the two-level covariate. Similarly, imputations for missing values at the third time point use the measurements at the second time point, both observed and imputed, as predictors, as well as the measurement at the first time point (always observed) and the dichotomous covariate. In contrast, an MCAR imputation model, using only the two-level covariate in the logistic regressions, is considered.

To assess the relative performance of the three approaches, various scenarios are considered. The methods are compared with respect to the effects of misspecification in the dropout mechanism and/or the measurement model. For instance, in modelling the missingness process, the use of an MAR dropout model for WGEE, or an MAR imputation model for MI-GEE and MI-transition, will be consistent with the dropout part of the data-generating model from the first stage. On the other hand, using the MCAR assumption instead yields a misspecification of the dropout model compared to the MAR mechanism assumed for the data-generating model. Further, misspecification of the measurement model will also be considered by either over- or underspecifying the mean structure.

11.4.2 Results

We define the data-generating mechanisms for GM I and GM II in turn. Denote by t_j the time point at which measurement j is taken and by x_i the two-level factorial covariate. GM I is based on a Bahadur model, which follows general formulation ((11.2)) with

$$\pi_{ij} = P(Y_{ij} = 1|x_i, t_j) = \beta_0 + \beta_x\ x_i + \beta_t\ t_j + \beta_{xt}\ x_i\ t_j,$$

where we choose $\beta_0 = -0.25$, $\beta_x = 0.5$, $\beta_t = 0.2$, and $\beta_{xt} = -0.8$, and with two- and three-way correlation coefficients equal to $\rho_{ij_1j_2} = 0.2$ and $\rho_{ij_1j_2j_3} = 0$, respectively. In GM I, the missingness process is assumed to be MAR, and the probability of dropout at time point t_j given x_i and given the measurement at the previous time point t_{j-1} is modelled by a logistic regression

$$\text{logit}[P(D_i = t_j|x_i, y_{i,j-1})] = \psi_0 + \psi_x\ x_i + \psi_{\text{prev}}\ y_{i,j-1},$$

with $\psi_0 = -0.5$, $\psi_x = 0.3$, and $\psi_{\text{prev}} = 0.8$.

The same dropout model is used for the missingness process in GM II, but now combined with the AR(2) transition model:

$$P(x_i) = \mu_x,$$
$$\text{logit}[P(Y_{i1} = 1|x_i)] = \alpha_0 + \alpha_x\ x_i,$$
$$\text{logit}[P(Y_{i2} = 1|x_i, y_{i1})] = \phi_0 + \phi_x\ x_i + \phi_1 y_{i1},$$
$$\text{logit}[P(Y_{i3} = 1|x_i, y_{i1}, y_{i2})] = \gamma_0 + \gamma_x\ x_i + \gamma_1\ y_{i1} + \gamma_2\ y_{i2}.$$

where $\mu_x = 0.5$, $\alpha_0 = -0.2$, $\alpha_x = 0.3$, $\phi_0 = -0.1$, $\phi_x = 0.5$, $\phi_1 = 0.7$, $\gamma_0 = -0.25$, $\gamma_x = 0.35$, $\gamma_1 = 0.4$, and $\gamma_2 = 0.6$.

To compute the bias of the estimates resulting from MI-GEE and WGEE, we need to marginalize the above conditional model to obtain marginalized parameters, which then approximately describe a marginal logistic function. These parameters are $\beta_0 = -0.3658$, $\beta_x = 0.2673$, $\beta_t = 0.2265$, and $\beta_{xt} = 0.079$.

We first investigate the relative performance of WGEE and MI-GEE for both GM I and the marginalized version of GM II when the analysis model is correctly specified, that is, both the measurement model and the dropout model are correctly specified. Note that we use the SAS procedure MI to impute the missing values for MI-GEE, which employs a conditional logistic imputation model for binary outcomes. Since we consider here the analyses on GM I and the marginalized version of GM II, the imputation model in MI-GEE will not exactly match the generation models. The results are summarized in Table 11.1. Observe that WGEE yields asymptotically unbiased parameter estimates for GM I, as is expected since GEE methods are moment-based versions of the Bahadur model (Section 11.2.1). However, this is not the case for GM II. In contrast, MI-GEE leads to asymptotically biased results under both data-generating models. This can again be attributed to the fact that the imputation model used for MI-GEE is of a conditional form, as opposed to the marginal nature of the models used in data generation. In addition, the relative bias for MI-GEE under GM II is larger than that for WGEE for the two-level covariate and for its interaction with time. With respect to the asymptotic MSE, WGEE gives similar values for both generating models and these are much smaller than those obtained using MI-GEE.

Table 11.1   Parameter estimates, standard errors (s.e.), relative bias, and mean squared error (MSE) for WGEE and MI-GEE for the correctly specified analysis models, under both data-generation models (GM I, based on Bahadur model, and GM II, based on AR(2) model).

		WGEE				MI-GEE			
	Parameter	Estimate	s.e.	Relative bias	MSE	Estimate	s.e.	Relative bias	MSE
GM I	β_0	−0.25	(2.84)	0.00	8.07	−0.20	(4.38)	−0.19	19.18
	β_x	0.50	(4.18)	0.00	17.50	−0.17	(6.42)	−1.33	41.67
	β_t	0.20	(1.56)	0.00	2.44	0.10	(2.07)	−0.50	4.28
	β_{xt}	−0.80	(2.40)	0.00	5.75	−0.13	(3.15)	−0.84	10.38
GM II	β_0	−0.43	(2.85)	0.17	8.11	−0.42	(4.39)	0.15	19.32
	β_x	0.21	(4.07)	−0.20	16.57	−0.44	(6.34)	0.65	40.23
	β_t	0.26	(1.56)	0.16	2.45	0.19	(2.07)	−0.14	4.28
	β_{xt}	0.11	(2.27)	0.43	5.14	−0.19	(3.09)	−3.35	9.60

Table 11.2 Parameter estimates, standard errors (s.e.), relative bias, and mean squared error (MSE) for WGEE and MI-GEE for analysis models with misspecified mean structure, under both data-generation models (GM I, based on Bahadur model, and GM II, based on AR(2) model).

		WGEE				MI-GEE			
Parameter		Estimate	s.e.	Relative bias	MSE	Estimate	s.e.	Relative bias	MSE
GM I	β_0	0.34	(2.23)	−2.37	5.30	−0.12	(3.43)	−0.53	11.79
	β_x	−0.80	(1.69)	−2.60	4.54	−0.39	(2.50)	−1.77	7.02
	β_t	−0.16	(1.14)	−1.78	1.42	0.06	(1.48)	−0.72	2.20
	β_{xt}	0.00	(—)	−1.00	0.64	0.00	(—)	−1.00	0.64
GM II	β_0	−0.52	(2.21)	0.41	4.89	−0.24	(3.39)	−0.35	11.50
	β_x	0.40	(1.66)	0.49	2.78	0.08	(2.45)	−0.71	6.03
	β_t	0.32	(1.13)	0.40	1.29	0.10	(1.45)	−0.55	2.12
	β_{xt}	0.00	(—)	−1.00	0.01	0.00	(—)	−1.00	0.01

Misspecification of the mean structure of the measurement model results in biased parameter estimates for all cases (Table 11.2). Under GM I, although the relative biases are larger for WGEE than for MI-GEE, the MSEs are still smaller for WGEE. On the other hand, for GM II, WGEE still results in smaller MSEs, with the relative biases smaller under WGEE for some parameter estimates (β_x and β_{xt}) but larger for others.

When the dropout or imputation model is misspecified, parameter estimates are again asymptotically biased for all cases considered (see Table 11.3). Fortunately, for WGEE, these biases are relatively small for the two-level

Table 11.3 Parameter estimates, standard errors (s.e.), relative bias, and mean squared error (MSE) for WGEE and MI-GEE with misspecified dropout model, under both data-generation models (GM I, based on Bahadur model, and GM II, based on AR(2) model).

		WGEE				MI-GEE			
Parameter		Estimate	s.e.	Relative bias	MSE	Estimate	s.e.	Relative bias	MSE
GM I	β_0	−0.12	(2.09)	−0.54	4.38	−0.31	(4.36)	0.24	19.02
	β_x	0.50	(3.07)	−0.00	9.45	0.06	(6.26)	−0.88	39.36
	β_t	0.12	(1.25)	−0.41	1.56	0.21	(2.05)	0.07	4.19
	β_{xt}	−0.82	(1.95)	−0.02	3.79	−0.29	(2.94)	−0.64	8.87
GM II	β_0	−0.34	(2.10)	−0.07	4.41	−0.49	(4.38)	0.34	19.16
	β_x	0.15	(2.95)	−0.45	8.72	0.69	(6.25)	1.58	39.18
	β_t	0.22	(1.26)	−0.05	1.58	0.28	(2.05)	0.26	4.22
	β_{xt}	0.13	(1.81)	0.67	3.30	−0.23	(2.93)	−3.91	8.66

Table 11.4 Parameter estimates, standard errors (s.e.), relative bias, and mean squared error (MSE) for MI-transition for both correct specification and misspecification in the dropout model, under the AR(2) data-generation model GM II.

Parameter	Correctly specified				Misspecified dropout			
	Estimate	s.e.	Relative bias	MSE	Estimate	s.e.	Relative bias	MSE
α_0	−0.20	(8.08)	0.00	65.29	−0.20	(8.08)	0.00	65.29
α_x	0.30	(16.10)	0.00	259.22	0.30	(16.10)	0.00	259.22
ϕ_0	−0.19	(3.49)	0.89	12.20	−0.21	(3.56)	1.14	12.68
ϕ_x	−0.04	(4.21)	−1.08	17.98	0.61	(4.51)	0.22	20.38
ϕ_1	0.24	(4.18)	−0.65	17.71	0.69	(4.63)	−0.02	21.42
γ_0	0.67	(4.43)	−3.68	20.47	0.06	(4.05)	−1.24	16.50
γ_x	0.04	(5.39)	−0.89	29.11	−0.29	(4.50)	−1.83	20.65
γ_1	−0.29	(4.84)	−1.49	24.22	0.54	(4.74)	−0.11	22.43
γ_2	−0.76	(4.99)	−2.90	26.30	0.09	(4.53)	−0.77	20.57

covariate (β_x) and for its interaction with time (β_{xt}) for GM I, and for the intercept (β_0) and time (β_t) for GM II. For GM I, the relative biases under MI-GEE are smaller than those under WGEE for the intercept and time. Under GM II, the magnitudes of the relative bias are always smaller for WGEE than for MI-GEE. In terms of MSEs, MI-GEE leads to much larger values, with magnitudes about 2 to 4 times those of WGEE.

The results for the MI-transition approach under GM II for a correctly specified case and for the case of misspecified dropout are shown in Table 11.4. The first panel shows asymptotically unbiased parameter estimates since, for this outcome, Y_{i1}, data for all subjects are assumed available and are thus not imputed. In the second panel, it can be noted that whether or not the model is correctly specified, the parameter estimates are asymptotically biased. Noticeable are the smaller relative biases for all parameters (e.g., ϕ_x and ϕ_1) except the intercept (ϕ_0) when the dropout process is misspecified. The MSEs under correctly and incorrectly specified dropout are similar, with the latter slightly larger. For the last panel, for the outcome (Y_{i3}), relative biases are again smaller when dropout is misspecified for the parameters γ_1 and γ_2. Moreover, under a misspecified dropout model, the resulting MSEs are smaller than those in the correctly specified case.

11.5 CONCLUDING REMARKS

When the analysis of incomplete non-Gaussian (e.g., binary) longitudinal data is considered, several routes are available. Apart from likelihood-based methods, such as the generalized linear mixed-effects model (Section 7.5), non-likelihood methods are attractive, especially when a marginal analysis is required. Because standard generalized estimating equations (Section 10.3.2) are unbiased only under MCAR, a variety of modifications and alternatives to GEE have been proposed. An important route is through weighted estimating equations, as proposed by Robins *et al.* (1995) and discussed in Section 10.4. A combination of GEE and multiple imputation methods (MI-GEE) provides an alternative route. Once multiple imputation is considered an option, it has the merit of allowing for a variety of combinations of imputation and substantive models.

In any particular setting the choice of a particular analysis route will depend on a range of considerations. For example, we have not had to address the general inefficiency of unadjusted weighted estimating equations (see Section 10.7) in this chapter because empirical studies such as that given here suggest strongly that this is much less of a concern with missing *binary* outcomes. The substantive setting will often determine which substantive model is required, a common example being a final time point marginal treatment comparison. It is important that the route chosen is appropriate for the substantive model required, as apposed to choosing a (possibly inappropriate) substantive model because it is more convenient in the missing data setting. The two approaches explored here provide useful routes for this when a likelihood-based analysis is impractical for the required substantive model. We have provided quantitative evidence, based on asymptotic simulations, that should help in the decision-making process. We have considered WGEE, MI-GEE, and MI-transition. In the range of binary settings considered we have seen that often, but not always, the MSE is smallest for WGEE. Still, in such cases, the bias in the multiple imputation methods is sufficiently small to allow for its use, should other circumstances favour this route of analysis.

Obviously, a simulation study is unable to cover all possible alternatives. Nevertheless, they are sufficiently straightforward to conduct so as to allow interested users to run them for themselves. Example code to do so is available from the website associated with this book.

12

Likelihood-Based Frequentist Inference

12.1 INTRODUCTION

The fundamental ignorability result of Rubin (1976), presented in Section 3.5 above, is the main rationale for suggesting direct likelihood as the standard paradigm for analysing incomplete data in clinical studies, because of its broad validity combined with its ease of application. This is true under the conditions that all data, whether from completely or incompletely observed study subjects, are included for analysis and that the joint parameter space of the measurement and missingness model parameters is the Cartesian product of the two component spaces. The latter requirement is the so-called separability or parameter distinctness condition.

Following the original work of Rubin and Little, a general view has evolved that 'likelihood methods' that ignore the missing value mechanism are valid under an MAR process, where likelihood is interpreted in a frequentist sense. The availability of flexible standard software allowing for the analysis of incomplete data, such as the procedures MIXED, GLIMMIX, and NLMIXED in SAS, contributes to this point of view. This statement needs careful qualification, however. Kenward and Molenberghs (1998) provided an exposition of the precise sense in which frequentist methods of inference are justified under MAR processes.

In a strict sense, direct likelihood inference is defined as an 'inference that results solely from ratios of the likelihood function for various values of the parameter', in agreement with the definition in Edwards (1972). In the concluding section of his 1976 paper, Rubin remarks:

Missing Data in Clinical Studies   G. Molenberghs and M.G. Kenward
© 2007 John Wiley & Sons, Ltd

One might argue, however, that this apparent simplicity of likelihood and Bayesian inference really buries the important issues. . . . likelihood inferences are at times surrounded with references to the sampling distributions of likelihood statistics. Thus, practically, when there is the possibility of missing data, some interpretations of Bayesian and likelihood inference face the same restrictions as sampling distribution inference. The inescapable conclusion seems to be that when dealing with real data, the practicing statistician should explicitly consider the process that causes missing data far more often than he does.

In essence, the problem from a frequentist point of view is that of identifying and using the appropriate sampling distribution. This is obviously relevant for determining distributions of test statistics, expected values of the information matrix, and measures of precision. Little and Rubin (1987) discuss several aspects of this problem and propose, using the observed information matrix, to circumvent problems associated with the determination of the correct expected information matrix. Laird (1988) makes a similar point in the context of incomplete longitudinal data analysis.

In a variety of settings, several authors have re-expressed this preference for the observed information matrix and derived methods to compute it: Meng and Rubin (1991), the supplemented EM algorithm; Baker (1992), composite link models; Fitzmaurice *et al.* (1994), incomplete longitudinal binary data; and Jennrich and Schluchter (1986). A group of authors has used the observed information matrix without reference to the problems associated with the expected information: Louis (1982), Meilijson (1989), and Kenward *et al.* (1994). Others, while claiming validity of analysis under MAR mechanisms, have used expected information matrices and other measures of precision that do not account for the missingness mechanism (Murray and Findlay 1988; Patel 1991). Several references are given in Baker (1992). It is clear that the problem as identified in the initial work of Rubin (1976) is not fully appreciated in the more recent literature. An exception to this is Heitjan's (1994) clear restatement of the problem.

This issue is obviously of relevance for practice. Apart from valid point estimates, the researcher should be able to rely on standard errors, confidence intervals, test statistics, and their associated *p*-values. Therefore, based on Kenward and Molenberghs (1998), this problem will be explored and guidelines for practice given, including how standard statistical software ideally ought to be used.

The general relationship between observed and expected information in a likelihood context on the one hand and sampling distributions on the other hand is explored in Section 12.2, with specific focus on bivariate normal and bivariate binary data in Sections 12.3 and 12.4. The impact of these results on the use of standard statistical software is studied in Section 12.5. Apart from the insight derived from formal investigation and simulations, we present analysis of three sets of data. The fluvoxamine data, first introduced in Section 2.6, are analysed in Section 12.6. The Muscatine coronary heart study data form the subject of Section 12.7 and Crépeau's data (Crépeau *et al.* 1985) are analysed in Section 12.8.

12.2 INFORMATION AND SAMPLING DISTRIBUTIONS

In this section, we will drop the subject subscript i from the notation. We assume that the joint distribution of the full data (Y, R) is regular in the sense of Cox and Hinkley (1974, p. 281). We are concerned here with the sampling distributions of certain statistics under MCAR and MAR mechanisms. Under an MAR process, the joint distribution of Y^o (the observed components) and R factorizes as in (3.16). In terms of the log-likelihood function, we have

$$\ell(\boldsymbol{\theta}, \boldsymbol{\psi}; \boldsymbol{y}^o, \boldsymbol{r}) = \ell_1(\boldsymbol{\theta}; \boldsymbol{y}^o) + \ell_2(\boldsymbol{\psi}; \boldsymbol{r}, \boldsymbol{y}^o). \tag{12.1}$$

It is assumed that $\boldsymbol{\theta}$ and $\boldsymbol{\psi}$ satisfy the separability condition. This partition of the likelihood has, with important exceptions, been taken to mean that, under an MAR mechanism, likelihood methods based on ℓ_1 alone are valid for inferences about $\boldsymbol{\theta}$ *even when interpreted in the broad frequentist sense*. We now consider more precisely the sense in which the different elements of the frequentist likelihood methodology can be regarded as valid in general under the MAR mechanism. It is now well known that such inferences are valid under an MCAR mechanism (Rubin 1976, Section 6).

First, we note that under the MAR mechanism, $\boldsymbol{r}$ is *not* an ancillary statistic for $\boldsymbol{\theta}$ in the extended sense of Cox and Hinkley (1974, p. 35), where a statistic $S(Y, R)$ is termed ancillary for $\boldsymbol{\theta}$ if its distribution does not depend upon $\boldsymbol{\theta}$. Hence, we are not justified in restricting the sample space from that associated with the pair (Y, R). In considering the properties of frequentist procedures below, we therefore define the appropriate sampling distribution to be that determined by this pair. We call this the *unconditional* sampling framework. By working within this framework, we do need to consider the missing value mechanism. We shall be comparing this with the sampling distribution that would apply if $\boldsymbol{r}$ were fixed by design – that is, if we repeatedly sampled using the distribution $f(\boldsymbol{y}^o; \boldsymbol{\theta})$. If this sampling distribution were appropriate, this would lead directly to the use of ℓ_1 as the sole basis for inference. We call this the *naive* sampling framework.

Little (1976), in a comment on the paper by Rubin (1976), mentions explicitly the role played by the non-response pattern. He argues:

> For sampling based inferences, a first crucial question concerns when it is justified to condition on the observed pattern, that is on the event $R = r$. . . . A natural condition is that R should be ancillary. . . . Otherwise the pattern on its own carries at least some information about $\boldsymbol{\theta}$, which should in principle be used.

Certain elements of the frequentist methodology can be justified immediately from (12.1). The maximum likelihood estimator obtained from maximizing $l_1(\boldsymbol{\theta}; \boldsymbol{y}^o)$ alone is identical to that obtained from maximizing the complete log-likelihood function. Similarly, the maximum likelihood estimator of $\boldsymbol{\psi}$ is functionally independent of $\boldsymbol{\theta}$ and so any maximum likelihood ratio concerning $\boldsymbol{\theta}$, with common $\boldsymbol{\psi}$, will involve ℓ_1 only. Because these statistics are identical whether derived from ℓ_1 or the complete log-likelihood, it follows that they have the required properties under the naive sampling framework. See, for example, Rubin (1976), Little (1976), and Little and Rubin (1987, Section 5.2).

An important element of likelihood-based frequentist inference is the derivation of measures of precision of the maximum likelihood estimators from the information. For this, either the observed information, i_O, can be used, where

$$i_O(\theta_j, \theta_k) = -\frac{\partial^2 \ell(\cdot)}{\partial \theta_j \partial \theta_k}$$

or the expected information, i_E, where

$$i_E(\theta_j, \theta_k) = E[i_O(\theta_j, \theta_k)]. \tag{12.2}$$

The above argument, justifying the use of the maximum likelihood estimators from $\ell_1(\boldsymbol{\theta}; \boldsymbol{y}^o)$, applies equally well to the use of the inverse of the *observed* information derived from ℓ_1 as an estimate of the asymptotic variance–covariance matrix of these estimators. This has been pointed out by Little and Rubin (1987, Section 8.2.2) and Laird (1988, p. 307). In addition, there are other reasons for preferring the observed information matrix (Efron and Hinkley 1978).

The use of the expected information matrix is more problematical. The expectation in (12.2) needs to be taken over the *unconditional* sampling distribution (the *unconditional information* i_U) and, consequently, the use of the naive sampling framework (producing the *naive information* i_N) can lead to inconsistent estimates of precision. In the next section, we give an example of the bias resulting from the use of the naive framework. It is possible, however, as we show below, to calculate the unconditional information by taking expectations over the appropriate distribution and so correct this bias. Although this added complication is generally unnecessary in practice, given the availability of the observed information, it does allow a direct examination of the effect of ignoring the missing value mechanism on the expected information.

As part of the process of frequentist inference, we also need to consider the sampling distribution of the test statistics. Provided that use is made of the likelihood ratio, or Wald and score statistics based on the observed information, then reference to a null asymptotic χ^2 distribution will be appropriate because this is derived from the *implicit* use of the unconditional sampling framework.

Only in those situations in which the sampling distribution is explicitly constructed must care be taken to ensure that the unconditional framework is used; that is, account must be taken of the missing data mechanism.

12.3 BIVARIATE NORMAL DATA

For an incomplete multivariate normal sample, Little and Rubin (1987) state:

> If the data are MCAR, the expected information matrix of $\theta = (\mu, \Sigma)$ represented as a vector is block diagonal. . . . The observed information matrix, which is calculated and inverted at each iteration of the Newton–Raphson algorithm, is not block diagonal with respect to μ and Σ, so this simplification does not occur if standard errors are based on this matrix. On the other hand, the standard errors based on the observed information matrix are more conditional and thus valid when the data are MAR but not MCAR, and hence should be preferable to those based on [the expected information] in applications.

Suppose now that we have N independent pairs of observations (Y_{i1}, Y_{i2}), each with a bivariate Gaussian distribution with mean vector $\mu = (\mu_1, \mu_2)'$ and variance–covariance matrix

$$\Sigma = \begin{pmatrix} \sigma_{11} & \sigma_{12} \\ \sigma_{12} & \sigma_{22} \end{pmatrix},$$

exactly as in Section 4.4.1. It is assumed that d complete pairs and only the first member (Y_{i1}) of the remaining pairs are observed. This implies that the dropout process can be represented by a scalar indicator R_i which is 1 if the second component is observed and 0 otherwise. The log-likelihood can be expressed as the sum of the log-likelihoods for the complete and incomplete pairs:

$$\ell = \sum_{i=1}^{d} \ln f(y_{i1}, y_{i2} \mid \mu_1, \mu_2, \sigma_{11}, \sigma_{12}, \sigma_{22}) + \sum_{i=d+1}^{N} \ln f(y_{i1} \mid \mu_1, \sigma_{11}),$$

which, in the Gaussian setting, has kernel

$$\ell = -\frac{N-d}{2} \ln \sigma_{11} - \frac{d}{2} \ln |\Sigma| - \frac{1}{2\sigma_{11}} \sum_{i=d+1}^{N} (y_{i1} - \mu_1)^2$$

$$- \frac{1}{2} \sum_{i=1}^{d} \begin{pmatrix} y_{i1} - \mu_1 \\ y_{i2} - \mu_2 \end{pmatrix}' \begin{pmatrix} \sigma_{11} & \sigma_{12} \\ \sigma_{12} & \sigma_{22} \end{pmatrix}^{-1} \begin{pmatrix} y_{i1} - \mu_1 \\ y_{i2} - \mu_2 \end{pmatrix}.$$

Straightforward differentiation produces the elements of the observed information matrix that relate to $\boldsymbol{\mu}$:

$$i_O(\boldsymbol{\mu}, \boldsymbol{\mu}) = (N-d) \begin{pmatrix} \sigma_{11}^{-1} & 0 \\ 0 & 0 \end{pmatrix} + d\Sigma^{-1},$$

and

$$i_O(\mu_1, \sigma_{11}) = \sum_{i=d+1}^{N} \frac{y_{i1} - \mu_1}{\sigma_{11}^2}$$

$$+ \sum_{i=1}^{d} \boldsymbol{e}_1' \Sigma^{-1} E_{11} \Sigma^{-1} \begin{pmatrix} y_{i1} - \mu_1 \\ y_{i2} - \mu_2 \end{pmatrix} \tag{12.3}$$

and, when at least one of the indices j, k, or ℓ is different from 1,

$$i_O(\mu_j, \sigma_{k\ell}) = \sum_{i=1}^{d} \boldsymbol{e}_j' \Sigma^{-1} E_{kl} \Sigma^{-1} \begin{pmatrix} y_{i1} - \mu_1 \\ y_{i2} - \mu_2 \end{pmatrix} \tag{12.4}$$

for

$$\boldsymbol{e}_1 = \begin{pmatrix} 1 \\ 0 \end{pmatrix}, \ \boldsymbol{e}_2 = \begin{pmatrix} 0 \\ 1 \end{pmatrix}$$

and

$$E_{11} = \begin{pmatrix} 1 & 0 \\ 0 & 0 \end{pmatrix}, \ E_{12} = \begin{pmatrix} 0 & 1 \\ 1 & 0 \end{pmatrix}, \ E_{22} = \begin{pmatrix} 0 & 0 \\ 0 & 1 \end{pmatrix}.$$

For the naive information, we just take expectations of these quantities over $(Y_{i1}, Y_{i2})' \sim N(\boldsymbol{\mu}, \Sigma)$ for $i = 1, \ldots, d$, and $Y_{i1} \sim N(\mu_1, \sigma_{11})$ for $i = d+1, \ldots, N$. It follows at once that the cross-terms linking the mean and variance–covariance parameters vanish, establishing the familiar orthogonality property of these sets of parameters in the Gaussian setting. We now examine the behaviour of the expected information under the actual sampling process implied by the MAR mechanism.

We need to consider first the conditional expectation of these quantities given the occurrence of R, the dropout pattern. Because $(\boldsymbol{Y}, R)$ enters the expression for $i_U(\boldsymbol{\mu}, \boldsymbol{\mu})$ only through m, the naive and unconditional information matrices for $\boldsymbol{\mu}$ are effectively equivalent. However, Kenward and Molenberghs (1998) showed that this is not true for the cross-term elements of the information matrices. Define $\alpha_j = E(Y_{i1} \mid r_i = j) - \mu_1$, $j = 0, 1$, and let $\beta = \sigma_{12}\sigma_{11}^{-1}$. Kenward and Molenberghs (1998) obtained:

$$i_U(\boldsymbol{\mu}, \sigma_{11}) = \frac{N}{\sigma_{11}} \left\{ \frac{(1-\pi)\alpha_0}{\sigma_{11}} \begin{pmatrix} 1 \\ 0 \end{pmatrix} + \frac{\pi\alpha_1}{\sigma_{11}\sigma_{22} - \sigma_{12}^2} \begin{pmatrix} \sigma_{22} \\ -\sigma_{12} \end{pmatrix} \right\}, \tag{12.5}$$

$$i_U(\boldsymbol{\mu}, \sigma_{12}) = \frac{N\pi\alpha_1}{\sigma_{11}\sigma_{22} - \sigma_{12}^2} \begin{pmatrix} -\beta \\ 1 \end{pmatrix}, \tag{12.6}$$

$$i_U(\boldsymbol{\mu}, \sigma_{22}) = \begin{pmatrix} 0 \\ 0 \end{pmatrix}, \tag{12.7}$$

for $\pi = P(r_i = 1)$. In contrast to the naive information, these cross-terms do not all vanish, and the orthogonality of mean and variance–covariance parameters is lost under the MAR mechanism. One implication of this is that although the information relating to the linear model parameters alone is not affected by the move from an MCAR to an MAR mechanism, the asymptotic variance–covariance matrix *is* affected due to the induced non-orthogonality and, therefore, the dropout mechanism cannot be regarded as ignorable as far as the estimation of precision of the estimators of the linear model parameters is concerned. It can also be shown that the expected information for the variance–covariance parameters is not equivalent under the MCAR and MAR dropout mechanisms, but the expressions are more involved. Assuming that π is non-zero, it can be seen that the necessary and sufficient condition for the terms in (12.5) and (12.6) to be equal to zero is that $\alpha_0 = \alpha_1 = 0$, the condition defining, as expected, an MCAR mechanism.

We now illustrate these findings with a few numerical results. The off-diagonal unconditional information elements (12.5)–(12.7) are computed for sample size $N = 1000$, mean vector $(0,0)'$, and two covariance matrices: (1) $\sigma_{11} = \sigma_{22} = 1$ and correlation $\rho = \sigma_{12} = 0.5$, and (2) $\sigma_{11} = 2$, $\sigma_{33} = 3$, and $\rho = 0.5$ leading to $\sigma_{12} = \sqrt{6}/2$. Further, two MAR dropout mechanisms are considered. They are both of the logistic form

$$P(R_1 = 0|y_{i1}) = \frac{\exp(\gamma_0 + \gamma_1 y_{i1})}{1 + \exp(\gamma_0 + \gamma_1 y_{i1})}.$$

We choose $\gamma_0 = 0$ and (a) $\gamma_1 = 1$ or (b) $\gamma_1 = -\infty$. The latter mechanism implies $r_i = 0$ if $y_{i1} \geq 0$ and $r_i = 1$ otherwise. Both dropout mechanisms yield $\pi = 0.5$. In all cases, $\alpha_1 = -\alpha_0$, with α_1 equal, in the four possible combinations of covariance and dropout parameters, to (1a) 0.4132, (1b) 0.7263, (2a) $\sqrt{2/\pi}$, and (2b) $2/\sqrt{\pi}$. Numerical values for (12.5)–(12.7) are presented in Table 12.1, as well as the average from the observed information matrices in a simulation with 500 replicates.

Obviously, these elements are far from zero, as would be found with the naive estimator. They are of the same order of magnitude as the upper left block of the information matrix (pertaining to the mean parameters), given by

$$\begin{pmatrix} 1166.67 & -333.33 \\ -333.33 & 666.67 \end{pmatrix}.$$

Table 12.1 Bivariate normal data. Computed and simulated values for the off-diagonal block of the unconditional information matrix. Sample size is $N = 1000$ (500 replications). (The true model has zero mean vector. Two true covariances Σ and two dropout parameters γ_1 are considered.)

Parameters			Unconditional $i_U(\mu, \cdot)$			Simulated $\widehat{i}_0(\mu, \cdot)$		
Σ	γ_1		σ_{11}	σ_{12}	σ_{22}	σ_{11}	σ_{12}	σ_{22}
1	0.5	1	-68.87	137.75	0.00	-69.36	137.95	-0.04
0.5	1		137.75	-275.49	0.00	137.88	-276.83	-0.04
2	$\sqrt{6}/2$	1	-30.26	49.42	0.00	-30.21	49.54	0.04
$\sqrt{6}/2$	3		49.42	-80.70	0.00	49.52	-81.31	0.06
1	0.5	$-\infty$	132.98	-265.96	0.00	135.67	-267.66	0.16
0.5	1		-265.96	531.92	0.00	-267.73	537.58	-0.02
2	$\sqrt{6}/2$	$-\infty$	47.02	-76.78	0.00	49.52	-78.73	-0.02
$\sqrt{6}/2$	3		-76.78	125.38	0.00	-78.58	126.91	0.02

Kenward and Molenberghs (1998) performed a limited simulation study to verify the coverage probability for the Wald tests under the unconditional and a selection of conditional frameworks. The hypotheses considered are $H_{01} : \mu_1 = 0$, $H_{02} : \mu_2 = 0$, and $H_{03} : \mu_1 = \mu_2 = 0$. The simulations have been restricted to the first covariance matrix used in Table 12.1 and to the second dropout mechanism ($\gamma_1 = -\infty$). Results are reported in Table 12.2. The coverages for the unconditional framework are in good agreement with a χ^2 reference distribution; the first naive framework (500 complete cases) leads to a conservative procedure, whereas the second and the third lead to extreme liberal behaviour, that is most marked for hypotheses H_{01} and H_{03}. This is to be expected because by fixing $m = 500$, the proportion of positive first outcomes is constrained to be equal to its predicted value. This has the effect of reducing the variability of $\hat{\mu}_1$. The second and the third frameworks also suppress the variability, but introduce bias at the same time. The comparative insensitivity of the behaviour of the test for H_{02} to the sampling framework is because μ_1 has only an indirect influence through the correlation between

Table 12.2 Bivariate normal data. True values are as in the third model of Table 12.1. Coverage probabilities ($\times 1000$) for Wald test statistics. Sample size is $N = 1000$ (500 replications). The null hypotheses are $H_{01} : \mu_1 = 0$, $H_{02} : \mu_2 = 0$, $H_{03} : \mu_1 = \mu_2 = 0$. For the naive sampling frameworks, m denotes the fixed number of complete cases.

Hypothesis	Unconditional	$m = 500$	$m = 450$	$m = 400$
H_{01}	933	996	187	0
H_{02}	953	952	913	830
H_{03}	952	992	338	0

the outcomes on both occasions. It should be noted that, due to numerical problems, not all simulations led to 500 successful estimations. On average, 489 convergencies were observed, the lowest value being 460 for H_{02} in the first naive sampling frame.

12.4 BIVARIATE BINARY DATA

Suppose that each member of the pair of observations (Y_{i1}, Y_{i2}), from unit i, $i = 1, \ldots N$, is a binary random variable, with associated probabilities $P(Y_{i1} = 1) = \lambda$ and $P(Y_{i2} = 1) = \theta$. It is assumed that an MAR mechanism is operating with respect to the second observation, that is, the probability of Y_{i2} being missing depends on Y_{i1} alone. It follows that Y_{i1} is always observed. We want to compare the naive information i_N with the unconditional information i_U for this set-up. We begin by assuming that Y_{i1} and Y_{i2} are independent. The joint distribution of Y_{i1}, Y_{i2}, and R_i can then be partitioned as follows: $f(y_{i1}, y_{i2}, r_i) = f(y_{i1})f(y_{i2})f(r_i \mid y_{i1})$. It follows at once that the observed information for θ can be expressed as

$$i_O(\theta, \theta) = \frac{1}{\theta^2} \sum_{i=1}^{d} y_{i2} + \frac{1}{(1-\theta)^2} \left(d - \sum_{i=1}^{d} y_{i2} \right), \tag{12.8}$$

where d denotes the number of observations made on the second occasion. The other elements of the information matrix are not relevant to the development.

The naive information is obtained from (12.8) by taking expectations over the joint distribution of d independent binary random variables with parameter θ, that is, we take expectations over the observed pattern of observations but not conditional on r, the realization of the random variable R associated with the occurrence of that particular pattern. Hence from (12.8) we get $i_N(\theta, \theta) = d\theta^{-1}(1-\theta)^{-1}$.

The unconditional information is derived in two steps. First we obtain the conditional expectation of (12.8) with respect to $Y \mid R$. For this we need

$$E_{Y \mid r_i = 1}(Y_{i2}) = P(Y_{i2} = 1 \mid r_i = 1)$$
$$= P(Y_{i2} = 1) = \theta,$$

because of the independence of Y_{i1} and Y_{i2} under the MAR mechanism. It follows that

$$E_{Y \mid R}\{i_O(\theta, \theta)\} = d\theta^{-1}(1-\theta)^{-1},$$

for d the number of observations on the second occasion. We are now treating d as the realization of a random variable M, over which we take expectations to obtain the unconditional information. Setting $\pi = P(R_i = 1)$, we have

$$i_U(\theta, \theta) = E_R \left(d \frac{1}{\theta(1-\theta)} \right) = \frac{E_R(d)}{\theta(1-\theta)} = \frac{N\pi}{\theta(1-\theta)}.$$

Replacing π by the estimate d/N, it can be seen that in practice the naive and unconditional information are equivalent and sampling-based inferences that use the naive information are valid. Under independence, the data are *observed at random* (OAR) and the result above is just a manifestation of the general validity of sampling-based methods under the combination of MAR and OAR, or equivalently MCAR, as pointed out by Heitjan (1994, p. 706).

We now introduce dependence between Y_{i1} and Y_{i2}. This can be expressed through the conditional success probabilities of Y_{i2}: $\theta_1 = P(Y_{i2} = 1 \mid y_{i1} = 1)$ and $\theta_0 = P(Y_{i2} = 1 \mid y_{i1} = 0)$. The off-diagonal elements of the observed information matrix are zero, so we need consider only the information for one of θ_0 and θ_1 to contrast the naive and unconditional forms of the expected information. For θ_1 the observed information reads

$$i_0(\theta_1, \theta_1) = \frac{1}{\theta_1^2} \sum_{i=1}^{d} y_{i1} y_{i2} + \frac{1}{(1 - \theta_1)^2} \sum_{i=1}^{d} y_{i1}(1 - y_{i2}). \tag{12.9}$$

For the naive information it follows at once, taking expectations in (12.9), that

$$i_N(\theta_1, \theta_1) = \frac{d\lambda}{\theta_1(1 - \theta_1)}. \tag{12.10}$$

For the unconditional information, Kenward and Molenberghs (1998) derived

$$i_U(\theta_1, \theta_1) = \frac{N\lambda\eta_1}{\theta_1(1 - \theta_1)}, \tag{12.11}$$

with a similar expression for $i_U(\theta_0, \theta_0)$.

We are now in a position to consider the conditions under which the naive and unconditional expectations are equivalent. From (12.10) and (12.11), it can be seen that conditions for $E_R(i_N(\theta_1, \theta_1)) = i_U(\theta_1, \theta_1)$ and $E_R(i_N(\theta_0, \theta_0)) = i_U(\theta_0, \theta_0)$ are $E_R(d/N) = \eta_1 = \eta_0$ and hence $\eta = \eta_1 = \eta_0$, the requirement for an MCAR mechanism to operate. It follows, as expected, that the MCAR mechanism is both a necessary and sufficient condition for the equivalence of the two forms of information.

These findings are illustrated with some numerical results. It is necessary to consider only the diagonal elements of i_N and i_U because the off-diagonal elements are all zero. Take a sample of size $N = 1000$ and consider various settings for the parameters (as shown in Table 12.3). A simulation run of 500 replicates was performed for each setting. Results are presented in Table 12.4. The simulations agree very closely with the unconditional information. Although not reported here, simulation runs with larger sample sizes produced similar results, with improved agreement between theoretical and simulated values.

Table 12.3 Bivariate binary data. Parameter settings.

Model	λ	θ_1	θ_0	η_1	η_0
1	0.50	0.25	0.75	0.75	0.25
2	0.50	0.25	0.75	0.25	0.75
3	0.25	0.40	0.60	0.40	0.60
4	0.25	0.40	0.60	0.60	0.40

Table 12.4 Bivariate binary data. Diagonal of the information matrix: naive, unconditional, and simulated. Sample size is $N = 1000$ (500 replications).

	Naive $i_N(.,.)$			Unconditional $i_U(.,.)$			Simulated $\widehat{i}_0(.,.)$		
Model	λ	θ_1	θ_0	λ	θ_1	θ_0	λ	θ_1	θ_0
1	4000	1333	1333	4000	2000	667	4004	2001	678
2	4000	1333	1333	4000	667	2000	4004	672	2014
3	5333	573	1719	5333	417	1875	5349	420	1879
4	5333	469	1406	5333	625	1250	5348	631	1259

To illustrate that basing the computation of test statistics on either the observed information matrix or the unconditional expectation is sufficient in order to obtain valid inference, we consider three Wald test statistics. The null hypotheses $H_{01} - H_{03}$ are that each of the three parameters λ, θ_1, and θ_0 is equal to the true value. The four parameter settings displayed in Table 12.3 are revisited under both the unconditional sampling framework (i.e., with m, the number of complete cases, varying at random), as well as under a few naive frameworks, fixing d (1) at its expected value, (2) about two standard deviations below its expected value, (3) at a value well below the minimal m observed under the unconditional sampling scheme (Table 12.5). Should the correct reference distribution be χ^2 with 1 degree of freedom, then the coverage probability, for 500 replicates, has probability interval [93.05,96.95]%. Clearly, the values obtained under the unconditional framework are in agreement. Combining all 12 coverages leads to 94.88%, well within the interval [94.44,95.56]%. In fact, the first naive framework, where m equals its expected value, shows an only slightly increased dispersion. However, suspicion is raised for the second naive framework, while the third one is dramatically different. As expected, the behaviour of hypothesis tests concerning θ_1 and θ_0 is much less affected by the choice of sampling framework. These conclusions are supported by QQ plots (not shown) for the Wald test statistics against the quantiles of a χ^2 reference distribution.

Table 12.5 Bivariate binary data. Coverage probabilities ($\times 1000$) for Wald test statistics. Sample size is $N = 1000$ (500 replications). The null hypotheses are $H_{01} : \hat{\lambda} = \lambda$, $H_{02} : \hat{\theta}_1 = \theta_1$, $H_{03} : \hat{\theta}_0 = \theta_0$. For the naive sampling frameworks, d denotes the fixed number of complete cases.

Model	d	H_{01}	H_{02}	H_{03}	d	H_{01}	H_{02}	H_{03}
		Unconditional				**Naive(1)**		
1		946	944	948	500	968	964	928
2		946	948	954	500	972	932	956
3		954	936	956	550	938	942	940
4		954	942	958	540	960	966	936
		Naive(3)				**Naive(4)**		
1	470	884	958	954	400	68	952	942
2	470	894	942	962	400	54	962	950
3	520	952	938	954	450	822	940	960
4	420	944	936	958	350	778	954	944

12.5   IMPLICATIONS FOR STANDARD SOFTWARE

The literature indicates an early awareness of problems with conventional likelihood-based frequentist inference in the MAR setting. Specifically, several authors point to the use of the observed information matrix as a way to circumvent issues with the expected information matrix. In spite of this, it seems that a broad awareness of this problem has diminished somewhat, while the number of methods formulated to deal with the MAR situation has risen dramatically in recent years. For example, the SAS procedures MIXED, NLMIXED, and GLIMMIX can be used to perform a direct likelihood analysis.

The MIXED procedure allows both Newton–Raphson and Fisher scoring algorithms. Specifying the 'scoring' option in the PROC MIXED statement requests the Fisher scoring algorithm in conjunction with the method of estimation for a specified number of iterations (1 by default). If convergence is reached before scoring is stopped, then the expected Hessian is used to compute approximate standard errors rather than the observed Hessian. In both cases, the standard errors for the fixed effects are based on inverting the upper left-hand block of the Hessian matrix. Since we have shown in Section 12.3 that the off-diagonal block, pertaining to the covariance between the fixed-effects and covariance parameters, does not have expectation zero, this procedure is, strictly speaking, incorrect. Correction factors to overcome this problem have been proposed (e.g., Prasad and Rao 1990), but they tend to be small for fairly well-balanced data sets. It has to be noted that a substantial amount of (randomly)

Table 12.6 Orthodontic growth data. Maximum likelihood estimates and standard errors (in parentheses) for the parameters in model 7 (complete data set and ignorable analysis).

Parameter	Complete data Estimate (s.e.;[a] s.e.[b])	Ignorable Estimate (s.e.;[a] s.e.[b])
β_0	17.3727 (1.1615; 1.1645)	17.2218 (1.2220; 1.2207)
β_{01}	−1.0321 (1.5089; 1.5156)	−0.9188 (1.5857; 1.5814)
β_{10}	0.4795 (0.0923; 0.0925)	0.4890 (0.0969; 0.0968)
β_{11}	0.7844 (0.0765; 0.0767)	0.7867 (0.0802; 0.0801)
σ^2	1.8746 (0.2946; 0.2946)	2.0173 (0.3365; 0.3365)
d	3.0306 (0.9552; 0.9550)	3.0953 (1.0011; 1.0011)

[a] Standard error based on the Newton–Raphson algorithm of PROC MIXED.
[b] Standard error obtained from inverting the entire observed information matrix.

missing data will destroy this balance. Kenward and Molenberghs (1998) showed, using the orthodontic growth data set, that differences in practice may be negligible. In Table 12.6, model 7 for the orthodontic growth data (Section 5.2) is reconsidered for both the complete data set, and the incomplete data on the basis of an ignorable analysis. The fixed-effects parameters are described by the relationship

$$Y_{ij} = \beta_0 + \beta_{01}x_i + \beta_{10}t_j(1 - x_i) + \beta_{11}t_jx_i + \varepsilon_{ij},$$

where $x_i = 1$ for girls and 0 for boys, $t_j = 8, 10, 12, 14$ is the time of measurement, and Y_{ij} is the growth measurement at occasion j for child i. The variance of ε_{ij} is $\sigma^2 + d$, and the covariance between ε_{ij} and $\varepsilon_{ij'}$, for $j \neq j'$, is d. Apart from the parameter estimates, two sets of standard errors are shown in Table 12.6: (1) taken from inverting the fixed-effects block from the observed Hessian and (2) taken from inverting the entire observed Hessian. The first set is found from the MIXED output, whereas the second one is constructed using the numerical optimizer OPTMUM of the GAUSS package.

Clearly, there are only minor differences between the two sets of standard errors, and the analysis on an incomplete set of data does not seem to widen the gap.

When the GLIMMIX procedure is employed to fit a generalized linear mixed model, the same cautionary remarks apply as with the MIXED procedure. Thus, even though the observed Hessian matrix can be employed, as an alternative to using the expected Hessian matrix, the variability in the variance components is not taken into account when computing the precision of the fixed effects. For the specific case of a linear mixed model fitted with the GLIMMIX procedure, exactly the same results obtain as with the MIXED procedure. In non-Gaussian, especially binary cases, the MQL and PQL expansion methods, owing to their approximate nature, are prone to considerable bias (Section 7.5). Arguably, the latter component of bias is considerable larger than that resulting from inaccurate use of the Hessian matrix.

In contrast, in the SAS procedure NLMIXED, the full Hessian matrix is employed for both numerical optimization and the computation of precision estimates. Hence, this tool is fully consistent with direct likelihood.

We can conclude from this that, with the exception of the expected information matrix, conventional likelihood-based frequentist inference, including standard hypothesis testing, is applicable in the MAR setting. Standard errors based on inverting the *entire* Hessian are to be preferred, a possibility with the NLMIXED procedure in SAS, but not fully with the MIXED and GLIMMIX procedure, even though differences are typically too small to be of concern.

12.6   ANALYSIS OF THE FLUVOXAMINE TRIAL

The first example we consider is the fluvoxamine trial, introduced in Section 2.6. We will first study two dichotomized versions (category 1 versus higher categories 2, 3, and 4; and categories 1 and 2 versus 3 and 4) of side effects and therapeutic effects at the first and the last measurement occasions. The data are shown in Table 12.7. The model of Section 12.4 is fitted to all four tables, which is particularly illustrative because naive and unconditional standard error estimates for λ coincide, concentrating potential differences between both estimators in the parameters θ_0 and θ_1 (Table 12.8). For the first analysis of side effects, there are only small differences, and inference at a common significance level is unaffected. This is different in setting 2. Indeed, the naive significance probability for $H_0 : \theta_0 = 0.5$ is 0.0319, while the unconditional version is 0.1306. Note that θ_1 is substantially different from θ_0 and, more importantly, that the missingness probabilities η_1 and η_0 are very different. For therapeutic effect, neither of the two settings leads to differences in standard errors of any importance.

The analysis considered above is based on a simple Markov type model. It concentrates the discrepancy between the naive and robust frameworks in the conditional probabilities $\theta_j (j = 0, 1)$. Other parameterizations are less sensitive

Table 12.7   Fluvoxamine trial. Dichotomized therapeutic effect outcome at first and last measurement occasions.

Setting	Outcome	Dichotomized	(0, 0)	(0, 1)	(1, 0)	(1, 1)	(0, *)	(1, *)
1	side	1/234	89	13	57	65	26	49
2	side	12/34	203	5	14	2	48	27
3	therapeutic	1/234	11	1	124	88	7	68
4	therapeutic	12/34	77	9	119	19	28	47

Table 12.8 Fluvoxamine trial. Analysis of the data in Table 12.7. Parameter estimates (naive standard errors; unconditional standard errors) are shown.

Parameter	1/234	12/34
Side effects		
λ	0.572 (0.029; 0.029)	0.144 (0.020; 0.020)
θ_1	0.533 (0.044; 0.045)	0.125 (0.058; 0.083)
θ_0	0.128 (0.034; 0.033)	0.024 (0.011; 0.011)
η_1	0.714	0.372
η_0	0.797	0.813
Therapeutic effect		
λ	0.937 (0.014; 0.014)	0.619 (0.028; 0.028)
θ_1	0.415 (0.034; 0.034)	0.138 (0.029; 0.029)
θ_0	0.083 (0.073; 0.080)	0.105 (0.033; 0.033)
η_1	0.757	0.746
η_0	0.632	0.754

to the (mis)use of the naive framework. As an illustration, we analyse side effects at the first, second, and fourth measurement occasion, on a three-category scale (with original categories 3 and 4 combined). A trivariate odds ratio model (Molenberghs and Lesaffre 1994) is adopted. Briefly, marginal cumulative logits for each outcome are combined with global marginal log odds ratios for the pairwise and third-order interactions in order to specify the joint distribution. The marginal logits are assumed to depend on *duration*, whereas the log odds ratios are assumed constant. Molenberghs, Kenward, and Lesaffre (1997) observed that dropout in the side-effects outcome depends both on the previous measurement, as well as on the value of *duration*. We analysed the set of 222 complete cases as well as all available data. Table 12.9 reports

Table 12.9 Fluvoxamine trial. Side effects at times 1, 2, and 4. Wald test statistics for the completers only and for an MAR analysis.

Hypothesis	d.f.	Compl. cases Expected	Observed	MAR Expected	Observed
Common duration effect	2	1.36	1.19	2.54	2.44
No duration effect	3	2.98	2.54	12.90	11.13
Common two-way association	2	10.70	9.99	11.48	9.13
Intercepts equal across times	4	28.73	28.83	34.96	33.44
Common diff. between intercepts	2	0.16	0.16	2.07	1.48
Linear trend in first intercept	1	0.0099	0.0099	0.16	0.18
Linear trend in second intercept	1	0.020	0.018	1.15	0.85
Linear trend in both intercepts	2	0.034	0.033	1.18	0.91

on the value of the (naive and unconditional) Wald statistic for a number of hypotheses. Although not spectacular, the differences between expected and observed information based tests is larger for the MAR analysis than for the complete case analysis. In particular, the *p*-value for the hypothesis of no *duration* effect (MAR) changes from 0.0049 with the expected information to 0.0110 with the observed information. In this example it was seen consistently that in MAR analyses the observed information yielded smaller test statistics than the expected information. For completers-only analyses this was not always the case.

12.7   THE MUSCATINE CORONARY RISK FACTOR STUDY

In the previous study of moderate size, for which there existed some preliminary evidence for an MAR mechanism in the side effects, differences appeared between inferences based on observed and expected information. Woolson and Clarke (1984) analysed data from the Muscatine coronary risk factor Study, a longitudinal study of coronary risk factors in school children (1971–1981). These authors analysed classifications of the children as obese or not obese made in 1977, 1979, and 1981. Apart from the outcome, the sex of the child and the age stratum (8, 10, 12, or 14) was recorded. All possible missingness patterns occur. There is no evidence that the missing data mechanism would be more complex than MCAR. We have fitted an odds ratio model, with the logit of each measurement depending on sex and age (linear trend). Categorization of age gave very similar results. Table 12.10 presents the Wald test statistics: the differences between statistics in the completers' analysis are very small. Although differences are slightly larger in the MAR analyses, there is no qualitative difference in the inference based on these tests.

Table 12.10 Muscatine coronary risk factor study. Wald test statistics for the completers only and for an MAR analysis.

Hypothesis	d.f.	Complete cases		MAR	
		Expected	Observed	Expected	Observed
Common sex effect	2	5.55	5.54	1.50	1.49
No sex effect	3	5.56	5.55	6.84	6.82
Common age effect	2	22.20	21.37	40.03	38.59
No age effect	3	22.40	21.66	46.17	45.39
Common two-way association	2	15.99	16.08	17.26	16.63
Common intercept across time	2	22.27	21.72	45.55	45.56
Linear trend in intercepts	1	0.10	0.10	2.16	2.09

12.8   THE CRÉPEAU DATA

Kenward and Molenberghs (1998) considered a relatively small example with a continuous response, analysed in Crépeau *et al.* (1985). Fifty-four rats were divided into five treatment groups corresponding to exposure to increasing doses of halothane (0%, 0.25%, 0.5%, 1%, and 2%). The groups were of sizes 11, 10, 11, 11, and 11 rats, respectively. Following an induced heart attack in each rat, the blood pressure was recorded on nine unequally spaced occasions. A number of rats died during the course of the experiment, including all rats from group 5 (2% halothane). Following the original authors, we omit this group from the analysis since they contribute no information at all, leaving 43 rats, of which 23 survived the experiment.

Examination of the data from these four groups does not provide any evidence of an MAR dropout process, although this observation must be considered in the light of the small sample size. A Gaussian multivariate linear model with an unconstrained covariance matrix was fitted to the data. There was very little evidence of a treatment-by-time interaction, and the following results are based on the use of a model with additive effects for treatment and time. The Wald statistics for the treatment main effect on 3 degrees of freedom are equal to 46.95 and 30.82 respectively, using the expected and observed information matrices. Although leading to the same qualitative conclusions, the figures are notably discrepant. A first reaction may be to attribute this difference to the incompleteness of the data. However, the lack of evidence for an MAR process, together with the relatively small sample size, points to another cause. The equivalent analysis of the 24 completers produces Wald statistics of 45.34 and 26.35, respectively; that is, the effect can be attributed to a combination of small-sample variation and possible model misspecification. A theoretical reason for this difference might be that the expected value of the off-diagonal block of the information matrix of the maximum likelihood estimates (describing covariance between mean and covariance parameters) has expectation zero but is likely to depart from this in small samples. As a consequence, the variances of the estimated treatment effects will be higher when derived from the observed information, thereby reducing the Wald statistic.

To summarize, this example provides an illustration of an alternative source of discrepancy between the expected and observed information matrices, which is likely to be associated with the use, in smaller samples, of covariance matrices with many parameters.

12.9   CONCLUDING REMARKS

In this chapter, following Kenward and Molenberghs (1998), we have re-explored the issues that surround conventional likelihood-based analyses of incomplete data under MAR when frequentist methods are used. We have restated and illustrated the fact that under MAR the *observed* information matrix produces consistent estimators of precision, in addition to the valid point estimators produced by maximum likelihood. The use of these leads in turn to valid frequentist inferences, for example those based on likelihood ratio, Wald and score test statistics. In contrast, the use of the *expected* information matrix is in principle to be discouraged, as it is biased unless the expectation is taken jointly over the outcome and missingness distributions. Our simulations and data analyses suggest, however, that even when the expected information matrix is used, differences are not likely to be spectacular, although there will of course be exceptions to this. We noted that in some software tools, such as the SAS procedures MIXED and GLIMMIX, the Hessian matrix used is an approximation only, since it ignores variability in the variance components. This, too, may yield generally small differences with the proper standard errors. The procedure NLMIXED, in contrast, uses the proper Hessian matrix.

Analysis of the Age-Related Macular Degeneration Trial

13.1 INTRODUCTION

In this chapter we analyse the age-related macular degeneration data introduced in Section 2.8. Recall that there are 240 subjects, 188 of which have complete follow-up. In line with guidelines in the current and previous parts of the book, it is therefore advisable to consider all subjects for inclusion in the analysis. Note that of the 52 subjects with incomplete follow-up, 8 exhibit a non-monotone pattern. While this does not hamper direct likelihood analyses, it is a challenge for WGEE. One way forward is to monotonize missingness patterns by means of multiple imputation and then conduct WGEE, or to switch to MI-GEE (Chapter 11) altogether.

As explained in Section 2.8, the original outcome, the number of letters correctly read on a vision chart or its difference from the baseline reading, can be considered continuous for practical purposes. This outcome is analysed in Section 13.2 using direct likelihood machinery. The derived dichotomous outcome, defined as increase or decrease in number of letters read compared with baseline, is analysed in Section 13.3 using WGEE and in Section 13.4 by means of generalized linear mixed models, falling within the direct likelihood framework. The use of multiple imputation is explored in Section 13.5.

Missing Data in Clinical Studies   G. Molenberghs and M.G. Kenward
© 2007 John Wiley & Sons, Ltd

13.2 DIRECT LIKELIHOOD ANALYSIS OF THE CONTINUOUS OUTCOME

We consider first a simple multivariate normal model, with unconstrained time trend under placebo, an occasion-specific treatment effect, and a 4×4 unstructured variance–covariance matrix. Thus,

$$Y_{ij} = \beta_{j1} + \beta_{j2} T_i + \varepsilon_{ij}, \tag{13.1}$$

where $T_i = 0$ for placebo and $T_i = 1$ for interferon-α. The direct likelihood analysis is contrasted with LOCF and CC, and parameter estimates (standard errors) for the eight mean model parameters are presented in Table 13.1.

While there is no overall treatment effect, and the p-values between the three methods do not vary too much, the picture is different for the occasion-specific treatment effects. At week 4, all three p-values indicate significance. While this is the only significant effect when only the completers are analysed, there is one more significant effect with LOCF (week 12) and two more when direct likelihood is employed (weeks 12 and 52). Once more, CC and LOCF miss important treatment differences, the most important one being that at week 52, the end of the study.

Table 13.1 Age-related macular degeneration trial. Parameter estimates (standard errors) for the linear mixed models, fitted to the continuous outcome of the difference between the number of letters read and baseline. CC, LOCF, and direct likelihood (observed data). p-values are given for treatment effect at each of the four times separately, as well as for all four times jointly.

Effect	Parameter	CC	LOCF	Observed data
Parameter estimates (standard errors)				
Intercept 4	β_{11}	−3.24 (0.77)	−3.48 (0.77)	−3.48 (0.77)
Intercept 12	β_{21}	−4.66 (1.14)	−5.72 (1.09)	−5.85 (1.11)
Intercept 24	β_{31}	−8.33 (1.39)	−8.34 (1.30)	−9.05 (1.36)
Intercept 52	β_{41}	−15.13 (1.73)	−14.16 (1.53)	−16.21 (1.67)
Treatment effect 4	β_{12}	2.32 (1.05)	2.20 (1.08)	2.20 (1.08)
Treatment effect 12	β_{22}	2.35 (1.55)	3.38 (1.53)	3.51 (1.55)
Treatment effect 24	β_{32}	2.73 (1.88)	2.41 (1.83)	3.03 (1.89)
Treatment effect 52	β_{42}	4.17 (2.35)	3.43 (2.15)	4.86 (2.31)
p-values				
Treatment effect 4	β_{12}	0.0282	0.0432	0.0435
Treatment effect 12	β_{22}	0.1312	0.0287	0.0246
Treatment effect 24	β_{32}	0.1491	0.1891	0.1096
Treatment effect 52	β_{42}	0.0772	0.1119	0.0366
Treatment effect (overall)		0.1914	0.1699	0.1234

13.3 WEIGHTED GENERALIZED ESTIMATING EQUATIONS

We now switch to the binary outcome, which indicates whether the number of letters correctly read at a follow-up occasion is higher or lower than the corresponding number of letters at baseline. A population-averaged (or marginal) model is used. In line with the previous section, we compare analyses performed on the completers only (CC), on the LOCF imputed data, as well as on the observed data. In all cases, standard GEE (Section 10.3.2) and linearization-based GEE (Section 10.3.3) will be considered. For the observed, partially incomplete data, GEE is supplemented with WGEE (Section 10.4).

The GEE analyses are reported in Table 13.2. In all cases, we use the logit link, and the model takes the form

$$\text{logit}[P(Y_{ij} = 1 | T_i, t_j)] = \beta_{j1} + \beta_{j2} T_i, \tag{13.2}$$

Table 13.2 Age-Related Macular Degeneration Trial. Parameter estimates (model-based standard errors; empirically corrected standard errors) for the marginal models: standard and linearization-based GEE on the CC and LOCF population, and on the observed data. In the latter case, WGEE is also used.

Effect	Parameter	CC	LOCF	Observed data Unweighted	WGEE
Standard GEE					
Intercept 4	β_{11}	−1.01 (0.24; 0.24)	−0.87 (0.20; 0.21)	−0.87 (0.21; 0.21)	−0.98 (0.10; 0.44)
Intercept 12	β_{21}	−0.89 (0.24; 0.24)	−0.97 (0.21; 0.21)	−1.01 (0.21; 0.21)	−1.78 (0.15; 0.38)
Intercept 24	β_{31}	−1.13 (0.25; 0.25)	−1.05 (0.21; 0.21)	−1.07 (0.22; 0.22)	−1.11 (0.15; 0.33)
Intercept 52	β_{41}	−1.64 (0.29; 0.29)	−1.51 (0.24; 0.24)	−1.71 (0.29; 0.29)	−1.72 (0.25; 0.39)
Treatment 4	β_{12}	0.40 (0.32; 0.32)	0.22 (0.28; 0.28)	0.22 (0.28; 0.28)	0.80 (0.15; 0.67)
Treatment 12	β_{22}	0.49 (0.31; 0.31)	0.55 (0.28; 0.28)	0.61 (0.29; 0.29)	1.87 (0.19; 0.61)
Treatment 24	β_{32}	0.48 (0.33; 0.33)	0.42 (0.29; 0.29)	0.44 (0.30; 0.30)	0.73 (0.20; 0.52)
Treatment 52	β_{42}	0.40 (0.38; 0.38)	0.34 (0.32; 0.32)	0.44 (0.37; 0.37)	0.74 (0.31; 0.52)
Correlation	ρ	0.39	0.44	0.39	0.33
Linearization-based GEE					
Intercept 4	β_{11}	−1.01 (0.24; 0.24)	−0.87 (0.21; 0.21)	−0.87 (0.21; 0.21)	−0.98 (0.18; 0.44)
Intercept 12	β_{21}	−0.89 (0.24; 0.24)	−0.97 (0.21; 0.21)	−1.01 (0.22; 0.21)	−1.78 (0.26; 0.42)
Intercept 24	β_{31}	−1.13 (0.25; 0.25)	−1.05 (0.21; 0.21)	−1.07 (0.23; 0.22)	−1.19 (0.25; 0.38)
Intercept 52	β_{41}	−1.64 (0.29; 0.29)	−1.51 (0.24; 0.24)	−1.71 (0.29; 0.29)	−1.81 (0.39; 0.48)
Treatment 4	β_{12}	0.40 (0.32; 0.32)	0.22 (0.28; 0.28)	0.22 (0.29; 0.29)	0.80 (0.26; 0.67)
Treatment 12	β_{22}	0.49 (0.31; 0.31)	0.55 (0.28; 0.28)	0.61 (0.28; 0.29)	1.85 (0.32; 0.64)
Treatment 24	β_{32}	0.48 (0.33; 0.33)	0.42 (0.29; 0.29)	0.44 (0.30; 0.30)	0.98 (0.33; 0.60)
Treatment 52	β_{42}	0.40 (0.38; 0.38)	0.34 (0.32; 0.32)	0.44 (0.37; 0.37)	0.97 (0.49; 0.65)
	σ^2	0.62	0.57	0.62	1.29
	τ^2	0.39	0.44	0.39	1.85
Correlation	ρ	0.39	0.44	0.39	0.59

similar in spirit to (13.1). A working exchangeable correlation matrix is considered. For the WGEE analysis, the following weight model is assumed:

$$\text{logit}[P(D_i = j | D_i \geq j)] = \psi_0 + \psi_1 y_{i,j-1} + \psi_2 T_i + \psi_{31} L_{1i}$$
$$+ \psi_{32} L_{2i} + \psi_{34} L_{3i}$$
$$+ \psi_{41} I(t_j = 2) + \psi_{42} I(t_j = 3), \qquad (13.3)$$

where $y_{i,j-1}$ is the binary outcome at the previous time $t_{i,j-1} = t_{j-1}$, $L_{ki} = 1$ if the patient's eye lesion is of level $k = 1, \ldots, 4$ (since one dummy variable is redundant, only three are used), and $I(\cdot)$ is the indicator function. Parameter estimates and standard errors for the dropout model are given in Table 13.3. Intermittent missingness will be ignored. Covariates of importance are treatment assignment, the level of lesions at baseline (a four-point categorical variable, for which three indicator variables are needed), and time at which dropout occurs. For the latter covariates, there are three levels, since dropout can occur at times 2, 3, or 4. Hence, two indicator variables are included. Finally, the previous outcome does not have a significant impact, but will be kept in the model nevertheless.

From Table 13.3 it is clear that there is very little difference between the standard GEE and linearization-based GEE results. This is undoubtedly the case for CC, LOCF, and unweighted *GEE* on the observed data. For these three cases, the model-based and empirically corrected standard errors also agree extremely well, owing to the unstructured nature of the full time by treatment mean structure. However, we do observe differences in the WGEE analyses. Not only do the parameter estimates differ a little between the two GEE versions, but there is a dramatic difference between the model-based and empirically corrected standard errors. This is entirely due to the weighting scheme. The weights were not calibrated to add up to the total sample size, which is reflected in the model-based standard errors. In the linearization-based case, part of the effect

Table 13.3 Age-related macular degeneration trial. Parameter estimates (standard errors) for a logistic regression model to describe dropout.

Effect	Parameter	Estimate (s.e.)
Intercept	ψ_0	0.14 (0.49)
Previous outcome	ψ_1	0.04 (0.38)
Treatment	ψ_2	−0.86 (0.37)
Lesion level 1	ψ_{31}	−1.85 (0.49)
Lesion level 2	ψ_{32}	−1.91 (0.52)
Lesion level 3	ψ_{33}	−2.80 (0.72)
Time 2	ψ_{41}	−1.75 (0.49)
Time 3	ψ_{42}	−1.38 (0.44)

is captured as overdispersion. This can be seen from adding the parameters σ^2 and τ^2. In all other analyses, the sum is close to one, as it should be when there is no residual overdispersion, but in the last column it is 3.14. Nevertheless, the two sets of empirically corrected standard errors agree very closely, which is reassuring.

In spite of there being no strong evidence for MAR, the results between GEE and WGEE differ in a non-trivial way. It is noteworthy that at 12 weeks, a treatment effect is observed with WGEE which is undetected when using the other marginal analyses. This finding is confirmed to some extent by the subject-specific random-intercept model, presented in the next section, when the data are used as observed.

When comparing parameter estimates across CC, LOCF, and observed data analyses, it is clear that LOCF has the effect of artificially increasing the correlation between measurements. The effect is mild in this case. The parameter estimates of the observed data GEE are close to the LOCF results for earlier time points and close to CC for later time points. This is to be expected, as at the start of the study the LOCF and observed populations are very similar, with the same holding between CC and observed populations near the end of the study. Note also that the treatment effect under LOCF, especially at 12 weeks and after 1 year, is biased downwards in comparison to the GEE analyses.

13.4 DIRECT LIKELIHOOD ANALYSIS OF THE BINARY OUTCOME

Let us now turn to a random-intercept logistic model, similar in spirit to (13.2):

$$\text{logit}[P(Y_{ij} = 1|T_i, t_j, b_i)] = \beta_{j1} + b_i + \beta_{j2}T_i, \tag{13.4}$$

with notation as before and $b_i \sim N(0, \tau^2)$. Both PQL and numerical integration are used for model fitting. The results for this model are given in Table 13.4. We observe the usual downward bias in the PQL compared to numerical integration analysis, as well as the usual relationship between the marginal parameters of Table 13.2 and their random-effects counterparts. Note also that the random-intercepts variance is largest under LOCF, underscoring again that this method artificially increases the association between measurements on the same subject. In this case, in contrast to marginal models, both LOCF and CC considerably overestimate the treatment effect at certain times, by varying degrees ranging from trivial to important, in particular at 4 and 24 weeks (unlike the continuous case; see Section 13.2).

Table 13.4 Age-related macular degeneration trial. Parameter estimates (standard errors) for the random-intercept models: PQL and numerical integration based fits on the CC and LOCF population, and on the observed data (direct likelihood).

Effect	Parameter	CC	LOCF	Direct likelihood
PQL				
Intercept 4	β_{11}	−1.19 (0.31)	−1.05 (0.28)	−1.00 (0.26)
Intercept 12	β_{21}	−1.05 (0.31)	−1.18 (0.28)	−1.19 (0.28)
Intercept 24	β_{31}	−1.35 (0.32)	−1.30 (0.28)	−1.26 (0.29)
Intercept 52	β_{41}	−1.97 (0.36)	−1.89 (0.31)	−2.02 (0.35)
Treatment 4	β_{12}	0.45 (0.42)	0.24 (0.39)	0.22 (0.37)
Treatment 12	β_{22}	0.58 (0.41)	0.68 (0.38)	0.71 (0.37)
Treatment 24	β_{32}	0.55 (0.42)	0.50 (0.39)	0.49 (0.39)
Treatment 52	β_{42}	0.44 (0.47)	0.39 (0.42)	0.46 (0.46)
Random-intercept s.d.	τ	1.42 (0.14)	1.53 (0.13)	1.40 (0.13)
Random-intercept var.	τ^2	2.03 (0.39)	2.34 (0.39)	1.95 (0.35)
Numerical integration				
Intercept 4	β_{11}	−1.73 (0.42)	−1.63 (0.39)	−1.50 (0.36)
Intercept 12	β_{21}	−1.53 (0.41)	−1.80 (0.39)	−1.73 (0.37)
Intercept 24	β_{31}	−1.93 (0.43)	−1.96 (0.40)	−1.83 (0.39)
Intercept 52	β_{41}	−2.74 (0.48)	−2.76 (0.44)	−2.85 (0.47)
Treatment 4	β_{12}	0.64 (0.54)	0.38 (0.52)	0.34 (0.48)
Treatment 12	β_{22}	0.81 (0.53)	0.98 (0.52)	1.00 (0.49)
Treatment 24	β_{32}	0.77 (0.55)	0.74 (0.52)	0.69 (0.50)
Treatment 52	β_{42}	0.60 (0.59)	0.57 (0.56)	0.64 (0.58)
Random-intercept s.d.	τ	2.19 (0.27)	2.47 (0.27)	2.20 (0.25)
Random-intercept var.	τ^2	4.80 (1.17)	6.08 (1.32)	4.83 (1.11)

13.5 MULTIPLE IMPUTATION

In Sections 13.3 and 13.4, the data were analysed using GEE and generalized linear mixed models, on the complete cases, the LOCF imputed data, and using the observed data. In the latter case, WGEE was also considered. For the generalized estimating equations, both classical GEE and linearization-based GEE were considered. The generalized linear mixed models were fitted with PQL and based on numerical integration.

One complication with WGEE is that the calculation of the weights is difficult with non-monotone missingness. Standard GEE on the incomplete data is valid only when the missing data are MCAR. It is precisely at this point that multiple imputation provides an appealing alternative, as outlined in Section 9.7.

The binary indicators were created by dichotomizing the continuous visual acuity outcomes as negative or non-negative. The continuous outcomes were defined as the change from baseline in number of letters read. One possible approach here, therefore, is to base multiple imputation on the underlying continuous outcomes. Ten multiply-imputed data sets were created. The imputation model included, apart from the four continuous outcome variables, the four-point categorical variable 'lesions' as well. For simplicity, the latter was treated as continuous. Separate imputations were conducted for each of the two treatment groups. These choices imply that the imputed values depend on lesions and treatment assignment, and hence analysis models that include one or both of these effects are *proper* in the sense of Rubin (1987). This means, broadly speaking, that the model used for imputation should include all relationships that later will be considered in the analysis and inference tasks. The added advantage of including 'lesions' in the imputation model is that even individuals for whom none of the four follow-up measurements is available are still imputed. Using the SAS procedure MI, the MCMC method was used, with EM starting values, and a single chain for all imputations.

Upon imputation, the same marginal GEE and random-intercept models as in Sections 13.3 and 13.4 were fitted to the completed data sets. The final results obtained following appropriate combination using Rubin's rules are reported in Table 13.5. The parameter estimates and standard errors are very similar to their counterparts in Tables 13.2 and 13.4. Of course, in the GEE case, there is no direct counterpart, since the WGEE method is different from GEE after multiple imputation, even though both are valid under MAR. However, in particular the similarity with the direct likelihood method (bottom right-hand column of Table 13.4) is clear, with only a minor deviation in estimate for the treatment effect after 1 year.

Table 13.5 Age-related macular degeneration trial. Parameter estimates (standard errors) for the standard GEE and numerical-integration based random-intercept models (generalized linear mixed models: GLMM), after generating 10 multiple imputations.

Effect	Parameter	GEE (13.2)	GLMM (13.4)
Intercept 4	β_{11}	-0.84 (0.20)	-1.46 (0.36)
Intercept 12	β_{21}	-1.02 (0.22)	-1.75 (0.38)
Intercept 24	β_{31}	-1.07 (0.23)	-1.83 (0.38)
Intercept 52	β_{41}	-1.61 (0.27)	-2.69 (0.45)
Treatment 4	β_{12}	0.21 (0.28)	0.32 (0.48)
Treatment 12	β_{22}	0.60 (0.29)	0.99 (0.49)
Treatment 24	β_{32}	0.43 (0.30)	0.67 (0.51)
Treatment 52	β_{42}	0.37 (0.35)	0.52 (0.56)
Random-intercept s.d.	τ		2.20 (0.26)
Random-intercept var.	τ^2		4.85 (1.13)

13.6   CONCLUDING REMARKS

In this chapter we have analysed visual acuity, as recorded in the age-related macular degeneration trial. Both the continuous as well as a dichotomous change from baseline are considered. In all cases, CC and LOCF are contrasted with analyses on the observed data. For the linear and generalized linear mixed models, direct likelihood methods are employed. With generalized estimating equations, both the unweighted and weighted versions have been considered. In addition, multiple imputation is combined with GEE, at the same time enabling the use of the continuous outcome for the imputation task, even when the analysis task involves the binary outcome, and alleviating the issues surrounding non-monotone missingness.

In all analyses, it is clear that CC and LOCF may differ, in a potentially unforeseeable way, from the direct likelihood and standard, weighted, or MI-based GEE analyses. This underscores, once again, that the latter analyses are to be considered as candidates for primary analysis.

In Chapter 25, we will return to these data, employing methods for non-random missingness (Part IV) and sensitivity analysis (Part V).

14

Incomplete Data and SAS

14.1 INTRODUCTION

In this chapter SAS implementations for the direct likelihood, GEE, WGEE and MI-GEE methods, as well as their CC and LOCF counterparts, are presented. In Section 14.2 complete case analysis is discussed. In Section 14.3 we show how to conduct last observation carried forward. MAR-based methods are discussed in Section 14.4, which is devoted to likelihood methods, and in Section 14.5, which considers generalized estimating equations. Multiple imputation is dealt with in Section 14.6. Several macros have been developed and will be introduced in the following. These are available from the authors.

14.2 COMPLETE CASE ANALYSIS

The only step required to perform a complete case analysis is deletion of subjects for which not all designed measurements have been obtained. When the data are organized 'horizontally' – one record per subject – this is particularly easy. With 'vertically' organized data, slightly more data manipulation is needed and the SAS macro prepared by Caroline Beunckens can be used.

For example, for the age-related macular degeneration trial, running the following statement produces the complete case CC data set for the continuous outcome:

```
%cc(data=armd155,id=subject,time=time,
    response=diff,out=armdcc2);
```

Missing Data in Clinical Studies   G. Molenberghs and M.G. Kenward
© 2007 John Wiley & Sons, Ltd

and for the binary outcome:

```
%cc(data=armd111,id=subject,time=time,
    response=bindif,out=armdcc);
```

Clearly, the CC macro requires four arguments. The `data=` argument is the data set to be analysed. If not specified, the most recent data set is used. The name of the variable in the data set that contains the identification variable is specified by `id=`, and `time=` specifies the variable indicating the time ordering within a subject. The outcome variable is passed on by means of the `response=` argument and the name of the output data set, created with the macro, is defined through `out=`.

After performing this data pre-processing, a complete case analysis follows of any type requested by the user, including, but not limited to, longitudinal analysis. The choice of appropriate analysis is another matter entirely.

The macro requires records, corresponding to missing values, to be present in the data set. Otherwise, it is assumed that a measurement occasion not included is missing by design.

Upon creation of the new data set, the code for model (13.1) is given by:

```
proc mixed data=armdcc2 method=ml;
title 'CC - continuous';
class time treat subject;
model diff = time treat*time / noint solution ddfm=kr;
repeated time / subject=subject type=un;
run;
```

When, in contrast, GEE of the form (13.2) is applied to the completers, the following code can be used for standard GEE:

```
proc genmod data=armdcc;
title 'CC - GEE';
class time treat subject;
model bindif = time treat*time / noint dist=binomial;
repeated subject=subject / withinsubject=time type=exch modelse;
run;
```

Alternatively, for the linearized version of GEE, with empirically corrected standard errors, one can use:

```
proc glimmix data=armdcc empirical;
title 'CC - GEE - linearized version - empirical';
nloptions maxiter=50 technique=newrap;
class time treat subject;
model bindif = time treat*time / noint solution dist=binary;
random _residual_ / subject=subject type=cs;
run;
```

For the generalized linear mixed model (13.4), with PQL, the following code is useful:

```
proc glimmix data=armdcc method=rspl;
title 'CC - mixed - PQL';
nloptions maxiter=50 technique=newrap;
class time treat subject;
model bindif = time treat*time / noint solution dist=binary;
random intercept / subject=subject type=un g gcorr;
run;
```

When numerical integration, for example with adaptive Gaussian quadrature, is envisaged, one could use:

```
data help;
set armdcc;
time1=0; if time=1 then time1=1;
time2=0; if time=2 then time2=1;
time3=0; if time=3 then time3=1;
time4=0; if time=4 then time4=1;
run;

proc nlmixed data=help qpoints=20 maxiter=100 technique=newrap;
title 'CC - mixed - numerical integration';
eta = beta11*time1+beta12*time2+beta13*time3+beta14*time4+b
    +(beta21*time1+beta22*time2+beta23*time3+beta24*time4)
    *(2-treat);
p = exp(eta)/(1+exp(eta));
model bindif ~ binary(p);
random b ~ normal(0,tau*tau) subject=subject;
estimate 'tau^2' tau*tau;
run;
```

Note that the DATA step in the above program merely creates dummy variables for each of the four measurement times.

14.3 LAST OBSERVATION CARRIED FORWARD

Similar steps to those for a complete case analysis need to be performed when LOCF is the goal. For a vertically organized data set, the following macro, also written by Caroline Beunckens, can be used, in the continuous case:

```
%locf(data=armd155,id=subject,time=time,
    response=diff,out=armdlocf2);
```

or in the dichotomous case:

```
%locf(data=armd111,id=subject,time=time,
    response=bindif,out=armdlocf);
```

The arguments are exactly the same and have the same meaning as in the CC macro of the previous section. Note that there now is a *new* response variable created, named `locf`, which should be used in the corresponding analysis programs. Thus, all SAS procedure MIXED, GENMOD, GLIMMIX, and NLMIXED code of the previous section remains valid, upon replacing the response variables `diff` and `bindiff` by `locf` and, of course, by appropriately changing the names of the data sets.

14.4   DIRECT LIKELIHOOD

In contrast to CC and LOCF, no extra data processing is necessary when a direct likelihood analysis is envisaged, provided the software tool used for analysis is able to handle measurement sequences of unequal length. This is the case for virtually all longitudinal data analysis tools, including the SAS procedures MIXED, NLMIXED, and GLIMMIX.

One note of caution is relevant, however. When residual correlation structures are used for which the order of the measurements within a sequence is important, such as unstructured and AR(1), but not simple or compound symmetry, and intermittent missingness occurs, care must be taken to ensure the *design* order within the sequence, and not the *apparent* order, is passed on. In the SAS procedure MIXED, a statement such as

```
repeated / subject=subject type=un;
```

is fine when every subject has, say, four designed measurements. However, when for a particular subject the second measurement is missing, there is a risk that the remaining measurements are considered the first, second, and third, rather than the first, third, and fourth. Thus, it is sensible to replace the above statement by:

```
repeated time / subject=subject type=un;
```

For the GENMOD procedure, the option `withinsubject=time` of the REPEATED statement can be used. Note that this produces GEE and not direct likelihood. For the GLIMMIX procedure, there is no such feature.

In all cases, especially when GLIMMIX is used, the proper order is passed on when a record is included, even for the missing measurements.

When the NLMIXED procedure is used, only random effects can be included, and in such a case all relevant information is contained in the actual effects that define the random-effects structure. For example, the order is immaterial for a random-intercepts model, and for a random slope in time, all information needed about time is passed on, for example, by the RANDOM statement:

```
random intercept time / subject=subject type=un;
```

Thus, in conclusion, all code for likelihood-based analyses, listed in Section 14.2, can be used, provided the original data sets (`armd155.sas7bdat` and `armd111.sas7bdat`) are passed on, and not the derived ones. Thus generally, with only a minimal amount of care, a direct likelihood analysis is no more complex than the corresponding analysis on a set of data that is free of missingness. The same holds for GEE-based analyses when, for example, the GENMOD procedure is used.

14.5 WEIGHTED ESTIMATING EQUATIONS

We illustrate WGEE by means of the analysis of the age-related macular degeneration trial discussed in Section 13.3.

A GENMOD program for the standard GEE analysis would be:

```
proc genmod data=armdwgee;
class time treat subject;
model bindif = time treat*time / noint dist=binomial;
repeated subject=subject / withinsubject=time type=exch modelse;
run;
```

Likewise, the linearization-based version listed in Section 14.2 can be used without any problem.

Let us now sketch the steps to be taken when conducting a weighted GEE analysis. To compute the weights, one first has to fit the dropout model using, for example, logistic regression. The outcome `dropout` is binary and indicates whether or not dropout occurs at a given time from the start of the measurement sequence until the time of dropout or the end of the sequence. Covariates in the model are the outcomes at previous occasions (`prev`), supplemented with genuine covariate information. The DROPOUT macro, constructed by Caroline Beunckens, is used to construct the variables 'dropout' and 'prev'.

Likewise, once a logistic regression has been fitted, these need to be translated into weights. These weights are defined at the individual measurement level and are equal to the product of the probabilities of not dropping out up to the measurement occasion. The last factor is the probability of either dropping out at that time or continuing the study. This task can be performed with the DROPWGT macro. The arguments are the same as in the DROPOUT macro, except that now also the predicted values from the logistic regression have to be passed on through the `pred=` argument, and the dropout indicator is passed on through the `dropout=` argument.

Using these macros, the following code can be used to prepare for a WGEE analysis:

```
%dropout(data=armd111,id=subject,time=time,
         response=bindif,out=armdhlp);

proc genmod data=armdhlp descending;
class trt prev lesion time;
model dropout = prev trt lesion time / pred dist=binomial;
```

```
ods output obstats=pred;
run;

data pred;
set pred;
keep observation pred;
run;

data armdhlp;
merge pred armdhlp;
run;

%dropwgt(data=armdhlp,id=subject,time=time,pred=pred,
        dropout=dropout,out=armdwgee);
```

To sum up, the dropout indicator and previous outcome variable are defined using the DROPOUT macro, whereupon an ordinary logistic regression is performed. Predicted values are first saved and then merged with the original data. Finally, the predicted values are translated into proper weights using the DROPWGT macro.

After these preparatory steps, we need only include the weights through the WEIGHT (or, equivalently, SCWGT) statement within the GENMOD procedure. This statement identifies a variable in the input data set to be used as the exponential family dispersion parameter weight for each observation. The exponential family dispersion parameter is divided by the WEIGHT variable value for each observation. Whereas the inclusion of the REPEATED statement turns a univariate exponential family model into GEE, the addition of WEIGHT further switches to WGEE. In other words, we just need to add:

```
weight wi;
```

Note that the WEIGHT statement can also be used in the GLIMMIX procedure, thus implying that a weighted version of the linearization-based GEE method is feasible.

14.6   MULTIPLE IMPUTATION

Multiple imputation was introduced in Chapter 9 and its use in a GEE setting exemplified using the age-related macular degeneration trial in Section 13.5.

The three tasks of multiple imputation, imputation, analysis, and inference, can be conducted within SAS. Two key procedures are MI and MIANALYZE. We will discuss each of the tasks in turn. One particular use of the MI procedure is to change non-monotone missingness into monotone missingness. We will devote some attention to this specific job as well.

14.6.1 The MI procedure for the imputation task

PROC MI is used to generate the imputations. It creates M imputed data sets from an input data set, physically stored in a single data set with indicator variable _imputation_ to separate the imputed copies.

There are a variety of imputation mechanisms available (Section 9.6), distinguishing between non-monotone and monotone sequences, and between continuous and categorical variables.

For imputations from a multivariate Gaussian imputation model the following MI program can be used:

```
proc mi data=armd13 seed=486048 out=armd13a
      simple nimpute=10 round=0.1;
var lesion diff4 diff12 diff24 diff52;
by treat;
run;
```

We consider now some of the options available in the PROC MI statement, and used above. The option `simple` displays simple descriptive statistics and pairwise correlations based on available cases in the input data set. The number of imputations is specified by the option `nimpute=`, with a default of 5. The option 'round=' controls the number of decimal places in the imputed values, with no rounding by default. For example, 'round = 0.1' requests a single decimal place. If more than one number is specified, one should use a VAR statement, and the specified numbers must correspond to the number of variables in the VAR statement. The 'seed—' option is used to specify a positive integer which is used by PROC MI to start the pseudo-random number generator. The default is a value generated from the time of day from the computer's clock. Although not essential, it is useful when an analysis needs to be checked afterwards or when a seed is specified by an external source such as a regulatory authority.

The imputation task is carried out separately for each level of the variables specified in the BY statement. For example, when there are several treatment arms, imputation can be done for each arm separately, thus not constraining the imputations in any way with respect to the relevant covariate, such as treatment assignment.

In PROC MI one can choose between one of the three imputation mechanisms. These were discussed in Section 9.6. When missingness is confined to dropout, the MONOTONE statement can, but need not, be used. The parametric regression method `method=reg` as well as the non-parametric propensity score method (`method=propensity`) are available. For general patterns of missingness, the MCMC statement can be used, which is the default as well.

In all cases, especially with MCMC, a number of options are available to flexibly control the imputation task. For example, `ngroups=` specifies the number of groups based on propensity scores when the propensity scores method is used. For the MCMC method, one can give the initial mean and covariance estimates to start the MCMC process by using the `initial=` option. The 'pmm' option in the MCMC statement uses the predictive mean matching method to impute an observed value that is closest to the predicted value in the MCMC method. The `regpmm` option in the MONOTONE statement uses the predictive mean matching method to impute an observed value that is closest to the predicted value for data sets with monotone missingness. One can specify more than one method in the MONOTONE statement, and for each imputed variable the covariates can be specified separately.

Whereas such methods as `propensity` and `regression` are used for incomplete continuous outcomes, incomplete categorical outcomes can be imputed by including them into the CLASS statement, in addition to their inclusion in the VAR statement. In such a case, the MONOTONE option should be used, and one can make use of logistic regression and discriminant analysis imputation by means of the options `logistic` and `discrim`, respectively.

With the (default) `initial=EM` option, the procedure uses the means and standard deviations from available cases as the initial estimates for the EM algorithm. The final estimates after applying the EM algorithm are then used to start the MCMC process. One can also specify `initial=` input SAS-data-set to use an SAS data set with the initial estimates of the mean and covariance matrix for each imputation. Further, the `niter=` option specifies the number of iterations between imputations in a single chain, the default being 100.

Note that, after carrying out the imputation task, the data are in horizontal format and need to put in the longitudinal, or vertical, format again.

We are now ready to continue with the analysis task.

14.6.2   The analysis task

The imputed data sets are then analysed using a standard complete data procedure. It is important to ensure that the BY statement is used to ensure that a separate analysis is carried out for each completed data set:

```
by_imputation_;
```

Parameter estimates and their estimated covariance matrices need to be stored in appropriate output data sets, so they can be passed on to the MIANALYZE procedure which effectively implements Rubin's combination formulae (Section 14.6.3). The MIANALYZE procedure has a generic form, but some care is needed when using it because estimates and accompanying covariance matrices have different names in different SAS procedures, and the output data sets corresponding to these may also be organized somewhat differently. The procedure is able to handle CLASS effects as well, even though a number of columns in the corresponding output data sets are then needed to multi-index the effect.

In spite of this CLASS feature of the MIANALYZE procedure, we recommend creating appropriate indicator variables for categorical effects and interactions, as a form of defensive programming, that is, removing one potential source of error. This also facilitates direct mapping between GEE and generalized linear mixed model parameters, using, respectively, the GENMOD and NLMIXED procedures.

To prepare for the analysis, indicator variables are created and then the data are sorted by imputation number.

```
data armd13c;
set armd13b;
time1=0;
time2=0;
time3=0;
time4=0;
trttime1=0;
trttime2=0;
trttime3=0;
trttime4=0;
if time=1 then time1=1;
if time=2 then time2=1;
if time=3 then time3=1;
if time=4 then time4=1;
if (time=1 & treat=1) then trttime1=1;
if (time=2 & treat=1) then trttime2=1;
if (time=3 & treat=1) then trttime3=1;
if (time=4 & treat=1) then trttime4=1;
run;

proc sort data=armd13c;
by _imputation_ subject time;
run;
```

The GENMOD procedure can then be called for a GEE analysis, similar to the one presented at the start of Section 14.5:

```
proc genmod data=armd13c;
class time subject;
by _imputation_;
model bindif = time1 time2 time3 time4
            trttime1 trttime2 trttime3 trttime4
   / noint dist=binomial covb;
repeated subject=subject
         / withinsubject=time type=exch modelse;
ods output ParameterEstimates=gmparms
           parminfo=gmpinfo CovB=gmcovb;
run;
```

Apart from an otherwise irrelevant change to user-defined coding indicator variables for the categorical covariates in the model, the BY statement has been added, as well as the ODS statement, to store the parameter estimates and the covariance parameters. For the latter, the `parminfo=` option is used next to the `covb=` option, to ensure the proper names of the covariate effects are mapped to abbreviations of type `Prm1`, etc. Note that the `covb=` output option works only because the `covb` option was included in the MODEL statement. The parameter estimates are generated by default. The direct output of the GENMOD procedure will be a GEE analysis for each of the ten imputed data sets. As such, they represent an intermediate step in the full multiple imputation analysis and are of no direct scientific interest. Formal inference needs to be conducted only using the results from the inference task (Section 14.6.3).

Because the `noint` option was included, the effect `Prm1` formally exists but it is unavailable as a parameter estimate. It is therefore prudent to delete it from the parameter information:

```
data gmpinfo;
set gmpinfo;
if parameter='Prm1' then delete;
run;
```

Analogously, the generalized linear mixed model analysis can be conducted on the multiply-imputed data sets:

```
proc nlmixed data=armd13c qpoints=20 maxiter=100
     technique=newrap cov ecov;
by _imputation_;
eta = beta11*time1+beta12*time2+beta13*time3+beta14*time4+b
     +beta21*trttime1+beta22*trttime2
     +beta23*trttime3+beta24*trttime4;
p = exp(eta)/(1+exp(eta));
model bindif ~ binary(p);
random b ~ normal(0,tau*tau) subject=subject;
estimate 'tau2' tau*tau;
ods output ParameterEstimates=nlparms
          CovMatParmEst=nlcovb
          AdditionalEstimates=nlparmsa
          CovMatAddEst=nlcovba;
run;
```

Apart from the BY statement, four output data sets are generated using the ODS statement. For the standard model parameters, we only need the `parameterestimates=` and `covmatparmest=` options. If, in addition, multiple imputation inference is requested about additional estimates, then they can be saved as well using the `additionalestimates=` and `covmataddest=` options. However, it is probably better to calculate the additional estimates directly from the results of the inference task, that is, to conduct multiple imputation inference and then calculate additional estimates, rather than the other way around. For both covariance matrices to be generated, the options `cov` and `ecov`, respectively, need to be included into the PROC NLMIXED statement.

For both models, we can now conduct the multiple imputation inference, following Rubin's combination rules as explained in Section 9.2.

14.6.3   The inference task

Finally, PROC MIANALYZE combines the M inferences into a single one, by making use of Rubin's formulae as set out in Section 9.2. Parameter and standard errors are passed on through a combination of the `data=`, `parms=`, `covb=`, and/or `xpxi=` options to the PROC MIANALYZE statement. Using `data=`, data sets of types COV, CORR, or EST can be passed on, as well as a data set containing parameter estimates and standard errors. When one wishes to pass on parameter estimates and variance–covariance matrices instead, it is better to use `parms=` and `covb=` or `parms=` and `xpxi=`. When the `covb=` matrices contain generic names (`Prm1,...`), the mapping between generic and actual parameter names is passed on using `parminfo=`.

Several options for fine-tuning are also available in PROC MIANALYZE. For example, the within-imputation, between-imputation, and total covariance matrices are printed upon including the `wcov`, `bcov`, and `tcov` options, respectively.

The parameters or effects for which multiple imputation inference is needed are passed on by means of the MODELEFFECTS statement (previously VAR statement). Categorical effects are handled as well, after including them in the CLASS statement. As stated earlier, it is safer to create appropriate indicator variables and avoid the use of the CLASS statement, as sometimes the mapping between parameter estimates and the corresponding precision parameters is not straightforward. In principle, the MIANALYZE procedure works after applying any standard analysis, using an SAS procedure, in the analysis task, from SAS Version 9.1 onwards.

The TEST statement allows testing for hypotheses about linear combinations of the parameters. The statement is based on Rubin (1987), and uses a t distribution which is the univariate version of the work by Li *et al.* and Rubin (1991), described in Section 9.4.

Applying the procedure to the GEE analysis on the age-related macular degeneration data, presented in Section 14.6.2, can be done using the following code:

```
proc mianalyze parms=gmparms covb=gmcovb
              parminfo=gmpinfo wcov bcov tcov;
modeleffects time1 time2 time3 time4
             trttime1 trttime2 trttime3 trttime4;
run;
```

Compared to the MI procedure, the MIANALYZE procedure is rather simple, in line with the simplicity and elegance of the pooling method of Section 9.4.

Conducting multiple imputation inference for the NLMIXED analysis, presented in Section 14.6.2, is done as follows:

```
proc mianalyze parms=nlparms covb=nlcovb
                wcov bcov tcov;
modeleffects beta11 beta12 beta13 beta14
              beta21 beta22 beta23 beta24;
run;
```

14.6.4 The MI procedure to create monotone missingness

When missingness is non-monotone, it is likely that several mechanisms operate simultaneously: for example, a simple (MCAR or MAR) mechanism for the intermediate missing values and a more complex (MNAR) mechanism for the missing data past the moment of dropout. However, analysing such data is complicated because many model strategies, especially those under the assumption of MNAR, but also WGEE, have been developed for dropout only or at least work in a considerably simpler way under monotone missingness. Therefore, a solution might be to generate multiple imputations that render the data sets monotone missing, by including in PROC MI:

```
mcmc impute = monotone;
```

and then to apply a method of choice to the multiple sets of data thus completed. Note that this is different from the monotone method in the MI procedure. The latter in fact does the opposite: it fully completes already monotone sets of data.

The other value for the `impute=` option is `impute=full`, which is also the default. This method implies that all missing values are imputed, whether monotone or non-monotone.

Part IV
Missing Not at Random

15

Selection Models

15.1 INTRODUCTION

Even though the assumption of likelihood ignorability encompasses both MAR
and the more stringent and often implausible MCAR mechanisms, in most real
settings it is impossible to exclude the possibility of a more general missingness
mechanism. One solution is to fit an MNAR model as proposed, for example,
by Diggle and Kenward (1994) who fitted models to the full data using the
simplex algorithm (Nelder and Mead 1965). This model, devised for Gaussian
outcomes, as well as counterparts for the non-Gaussian case, are presented
in this chapter. However, it is important to realize, as pointed out by several
authors (discussion to Diggle and Kenward 1994; Verbeke and Molenberghs
2000, Chapter 18; Molenberghs and Verbeke 2005, Chapter 31), that one has
to be extremely careful in interpreting evidence for or against MNAR using only
the data under analysis.

A sensible compromise between blindly shifting to MNAR models and
ignoring them altogether is to make them a component of a sensitivity
analysis. Such analyses typically will explore the dependence of conclusions
on assumptions that cannot be assessed from the data under analysis, which
usually means departures from the MAR assumption. In that sense, it is
important to consider the effect on key parameters such as treatment effect, or
evolution over time. We will return to sensitivity analysis in Part V.

In Section 15.2 we present the aforementioned model of Diggle and Kenward
(1994), together with some remarks on sensitivity analysis. The method
is illustrated, along with its implementation in SAS, in Section 15.3. In
Section 15.4 a counterpart for categorical data, introduced by Molenberghs *et al.*
(1997) is described. Both of these models have been constructed for monotone

Missing Data in Clinical Studies   G. Molenberghs and M.G. Kenward
© 2007 John Wiley & Sons, Ltd

missingness. A version of the categorical data model by Baker *et al.* (1992), able to cope with general missingness, is discussed in Section 15.5.

15.2   THE DIGGLE–KENWARD MODEL FOR CONTINUOUS OUTCOMES

We assume that for subject i, $i = 1, \ldots, N$, a sequence of measurements Y_{ij} is designed to be measured at time points t_{ij}, $j = 1, \ldots, n_i$, resulting in a vector $Y_i = (Y_{i1}, \ldots, Y_{in_i})'$ of measurements for each participant. If dropout occurs, Y_i is only partially observed. We denote the occasion at which dropout occurs by $D_i > 1$, and Y_i is split into the $(D_i - 1)$-dimensional observed component Y_i^o and the $(n_i - D_i + 1)$-dimensional missing component Y_i^m. In the case of no dropout, we let $D_i = n_i + 1$, and Y_i equals Y_i^o. The likelihood contribution of the ith subject, based on the observed data (y_i^o, d_i), is proportional to the marginal density function

$$f(y_i, d_i | \theta, \psi) = \int f(y_i, d_i | \theta, \psi) \, dy_i^m$$

$$= \int f(y_i | \theta) f(d_i | y_i, \psi) \, dy_i^m, \qquad (15.1)$$

in which a marginal model for Y_i is combined with a model for the dropout process, conditional on the response, and where θ and ψ are vectors of unknown parameters in the measurement model and dropout model, respectively.

Let $h_{ij} = (y_{i1}, \ldots, y_{i,j-1})$ denote the observed history of subject i up to time $t_{i,j-1}$. The Diggle–Kenward model for the dropout process allows the conditional probability for dropout at occasion j, given that the subject was still observed at the previous occasion, to depend on the history h_{ij} and the possibly unobserved current outcome y_{ij}, but not on future outcomes y_{ik}, $k > j$. These conditional probabilities $P(D_i = j | D_i \geq j, h_{ij}, y_{ij}, \psi)$ can now be used to calculate the probability of dropout at each occasion:

$$P(D_i = j | y_i, \psi) = P(D_i = j | h_{ij}, y_{ij}, \psi)$$

$$= \begin{cases} P(D_i = j | D_i \geq j, h_{ij}, y_{ij}, \psi) & j = 2 \\ P(D_i = j | D_i \geq j, h_{ij}, y_{ij}, \psi) \\ \quad \times \prod_{k=2}^{j-1} [1 - P(D_i = k | D_i \geq k, h_{ik}, y_{ik}, \psi)] & j = 3, \ldots, n_i \quad (15.2) \\ \prod_{k=2}^{n_i} [1 - P(D_i = k | D_i \geq k, h_{ik}, y_{ik}, \psi)] & j = n_i + 1. \end{cases}$$

Diggle and Kenward (1994) combine a multivariate normal model for the measurement process with a logistic regression model for the dropout process. More specifically, the measurement model assumes that the vector

Y_i of repeated measurements for the ith subject satisfies the linear regression model $Y_i \sim N(X_i\boldsymbol{\beta}, V_i)$, $i = 1, \ldots, N$. The matrix V_i can be left unstructured or assumed to be of a specific form, for example, resulting from a linear mixed model, a factor-analytic structure, or spatial covariance structure (Verbeke and Molenberghs 2000). A commonly used version of such a logistic dropout model is

$$\text{logit}\left[P(D_i = j \mid D_i \geq j, \boldsymbol{h}_{ij}, y_{ij}, \boldsymbol{\psi})\right] = \psi_0 + \psi_1 y_{ij} + \psi_2 y_{i,j-1}. \tag{15.3}$$

More general models can easily be constructed by including the complete history $\boldsymbol{h}_{ij} = (y_{i1}, \ldots, y_{i,j-1})$, as well as external covariates, in the above conditional dropout model. Note also that, strictly speaking, one could allow dropout at a specific occasion to be related to all future responses as well. However, in many settings this is rather counterintuitive. Moreover, including future outcomes seriously complicates the calculations since computation of the likelihood (15.1) then requires evaluation of a possibly high-dimensional integral. The special cases of model (15.3) corresponding to MAR and MCAR are obtained from setting $\psi_1 = 0$ or $\psi_1 = \psi_2 = 0$, respectively. In the first case, dropout is no longer allowed to depend on the current measurement, and in the second case, dropout is independent of the outcome altogether.

Diggle and Kenward (1994) obtained parameter and precision estimates by means of maximum likelihood. The likelihood involves marginalization over the unobserved outcomes Y_i^m. In practice, this involves relatively tedious and computationally demanding forms of numerical integration. This, combined with likelihood surfaces tending to be rather flat or otherwise awkward in shape, makes the model difficult to use. These issues are related to the problems to be discussed next.

Apart from the technical difficulties encountered during parameter estimation, there are further important issues surrounding MNAR-based models. Even when the measurement model (e.g., the multivariate normal model) would be the choice for describing the measurement process *should the data be complete*, the analysis of the actually observed, incomplete version is, in addition, subject to further untestable modelling assumptions. As such, a particular MNAR model should not be used to provide definitive conclusions from a trial, rather each can be used to produce conclusions that would apply if certain specific (untestable) assumptions about the dropout mechanism were true.

When missingness is MAR, the problems are less complex, since it has been shown that, in a likelihood or Bayesian framework, it is sufficient to analyse the observed data, without explicitly modelling the dropout process (Rubin 1976; Verbeke and Molenberghs 2000). However, the very assumption of MAR is itself untestable, an issue taken up in Chapter 19. Therefore, ignoring MNAR models is no different an option than shifting to one particular MNAR model, it is just much more convenient. A sensible compromise between considering a single MNAR model, on the one hand, and excluding such models from consideration, on the other hand, is to study the nature of such sensitivities and, building on this knowledge, formulate ways for conducting sensitivity analyses. Indeed, a strong conclusion, arising from most sensitivity analysis work, is that MNAR models have to be approached cautiously. This was made clear by several discussants to the original paper by Diggle and Kenward (1994), in particular Laird, Little, and Rubin, and similar points have been made by many since, among them Scharfstein *et al.* (1999).

One related issue is that formal tests for the null hypothesis of MAR versus the alternative of MNAR should be approached with the utmost caution, a topic studied in detail by Jansen *et al.* (2006b). This point is elaborated on in Chapter 20 below. Verbeke *et al.* (2001a) have shown, in the context of an onychomycosis study, that excluding a small amount of measurement error can change drastically the likelihood ratio test statistics for the MAR null hypothesis; see also Verbeke and Molenberghs (2000, Chapter 17). Kenward (1998) revisited the analysis of the mastitis data performed by Diggle and Kenward (1994). In this study, the milk yields of 107 cows were to be recorded for two consecutive years. While the data were complete in the first year, 27 animals were missing in the second year because they developed mastitis and their milk yield was no longer of use. While in Diggle and Kenward (1994) there was some evidence for MNAR, Kenward (1998) showed that removing two out of 107 anomalous profiles completely negated this evidence. In addition, he showed that changing the conditional distribution of the year 2 yield, given the year 1 yield, from a normal distribution to a heavy-tailed t also led to the same result of no residual evidence for MNAR; see also Section 22.3. This particular conditional distribution is of great importance, because a subject with missing data does not contribute to it, and hence is a source of sensitivity issues. Once more, the conclusion is that fitting an MNAR model should be subject to careful scrutiny.

We will return to these issues, at length, in Part V. Such issues concerning the use of MNAR models should be borne in mind throughout the following development.

15.3 ILLUSTRATION AND SAS IMPLEMENTATION

Consider a heart failure study in which the primary efficacy endpoint is based upon the ability to do physical exercise, measured as the number of seconds a subject is able to ride an exercise bike. There are 25 subjects assigned to placebo and 25 to treatment. The treatment consisted of the administration of angiotensin-converting enzyme inhibitors. Four measurements were taken, at monthly intervals. Table 15.1 presents outcome scores, transformed to normality. We will refer to them as the exercise bike data. All 50 subjects are observed at the first occasion, whereas there are 44, 41, and 38 subjects

Table 15.1 Exercise bike data.

Placebo				Treatment			
1	2	3	4	1	2	3	4
0.43	0.94	4.32	4.51	−2.54	−0.20	−0.15	3.53
3.10	5.82	5.59	6.32	4.33	5.57	6.86	6.87
0.56	2.21	1.18	1.54	−2.46	—	—	—
−1.18	−0.30	2.48	2.67	2.30	4.64	7.37	7.99
1.24	2.83	1.98	3.21	0.73	3.29	5.23	6.12
−1.87	−0.06	1.16	1.84	0.38	1.25	2.91	4.71
−0.28	1.30	—	—	1.51	4.00	5.98	—
2.93	—	—	—	0.38	0.94	3.28	4.05
−0.20	3.34	3.71	3.69	0.42	2.53	—	—
−0.12	2.01	2.35	2.70	2.41	4.24	4.79	8.14
−1.60	1.42	0.41	0.72	0.12	1.48	3.12	3.69
0.64	—	—	—	−3.46	−0.93	2.78	3.02
−1.14	−1.20	0.09	2.39	−0.55	—	—	—
2.24	2.12	3.00	1.52	0.74	2.40	4.04	5.61
−0.44	0.88	2.83	1.47	2.37	2.79	4.05	5.91
0.39	1.77	3.62	4.35	1.94	5.05	3.06	5.89
−4.37	−2.43	−0.43	−0.13	0.77	2.46	—	—
0.20	2.05	3.18	5.13	1.32	—	—	—
1.31	3.82	2.70	3.59	2.15	4.84	7.70	8.29
−0.38	−1.92	−0.12	−0.40	−0.09	2.02	4.68	5.29
−0.78	—	—	—	2.10	4.91	7.48	8.91
−0.48	0.32	0.66	3.03	1.36	0.62	1.87	—
−0.64	1.53	1.29	—	3.14	5.79	5.95	7.50
0.88	2.10	1.90	3.51	−0.94	−0.08	3.57	3.80
2.02	3.10	4.93	4.76	0.89	1.51	3.14	5.96

seen at the second, third, and fourth visits, respectively. Individual and mean profiles by treatment arm are shown in Figures 15.1 and 15.2, respectively. The percentage of patients that are still in the study after each visit is tabulated in Table 15.2 by treatment arm.

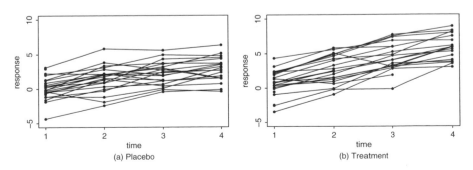

(a) Placebo   (b) Treatment

Figure 15.1 Exercise bike data. Individual profiles by treatment arm.

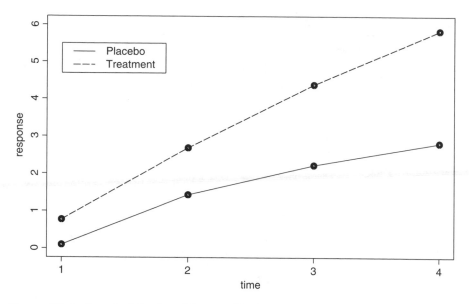

Figure 15.2   Exercise bike data. Mean profiles by treatment arm.

Table 15.2   Exercise bike data. Percentage of patients still in study, by treatment arm.

Visit	Placebo	Treatment
1	100	100
2	88	88
3	84	80
4	80	72

A SAS program has been written by Caroline Beunckens that maximizes the log-likelihood for this model using PROC IML. This has also been reported in Dmitrienko *et al.* (2005). A linear mixed model is used for the measurement process (Section 7.3) that allows the inclusion of a variety of fixed effects, a random intercept, and Gaussian serial correlation. This implies the marginal variance–covariance matrix V_i becomes

$$V_i = dJ_n + \sigma^2 I_n + \tau^2 H_i, \tag{15.4}$$

where J_n is an $n \times n$ matrix with all elements equal to 1, I_n is the $n \times n$ identity matrix, and H_i is determined through the autocorrelation function $\rho^{u_{jk}}$, with u_{jk} the Euclidean distance between t_{ij} and t_{ik}:

$$H_i = \begin{pmatrix} 1 & \rho^{u_{12}} & \cdots & \rho^{u_{1n}} \\ \rho^{u_{12}} & 1 & \cdots & \rho^{u_{2n}} \\ \vdots & \vdots & \ddots & \vdots \\ \rho^{u_{1n}} & \rho^{u_{2n}} & \cdots & 1 \end{pmatrix}.$$

The program can easily be adapted for alternative model forms by merely changing the V_i matrix. A general, flexible macro is available.

The program needs matrices x and z, which contain all the X_i and Z_i design matrices $(i = 1, \ldots, N)$, and the vector y of all Y_i response vectors $(i = 1, \ldots, N)$. Next, initial is a vector of initial values for the parameters in the model. Finally, nsub and ntime are the number of subjects N and the number of time points n, respectively.

In the program, the module integr calculates the integral over the missing data. Next, the module loglik evaluates the log-likelihood function $L(\theta, \psi)$ and maximizes over it. Diggle and Kenward (1994) used the simplex algorithm (Nelder and Mead 1965) for this purpose; however, here we use the Newton–Raphson ridge optimization method (call nlpnrr), since it combines stability and speed. However, in other analyses, it may be necessary to try (several) other optimization methods, and several alternatives are available in SAS.

The program calls nlpnrr as follows:

```
call nlpnrr(rc,xr,"loglik",initial,opt,con);
```

Here, "loglik" is the module of the function we want to maximize. The initial values to start the optimization method are listed in initial. The opt argument indicates an options vector that specifies details of the optimization process. Maximization instead of minimization is indicated by opt[1]=1. The output printed is controlled by opt[2], which will yield summaries for the optimization start and termination, the iteration history, and initial as well as final parameter estimates. A constraint matrix is specified in con, defining lower and upper bounds for the parameters in the first two rows. Constraints, necessary in this case, are $d > 0$, $\tau^2 > 0$, and $\sigma^2 > 0$. Finally, all optimization methods return the following results: the scalar return code rc and a row vector xr. The return code rc indicates the reason for the termination of the optimization process. A positive return code indicates successful termination, whereas a negative one indicates unsuccessful termination, that is, that the result xr is unreliable. The row vector xr contains the optimal point when the return code is positive.

The program also calls nlpfdd, which is a subroutine for approximating derivatives by finite-difference methods:

```
call nlpfdd(maxlik,grad,hessian,"loglik",est);
```

Here, again "loglik" is the module of the log-likelihood function. The vector specifying the point at which the functions and derivatives should be computed is `est`. This subroutine computes the function values `maxlik` (which is in this case the maximum likelihood, since `est` is the maximum likelihood estimate), the gradient vector `grad`, and the Hessian matrix `hessian` (which is needed to calculate the information matrix, and thus the standard errors `stde`).

We now fit the Diggle–Kenward model under MCAR, MAR, and MNAR to the exercise bike data. Dropout will also be allowed to depend on covariates.

To obtain initial values for the parameters of the measurement model, we fit a linear mixed model to the exercise bike data using the SAS procedure MIXED. We assume a linear trend within each treatment group. This implies that each profile can be described using an intercept and a slope. For subject $i = 1, \ldots, 50$ at time point $j = 1, \ldots, 4$, the model can be expressed as

$$Y_{ij} = \beta_0 + \beta_1 (\text{group}_i - 1) + \beta_2 t_j (\text{group}_i - 1) + \beta_3 t_j \text{group}_i + \varepsilon_{ij},$$

where $\varepsilon_i \sim N(\mathbf{0}, V_i)$ and $V_i = dJ_4 + \sigma^2 I_4 + \tau^2 H_i$, with

$$H_i = \begin{pmatrix} 1 & \rho & \rho^2 & \rho^3 \\ \rho & 1 & \rho & \rho^2 \\ \rho^2 & \rho & 1 & \rho \\ \rho^3 & \rho^2 & \rho & 1 \end{pmatrix}.$$

The intercept for the placebo group is $\beta_0 + \beta_1$, and the intercept for the treatment group is β_0. The slopes are β_2 and β_3, respectively. The following code can be used:

```
proc mixed data=b.bike method=ml;
class group id;
model y = group time*group / solution;
repeated / type=ar(1) local subject=id;
random intercept / type=un subject=id;
run;
```

The resulting initial values are shown in Table 15.3.

The general dropout mechanism takes the form:

$$\text{logit} \left[P(D_i = j \mid D_i \geq j, \mathbf{h}_{ij}, y_{ij}, \boldsymbol{\psi}) \right] = \psi_0 + \psi_1 y_{i,j-1} + \psi_2 y_{ij} + \gamma \, \text{group}_i. \quad (15.5)$$

The general expression allows for missingness to be MNAR and to depend on group. Simpler dropout mechanisms follow in obvious ways. For example, when no covariates are allowed to influence dropout, $\gamma \equiv 0$. MAR is implied by $\psi_2 \equiv 0$, and finally, for MCAR, $\psi_1 \equiv 0$ in addition. Parameter estimates resulting from the model fit under the three missingness mechanisms, together with the estimates of the ignorable analysis using the MIXED procedure, are listed in Table 15.4.

The results of the measurement model should be the same under the ignorable, MCAR, and MAR assumptions. As we can see from Table 15.4, this is

Table 15.3 Exercise bike data. Parameter estimates of the linear mixed model, used as initial values for the Diggle–Kenward model.

Effect	Parameter	Estimate	Rounded to initial value
Treatment intercept	β_0	−0.8233	−0.82
Difference intercepts	β_1	0.1605	0.16
Placebo slope	β_2	0.9227	0.92
Treatment slope	β_3	1.6451	1.65
Random-intercept variance	d	2.0811	2.08
Serial process variance	τ^2	0.7912	0.79
Serial process correlation	ρ	0.4639	0.46
Measurement error variance	σ^2	0.2311	0.23

Table 15.4 Exercise bike data. Parameter estimates (standard errors) under ignorable, MCAR, MAR, and MNAR assumptions, with and without covariate in the dropout model for the latter case.

Parameter	Ignorable	MCAR	MAR	MNAR	MNAR+ Covariate
β_0	−0.82 (0.39)	−0.82 (0.40)	−0.82 (0.40)	−0.83 (0.40)	−0.82 (0.40)
β_1	0.16 (0.56)	0.16 (0.56)	0.16 (0.56)	0.17 (0.56)	0.16 (0.56)
β_2	0.92 (0.10)	0.92 (0.10)	0.92 (0.10)	0.93 (0.10)	0.92 (0.10)
β_3	1.65 (0.10)	1.65 (0.10)	1.65 (0.10)	1.66 (0.11)	1.64 (0.11)
d	2.08 (0.90)	2.08 (0.91)	2.08 (0.90)	2.09 (0.85)	2.07 (0.96)
τ^2	0.79 (0.54)	0.79 (0.55)	0.79 (0.55)	0.80 (0.70)	0.79 (0.45)
ρ	0.46 (1.10)	0.46 (1.13)	0.46 (1.12)	0.44 (1.12)	0.49 (1.13)
σ^2	0.23 (1.08)	0.23 (1.11)	0.23 (1.11)	0.21 (1.24)	0.25 (1.02)
ψ_0		−2.33 (0.30)	−2.17 (0.36)	−2.42 (0.88)	−1.60 (1.14)
ψ_1			−0.10 (0.14)	−0.24 (0.43)	−0.02 (0.47)
ψ_2				0.16 (0.47)	−0.13 (0.54)
γ					−0.66 (0.79)
-2ℓ		641.77	641.23	641.11	640.44

more or less the case, except for some of the variance components, due to slight numerical variation. This points to the numerical instabilities brought about by fitting the Diggle–Kenward model, a common occurrence with MNAR selection models. Adding the covariate to the dropout model results in a deviance change of 0.67, which means the covariate is not significant ($p = 0.413$). A likelihood ratio test for the MAR versus MNAR assumption ($\psi_2 = 0$ or not), cannot be compared to the usual conventional reference χ^2 distribution (Jansen *et al.* 2006b). We return to this issue in Chapter 20. Under the MNAR assumption, the estimates for ψ_1 and ψ_2 are more or less equal, but with different signs. This feature is commonly observed, as it is in Diggle and Kenward's original paper. We will see further instances in Chapters 20 and 22, when analysing the mastitis data set, and in Chapter 26, when the vorozole data are analysed.

The interpretation is that missingness depends on the increment of the outcome between two subsequent measurements, rather than on the size, for example captured by means of the average of two subsequent measurements.

The macros used are discussed in more detail in Dmitrienko *et al.* (2005). They can be found on the authors' website.

15.4   AN MNAR DALE MODEL

Molenberghs *et al.* (1997) proposed a model for longitudinal ordinal data with non-random dropout, similar in spirit to the Diggle–Kenward model presented in the previous section. Rather than using a normal distribution, the vector of repeated ordinal measures is assumed to follow a multivariate Dale model (Dale 1986; Molenberghs and Lesaffre 1994; Molenberghs and Verbeke 2005, Section 7.7). The resulting likelihood can be maximized relatively easily using the EM algorithm, because all outcomes are of a categorical type. It means that the integration over the missing data, needed to maximize the likelihood of Diggle and Kenward (1994), is replaced by a finite sum.

15.4.1   Likelihood function

We derive a general form for the likelihood for longitudinal data with non-random dropout and introduce particular functional forms for the response, using the multivariate Dale model developed by Molenberghs and Lesaffre (1994), and for the dropout process, using a simple logistic regression formulation.

Assume we have $r = 1, \ldots, N$ design levels in the study, characterized by covariate information X_r. Let there be N_r subjects at design level r. Let the outcome for subject i at level r be a c-level ordinal categorical outcome designed to be measured at occasions $j = 1, \ldots, n$, and denoted by Y_{rij}. We could allow the number of measurement occasions to be different across subjects, but in an incomplete data setting it is often sensible to assume that the number of measurements at the design stage is constant. Extension to the more general case is straightforward.

The outcomes at level r are grouped into a contingency table $Z_r^{c*}(k_1 \ldots k_n)$. The cumulative version is $Z_r^c(k_1 \ldots k_n)$, defined by

$$Z_r^c(\boldsymbol{k}) = \sum_{\boldsymbol{\ell} \leq \boldsymbol{k}} Z_r^{c*}(\boldsymbol{\ell}),$$

in which $\boldsymbol{\ell} \leq \boldsymbol{k}$ can be written out as $(l_1, \ldots, l_n) \leq (k_1, \ldots, k_n)$, meaning that $l_j \leq k_j, j = 1, \ldots, n$. The superscript c refers to the, possibly hypothetical, complete data. The corresponding cell probabilities are $\mu_r^{c*}(\boldsymbol{k})$ and $\mu_r^c(\boldsymbol{k})$. The corresponding vectors are $\boldsymbol{Z}^{c*}$, $\boldsymbol{Z}^c$, $\boldsymbol{\mu}^{c*}$, and $\boldsymbol{\mu}^c$, respectively.

Any full model for the vector of outcomes can be used. At the heart of the model is a set of link functions:

$$\eta_r^c(\mu_r^c) = X_r^c \beta. \tag{15.6}$$

We also need to model the missingness or, in this particular case, the dropout process. Assume the random variable D can take values $2, \ldots, n+1$, the time at which a subject drops out, where $D = n+1$ indicates no dropout. The value $D = 1$ is not included since we assume at least one follow-up measurement is available. The hypothetical full data consist of the complete data and the dropout indicator. The full data, $\mathbf{Z}_r^{c*}$, contain components $Z_{rdk_1 \ldots k_n}^{c*}$ with joint probabilities

$$\nu_{rdk_1 \ldots k_n}^{c*} = \mu_{rk_1 \ldots k_n}^{c*}(\boldsymbol{\beta}) \, \phi_{rd|k_1 \ldots k_n}(\boldsymbol{\psi}), \tag{15.7}$$

where the $\boldsymbol{\psi}$ parameterizes the dropout probabilities $\phi_{rd|k_1 \ldots k_n}$. We typically assume both parameters are distinct but this is, strictly speaking, not necessary.

Assume that the distribution of D may depend both on the past history of the process, denoted by $H_d = (k_1, \ldots, k_{d-1})$ for $D = d$, and the current outcome category k_d, but not on the process after that time. The advantage in modelling terms is that the set of unobserved outcomes, relevant to the modelling task, is a singleton. Also, it is usually deemed plausible in time-ordered longitudinal data that there is no a additional information on the dropout process in the future measurements, given the history and the current, possibly unobserved, measurement.

The factorization (15.7) was done in terms of cell probabilities, superscripted with $*$. The factorization in terms of cumulative probabilities is identical and obtained upon dropping the superscript $*$. Consequently,

$$\phi_{rd|k_1 \ldots k_n}^{c*}(\boldsymbol{\psi}) = \phi_{rd|k_1 \ldots k_d}^{c*}(\boldsymbol{\psi})$$

$$= \begin{cases} \prod_{t=2}^{d-1} [1 - p_{rt}(H_t, k_t; \boldsymbol{\psi})] \, p_{rd}(H_d, k_d; \boldsymbol{\psi}) & \text{if } D \leq n, \\ \prod_{t=2}^{n} [1 - p_{rt}(H_t, k_t; \boldsymbol{\psi})] & \text{if } D = n+1. \end{cases} \tag{15.8}$$

where

$$p_{rd}(H_d, k_d; \boldsymbol{\psi}) = P(D = d | D \geq d, H_d, k_d; W_r; \boldsymbol{\psi}).$$

Here, W_r is a set of covariates, used to model the dropout process. Expression (15.8) is similar to the ones in Section 10.4 used in the context of weighted generalized estimating equations. The difference is that here dropout is allowed to depend on the current, possibly unobserved, measurement.

Molenberghs *et al.* (1997) specified the model for the dropout probabilities by logit links in the same way as in the Diggle–Kenward model, assuming a linear relationship between the log odds and the original response. However, the latter is not necessary. For example, non-linear relations and ones involving interactions between the response variables and the covariates could be used. In the following formulation, we expect that dropout does not depend on observations preceding k_{d-1}, and thus only depends on k_{d-1} and k_d, but an extension would be straightforward:

$$\text{logit}[p_{rd}(H_d, k_d; \boldsymbol{\psi})] = \psi_0 + \psi_1 k_{d-1} + \psi_2 k_d.$$

This model can also be extended by allowing dependence on covariates W_r. The case $\psi_2 = 0$ corresponds to an MAR dropout process and the case $\psi_1 = \psi_2 = 0$ to an MCAR dropout process.

When dropout occurs, $\mathbf{Z}_r^c$ will not be observed but only $\mathbf{Z}_r$, a partially classified table, with corresponding probabilities $\boldsymbol{\nu}_r$. The components of $\boldsymbol{\nu}_r$ are simple linear functions of the components of $\boldsymbol{\nu}_r^c$. This is true for both the cell counts and the cumulative counts.

The multinomial log-likelihood is

$$\ell(\boldsymbol{\beta}, \boldsymbol{\psi}; \mathbf{Z}^*) = \ln\left(\frac{1}{\prod_1^N \mathbf{Z}_r^*!}\right) + \sum_{r=1}^N (\mathbf{Z}_r^*)' \ln(\boldsymbol{\nu}_r), \tag{15.9}$$

with the components of $\boldsymbol{\nu}_r$ summing to one. The kernel of the log-likelihood is the sum of two contributions. For the complete sequences we have

$$\ell_1(\boldsymbol{\beta}, \boldsymbol{\psi}; \mathbf{Z}^*) = \sum_{r=1}^N \sum_{(k_1,\ldots,k_n)} Z_{r,n+1,k_1,\ldots,k_n}^*$$

$$\times \log\left\{\mu_{rk_1\ldots k_n}^*(\boldsymbol{\beta}) \prod_{t=2}^n [1 - p_{rt}(H_t, k_d; \boldsymbol{\psi})]\right\},$$

and similarly for the incomplete sequences (say, $r = N_1 + 1, \ldots, N = N_1 + N_2$)

$$\ell_2(\boldsymbol{\beta}, \boldsymbol{\psi}; \mathbf{Z}^*) = \sum_{r=1}^N \sum_{d=2}^n \sum_{(k_1,\ldots,k_{d-1})} Z_{rdk_1\ldots k_{d-1}}^*$$

$$\times \ln\left\{\prod_{t=2}^{d-1} [1 - p_{rt}(H_t, k_t; \boldsymbol{\psi})] \sum_{k_d=1}^c \mu_{rk_1\ldots k_d}^* p_{rd}(H_d, k_d; \boldsymbol{\psi})\right\}.$$

We note that, when the probability of dropout does not depend on k_d, that is, when the dropout process is MAR, the second part of the likelihood partitions into two components, the first for the response process involving $\boldsymbol{\beta}$ only and the second for the dropout process involving $\boldsymbol{\psi}$ only. When the missingness mechanism is MNAR, the resulting likelihood is complex, but the processes of maximization for $\boldsymbol{\beta}$ and for $\boldsymbol{\psi}$ can be separated through the use of the EM algorithm (Dempster *et al.* 1977; see Chapter 8 above). Details are provided in Molenberghs *et al.* (1997) and in Molenberghs and Verbeke (2005, Section 29.2.2).

15.4.2 Analysis of the fluvoxamine trial

These data were introduced in Section 2.6 and then analysed in Section 12.6. From the initially recruited subjects, 14 were not observed at all after the start, 31 and 44 patients respectively were observed on the first only and first and second occasions, and 224 had complete observations. We omit from the current analyses two patients with non-monotone missing values, leaving 299 in the current analyses. We summarize the therapeutic and side-effects results in two sets of contingency tables, Tables 15.5 and 15.6.

For the data on therapeutic effect as well as on side effects we present four sets of parameter estimates. Each set is the result of fitting a marginal proportional odds model to the response and, for MNAR models, a logistic regression model to the dropout process. In the first set, the response model alone is fitted to the data from those subjects with complete records. Such an analysis will be

Table 15.5 Fluvoxamine trial. Summary of the ordinal therapeutic outcomes at three follow-up times. (For example, category 241 corresponds to a classification of 2 on the first visit, 4 on the second visit, and 1 on the third visit; a * in one of the positions indicates dropout.)

Category	No.	Category	No.	Category	No.	Category	No.
Completers							
111	10	211	32	311	12	411	1
112		212	1	312	1	412	
113		213		313		413	
114		214	1	314		414	
121	1	221	13	321	35	421	5
122		222	16	322	14	422	5
123	1	223	1	323	1	423	
124		224	3	324	1	424	1
131		231	1	331	6	431	13
132		232	2	332	5	432	13
133		233	2	333	3	433	5
134		234		334	1	434	
141		241	1	341	1	441	4
142		242		342	2	442	2
143		243	1	343		443	4
144		244		344		444	3
Dropout after 2nd visit							
11*	3	21*	3	31*		41*	
12*		22*	7	32*	7	42*	2
13*		23*	3	33*	3	43*	5
14*		24*	2	34*	1	44*	8
Dropout after 1st visit							
1**	4	2**	6	3**	9	4**	12

Table 15.6 Fluvoxamine trial. Summary of the ordinal side-effects outcomes at three follow-up times. (Categories as in Table 15.5.)

Category	No.	Category	No.	Category	No.	Category	No.
Completers							
111	86	211	25	311	1	411	2
112	5	212	6	312		412	1
113	1	213		313		413	
114		214		314		414	
121	3	221	28	321	1	421	
122		222	39	322	5	422	1
123	7	223	4	323		423	
124		224		324		424	
131		231		331		431	
132		232	4	332	3	432	
133		233		333	2	433	
134		234		334		434	
141		241		341		441	
142		242		342		442	
143		243		343		443	
144		244		344		444	
Dropout after 2nd visit							
11*	13	21*	3	31*	1	41*	
12*	4	22*	9	32*	1	42*	
13*		23*	3	33*	5	43*	
14*		24*	1	34*	2	44*	2
Dropout after 1st visit							
1**	9	2**	6	3**	7	4**	9

consistent with an analysis of the full data set if the dropout process is completely random. The remaining three sets of estimates are obtained from fitting models with non-random, random, and completely random dropout, defined in terms of constraints on the ψ parameters.

We consider first the analysis of the side-effects data (Table 15.7). Covariates have been included in the response component of the model. The relationships with two covariates, sex and age, have been held constant across visits, the relationships with the other two covariates, duration and severity, have been allowed to differ among visits.

Conditional on acceptance of the validity of the overall model, we can, by examining the statistical significance of the parameters in the dropout model, test for different types of dropout process. Three statistics, likelihood ratio, Wald, and score, can be computed for each null hypothesis, and we present each one in Table 15.8 for comparisons of MNAR versus MAR and of MAR versus MCAR. In line with Diggle and Kenward (1994) and Molenberghs *et al.* (1997), it is tempting to assume both statistics follow a null asymptotic χ_1^2 distribution. As

Table 15.7 Fluvoxamine trial. Maximum likelihood estimates (standard errors) for side effects.

Parameter	Completers	MCAR	MAR	MNAR
Measurement model				
Intercept 1	1.38 (1.00)	−0.60 (0.82)	−0.60 (0.82)	−0.78 (0.79)
Intercept 2	4.42 (1.04)	1.59 (0.83)	1.59 (0.83)	1.31 (0.80)
Intercept 3	6.32 (1.14)	2.90 (0.85)	2.90 (0.85)	2.51 (0.82)
Age	−0.22 (0.08)	−0.20 (0.07)	−0.20 (0.07)	−0.19 (0.07)
Sex	−0.35 (0.25)	−0.03 (0.22)	−0.03 (0.22)	0.00 (0.21)
Duration (visit 1)	0.05 (0.08)	−0.13 (0.05)	−0.13 (0.05)	−0.12 (0.05)
Duration (visit 2)	−0.10 (0.08)	−0.20 (0.06)	−0.20 (0.06)	−0.21 (0.05)
Duration (visit 3)	−0.13 (0.08)	−0.19 (0.07)	−0.19 (0.07)	−0.23 (0.06)
Severity (visit 1)	0.00 (0.16)	0.26 (0.13)	0.26 (0.13)	0.28 (0.12)
Severity (visit 2)	0.09 (0.16)	0.33 (0.13)	0.33 (0.13)	0.34 (0.13)
Severity (visit 3)	0.17 (0.16)	0.41 (0.13)	0.41 (0.13)	0.40 (0.13)
Association				
Visits 1 and 2	2.89 (0.33)	3.12 (0.30)	3.12 (0.30)	3.26 (0.29)
Visits 1 and 3	2.06 (0.32)	2.33 (0.35)	2.33 (0.35)	2.30 (0.32)
Visits 2 and 3	2.86 (0.34)	3.16 (0.37)	3.16 (0.37)	3.18 (0.36)
Visits 1, 2, and 3	0.45 (0.76)	0.48 (0.79)	0.48 (0.79)	0.61 (0.71)
Dropout model				
ψ_0		−1.90 (0.13)	−3.68 (0.34)	−4.26 (0.48)
ψ_1				1.08 (0.54)
ψ_2			0.94 (0.15)	0.18 (0.45)
−2 log-likelihood		1631.97	1591.98	1587.72

Table 15.8 Fluvoxamine trial. Side effects. Test statistics for dropout mechanism.

	MNAR v. MAR		MAR v. MCAR	
Wald	4.02	($p = 0.045$)	38.91	($p < 0.001$)
Likelihood ratio	4.26	($p = 0.039$)	39.99	($p < 0.001$)
Score	4.24	($p = 0.040$)	45.91	($p < 0.001$)

mentioned on page 374 above, Jansen *et al.* (2006b) show that great care has to be taken with the test for MNAR against MAR (see Chapter 20).

All tests provide weak evidence for MNAR in the context of the assumed model. They also strongly support MAR over MCAR. But again, one has to be very cautious with such conclusions, a central theme in Part V.

The estimated dropout model is, with simplified notation,

$$\text{logit}[P(\text{dropout})] = -4.26 + 1.08Y_c + 0.18Y_{pr}$$

for Y_{pr} and Y_c the previous and current observations, respectively. It is instructive to rewrite this in terms of the increment and sum of the successive measurements:

$$\text{logit}[P(\text{dropout})] = -4.26 + 0.63[0.08](Y_c + Y_{pr}) + 0.45[0.49](Y_c - Y_{pr}).$$

Standard errors of the estimated parameters have been added in square brackets. It can be seen that the estimated probability of dropout increases greatly with large side effects. The corresponding standard error is comparatively small. Although the coefficient of the increment does not appear negligible in terms of its absolute size, in the light of its standard error it cannot be said to be significantly different from zero. This reflects the lack of information in these data on the coefficient of the increment in the dropout model.

Although the evidence of dependence of the dropout process on previous observation is overwhelming, that for MNAR is borderline.

It is worth noting that there are substantial differences between the analyses of the completers only and full data sets with respect to the parameter estimates of the response model. In the presence of an MAR and MNAR process, the former analysis produces inconsistent estimators. Given the clear association of side-effect occurrence and the covariates age, duration, and severity, we investigated the relationship between these and dropout, but found only marginal evidence for a dependence on sex and severity.

In Table 15.9 the results from the analyses of the therapeutic effect are presented. Here, apart from overall effects of time, no covariates are included because all showed negligible association with the response. Interestingly, the comparison of the three dropout models (Table 15.10) produces somewhat different conclusions about the dropout mechanism, when compared to those of the side-effects analysis (Table 15.8).

Here, the three classes of tests again behave consistently. The evidence for MNAR is strong, but the same warnings about the sensitivity of the MNAR model to modelling assumptions apply here. The tests comparing the MAR and MCAR processes show only moderate evidence of a difference. The latter tests are not strictly valid, however, in the presence of MNAR missingness. It is interesting that a comparison of the MCAR and MAR models, which is much easier to accomplish than the comparison of MAR and MNAR, gives little suggestion that such a relationship might exist between dropout and response. This is partly a consequence of the nature of the dropout relationship in this example. With the side effects the association between dropout and response was dominated by the average response. With the therapeutic observations, however, dependence of dropout probability is largely on the measurement increment, also a feature of the analyses in Diggle and Kenward (1994). From the fitted MNAR model we have

$$\text{logit}\{P(\text{dropout})\} = -2.00 - 1.11Y_c + 0.77Y_{pr}$$
$$= -2.00 - 0.17[0.17](Y_c + Y_{pr}) - 0.94[0.28](Y_c - Y_{pr}).$$

Table 15.9 Fluvoxamine trial. Maximum likelihood estimates (standard errors) for therapeutic effect.

Parameter	Completers	MCAR	MAR	MNAR
Measurement model				
Intercept 1	−2.36 (0.17)	−2.32 (0.15)	−2.32 (0.15)	−2.33 (0.14)
Intercept 2	−0.53 (0.13)	−0.53 (0.12)	−0.53 (0.11)	−0.52 (0.10)
Intercept 3	1.03 (0.14)	0.90 (0.11)	0.90 (0.12)	0.90 (0.09)
Visit 2 − Visit 1	1.38 (0.12)	1.22 (0.10)	1.22 (0.10)	1.32 (0.11)
Visit 3 − Visit 1	2.70 (0.19)	2.58 (0.18)	2.58 (0.18)	2.83 (0.19)
Association				
Visits 1 and 2	2.58 (0.24)	2.57 (0.22)	2.57 (0.22)	2.46 (0.20)
Visits 1 and 3	0.85 (0.23)	0.86 (0.24)	0.86 (0.24)	0.77 (0.19)
Visits 2 and 3	1.79 (0.25)	1.79 (0.25)	1.79 (0.25)	1.59 (0.20)
Visits 1, 2 and 3	0.39 (0.52)	0.27 (0.52)	0.27 (0.52)	0.22 (0.23)
Dropout model				
ψ_0		−1.88 (0.13)	−2.56 (0.37)	−2.00 (0.48)
ψ_1				−1.11 (0.42)
ψ_2			0.26 (0.13)	0.77 (0.19)
−2 log-likelihood		2156.91	2152.87	2145.93

Table 15.10 Fluvoxamine trial. Therapeutic effect. Test statistics for dropout mechanism.

	MNAR v. MAR		MAR v. MCAR	
	Statistic	*p*-value	Statistic	*p*-value
Wald	6.98	0.008	3.98	0.046
Likelihood ratio	6.94	0.008	4.03	0.044
Score	9.31	0.002	4.02	0.045

A plausible interpretation would be that dropout decreases when there is a favourable change in therapeutic effect, and increases only comparatively slightly when there is little therapeutic effect. Larger differences can also be seen among the parameter estimates of the response component, between the MCAR and MAR models on the one hand and the non-random dropout model on the other, than are apparent in the analysis of the side effects. The estimated differences between visits are greater in the MNAR model; in the MAR analysis no account is taken of the dependence of dropout on increment, so the sizes of the changes between visits are biased downwards. These differences are, however, of little practical importance given the sizes of the associated standard errors. Similarly, the statistical dependence between repeated measurements as measured by the log odds ratios is smaller under the MNAR model, possibly because of the effect of selection under the MAR model.

15.4.3　The tinea pedis study

The tinea pedis study is a multicentre trial on the treatment of foot infection. There were respectively 91 and 102 patients on each of the two treatment arms. The outcome of interest is the severity of lesions reported on three occasions

Table 15.11　The tinea pedis study. Summary of severity of lesions outcome from the Tina Pedes study. (For example, category 231 corresponds to a classification of 2 on the first visit, 3 on the second visit, and 1 on the third visit; a * in one of the positions indicates dropout.)

| | Treatment arm | | |
Outcome	1	2	Total
Completers			
111	7	7	14
112		1	1
211	10	7	17
212		1	1
213			
221	1	4	5
222	2	1	3
223	1	2	3
231	1		1
...			
311	22	21	43
312		3	3
313		1	1
321	25	17	42
322		4	4
323		2	2
331	5	10	15
332	3	4	7
333	1	4	5
Dropout after 2nd visit			
21*	1	1	2
22*	1		1
23*		2	2
31*	3	3	6
32*	4	2	6
33*		2	2
Dropout after 1st visit			
1**	1		1
2**			
3**	3	2	5
Total	91	101	192

on a three-point ordinal scale: absent/minimal, mild and moderate/severe. Of the 193 patients who began the study, 6 and 19 dropped out after one and two visits, respectively. There was one subject with a non-monotone missing value who has been omitted from the analysis. The original data are summarized in Table 15.11. Again we are interested in whether there is dependence of dropout on the previous and/or current measure of severity and, particularly given the relatively low dropout rate, whether there is sufficient information to provide answers to these questions. In the fitted model for the response variable, the treatment effect is allowed to change with time.

We fit three models, corresponding to MCAR, MAR, and MNAR. The results are summarized in Table 15.12. The comparison of the MCAR and MAR models produces a likelihood ratio test statistic of 1.25 and shows little evidence of dependence of dropout mechanism on previous value. For the MNAR dropout case a boundary solution is obtained: the value of β_1^{241} approaches $-\infty$. This can be seen from a profile likelihood or from the imputation table obtained in the EM algorithm. This is presented as Table 15.13. Under MCAR and MAR, the unobserved outcomes are predicted to come from lower categories under treatment 1 than under treatment 2, although differences are modest. Note that all imputed observations under the MNAR model fall in category 1.

Table 15.12 Tinea pedis study. Maximum likelihood estimates for the response.

Parameter	MCAR	MAR	MNAR
Marginal mean model			
Intercept 1	−2.31	−2.31	−2.20
Intercept 2	−0.82	−0.82	−0.72
Visit 2 − Visit 1	2.73	2.73	2.64
Visit 3 − Visit 1	5.78	5.78	5.82
Treatment effect, visit 1	−0.10	−0.10	−0.16
Treatment effect, visit 2	−0.32	−0.32	−0.29
Treatment effect, visit 3	−1.24	−1.24	−1.22
Association (odds ratios)			
Visits 1 and 2	1.53	1.53	1.48
Visits 1 and 3	0.06	0.06	0.08
Visits 2 and 3	1.59	1.59	1.52
Visits 1, 2, and 3	0.39	0.39	−0.53
Dropout model			
ψ_0	−2.65	−2.07	—
ψ_1			−∞
ψ_2		−0.27	—
−2 log-likelihood	1033.08	1031.83	—

Table 15.13 Tinea pedis study. Imputation for severity of lesion. The row classification indicates observed categories; for example, category 32 corresponds to a classification of 3 on the first category and 2 on the second category. The column classification corresponds to imputation in one of the three categories at the time of dropout.

Category	Observed t_1	Observed t_2	Imputed t_1 1	Imputed t_1 2	Imputed t_1 3	Imputed t_2 1	Imputed t_2 2	Imputed t_2 3
MCAR and MAR								
11								
12								
13								
21	1	1	96	3	1	88	11	1
22	1		80	18	2			
23		2				30	52	18
31	3	3	97	3	0	91	9	1
32	4	2	90	9	1	73	24	3
33		2				43	46	11
1	1		82	16	2			
2								
3	3	2	36	50	14	29	59	12
MNAR								
11								
12								
13								
21	1	1	100	0	0	100	0	0
22	1		100	0	0			
23		2				100	0	0
31	3	3	100	0	0	100	0	0
32	4	2	100	0	0	100	0	0
33		2				100	0	0
1	1		100	0	0			
2								
3	3	2	100	0	0	100	0	0

15.5   A MODEL FOR NON-MONOTONE MISSINGNESS

In Section 15.4 we presented a model for ordinal data but confined missingness to the dropout type. Here, general missingness will be studied, in the specific context of a bivariate binary outcome. Baker *et al.* (1992) considered a log-linear type of model for two binary outcomes subject to incompleteness. A main advantage of this method is that it can easily deal with non-monotone missingness.

$\pi_{11,11}$	$\pi_{11,12}$
$\pi_{11,21}$	$\pi_{11,22}$

$\pi_{10,11}$	$\pi_{10,12}$
$\pi_{10,21}$	$\pi_{10,22}$

$\pi_{01,11}$	$\pi_{01,12}$
$\pi_{01,21}$	$\pi_{01,22}$

$\pi_{00,11}$	$\pi_{00,12}$
$\pi_{00,21}$	$\pi_{00,22}$

$\downarrow$　　　　$\downarrow$　　　　$\downarrow$　　　　$\downarrow$

$\pi_{11,11}$	$\pi_{11,12}$
$\pi_{11,21}$	$\pi_{11,22}$

$\pi_{10,1+}$
$\pi_{10,2+}$

$\pi_{01,+1}$	$\pi_{01,+2}$

$\pi_{00,++}$

Figure 15.3 Theoretical distribution over complete and observed cells of a bivariate binary outcome. Tables correspond to completely observed subjects and subjects with the second, the first, and both measurements missing, respectively.

As in Section 15.4, let $r = 1, \ldots, N$ index distinct covariate levels. In this section, the index r will be suppressed. Let $j, k = 1, 2$ correspond to the outcome categories of the first and second measurement respectively, and let $r_1, r_2 = 0, 1$ correspond to the missingness indicators (1 for an observed and 0 for a missing measurement). Such a set-up leads to a four-way classification. The complete data and observed data cell probabilities $\pi_{r_1 r_2,jk}$ for this setting are presented in Figure 15.3.

To accommodate (possibly continuous) covariates, as proposed by Jansen *et al.* (2006b), we will use a parameterization, different from and extending the original one, which belongs to the selection model family (Little 1994a):

$$\pi_{r_1 r_2,jk} = p_{jk} q_{r_1 r_2 | jk}, \tag{15.10}$$

where p_{jk} parameterizes the measurement process and $q_{r_1 r_2 | jk}$ describes the missingness mechanism, conditional on the measurements. In particular, we will assume that

$$p_{jk} = \frac{\exp(\theta_{jk})}{\sum_{j,k=1}^{2} \exp(\theta_{jk})}, \tag{15.11}$$

$$q_{r_1 r_2 | jk} = \frac{\exp[\beta_{jk}(1 - r_2) + \alpha_{jk}(1 - r_1) + \gamma(1 - r_1)(1 - r_2)]}{1 + \exp(\beta_{jk}) + \exp(\alpha_{jk}) + \exp(\beta_{jk} + \alpha_{jk} + \gamma)}, \tag{15.12}$$

for unknown parameters θ_{jk}, β_{jk}, α_{jk}, and γ. A priori, no ordering is imposed on the outcomes. The advantage is that genuine multivariate settings (e.g., several questions in a survey) can be handled as well. When deemed necessary, the implications of time-ordering can be imposed by considering specific models and leaving out others. For example, one may want to avoid dependence of missingness on future observations. In the current bivariate case, the index k

would have to be removed from α in the above model. To identify the model, we set $\theta_{22} = 0$ and further $\theta_{jk} = X_{jk}\boldsymbol{\eta}$. This allows the inclusion of covariate effects that, together with (15.11), is similar in spirit to the multigroup logistic model (Albert and Lesaffre 1986). Even though the parameters $\boldsymbol{\eta}$ are conditional in nature and therefore somewhat difficult to directly interpret when planned sequences are of unequal length (but not in the case considered here), (15.11) allows easy calculation of the joint probabilities. Such computational advantages become increasingly important as the length of the response vector grows. If necessary, specific functions of interest, such as a marginal treatment effect, can be derived. They will typically take the form of non-linear functions. Arguably, a model of the type here can be most useful as a component of a sensitivity analysis, in conjunction with the use of different (e.g., marginal) models.

In many examples, the design matrices X_{jk} will be equal to each other. Stacking all parameters will lead to the following design:

$$\boldsymbol{\theta} = X\boldsymbol{\eta}. \tag{15.13}$$

Likewise, a design can be constructed for the non-response model parameters:

$$\boldsymbol{\delta} = W\boldsymbol{\psi}, \tag{15.14}$$

where the vector $\boldsymbol{\delta}$ stacks the β_{jk}, α_{jk} and γ, and W is an appropriate design matrix. The vector $\boldsymbol{\psi}$ groups the parameters of interest. For example, if MCAR is considered, the α and β parameters do not depend on either j or k and then $\boldsymbol{\psi}' = (\alpha, \beta, \gamma)$. Both designs (15.13) and (15.14) can be combined into one, using $\boldsymbol{\xi} = (\boldsymbol{\theta}', \boldsymbol{\delta}')'$,

$$T = \begin{pmatrix} X & 0 \\ 0 & W \end{pmatrix},$$

and

$$\boldsymbol{\phi} = (\boldsymbol{\eta}', \boldsymbol{\psi}')'. \tag{15.15}$$

The corresponding log-likelihood function can be written as:

$$\ell = \sum_{j,k=1}^{2} y_{11jk} \ln \pi_{11,jk} + \sum_{j=1}^{2} y_{10j+} \ln(\pi_{10,j1} + \pi_{10,j2}) + \sum_{k=1}^{2} y_{01+k} \ln(\pi_{01,1k} + \pi_{01,2k})$$

$$+ y_{00++} \ln(\pi_{00,11} + \pi_{00,12} + \pi_{00,21} + \pi_{00,22})$$

$$= \sum_{j,k=1}^{2} \sum_{s=1}^{y_{11jk}} \ln \pi_{11,jk} + \sum_{j=1}^{2} \sum_{s=1}^{y_{10j+}} \ln \pi_{10,j+} + \sum_{k=1}^{2} \sum_{s=1}^{y_{01+k}} \ln \pi_{01,+k} + \sum_{s=1}^{y_{00++}} \ln \pi_{00,++}.$$

Computation of derivatives, needed for optimization and for the calculation of influence measures, is straightforward.

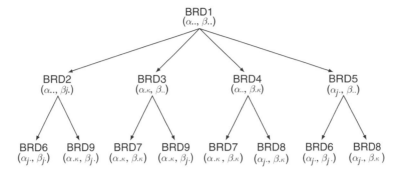

Figure 15.4 Graphical representation of the Baker *et al.* model nesting structure.

To include covariates, the design level $r = 1, \ldots, N$ needs to be introduced again. In particular, with subject-specific covariates, it may be sensible to use $i = 1, \ldots, N$ to index individuals.

Baker *et al.* (1992) consider nine identifiable models, BRD_i, $i = 1, \ldots, 9$, based on setting α_{jk} and β_{jk} constant in one or more indices. An overview, together with the nesting structure, is given in Figure 15.4. Whereas these authors considered the nine models in terms of the original parameterization, they do carry these over to parameterization (15.12). Interpretation is straightforward. For example, BRD1 is MCAR, while in BRD4 missingness in the first variable is constant, while missingness in the second variable depends on its value. Two of the main advantages of this family are ease of computation in general, and the existence of a closed-form solution for several of its members (BRD2 to BRD9).

15.5.1 Analysis of the fluvoxamine trial

Let us return to the fluvoxamine data, analysed earlier in Sections 12.6 and 15.4.2. In the analysis, all patients with known duration level are considered, leaving a total of 310 out of 315 subjects in the study. In the measurement model, the effect of duration is held constant over both visits. Regarding the missingness model, an effect of duration is assumed in both the α and the β parameters. Each of the nine models is represented by a specific choice for the design. For example, for BRD1, and using the index i for individual, we obtain:

$$\phi = (\eta_1, \eta_2, \eta_3, \eta_4, \alpha, \alpha_{\text{dur}}, \beta, \beta_{\text{dur}}, \gamma)',$$

$$X_i = \begin{pmatrix} 1 & 0 & 0 & \text{duration}_i \\ 0 & 1 & 0 & \text{duration}_i \\ 0 & 0 & 1 & \text{duration}_i \end{pmatrix},$$

and

$$
W_i = \begin{pmatrix}
1 & \text{duration}_i & 0 & 0 & 0 \\
1 & \text{duration}_i & 0 & 0 & 0 \\
1 & \text{duration}_i & 0 & 0 & 0 \\
1 & \text{duration}_i & 0 & 0 & 0 \\
0 & 0 & 1 & \text{duration}_i & 0 \\
0 & 0 & 1 & \text{duration}_i & 0 \\
0 & 0 & 1 & \text{duration}_i & 0 \\
0 & 0 & 1 & \text{duration}_i & 0 \\
0 & 0 & 0 & 0 & 1
\end{pmatrix}.
$$

The matrix X_i includes a time-dependent intercept and a time-independent effect of duration. The W_i matrix indicates which of the nine BRD models is considered; changing the model also changes the vector $\boldsymbol{\psi}$.

We will consider three sets of BRD models in some detail. Table 15.14 presents models (parameter estimates, standard errors, negative log-likelihoods) without duration. In Table 15.15 duration is added as a covariate to the measurement model but not yet to the missingness model, whereas in Table 15.16 the effect of duration is included in both measurement and missingness parts of the model. Sampling zeroes in some of the cells forces some parameters to lie on the boundary of their corresponding parameter space which, due to the parameterization, is equal to ∞. This should not be seen as a disadvantage of our model, as boundary solutions are a well-known feature of MNAR models (Rubin 1996). The advantage of our parameterization is that either an interior or a boundary solution is obtained, and never an invalid solution.

From Table 15.14 we learn that likelihood ratio tests fail to reject BRD1 in favour of a more complex model, implying that the simplest mechanism, MCAR, would be adequate. However, this conclusion changes when duration is included in the measurement model (Table 15.15). The effect of duration is highly significant, whichever of the nine BRD models is chosen to conduct a likelihood ratio test. In addition, within Table 15.15, BRD4 rather than BRD1 provides the most adequate description. The likelihood ratio test statistic for comparing BRD1–4 equals 7.10, while those for BRD4–7 and BRD4–8 are 2.10 and 1.52, respectively. Thus, from this set of models, one observes that duration improves the fit and, moreover, one would be inclined to believe that duration, included in the measurement model, has the effect of changing the nature of the missingness mechanism, by making it more complex, even though it is often believed that including explanatory variables (either in the model for the outcomes or in the missingness model) may help to explain structure in the missingness mechanism. BRD4 states that missingness at the second occasion depends on the (possibly unobserved) value at that same occasion, a so-called type I model, in the typology of Baker (2000), in contrast to type II models, where missingness in a variable depends also at least on other, possibly

Table 15.14 Fluvoxamine trial. Maximum likelihood estimates and standard errors of BRD models. All observations included. No covariates.

Effect	BRD1	BRD2	BRD3	BRD4	BRD5	BRD6	BRD7	BRD8	BRD9
Measurement model									
Intercept$_{11}$	0.22 (0.15)	0.20 (0.15)	0.28 (0.15)	0.03 (0.17)	0.32 (0.15)	0.32 (0.15)	0.14 (0.16)	0.16 (0.17)	0.27 (0.15)
Intercept$_{12}$	−1.72 (0.30)	−1.74 (0.30)	−1.72 (0.30)	−1.61 (0.30)	−1.62 (0.30)	−1.62 (0.30)	−1.61 (0.30)	−1.44 (0.32)	−1.72 (0.30)
Intercept$_{21}$	−0.12 (0.18)	−0.12 (0.18)	−0.05 (0.18)	−0.42 (0.23)	−0.13 (0.18)	−0.13 (0.18)	−0.31 (0.21)	−0.39 (0.22)	−0.04 (0.17)
Dropout model									
α	−4.72 (0.71)	−4.72 (0.71)		−4.72 (0.71)					
$\alpha_{1.}$					−3.87 (0.71)	−3.93 (0.71)		−3.93 (0.71)	
$\alpha_{2.}$					−∞	−∞		−∞	
$\alpha_{.1}$			−4.27 (0.71)				−4.29 (0.71)		−4.29 (0.71)
$\alpha_{.2}$			−∞				−∞		−∞
β	−1.09 (0.13)		−1.09 (0.13)		−1.09 (0.13)				
$\beta_{1.}$		−1.37 (0.22)				−1.37 (0.22)			−1.37 (0.22)
$\beta_{2.}$		−0.91 (0.17)				−0.91 (0.17)			−0.91 (0.17)
$\beta_{.1}$				−1.57 (0.38)			−1.57 (0.38)	−1.56 (0.37)	
$\beta_{.2}$				−0.55 (0.29)			−0.56 (0.29)	−0.56 (0.29)	
γ	3.04 (0.77)	3.04 (0.77)	3.04 (0.77)	3.04 (0.77)	3.04 (0.77)	3.31 (0.79)	3.51 (0.84)	3.31 (0.79)	3.11 (0.77)
−log-likelihood	565.96	564.55	565.07	564.55	565.34	563.97	563.70	563.97	563.70

Table 15.15 Fluvoxamine trial. Maximum likelihood estimates and standard errors of BRD models. All observations included. Duration as covariate in the measurement model.

Effect	BRD1	BRD2	BRD3	BRD4	BRD5	BRD6	BRD7	BRD8	BRD9
Measurement model									
Intercept$_{11}$	0.46 (0.17)	0.45 (0.17)	0.53 (0.17)	0.23 (0.20)	0.57 (0.17)	0.57 (0.17)	0.35 (0.18)	0.36 (0.19)	0.52 (0.18)
Intercept$_{12}$	−1.46 (0.31)	−1.48 (0.31)	−1.46 (0.31)	−1.26 (0.32)	−1.37 (0.31)	−1.37 (0.31)	−1.26 (0.32)	−1.06 (0.33)	−1.46 (0.31)
Intercept$_{21}$	0.10 (0.20)	0.10 (0.19)	0.17 (0.20)	−0.25 (0.23)	0.09 (0.21)	0.09 (0.20)	−0.13 (0.21)	−0.21 (0.22)	0.18 (0.20)
Duration	−0.02 (0.01)	−0.02 (0.01)	−0.02 (0.01)	−0.02 (0.01)	−0.02 (0.01)	−0.02 (0.01)	−0.02 (0.01)	−0.02 (0.01)	−0.02 (0.01)
Dropout model									
α	−4.71 (0.71)	−4.71 (0.71)							
$\alpha_{1.}$				−4.71 (0.71)	−3.85 (0.71)	−3.92 (0.71)			
$\alpha_{2.}$					$-\infty$	$-\infty$			
$\alpha_{.1}$			−4.24 (0.71)				−4.28 (0.71)	−3.94 (0.71)	−4.26 (0.71)
$\alpha_{.2}$			$-\infty$				$-\infty$	$-\infty$	$-\infty$
β	−1.11 (0.13)		−1.11 (0.13)		−1.11 (0.13)				
$\beta_{1.}$		−1.44 (0.23)				−1.44 (0.23)			−1.44 (0.23)
$\beta_{2.}$		−0.90 (0.17)				−0.90 (0.17)			−0.90 (0.17)
$\beta_{.1}$				−1.86 (0.45)			−1.87 (0.46)	−1.86 (0.45)	
$\beta_{.2}$				−0.43 (0.25)			−0.43 (0.25)	−0.43 (0.25)	
γ	2.98 (0.77)	2.98 (0.77)	2.98 (0.77)	2.98 (0.77)	2.98 (0.77)	3.31 (0.79)	3.74 (0.89)	3.39 (0.79)	3.07 (0.77)
−log-likelihood	550.15	548.31	549.12	546.60	549.39	547.57	545.55	545.84	547.30

Table 15.16 Fluvoxamine trial. Maximum likelihood estimates and standard errors of BRD models. All observations included. Duration as covariate in both measurement and missingness model.

Effect	BRD1	BRD2	BRD3	BRD4	BRD5	BRD6	BRD7	BRD8	BRD9
Measurement model									
Intercept_{11}	0.46 (0.18)	0.45 (0.17)	0.53 (0.18)	0.30 (0.20)	0.57 (0.17)	0.57 (0.17)	0.41 (0.18)	0.43 (0.19)	0.52 (0.18)
Intercept_{12}	−1.46 (0.31)	−1.48 (0.31)	−1.46 (0.31)	−1.37 (0.31)	−1.37 (0.31)	−1.37 (0.31)	−1.37 (0.31)	−1.22 (0.33)	−1.46 (0.31)
Intercept_{21}	0.10 (0.20)	0.10 (0.20)	0.17 (0.20)	−0.15 (0.24)	0.09 (0.20)	0.09 (0.21)	−0.04 (0.22)	−0.13 (0.23)	0.18 (0.20)
Duration	−0.02 (0.01)	−0.02 (0.01)	−0.02 (0.01)	−0.02 (0.01)	−0.02 (0.01)	−0.02 (0.01)	−0.02 (0.01)	−0.02 (0.01)	−0.02 (0.01)
Dropout model									
$\alpha_{..}$	−4.57 (0.72)	−4.57 (0.72)		−4.57 (0.72)					
$\alpha_{.1}$					−3.82 (0.73)	−3.87 (0.73)		−3.88 (0.73)	
$\alpha_{.2}$					−∞	−∞		−∞	
$\alpha_{1.}$			−4.20 (0.72)				−4.23 (0.73)		−4.22 (0.72)
$\alpha_{2.}$			−∞				−∞		−∞
α_{dur}	−0.02 (0.02) −1.40 (0.16)	−0.02 (0.02)	−0.01 (0.02) −1.40 (0.16)	−0.02 (0.02)	−0.01 (0.02) −1.40 (0.16)	−0.01 (0.02)	−0.01 (0.02)	−0.00 (0.02)	−0.01 (0.02)
$\beta_{..}$	−1.63 (0.24) −1.22 (0.20)	−1.63 (0.24) −1.22 (0.20)				−1.63 (0.24) −1.22 (0.20)			
$\beta_{.1}$				−1.79 (0.36)			−1.79 (0.36)	−1.77 (0.35)	
$\beta_{.2}$				−0.87 (0.33)			−0.88 (0.33)	−0.88 (0.33)	
$\beta_{1.}$									−1.63 (0.24)
$\beta_{2.}$									−1.22 (0.20)
β_{dur}	0.02 (0.01)	0.02 (0.01)	0.02 (0.01)	0.02 (0.01)	0.02 (0.01)	0.02 (0.01)	0.02 (0.01)	0.02 (0.01)	0.02 (0.01)
γ	3.10 (0.78)	3.10 (0.78)	3.10 (0.77)	3.10 (0.78)	3.09 (0.78)	3.33 (0.79)	3.50 (0.84)	3.32 (0.79)	3.16 (0.78)
−loglik	543.78	542.74	542.86	542.63	543.14	542.14	541.77	542.05	541.86
p^{a}	0.0017	0.0038	0.0019	0.0189	0.0019	0.0044	0.0228	0.0226	0.0043

[a] p-value for the comparison with the corresponding BRD model in Table 15.15, to test the null hypothesis of no effect of duration in the missingness model.

incomplete, assessments. As repeatedly emphasized, however, such conclusions are highly dependent on the untestable assumptions that underpin them.

A key conclusion is that, up to this point, no covariate effects have been considered on the missingness parameters. An analysis including duration in the missingness part of the model should be entertained and examined carefully. When Table 15.16 is considered, the conclusions do change drastically. First, all evidence for non-MCAR missingness disappears as, based on likelihood ratio tests, BRD1 comes out as the most adequate description of all nine models. Second, comparing corresponding BRD models between Tables 15.15 and 15.16 (*p*-values on the bottom line of Table 15.16), it is clear that the effect of duration on the missingness model cannot be neglected.

Important modelling and data-analytic conclusions can be drawn from this. First, it clearly does not suffice to consider covariate effects on the measurement model, but one has to carefully contemplate such effects on the missingness model as well. Therefore, the models in Table 15.16 should be regarded as the ones of primary interest. Second, it is found that a longer duration implies a less favourable side-effects outcome, as well as an increased change of missing visits. Obviously, duration acts as a confounding variable which, unless included in both parts of the model, may suggest a relationship between the measurement and missingness models, and thus one may erroneously be led to believe that the missing data are MNAR. Third, it should be noted that the parameter estimates of duration are remarkably stable. This implies that, if one is primarily interested in the effect of duration on the occurrence of side effects, all 18 models containing this effect provide very similar evidence. Although this need not be the case in general, it is a comforting aspect of this particular data analysis.

15.6   CONCLUDING REMARKS

In Section 15.2 a model for repeated Gaussian measures, subject to possibly MNAR missingness, was presented. Similarly, in Section 15.4 a modelling approach for incomplete ordinal outcomes with dropout was presented. The approach is very general and any measurement model can be used. In fact, it is easy enough to adapt the method to any type of outcome. Not only marginal models but also random-effects models can be used by way of measurement model. In Section 15.5 a model specifically for binary data, but with general missingness patterns, has been presented. The one limitation of the model in Section 15.4 is its suitability for dropout only. Several extensions of general missingness have been studied in the literature. Troxel *et al.* (1998) presented methods for non-ignorable non-monotone missingness. Baker (1995a) presented a modification of Diggle and Kenward (1994) to accommodate non-monotone missingness. Jansen and Molenberghs (2005) modify the model of Section 15.4 to account for non-monotone missingness by replacing the logistic regressions for dropout with a second multivariate Dale model to describe the vector of missingness indicators, given the outcomes.

Thus, a wide variety of selection models are available for incomplete longitudinal data, under MNAR and possibly also with non-monotone missingness. Nevertheless, care has to be taken with such models. As with all model fitting, the conclusions drawn are conditional on the appropriateness of the assumed model. Here especially, there are aspects of the model that are in a fundamental sense not testable, namely the relationship between dropout and the missing observations. It is assumed in the modelling approach taken here that the relationships among the measurements from a subject are the same whether or not some of these measurements are unobserved due to dropout. It is this assumption, combined with the adoption of an explicit model linking outcome and dropout probability, that allows us to infer something about the MNAR nature of the dropout process. Given the dependence of the inferences on untestable assumptions, care is needed in the interpretation of the analysis.

Even if evidence is found that an MNAR model fits the observed data better than the corresponding MAR model, this does not imply that the reason for the lack of fit of the MAR model corresponds to that represented in the MNAR model. The lack of fit may well be real but the cause of this does not necessarily follow from the non-random dropout process postulated. This is exemplified in Chapter 19.

On the other hand, the absence of evidence for non-random dropout may simply mean that a non-random dropout process is operating in a quite different manner, and in practice it is likely that many such processes are operating simultaneously.

Thus, the sensitivity of the posited model to modelling assumptions needs to be addressed with great caution. We refer to Part V for a discussion of sensitivity analysis in the non-Gaussian setting.

16

Pattern-Mixture Models

16.1 INTRODUCTION

Pattern-mixture models (PMMs) were introduced in Section 3.3 as one of the three major frameworks within which missing data models can be developed, alongside selection models (Chapter 15) and shared-parameter models (Chapter 17). Early references include Rubin (1977), who even mentioned the concept of a sensitivity analysis, Glynn *et al.* (1986) and Little and Rubin (1987). Important early development was provided by Little (1993, 1994a, 1995).

Pattern-mixture models can be considered for their own sake, typically because they are appropriate, in given circumstances, to answer a particular scientific question. Furthermore, a range of authors have considered PMM as a useful contrast to selection models either (1) to answer the same scientific question, such as marginal treatment effect or time evolution, based on these two rather different modelling strategies, or (2) to gain additional insight by supplementing the selection model results with those from a pattern-mixture approach. Pattern-mixture models also have a special role in some multiple imputation based sensitivity analyses.

Examples of pattern-mixture applications can be found in Verbeke *et al.* (2001a) or Michiels *et al.* (2002) for continuous outcomes, and Molenberghs *et al.* (1999b) or Michiels *et al.* (1999) for categorical outcomes. Further references include Cohen and Cohen (1983), Muthén *et al.* (1987), Allison (1987), McArdle and Hamagani (1992), Little and Wang (1996), Little and Yau (1996), Hedeker and Gibbons (1997), Hogan and Laird (1997), Ekholm and Skinner (1998), Molenberghs *et al.* (1998a), Verbeke and Molenberghs (2000), Thijs *et al.* (2002), and Molenberghs and Verbeke (2005).

Missing Data in Clinical Studies   G. Molenberghs and M.G. Kenward
© 2007 John Wiley & Sons, Ltd

Molenberghs *et al.* (1998b) and Kenward *et al.* (2003) studied the relationship between selection models and PMM within the context of missing data mechanisms (Section 3.4). The earlier paper presents the PMM counterpart of MAR, and the later one states how PMMs can be constructed such that dropout does not depend on future points in time.

An important feature of PMMs is that they are by construction underidentified, that is, overspecified. Little (1993, 1994a) addresses this through the use of identifying restrictions: inestimable parameters of the incomplete patterns are set equal to (functions of) the parameters describing the distribution of the completers. Identifying restrictions are not the only way to overcome underidentification, and we will discuss alternative approaches in Section 16.4. Although some authors perceive this underidentification as a drawback, we believe that it has, in a certain sense, important advantages. First, it helps us to understand the precise nature of sensitivity in selection models (Section 16.3 and Chapter 19). Second, and related to the previous point, the PMMs can serve important roles in a sensitivity analysis.

We begin with a simple illustration of the PMM framework for three Gaussian outcomes in Section 16.2. An apparent paradox, resulting from comparing selection and PMMs, is reviewed in Section 16.3. The various strategies to handle PMMs are mapped out in Section 16.4. Section 16.5 focuses on identifying restrictions strategies. The analysis of three data sets further illustrates the methodology. Section 16.6 analyses the vorozole study, introduced in Section 2.2. Further analyses are presented in Chapter 26. Section 16.7 is devoted to the analysis of a clinical trial conducted in Alzheimer's patients. Finally, the fluvoxamine trial is reanalysed from a PMM perspective in Section 16.8.

16.2   A SIMPLE GAUSSIAN ILLUSTRATION

We introduce the concept of pattern-mixture modelling using a trivariate normal setting. Adopting the pattern-mixture decomposition (3.4), suppressing dependence on covariates and restricting attention to dropout, we obtain, using (3.1),

$$f(\boldsymbol{y}_i, d_i | \boldsymbol{\theta}, \boldsymbol{\psi}) = f(\boldsymbol{y}_i | d_i, \boldsymbol{\theta}) f(d_i | \boldsymbol{\psi}). \tag{16.1}$$

Define $t_i = d_i - 1$, so that while d_i signifies the moment of dropout, t_i is the corresponding last occasion at which a measurement is obtained. Then (16.1) becomes

$$f(\boldsymbol{y}_i, t_i | \boldsymbol{\theta}, \boldsymbol{\psi}) = f(\boldsymbol{y}_i | t_i, \boldsymbol{\theta}) f(t_i | \boldsymbol{\psi}), \tag{16.2}$$

with t_i the realization of the dropout index T_i.

Consider a trivariate normal outcome, where T_i can take values 1 and 2 for dropouts and 3 for completers. A PMM implies a different distribution for each time of dropout. We can write

$$\boldsymbol{y}_i|t_i \sim N\{\boldsymbol{\mu}(t_i), \Sigma(t_i)\}, \tag{16.3}$$

where

$$\boldsymbol{\mu}(t) = \begin{pmatrix} \mu_1(t) \\ \mu_2(t) \\ \mu_3(t) \end{pmatrix} \quad \text{and} \quad \Sigma(t) = \begin{pmatrix} \sigma_{11}(t) & \sigma_{21}(t) & \sigma_{31}(t) \\ \sigma_{21}(t) & \sigma_{22}(t) & \sigma_{32}(t) \\ \sigma_{31}(t) & \sigma_{32}(t) & \sigma_{33}(t) \end{pmatrix},$$

for $t = 1, 2, 3$. Let $P(t) = \pi_t = f(t_i|\boldsymbol{\psi})$; then the marginal distribution of the response is a mixture of normals with overall mean

$$\boldsymbol{\mu} = \sum_{t=1}^{3} \pi_t \boldsymbol{\mu}(t).$$

The variance for an estimator of $\boldsymbol{\mu}$ can be derived by application of the delta method.

However, although the π_t can be simply estimated from the observed proportions in each dropout group, only 16 of the 27 response parameters can be identified from the data without making further assumptions. These 16 comprise all the parameters from the completers plus those from the following two submodels. For $t = 2$,

$$N\left(\begin{pmatrix} \mu_1(2) \\ \mu_2(2) \end{pmatrix}, \begin{pmatrix} \sigma_{11}(2) & \sigma_{21}(2) \\ \sigma_{21}(2) & \sigma_{22}(2) \end{pmatrix} \right),$$

is identified, and for $t = 1$,

$$N\left(\mu_1(1), \sigma_{11}(1) \right)$$

contains the estimable parameters. This is a *saturated* PMM and the above representation makes it very clear what information each dropout group provides and, consequently, the assumptions that need to be made if we are to predict the behaviour of the unobserved responses, and so obtain marginal models for the response. If the three sets of parameters $\boldsymbol{\mu}(t)$ are simply equated, with the same holding for the corresponding variance components, then this implies that dropout is MCAR. Progress can be made with less stringent restrictions, however, such as CCMV, ACMV, and NCMV, as introduced in Section 3.6.

Practically speaking, the choice of precisely which restrictions will be used ought to be guided by the context. In addition, a more structured model for the response with the incorporation of covariates might be called for. Hence, models for $f(t_i|\psi)$ can be constructed in many ways. Most authors assume that the dropout process is fully observed and that T_i satisfies a parametric model (Wu and Bailey 1988, 1989; Little 1993; DeGruttola and Tu 1994). Hogan and Laird (1997) extend this to cases where the dropout time is allowed to be right censored and no parametric restrictions are put on the dropout times. Their conditional model for Y_i^o given T_i is a linear mixed model with dropout time as one of the covariates in the mean structure. Owing to the right censoring, the estimation method must handle incomplete covariates. Hogan and Laird (1997) use the EM algorithm (Dempster *et al.* 1977) for maximum likelihood estimation.

At this point, a distinction between so-called *outcome-based* and *random-coefficient-based* models is useful. In the context of the former, Little (1995) and Little and Wang (1996) consider the restrictions implied by a selection dropout model in the pattern-mixture framework. We return to such connections between both frameworks in Section 16.3. For example, with two time points and a Gaussian response, Little proposes a general form of dropout model,

$$P(\text{dropout}\,|\,\boldsymbol{y}) = g(y_1 + \lambda y_2), \qquad (16.4)$$

with the function $g(\cdot)$ left unspecified. In a selection modelling context, (16.4) is often assumed to have a logistic form (see, for example, Section 15.2). This relationship implies that the conditional distribution of Y_1 given $Y_1 + \lambda Y_2$ is the same for those who drop out and those who do not. With this restriction and given λ, the parameters of the full distribution of the dropouts is identified. The 'weight' λ can then be used as a sensitivity parameter, its size determining dependence of dropout on the past and present, as in the selection models. Such a procedure can be extended to more general problems (Little 1995; Little and Wang 1996). It is instructive in this very simple setting to compare the sources of identifiability in the pattern-mixture and selection models. In the former, the information comes from the assumption that the dropout probability is some function of a linear combination of the two observations with known coefficients. In the latter, it comes from the shape of the assumed conditional distribution of Y_2 given Y_1 (typically Gaussian), together with the functional form of the dropout probability. The difference is highlighted if we consider a sensitivity analysis for the selection model that varies λ in the same way as with the pattern-mixture model. Such sensitivity analysis is much less convincing because the data can, through the likelihood, distinguish between the fit associated with different values of λ.

Therefore, identifability problems in the selection context tend to be masked. Indeed, there are always unidentified parameters, although a related 'problem' seems absent in the selection model. This apparent paradox has been observed by Glynn *et al.* (1986). Let us now consider their paradox.

16.3 A PARADOX

We assume that there are two measurements, of which Y_1 is always observed and Y_2 is either observed ($t = 2$) or missing ($t = 1$). The notation is simplified further by suppressing dependence on parameters and additionally adopting the following definitions:

$$g(t|y_1, y_2) := f(t|y_1, y_2),$$
$$p(t) := f(t),$$
$$f_t(y_1, y_2) := f(y_1, y_2|t).$$

Equating the selection model and pattern-mixture model factorizations yields

$$f(y_1, y_2)g(t = 2|y_1, y_2) = f_2(y_1, y_2)p(t = 2),$$
$$f(y_1, y_2)g(t = 1|y_1, y_2) = f_1(y_1, y_2)p(t = 1).$$

Since we have only two patterns, this obviously simplifies further to

$$f(y_1, y_2)g(y_1, y_2) = f_2(y_1, y_2)p,$$
$$f(y_1, y_2)[1 - g(y_1, y_2)] = f_1(y_1, y_2)[1 - p],$$

of which the ratio produces

$$f_1(y_1, y_2) = \frac{1 - g(y_1, y_2)}{g(y_1, y_2)} \frac{p}{1 - p} f_2(y_1, y_2).$$

All selection model factors are identified, as are the pattern-mixture quantities on the right-hand side. However, the left-hand side is not entirely identifiable. We can further separate the identifiable from the non-identifiable quantities:

$$f_1(y_2|y_1) = f_2(y_2|y_1) \frac{1 - g(y_1, y_2)}{g(y_1, y_2)} \frac{p}{1 - p} \frac{f_2(y_1)}{f_1(y_1)}. \tag{16.5}$$

In other words, the conditional distribution of the second measurement given the first, *in the incomplete first pattern*, about which there is no information in the data, is identified by equating it to its counterpart from the complete pattern, modulated via the ratio of the 'prior' and 'posterior' odds for dropout ($p/(1-p)$ and $g(y_1, y_2)/(1 - g(y_1, y_2))$, respectively) and via the ratio of the densities for the first measurement.

Thus, although an identified selection model is seemingly less arbitrary than a pattern-mixture model, it incorporates *implicit* restrictions. Indeed, it is precisely these that are used in (16.5) to identify the component for which there is no information.

16.4 STRATEGIES TO FIT PATTERN-MIXTURE MODELS

In Section 16.2 we referred to the identifying restrictions strategies, previously introduced in Section 3.6. In spite of their intrinsic underidentification, such restrictions are the first, and possibly the most important, of a variety of ways to fit PMMs. We will refer to such identifying restrictions as *Strategy 1*, and return to them in Section 16.5.

As an alternative to identifying restrictions, we can undertake model simplification to identify the parameters; we will refer to this as *Strategy 2*. The advantage of this strategy is that the number of parameters decreases, which is desirable since the length of the parameter vector is a general issue with pattern-mixture PMMs. Hogan and Laird (1997) noted that, to estimate the large number of parameters in general PMMs, one has to make the awkward requirement that each dropout pattern occurs sufficiently often. Broadly, we distinguish between two interconnected types of simplifications.

- *Strategy 2a*. Trends can be restricted to functional forms supported by the information available within a pattern. For example, a linear or quadratic time trend is easily extrapolated beyond the last obtained measurement. One merely needs to provide an *ad hoc* solution for the first or the first few patterns. To fit such models, a conventional model-building exercise is conducted within each of the patterns separately.
- *Strategy 2b*. Alternatively, one can choose to let the model parameters vary across patterns in a controlled parametric way. Thus, rather than estimating a separate time trend within each pattern, one might, for example, assume that the time evolution within a pattern is unstructured, but parallel across patterns. This can be done by treating pattern as a covariate. The available data can be used to assess whether such simplifications are supported over the time ranges for which information is collected.

While Strategy 2 is computationally the simpler, there is a price to pay. Such simplified models, qualified as 'assumption-rich' by Sheiner *et al.* (1997), are also making untestable assumptions, exactly as in the selection model case. Using the fitted profiles to predict their evolution beyond the time of dropout is nothing but extrapolation. It is possible only by making the models sufficiently simple. It is, for example, not possible to assume an unstructured time trend in incomplete patterns and then still extrapolate in an unambiguous fashion. In contrast, assuming a linear time trend allows estimation in all patterns containing at least two measurements. However, it is less obvious what the precise nature of the dropout mechanism is. In Section 3.6 it was made clear that, unless due care is taken, dropout may depend on future, unobserved measurements or may have other undesirable properties. In many cases such future dependence will be an undesirable feature, but this can be avoided through the use of an appropriate set of identifying restrictions. Other unwanted features may be less easy to control from the pattern-mixture framework.

A final observation, applying to both strategies, is that PMMs do not always automatically provide estimates and standard errors of marginal quantities of interest, such as overall treatment effect or overall time trend. Hogan and Laird (1997) provided a way to derive selection model quantities from the PMM. Multiple imputation and other sampling-based routes can be used for this. Several authors have followed this idea to formally compare the conclusions from a selection model with the selection model parameters in a PMM (Verbeke *et al.* 2001a; Michiels *et al.* 1999).

16.5 APPLYING IDENTIFYING RESTRICTIONS

In Section 3.6 we laid out the identifying-restrictions framework, as presented by Little (1993, 1994a) with CCMV, Molenberghs *et al.* (1998b) for a general framework, including NCMV and ACMV, and Kenward *et al.* (2003), who focus on restrictions avoiding dependence of dropout on measurements made at future occasions. Here, we will indicate how such restrictions can be used in practice.

The following sequence of steps is required.

1. Fit a model to the pattern-specific identifiable densities: $f_t(y_1, \ldots, y_t)$. This results in a parameter estimate, $\hat{\gamma}_t$.
2. Select an identification method of choice.
3. Using this identification method, determine the conditional distributions of the unobserved outcomes, given the observed ones:

$$f_t(y_{t+1}, \ldots, y_T | y_1, \ldots, y_t). \tag{16.6}$$

4. Using standard multiple imputation methodology (Rubin 1987; Schafer 1997; Verbeke and Molenberghs 2000; Minini and Chavence 2004a, 2004b; Chapter 9 above), draw multiple imputations for the unobserved components, given the observed outcomes and the correct pattern-specific density (16.6).
5. Analyse the multiply-imputed sets of data using the method of choice. This can be another pattern-mixture model, but also a selection model or any other desired model.
6. Inferences can be conducted in the standard multiple imputation way (Section 9.4 above; Rubin 1987; Schafer 1997).

We have seen how general identifying restrictions (3.18), with CCMV, NCMV, ACMV, and NFMV as special cases, lead to the conditional densities for the unobserved components, given the observed ones. This reduced to deriving expressions for ω, such as in (3.22) for ACMV. In addition, we need to draw imputations from the conditional densities.

We proceed by studying the special case of three measurements. We consider an identification scheme and, at first, avoid having to specify a parametric form for these densities. The following steps are required:

1. Estimate the parameters of the identifiable densities: from pattern 3, $f_3(y_1, y_2, y_3)$; from pattern 2, $f_2(y_1, y_2)$; and from pattern 1, $f_1(y_1)$.
2. To properly account for the uncertainty with which the parameters are estimated, we need to draw from them as is customarily done in multiple imputation. It will be assumed that in all densities from which we draw, this parameter vector is used.
3. For *pattern 2*, given an observation in this pattern, with observed values (y_1, y_2), calculate the conditional density $f_3(y_3|y_1, y_2)$ and draw from it.
4. For *pattern 1*, we now have to distinguish three sub-steps.

(a) There is now only one ω involved: for pattern 1, in order to determine $f_1(y_2|y_1)$, as a combination of $f_2(y_2|y_1)$ and $f_3(y_2|y_1)$. Every ω in the unit interval is valid. Specific cases are: for NCMV, $\omega = 1$; for CCMV, $\omega = 0$; for ACMV, ω identifies a linear combination across patterns. Note that, given y_1, this is a constant, depending on α_2 and α_3. For NFD1 and NFD2 (see Section 3.6) the first unidentified conditional density can be chosen freely; thereafter a system of ωs has to be chosen as well. To pick one of the two components f_2 or f_3, we need to generate a random uniform variate, U say, except in the boundary NCMV and CCMV cases.
(b) If $U \le \omega$, calculate $f_2(y_2|y_1)$ and draw from it. Otherwise, do the same based on $f_3(y_2|y_1)$.
(c) Given the observed y_1 and given y_2 which has just been drawn, calculate the conditional density $f_3(y_3|y_1, y_2)$ and draw from it.

All steps but the first have to be repeated M times, and further inferential steps proceed as in Section 9.2.

When the observed densities are assumed to have normal distributions, the corresponding conditional densities are particularly straightforward. However, in some cases, the conditional density is a mixture of normal densities. Then, an additional and straightforward draw from the components of the mixture is necessary. Similar developments are possible with categorical data, ensuring that draws from the proper conditional multinomial distributions are made.

16.6 PATTERN-MIXTURE ANALYSIS OF THE VOROZOLE STUDY

Here, we consider the special but insightful case of the three initial measurements from the vorozole study, introduced in Section 2.2. We return to the analysis of the data set in Chapter 26. In Section 16.6.1, we give further insight into the general modelling strategy, described in the previous section. These methods are then applied to the vorozole study. The relative simplicity of the method in this setting provides further insight into the technical aspects of the proposed procedure. The data analysis of three measurements will also lay the foundations for an efficient *full* analysis of the data over the entire study period, which is the subject of Section 26.4.

16.6.1 Derivations

In this setting, there are only three patterns, and identification (3.19) takes the following form:

$$f_3(y_1, y_2, y_3) = f_3(y_1, y_2, y_3),\tag{16.7}$$

$$f_2(y_1, y_2, y_3) = f_2(y_1, y_2)f_3(y_3|y_1, y_2),\tag{16.8}$$

$$f_1(y_1, y_2, y_3) = f_1(y_1)[\omega f_2(y_2|y_1) + (1 - \omega)f_3(y_2|y_1)] \times f_3(y_3|y_1, y_2).\tag{16.9}$$

Since $f_3(y_1, y_2, y_3)$ is completely identifiable from the data, and for $f_2(y_1, y_2, y_3)$ there is only one possible identification, given (3.18), the only place where a choice has to be made is pattern 1. Setting $\omega = 1$ corresponds to NCMV, while $\omega = 0$ implies CCMV. Using (3.22) in this particular case, ACMV corresponds to

$$\omega = \frac{\alpha_2 f_2(y_1)}{\alpha_2 f_2(y_1) + \alpha_3 f_3(y_1)}.\tag{16.10}$$

The conditional density $f_1(y_2|y_1)$ in (16.9) can be rewritten as

$$f_1(y_2|y_1) = \frac{\alpha_2 f_2(y_1, y_2) + \alpha_3 f_3(y_1, y_2)}{\alpha_2 f_2(y_1) + \alpha_3 f_3(y_1)}.$$

Drawing from the conditional density proceeds as set out in Section 16.5.

Let us turn to model specification. Assume that the observed densities are estimated using linear mixed models. Then, $f_3(y_1, y_2, y_3)$, $f_2(y_1, y_2)$, and $f_1(y_1)$ produce fixed-effects and variance parameters. Group all of them in γ and assume a draw is made from their distribution, γ^* say. To this end, their precision estimates need to be computed. These are easily obtained in most standard software packages, such as SAS.

We illustrate this for (16.8). Generally, we would opt for the linear mixed model (Section 7.3 above; Laird and Ware 1982; Verbeke and Molenberghs 2000). This development also builds upon Section 16.2. Writing β for the p-dimensional vector containing the fixed effects, and $\varepsilon_i \sim N(\mathbf{0}, \Sigma)$ as the vector of correlated error terms, the linear model is

$$Y_i = X_i\beta + \varepsilon_i.$$

In the pattern-mixture case, the parameters involved in this model will be allowed to depend on dropout pattern. Now, assume that the ith subject has only two measurements, and hence belongs to the second pattern. Let its design matrices be X_i and Z_i for the fixed effects and random effects, respectively. Its mean and variance for the *third* pattern are

$$\mu_i(3) = X_i \beta^*(3),\tag{16.11}$$

$$V_i(3) = Z_i D^*(3) Z_i' + \Sigma_i(3),\tag{16.12}$$

where (3) indicates that the parameters are specific to the third pattern.

Now, based on (16.11)–(16.12) and the observed values $y_i = (y_{i1}, y_{i2})'$, the parameters for the conditional density follow immediately:

$$\mu_{i,2|1}(3) = \mu_{i,2}(3) + V_{i,21}(3)[V_{i,11}(3)]^{-1}(y_i - \mu_{i,1}(3)),$$

$$V_{i,2|1}(3) = V_{i,22}(3) - V_{i,21}(3)[V_{i,11}(3)]^{-1}V_{i,12}(3),$$

where a subscript 1 indicates the first two components and a subscript 2 refers to the third component. Draws from every other conditional density can be obtained in essentially the same way.

16.6.2 Application to the vorozole study

We apply the proposed methodology to those subjects with 1, 2, and 3 follow-up measurements. One hundred ninety subjects are included, with subsample sizes 35, 86, and 69, respectively. The pattern-specific probabilities are

$$\widehat{\pi} = (0.184, 0.453, 0.363)',\tag{16.13}$$

with asymptotic covariance matrix

$$\widehat{\mathrm{var}}(\widehat{\pi}) = \begin{pmatrix} 0.000791 & -0.000439 & -0.000352 \\ -0.000439 & 0.001304 & -0.000865 \\ -0.000352 & -0.000865 & 0.001217 \end{pmatrix}.\tag{16.14}$$

These figures not only give us an indication of the patterns' relative importance, they are also needed to calculate the marginal treatment effect and to test for its importance, which was the primary goal of the analysis.

It is of interest to study the treatment-arm-specific pattern probabilities as well. For the vorozole arm, the subsample sizes are 18, 48, and 36, producing probabilities $\widehat{\pi}_v = (0.177, 0.471, 0.354)'$ with asymptotic covariance matrix

$$\widehat{\mathrm{var}}(\widehat{\pi}_v) = \begin{pmatrix} 0.001425 & -0.000814 & -0.000611 \\ -0.000814 & 0.002442 & -0.001628 \\ -0.000611 & -0.001628 & 0.002239 \end{pmatrix}.$$

For the megestrol acetate arm, the subsample sizes are 17, 38, and 33, giving probabilities $\widehat{\boldsymbol{\pi}}_m = (0.193, 0.432, 0.375)'$ and asymptotic covariance matrix

$$\widehat{\text{var}}(\widehat{\boldsymbol{\pi}}_m) = \begin{pmatrix} 0.001771 & -0.000948 & -0.000823 \\ -0.000948 & 0.002788 & -0.001840 \\ -0.000823 & -0.001840 & 0.002663 \end{pmatrix}.$$

The treatment-arm-specific probabilities do not significantly differ and a conventional χ^2 test produces $p = 0.864$. Hence, we will employ expressions (16.13) and (16.14).

Model fitting

The patients in this study drop out mainly because they relapse or die. This in itself poses specific challenges that can be addressed within the pattern-mixture framework much more easily than in the selection model framework. If one is prepared to assume that a patient who dies is representative of a subset of the population with the same characteristics and probability of death, then identifying restrictions (i.e., extrapolation beyond the time of death) is meaningful. In case one does not want to extrapolate beyond the moment of death, one can restrict modelling to the observed data only. The former viewpoint refers to <u>Strategy 1</u>, while the latter refers to <u>Strategy 2</u>. An intermediate approach would be to allow for extrapolation beyond relapse and not beyond death. Unfortunately, for the vorozole data set, the information needed in order to do so is unavailable. Note that, while this feature may seem a disadvantage of PMMs, we believe it is an asset, because it not only forces one to think about such issues, but also provides a modelling solution no matter which point of view is adopted.

For Strategy 1, we start by <u>fitting a model to the observed data</u>, including linear and quadratic time effects, as well as their interactions with baseline value. Furthermore, time-by-treatment interaction is included, for consistency with the original analysis plan. Because the profiles are forced to pass through the origin, all effects interact with time, as we are studying change versus baseline. An unstructured 3×3 covariance matrix is assumed for each pattern. Parameter estimates are presented in Table 16.1, in the 'initial' column. Obviously, not all effects are estimable in this initial model.

The model is graphically summarized in Figure 16.1. As there is one binary (treatment arm) and one continuous covariate (baseline level of FLIC score), insight can be obtained by plotting the models for selected values of baseline. We chose the minimum, average, and maximum values. Note that the extrapolation can have surprising effects, even with these relatively simple models. Thus, while this form of extrapolation is simple, its plausibility can be called into question.

This initial model provides a basis, and its graphical representation additional motivation, for considering <u>identifying restriction models</u>. Results are presented in Table 16.1. In all of the plots (Figures 16.2–16.7), the same mean response

[margin annotations: Strategy 2a; Strategy 1]

Table 16.1 Vorozole study. Multiple imputation estimates and standard errors for CCMV, NCMV, and ACMV restrictions.

Effect	Initial	CCMV	NCMV	ACMV
Pattern 1	$f_\lambda(y_\lambda)$			
Time	3.40 (13.94)	13.21 (15.91)	7.56 (16.45)	4.43 (18.78)
Time × base	−0.11 (0.13)	−0.16 (0.16)	−0.14 (0.16)	−0.11 (0.17)
Time × treat	0.33 (3.91)	−2.09 (2.19)	−1.20 (1.93)	−0.41 (2.52)
Time^2		−0.84 (4.21)	−2.12 (4.24)	−0.70 (4.22)
Time^2 × base		0.01 (0.04)	0.03 (0.04)	0.02 (0.04)
σ_{11}	131.09 (31.34)	151.91 (42.34)	134.54 (32.85)	137.33 (34.18)
σ_{12}		59.84 (40.46)	119.76 (40.38)	97.86 (38.65)
σ_{22}		201.54 (65.38)	257.07 (86.05)	201.87 (80.02)
σ_{13}		55.12 (58.03)	49.88 (44.16)	61.87 (43.22)
σ_{23}		84.99 (48.54)	99.97 (57.47)	110.42 (87.95)
σ_{33}		245.06 (75.56)	241.99 (79.79)	286.16 (117.90)
Pattern 2	$f_2(y_\lambda, y_2)$			
Time	53.85 (14.12)	29.78 (10.43)	33.74 (11.11)	28.69 (11.37)
Time × base	−0.46 (0.12)	−0.29 (0.09)	−0.33 (0.10)	−0.29 (0.10)
Time × treat	−0.95 (1.86)	−1.68 (1.21)	−1.56 (2.47)	−2.12 (1.36)
Time^2	−18.91 (6.36)	−4.45 (2.87)	−7.00 (3.80)	−4.22 (4.20)
Time^2 × base	0.15 (0.05)	0.04 (0.02)	0.07 (0.03)	0.05 (0.04)
σ_{11}	170.77 (26.14)	175.59 (27.53)	176.49 (27.65)	177.86 (28.19)
σ_{12}	151.84 (29.19)	147.14 (29.39)	149.05 (29.77)	146.98 (29.63)
σ_{22}	292.32 (44.61)	297.38 (46.04)	299.40 (47.22)	297.39 (46.04)
σ_{13}		57.22 (37.96)	89.10 (34.07)	99.18 (35.07)
σ_{23}		71.58 (36.73)	107.62 (47.59)	166.64 (66.45)
σ_{33}		212.68 (101.31)	264.57 (76.73)	300.78 (77.97)
Pattern 3	$f_3(y_\lambda, y_2, y_3)$			
Time	29.91 (9.08)	29.91 (9.08)	29.91 (9.08)	29.91 (9.08)
Time × base	−0.26 (0.08)	−0.26 (0.08)	−0.26 (0.08)	−0.26 (0.08)
Time × treat	0.82 (0.95)	0.82 (0.95)	0.82 (0.95)	0.82 (0.95)
Time^2	−6.42 (2.23)	−6.42 (2.23)	−6.42 (2.23)	−6.42 (2.23)
Time^2 × base	0.05 (0.02)	0.05 (0.02)	0.05 (0.02)	0.05 (0.02)
σ_{11}	206.73 (35.86)	206.73 (35.86)	206.73 (35.86)	206.73 (35.86)
σ_{12}	96.97 (26.57)	96.97 (26.57)	96.97 (26.57)	96.97 (26.57)
σ_{22}	174.12 (31.10)	174.12 (31.10)	174.12 (31.10)	174.12 (31.10)
σ_{13}	87.38 (30.66)	87.38 (30.66)	87.38 (30.66)	87.38 (30.66)
σ_{23}	91.66 (28.86)	91.66 (28.86)	91.66 (28.86)	91.66 (28.86)
σ_{33}	262.16 (44.70)	262.16 (44.70)	262.16 (44.70)	262.16 (44.70)

Strategy: ~~2a~~ ↗ ↗ ↗

scale as in Figure 16.1 was retained, illustrating that the identifying restriction strategies extrapolate much more closely to the observed data mean responses. There are some differences among the identifying restriction methods. Roughly speaking, CCMV extrapolates rather towards a rise whereas NCMV seems to

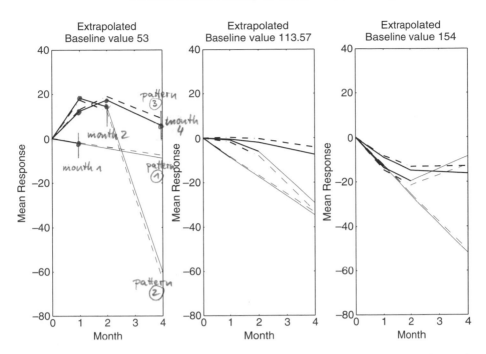

Figure 16.1 Vorozole study. Extrapolation based on initial model fitted to observed data (Strategy 2). For three levels of baseline value (minimum, average, maximum), plots of mean profiles over time are presented. (Thick lines run from baseline until the last obtained measurement, while thin lines represent extrapolations. Dashed lines refer to megestrol acetate; solid lines represent is the vorozole arm.)

predict more of a decline, at least for baseline value 53. Further, ACMV seems to indicate a steady state. For the other baseline levels, a status quo or a mild increase is predicted. This conclusion needs to be considered carefully. Since these patients drop out mainly because they relapse or die, it seems unreasonable to expect a rise in quality of life. Hence, it is likely that the dropout mechanism is not CCMV, since this strategy always refers to the 'best' group, that is, the one with the best prognosis. ACMV, which compromises between all strategies, may be more realistic, but here NCMV is likely to be better since information is borrowed from the nearest pattern.

Nevertheless, the NCMV prediction looks more plausible since the worst baseline value shows declining profiles, whereas the best one leaves room for improvement. Should one want to explore the effect of assumptions beyond the range of (3.18), one can allow ω_s to include components outside the unit interval. In this situation, one has to ensure that the resulting density is still non-negative over its entire support.

In Strategy 2b, *pattern* is included as a covariate. An initial model is considered with the following effects: time, the interaction between time and

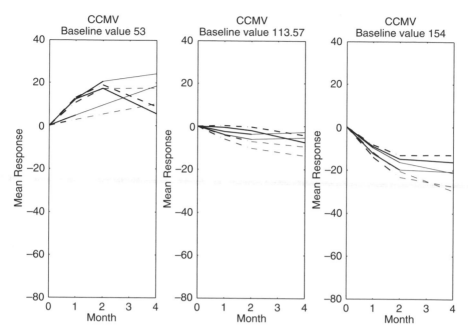

Figure 16.2 Vorozole study. Complete case missing value restrictions analysis. For three levels of baseline value (minimum, average, maximum), plots of mean profiles over time are presented. (Thick lines run from baseline until the last obtained measurement, while thin lines represent extrapolations. Dashed lines refer to megestrol acetate; the solid lines represent the vorozole arm.)

treatment, baseline value, pattern, treatment × baseline, treatment × pattern, and baseline × pattern. Further, a quadratic in time is included, as well as its interaction with baseline, treatment, and pattern. No interactions beyond the third order are included, and an unstructured covariance matrix is assumed common to all three patterns. This implies that the current model is *not* equivalent to a Strategy 1 model, where all parameters are pattern-specific. The estimated model parameters are presented in Table 16.2 and a graphical representations is given in Figure 16.8. It is clear that dropouts decline immediately, whereas those who stay longer in the study first show a rise and then a decline. However, this is less pronounced for higher baseline values. On the other hand, the extrapolation based on the fitted model is very unrealistic, rendering this deceptively simple approach a bad choice. These findings reinforce the need for careful reflection on the extrapolation method.

Hypothesis testing

We focus here on treatment effect. A by-product of the pattern-mixture strategy is that a pattern-specific treatment effect can result. This is the case for all five models in Tables 16.1 and 16.2. Since the main scientific interest is in the

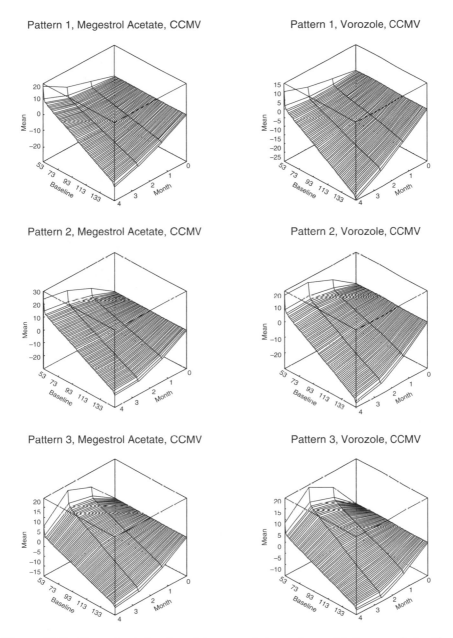

Figure 16.3 Vorozole study. Complete case missing value restrictions analysis. The mean response surface is shown as a function of time (month) and baseline value, by pattern and by treatment group.

Pattern 1, Megestrol Acetate, NCMV

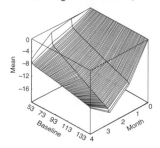

Pattern 1, Vorozole, NCMV

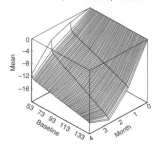

Pattern 2, Megestrol Acetate, NCMV

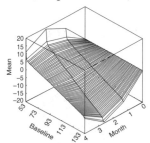

Pattern 2, Vorozole, NCMV

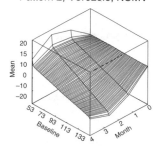

Pattern 3, Megestrol Acetate, NCMV

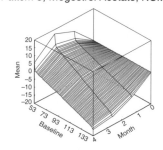

Pattern 3, Vorozole, NCMV

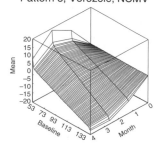

Figure 16.4 Vorozole study. Neighbouring case missing value restrictions analysis. The mean response surface is shown as a function of time (month) and baseline value, by pattern and by treatment group.

estimation of the *marginal treatment effect*, we can combine the pattern-specific effects into a pattern-averaged effect. We apply both of these approaches to the models in Tables 16.1 and 16.2.

We first indicate how a (treatment) effect, marginalized over patterns, can be computed. Let $\beta_{\ell t}$ represent the treatment effect parameter estimates $\ell = 1, \ldots, g$ (assuming there are $g \leq 1$ groups) in pattern $t = 1, \ldots, n$, and let π_t

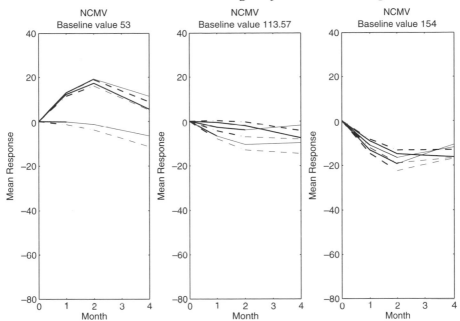

Figure 16.5 Vorozole study. Neighbouring case missing value restrictions analysis. For three levels of baseline value (minimum, average, maximum), plots of mean profiles over time are presented. (Thick lines run from baseline until the last obtained measurement, while thin lines represent part extrapolations. Dashed lines refer to megestrol acetate; solid lines represent the vorozole arm.)

be the proportion of patients in pattern t. Then, the estimates of the marginal treatment effects β_ℓ are

$$\beta_\ell = \sum_{t=1}^{n} \beta_{\ell t} \pi_t, \qquad \ell = 1, \ldots, g. \tag{16.15}$$

The variance is obtained using the delta method and assumes the form

$$\mathrm{var}(\beta_1, \ldots, \beta_g) = AVA', \tag{16.16}$$

where

$$V = \begin{pmatrix} \mathrm{var}(\beta_{\ell t}) & 0 \\ \hline 0 & \mathrm{var}(\pi_t) \end{pmatrix} \tag{16.17}$$

and

$$A = \frac{\partial(\beta_1, \ldots, \beta_g)}{\partial(\beta_{11}, \ldots, \beta_{ng}, \pi_1, \ldots, \pi_n)}. \tag{16.18}$$

Pattern 1, Megestrol Acetate, ACMV

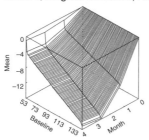

Pattern 1, Vorozole, ACMV

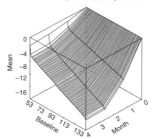

Pattern 2, Megestrol Acetate, ACMV

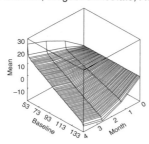

Pattern 2, Vorozole, ACMV

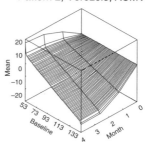

Pattern 3, Megestrol Acetate, ACMV

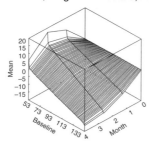

Pattern 3, Vorozole, ACMV

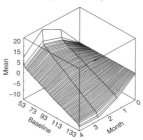

Figure 16.6 Vorozole study. Available case missing value restrictions analysis. The mean response surface is shown as a function of time (month) and baseline value, by pattern and by treatment group.

The estimate of the covariance matrix of the $\widehat{\boldsymbol{\beta}}_{\ell t}$ is easily obtained from statistical software (e.g., the `covb` option in the MODEL statement of the SAS procedure MIXED). The multinomial quantities are easy to obtain from the pattern-specific sample sizes. In the case of the vorozole data, these quantities are presented in (16.13) and (16.14). A Wald test statistic for the null hypothesis $H_0 : \beta_1 = \ldots = \beta_g = 0$ is then given by

$$\boldsymbol{\beta}_0'(AVA')^{-1}\boldsymbol{\beta}_0, \tag{16.19}$$

where $\boldsymbol{\beta}_0 = (\beta_1, \ldots, \beta_g)'$.

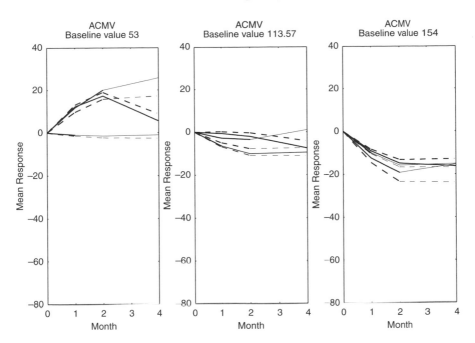

Figure 16.7 Vorozole study. Available case missing value restrictions analysis. For three levels of baseline value (minimum, average, maximum), plots of mean profiles over time are presented. (Thick lines run from baseline until the last obtained measurement, while thin lines represent extrapolations. Dashed lines refer to megestrol acetate; solid lines represent the vorozole arm.)

We now apply the above developments to each of the strategies. As the identifying restriction strategies are slightly more complicated than the others, we will consider the other strategies first.

For Strategy 2a, recall that the parameters are presented in Table 16.1 as the initial model. The treatment effect vector is $\boldsymbol{\beta} = (0.33, -0.95, 0.82)'$ with $V = \text{diag}(15.28, 3.44, 0.90)$, as the patterns are analysed separately. This leads to the test statistic $\boldsymbol{\beta}' V^{-1} \boldsymbol{\beta} = 1.02$ on 3 degrees of freedom, giving $p = 0.796$.

To calculate the marginal treatment effect, we apply (16.16)–(16.19). The marginal effect is estimated as $\hat{\beta}_0 = -0.07$ (s.e. 1.16). The corresponding asymptotic p-value is 0.95. Both approaches agree on the non-significance of the treatment effect.

For Strategy 2b, the parameters are presented in Table 16.2. The treatment effect vector is $\boldsymbol{\beta} = (5.25, 348, 3.44)'$ with non-diagonal covariance matrix:

$$V = \begin{pmatrix} 41.12 & 23.59 & 25.48 \\ 23.59 & 29.49 & 30.17 \\ 25.48 & 30.17 & 36.43 \end{pmatrix}.$$

Table 16.2 Vorozole study. Parameter estimates and standard errors for Strategy 2b. *Pattern used as covariate*

Effect	Pattern	Estimate (s.e.)
Time	1	7.29 (15.69)
Time	2	37.05 (7.67)
Time	3	39.40 (9.97)
Time × treat	1	5.25 (6.41)
Time × treat	2	3.48 (5.46)
Time × treat	3	3.44 (6.04)
Time × base	1	−0.21 (0.15)
Time × base	2	−0.34 (0.06)
Time × base	3	−0.36 (0.08)
Time × treat×base		−0.06 (0.04)
Time^2	1	
Time^2	2	−9.18 (2.47)
Time^2	3	−7.70 (2.29)
Time^2 × treat		1.10 (0.74)
Time^2 × base		0.07 (0.02)
σ_{11}		173.63 (18.01)
σ_{12}		117.88 (17.80)
σ_{22}		233.86 (26.61)
σ_{13}		89.59 (24.56)
σ_{23}		116.12 (34.27)
σ_{33}		273.98 (48.15)

The correlations are substantial. The reason for this is that some parameters, in particular the other treatment effects (three-way interaction with baseline and time, interaction with time squared), are common to all three patterns, hence inducing dependence across patterns. This leads to the test statistic $\boldsymbol{\beta}'V^{-1}\boldsymbol{\beta} = 0.70$ on 3 degrees of freedom, producing $p = 0.874$. Calculating the marginalized treatment effect, we obtain $\hat{\beta}_0 = 3.79$ (s.e. 5.44). The corresponding asymptotic p-value is 0.49. The different numerical value of the treatment effect, as compared to those obtained with the other strategies, is entirely due to the presence of a quadratic treatment effect which, for ease of exposition, is left out of the picture in testing here. It is straightforward to add this parameter to the contrast(s) being considered, should one want to do so.

For Strategy 1, we consider several approximate methods of inference. The CCMV case will be discussed in detail. The two other restriction types are dealt with in similar way. There are three treatment effects, one for each pattern. Hence, multiple imputation produces a vector of treatment effects and the within, between and total covariance matrices:

$$\boldsymbol{\beta}_{CC} = (-2.09, -1.68, 0.82)', \tag{16.20}$$

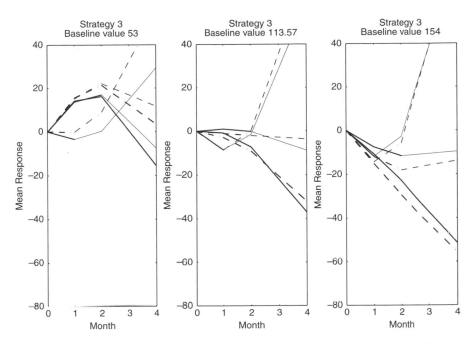

Figure 16.8 Vorozole study. Models with pattern used as a covariate (Strategy 2b). For three levels of baseline value (minimum, average, maximum), plots of mean profiles over time are presented. (Thick lines run from baseline until the last obtained measurement, while thin lines represent extrapolations. Dashed lines refer to megestrol acetate; solid lines represent the vorozole arm.)

$$W_{CC} = \begin{pmatrix} 1.67 & 0.00 & 0.00 \\ 0.00 & 0.59 & 0.00 \\ 0.00 & 0.00 & 0.90 \end{pmatrix}, \tag{16.21}$$

$$B_{CC} = \begin{pmatrix} 2.62 & 0.85 & 0.00 \\ 0.85 & 0.72 & 0.00 \\ 0.00 & 0.00 & 0.00 \end{pmatrix}, \tag{16.22}$$

and

$$T_{CC} = \begin{pmatrix} 4.80 & 1.02 & 0.00 \\ 1.02 & 1.46 & 0.00 \\ 0.00 & 0.00 & 0.90 \end{pmatrix}. \tag{16.23}$$

In a stratified analysis, we want to test the null hypothesis $H_0 : \boldsymbol{\beta} = \boldsymbol{0}$. Using (16.20)–(16.22), multiple imputation methods can be applied. Note that, even though the analysis is done by pattern, the between and total matrices have non-zero off-diagonal elements. This is because the imputation is based on information from *other* patterns, hence introducing inter-pattern dependence.

Table 16.3 Vorozole study. Tests of treatment effect for CCMV, NCMV, and ACMV restrictions.

Parameter	CCMV	NCMV	ACMV
Stratified analysis			
k	3	3	3
τ	12	12	12
Denominator d.f. w	28.41	17.28	28.06
r	1.12	2.89	1.14
F-statistic	1.284	0.427	0.946
p-value	0.299	0.736	0.432
Marginal analysis			
Marginal effect (s.e.)	-0.85 (0.77)	-0.63 (1.22)	-0.74 (0.85)
k	1	1	1
τ	4	4	4
Denominator d.f. w	4	4	4
r	1.49	4.57	1.53
F-statistic	0.948	0.216	0.579
p-value	0.385	0.667	0.489

Results are presented in Table 16.3. All p-values are far from significance, a result consistent with the evidence from Strategies 2a and 2b

For the marginal parameter, the situation is more complicated here than with Strategies 1a and 2b Indeed, classical theory often assumes inference is geared towards elements of the original vector, or contrasts among these. Formula (16.15) represents a non-linear transformation of the parameter vector and therefore needs further development. First, consider π to be part of the parameter vector. Since there is no missingness involved in this part, it contributes to the within matrix, but not to the between matrix. Then, using (16.16), the approximate within matrix for the marginal treatment effect is

$$W_0 = \pi' W \pi + \beta' \mathrm{Var}(\pi) \beta,$$

with, for the between matrix, simply

$$B_0 = \pi' B \pi.$$

The results are presented in the second panel of Table 16.3. All three p-values are in between those obtained for Strategies 2a and 2b. Of course, all five agree on the lack of significance of the treatment effect. The reason for the differences is to be found in the way the treatment effect is extrapolated beyond the period of observation. Indeed, the highest p-value is obtained for Strategy 2a and, from Figure 16.1, we learn that virtually no separation between both treatment arms is projected. On the other hand, wider separations are seen in Figure 16.8.

Finally, we note that all conclusions are conditional upon the unverifiable assumption that the posited restrictions (and hence, dropout mechanisms) are correct. This underscores the need for sensitivity analysis.

16.7 A CLINICAL TRIAL IN ALZHEIMER'S DISEASE

These data come from a three-arm clinical trial involving patients diagnosed with Alzheimer's disease (Reisberg *et al.* 1987), conducted by 50 investigators in 8 countries. The outcome is a dementia score ranging from 0 to 43. Treatment arm 1 is placebo, with 114 patients, while arms 2, with 115 patients, and 3, with 115 patients, involve active compounds. Of the patient population, 56.4% are female. There are 341 Caucasians, 2 Orientals and 1 black subject. Age ranges from 56 to 97 years, with a median of 81 years. Measurements are taken at baseline, at weeks 1, 2 and then every two weeks until week 12. Individual profiles are plotted in Figure 16.9. In agreement with the protocol, we will analyse change with respect to baseline. This outcome is sufficiently close to normality, in contrast to the raw score.

Attrition over time is fairly steady for each treatment arm. The sample size for each dropout pattern and treatment arm is displayed in Table 16.4. In each of the arms, about 40% of subjects drop out before the end of the study.

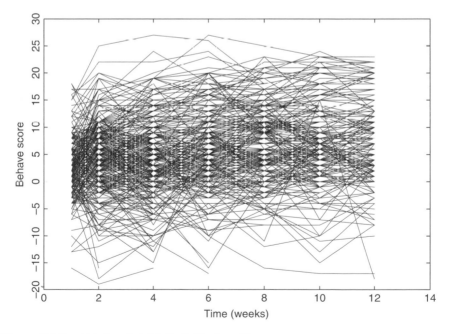

Figure 16.9 Alzheimer's trial. Individual profiles.

Table 16.4 Alzheimer's trial. Sample size by treatment arm and dropout pattern.

Pattern	1	2	3	4	5	6	7
Treatment 1	4	5	16	3	9	6	71
Treatment 2	4	9	7	6	3	5	81
Treatment 3	12	4	15	9	5	3	67

Unfortunately, very little is known about the reasons for this dropout. While such information is generally important, one also needs to be able to analyse incomplete data in the absence of such knowledge.

A linear mixed model (Section 7.3) was fitted to the outcomes, in which the variance structure was modelled by means of a random subject effect, an exponential serial correlation process and measurement error. The fixed effects considered in the model were, apart from treatment effect, those of age, time, investigator, and country, as well as two- and three-way interactions. From an initial model-selection exercise, only main effects of age, time, time^2, and treatment group were retained.

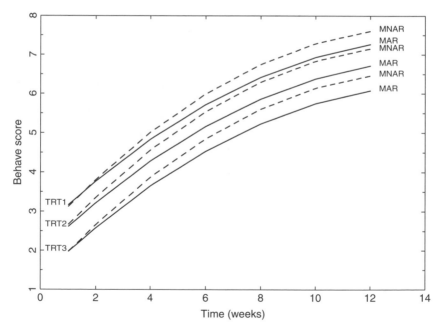

Figure 16.10 Alzheimer's trial. Selection models. Fitted average profiles. (TRT, treatment).

Scientific interest is in the effect of treatment. As there are three arms, we consider two treatment contrasts of the experimental arms versus the standard arm. Our focus here will be on estimates and standard errors for these contrasts as well as on tests for the null hypothesis of no treatment effect. We first consider the selection model approach. As in Section 15.2, we combine the measurement model with a logistic regression for dropout with (a) only an intercept, corresponding to MCAR; (b) with an intercept and an effect for previous outcome, corresponding to MAR; or (c) with an intercept and an effect of the current possibly unobserved measurement, corresponding to MNAR. The fitted average profiles are plotted in Figure 16.10. Parameter estimates and standard errors for the treatment contrasts, as well as the associated test results, are reported in Table 16.5. Treatment effects are non-significant. The likelihood ratio statistic for comparing the MAR and MNAR models is 5.4 on 2 degrees of freedom. Again, we cannot use the standard χ^2 reference distribution for this, and given the dependence on modelling assumptions, this must be treated with interpreted with due caution. We return to such issues in Chapter 19.

Next, we turn attention to the PMMs. Apart from ACMV, CCMV, and NCMV, we also consider NFD1 and NFD2 (see Section 3.6). As in the previous example (Section 16.6), both marginal and pattern-specific treatment effects and corresponding inferences are computed. The results of our analysis are reported in Tables 16.5 and 16.6. The marginal treatment effect assessments are all non-significant, in line with the results from the selection model analysis. However, all stratified treatment assessments produce significant p-values, although to various levels of strength. Strong evidence is obtained from the ACMV model. Of course, the CCMV analysis provides even stronger evidence, but this assumption may be unrealistic, since even patterns with few observations are completed using the set of completers, corresponding to pattern 7. Both of the other NFMV mechanisms, corresponding to cases 4 and 5, where dropout does not depend on future unobserved values, provide mild evidence for treatment effect. Importantly, we are in a position to consider which patterns are responsible for an identified treatment effect. Note that the contrasts are nowhere near significant in the complete

Table 16.5 Alzheimer's trial. Inference for treatment contrasts: selection models. For the contrasts, parameter estimates (and standard errors) are reported.

Contrast	MAR	MNAR
Marginal Analysis		
1	0.55 (0.71)	0.45 (0.71)
2	0.64 (0.71)	0.69 (0.71)
F value	2.82	2.68
p value	0.2446	0.2619

Table 16.6 Alzheimer's trial. Inference for treatment contrasts: pattern-mixture models. For the contrasts, parameter estimates (and standard errors) are reported. (ACMV, available case missing values; CCMV, complete case missing values; NCMV, neighbouring case missing values; FD1, case 4; FD2, case 5.)

Pattern	Contrast	ACMV	CCMV	NCMV	FD1	FD2
Stratified analysis						
1	1	9.27(6.42)	5.84(5.16)	−4.19(6.27)	4.90(8.29)	5.44(6.52)
	2	−8.19(6.58)	−6.92(6.15)	2.56(5.12)	−7.78(7.62)	−4.48(7.76)
2	1	2.78(4.75)	−0.00(2.90)	−4.43(3.54)	0.61(4.88)	−1.49(4.07)
	2	−3.57(4.53)	−5.08(3.92)	−1.37(4.12)	−6.48(5.22)	−4.54(5.46)
3	1	6.78(4.20)	6.95(2.66)	0.10(2.40)	4.18(2.64)	0.18(3.65)
	2	−1.75(2.76)	−3.44(2.12)	0.83(2.14)	−2.66(2.29)	−0.10(2.20)
4	1	11.05(3.21)	10.87(2.85)	6.59(3.09)	9.65(3.56)	9.97(2.90)
	2	−3.84(4.09)	−6.55(3.88)	−3.23(4.09)	−6.84(3.78)	−4.30(4.24)
5	1	0.15(5.71)	−2.05(6.29)	−5.60(6.46)	−3.02(5.92)	−6.13(6.42)
	2	−0.74(3.99)	−0.87(4.51)	0.92(4.68)	−0.53(4.24)	1.05(4.57)
6	1	14.16(3.75)	12.91(3.71)	13.44(3.72)	13.28(3.82)	12.72(3.79)
	2	−5.24(3.48)	−4.74(3.69)	−4.95(3.79)	−4.71(3.63)	−4.77(3.70)
7	1	−0.99(0.85)	−0.99(0.85)	−0.99(0.85)	−0.99(0.85)	−0.99(0.85)
	2	1.68(0.88)	1.68(0.88)	1.68(0.88)	1.68(0.88)	1.68(0.88)
F-value		2.45	2.96	1.76	1.92	1.77
p-value		0.0024	0.0002	0.0407	0.0225	0.0413
Marginal analysis						
	1	1.97(1.05)	1.47(0.87)	−0.48(0.85)	1.05(1.04)	0.37(0.96)
	2	−0.24(0.81)	−0.56(0.86)	0.91(0.77)	−0.59(1.01)	0.19(0.84)
F-value		2.15	1.23	0.66	0.52	0.19
p-value		0.1362	0.3047	0.5208	0.6043	0.8276

pattern 7, while patterns 4 and 6 seem to contribute to the effect, consistently across patterns. The first contrast of pattern 3 is significant only under CCMV, perhaps explaining why this strategy yields the most significant result.

Figure 16.11 provides a graphical summary the fit of these models for the first treatment arm; very similar displays for the other arms have been omitted. Clearly, the chosen identifying restrictions have a strong impact, especially for the patterns with earlier dropout. Of course, from Table 16.4 it is clear that the earlier patterns are rather sparsely filled. It is striking to see that the missing non-future dependence patterns are not all grouped together. An important and perhaps counterintuitive feature is that the fitted averages depend on the identification method chosen, even at time points prior to dropout. The reason for this is that, after imputation, a parametric model is fitted to the completed sequences as a whole, as opposed to, for example, change point models with change point at the time of dropout. Hence, the smoothing induced by the parametric model applies across the entire sequence, before and after dropout.

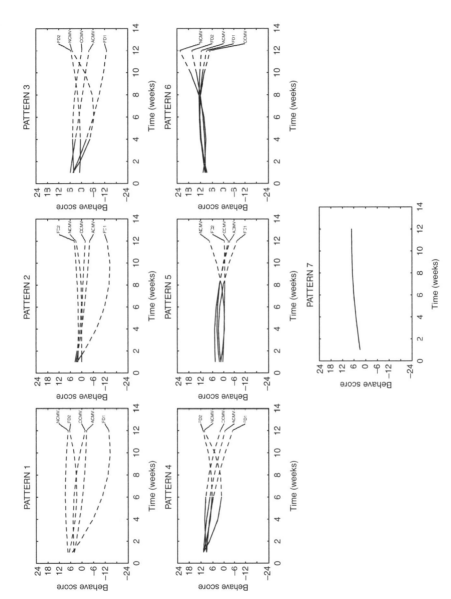

Figure 16.11 Alzheimer's trial. Pattern-mixture models. Fitted average profiles for each of the five identification strategies. Treatment arm 1. ACMV, CCMV, NCMV, NFD1, and NFD2.

16.8   ANALYSIS OF THE FLUVOXAMINE TRIAL

The fluvoxamine trial was introduced in Section 2.6 and later analysed in Sections 12.6, 15.4.2, and 15.5.1. A dichotomized version of side effects, at the first and last visits, will be considered, where category 1 (no side effect) is contrasted with the others for both outcomes (category 0). Hence, we model the probability of *no* side effects. There are 299 patients with at least one measurement, including 242 completers. We will start with selection models and then move on to pattern-mixture models. In all cases, a bivariate Dale model (Molenberghs and Lesaffre 1994; Molenberghs and Verbeke 2005, Section 7.7) will be considered for the bivariate binary outcome. This means each of the outcomes is described using logistic regression parameters, and the association between both is captured by means of a (log) odds ratio.

16.8.1   Selection modelling

Table 16.7 gives parameter estimates and asymptotic confidence intervals for a selection model that includes age, sex, and psychiatric antecedents, both in the marginal measurement model and the logistic model for dropout. Note that age is a continuous covariate, whereas the other two are dichotomous. To allow for MAR, the first response is also entered in the dropout model. The association is modelled in terms of a constant log odds ratio.

In the marginal model, sex and antecedents appear to have little effect, whereas age is borderline and its coefficients at both measurement occasions are very similar. Likewise, *age* and *antecedents* add little to the dropout model, and sex and the outcome at the first occasion are borderline, albeit at different

Table 16.7   Fluvoxamine trial. Selection model parameter estimates and 95% confidence intervals (full model).

Parameter	First measurement		Last measurement	
Intercept	0.786	[−0.083, 1.654]	1.432	[0.397, 2.467]
Age/30	−0.669	[−1.218, −0.119]	−0.676	[−1.318, −0.034]
Sex	−0.318	[−0.811, 0.175]	0.254	[−0.337, 0.846]
Antecedents	0.134	[−0.366, 0.633]	−0.057	[−0.649, 0.536]
Association				
Log odds ratio	2.038	[1.335, 2.740]		
Dropout model				
Intercept	1.583	[0.571, 2.595]		
Previous	−0.556	[−1.119, 0.007]		
Age/30	−0.261	[−0.874, 0.352]		
Sex	0.608	[0.052, 1.164]		
Antecedents	−0.254	[−0.836, 0.327]		

Table 16.8 Fluvoxamine trial. Selection model parameter estimates and 95% confidence intervals after model reduction.

Parameter	First measurement		Last measurement	
Intercept	0.661	[−0.043, 1.365]	1.560	[0.823, 2.297]
Common age (/30)	−0.664	[−1.141, −0.188]		
Association				
Log odds ratio	1.956	[1.270, 2.642]		
Dropout model				
Intercept	1.085	[0.547, 1.624]		
Previous	−0.584	[−1.140, −0.028]		
Sex	0.568	[0.025, 1.110]		

sides of the critical level. The association between both measurements, even with adjustment of the marginal regression for covariate effects, remains very high, with an odds ratio of $\exp(2.038) = 7.675$.

A backward selection procedure was performed on the measurement and dropout processes separately, based on the likelihood ratio test. Parameters were removed in the following order. For the measurement model: both antecedents effects and both sex effects were removed. Subsequently, the two age parameters were combined into a common age effect. For the dropout model, age and antecedents were removed. The result is shown in Table 16.8. From this model, it is seen that the probability of side effects is higher at the first measurement occasion than at the last one, and increases with *age*. In particular, for an increase of 1 year, the odds of side effects increase by a factor $\exp(0.664/30) = 1.022$, because age was divided by 30 for ease of display of the estimates. The probability of dropout is higher if side effects are observed at the first occasion, and is lower for males than for females. In particular, the dropout probabilities are 0.256 (0.161) for males with (without) previous side effects, and 0.377 (0.253) for females with (without) side effects. The association, as well as the other parameters, except for the intercept, are similar to those found in Table 16.7.

16.8.2 Pattern-mixture modelling

For the pattern-mixture approach, the parameter estimates and confidence intervals for the variables age, sex, and antecedents can be found in Table 16.9. The model is parameterized as follows: intercepts and covariate effects are given for the complete observations, together with the differences between effects for incomplete and complete observations. The latter ones would be zero if the distribution among completers equalled the distribution among dropouts. This model is used for the first as well as for the last observation. A constant

Table 16.9 Fluvoxamine trial. Pattern-mixture model. Profile likelihood (PL) and multiple imputation (MI) (full model).

Parameter	Method	First measurement		Last measurement	
Complete observations					
Intercept	PL	1.296	[0.289, 2.339]	1.664	[0.616, 2.767]
	MI	1.296	[0.268, 2.325]	1.663	[0.596, 2.731]
Age/30	PL	−0.849	[−1.519, −0.203]	−0.756	[−1.440, −0.091]
	MI	−0.849	[−1.500, −0.198]	−0.756	[−1.414, −0.097]
Sex	PL	−0.593	[−1.189, −0.007]	0.127	[−0.497, 0.739]
	MI	−0.593	[−1.182, −0.004]	0.127	[−0.483, 0.737]
Antecedents	PL	0.222	[−0.353, 0.805]	−0.016	[−0.634, 0.594]
	MI	0.222	[−0.357, 0.800]	−0.016	[−0.621, 0.589]
Incomplete minus complete observations					
Intercept	PL	−2.151	[−4.300, −0.084]	−0.913	[−4.376, 3.204]
	MI	−2.156	[−4.224, −0.087]	−1.018	[−4.393, 2.357]
Age/30	PL	0.869	[−0.396, 2.142]	0.366	[−1.845, 2.435]
	MI	0.871	[−0.396, 2.139]	0.395	[−1.503, 2.292]
Sex	PL	0.879	[−0.268, 2.050]	0.382	[−1.413, 2.236]
	MI	0.879	[−0.274, 2.033]	0.347	[−1.477, 2.171]
Antecedents	PL	−0.234	[−1.428, 0.986]	−0.107	[−2.271, 1.802]
	MI	−0.234	[−1.439, 0.970]	−0.012	[−1.858, 1.834]
Association					
Log odds ratio	PL	2.038	[1.354, 2.789]		
	MI	2.065	[1.346, 2.784]		
Dropout model, CI based on asymptotic variance (AV)					
Intercept	AV	1.390	[0.450, 2.370]		
Age/30	AV	−0.349	[−0.953, 0.255]		
Sex	AV	0.559	[0.010, 1.108]		
Antecedents	AV	−0.232	[−0.809, 0.345]		

log odds ratio is assumed for the association between both measurements. The confidence intervals are calculated using profile likelihood, as well as using multiple imputation. For the multiple imputation technique, the results are given for 100 imputations. As a check, Michiels *et al.* (1999) have also calculated the confidence intervals for 1000 and 4000 imputations, leading to negligible differences. Both methods to calculate confidence intervals (results not shown here) give approximately the same results. The same variables are used to fit the dropout model, and because the data needed to estimate this model are complete, we have calculated confidence intervals based on the asymptotic variance. Although multiple imputation is only performed to estimate the precision, we also display the corresponding parameter estimates as an extra indication for convergence of the algorithm.

Antecedents and sex have nearly no effect on the measurement model, but the *sex* parameter for the first measurement gives a borderline influence. *Age* has an effect on the measurement outcomes, but there is no difference between this effect for the complete and incomplete observations. The association between both measurements is very strong. The odds ratio is $\exp(2.038) = 7.675$. Age and antecedents have no effect on the dropout model, unlike sex.

The model was reduced using a backward selection procedure. For the measurement model, we dropped antecedents, the additional age effect for the incomplete observations, and all the sex effects. Finally, a joint age effect for both time points is assumed. In the dropout model, antecedents and age were removed. Sex was kept, although it is borderline. The final model can be found in Table 16.10.

From this model it can be seen that the probability of dropout is higher for males than for females: 0.253 and 0.168, respectively. The probability of having side effects is higher at the first occasion than at the last, and increases for those who did not show up at the last visit. This probability also increases with age. For an increase of 1 year, the odds of having side effects increase by a factor of 1.022. The association is similar to its value in the full model, shown in Table 16.9.

Note that the PMM assumed a common odds ratio among completers and dropouts. This implies that the conditional distribution of the missing second measure follows the same conditional distribution given the first variable as does the complete variable. This ACMV restriction, as discussed in Section 3.3, is equivalent to the MAR assumption in the selection model.

Table 16.10 Fluvoxamine trial. Pattern-mixture model. Profile likelihood (PL) and multiple imputation (MI) after model reduction.

Parameter	Method	First measurement	Last measurement
Complete observations			
Intercept	PL	0.762 [0.036, 1.478]	1.590 [0.846, 2.333]
	MI	0.747 [0.029, 1.466]	1.576 [0.836, 2.315]
Incomplete minus complete observations			
Intercept	PL	−0.499 [−1.065, 0.050]	−0.268 [−1.123, 0.704]
	MI	−0.499 [−1.055, 0.056]	−0.275 [−1.071, 0.521]
Common age effect (/30)			
	PL	−0.650 [−1.132, −0.162]	
	MI	−0.639 [−1.121, −0.158]	
Association			
Log odds ratio	PL	1.977 [1.291, 2.682]	
	MI	1.943 [1.263, 2.623]	
Dropout model, CI based on asymptotic variance (AV)			
Intercept	AV	0.766 [0.353, 1.179]	
Sex	AV	0.517 [−0.021, 1.056]	

16.8.3 Comparison

Both reduced models include age as a predictor for side effects. For the selection model, this effect is the same at both measurement occasions. The same is true for the PMM and for both subgroups, although it could in principle differ for completers and dropouts. As a result, the estimates of the age effects in both frameworks become comparable and their numerical values are very close indeed. By construction, the association parameters are also comparable; they are certainly of the same magnitude. Of course, the dropout models differ, since only in a selection model can measurements be included in the dropout part as covariates. The sex effect is similar in both models, but its effect is of borderline significance.

The PMM can yield valuable insight in its own right. Specifically, the probability of side effects, after adjusting for age, is higher in the dropout group than in the completers' group, both at the first as well as at the last measurement occasion. For someone aged 30, say, the probabilities of side effects at the first measurement occasion in the completers' group and the dropouts' groups are 0.4720 and 0.5956, respectively. At the last measurement occasion these probabilities are 0.2809 and 0.3380, respectively. These values can be obtained in a selection framework as well, albeit less straightforwardly. Another advantage of the PMM is that the model building can be done for the different dropout groups separately. For example, if sex were a prognostic factor for side effects in the dropout group but not in the completers' group, this could easily be incorporated in the pattern-mixture analysis.

16.9 CONCLUDING REMARKS

We have introduced a number of practical ways of using pattern-mixture models with clinical data, building on the formalism laid out in Section 3.6. We have distinguished between two rather different strategies. The first uses identifying restrictions. The second, broadly speaking, uses models that are sufficiently simple for extrapolations to be possible past the point of dropout within a particular pattern. The results from this second route depend greatly on the extrapolations made, which may of course be highly inappropriate, especially as they are typically based on low-order polynomials. At the same time the assumptions that these extrapolations imply concerning the dropout mechanism are far from transparent. Within the first strategy, it is possible to consider identification based on the completers (CCMV), the neighbours (NCMV), and by analogy with MAR (ACMV). Furthermore, one can ensure that any dropout depends on values at or before the time at which it occurs, but not on points later in time. Even when a PMM is assumed, it is possible to conduct conventional marginal inference, that is, marginalized over the patterns.

Due to the versatility of the framework, PMMs can be used in their own right, as well as for the purpose of contrast with other frameworks, in particular the selection model framework. Thus, they can be a valuable tool in the sensitivity analyst's toolkit.

It may even be possible, rather than choosing between selection models and PMMs, to combine aspects of both. Such a route was chosen by Molenberghs *et al.* (1998a).

We have illustrated the methodology on three sets of data, two continuous ones, the vorozole trial and a clinical trial conducted on Alzheimer's patients, and one with discrete, binary outcomes, the fluvoxamine trial.

17

Shared-Parameter Models

Interest in methods for joint modelling of longitudinal and survival time data has developed considerably in recent years (see, for example, Pawitan and Self 1993; DeGruttola and Tu 1994; Taylor *et al.* 1994; Faucett and Thomas 1996; Lavalley and DeGruttola 1996; Hogan and Laird 1997, 1998; Wulfsohn and Tsiatis 1997; Henderson *et al.* 2000; Xu and Zeger 2001). Broadly speaking, there are three main reasons for considering such models.

First, a time-to-event outcome may be measured in terms of a longitudinal covariate. Such a joint model then allows, in a natural way, for incorporation of measurement error present in the longitudinal covariate into the model.

Second, a number of researchers have used joint modelling methods to exploit longitudinal markers as surrogates for survival. Tsiatis *et al.* (1995), for instance, propose a model for the relationship of survival to longitudinal data measured with error and, using Prentice criteria, examine whether CD4 counts may serve as a useful surrogate marker for survival in patients with AIDS. Xu and Zeger (2001) investigate the issue of evaluating multiple surrogate endpoints and discuss a joint latent model for a time to clinical event and for repeated measures over time on multiple biomarkers that are potential surrogates. In addition, they propose two complementary measures to assess the relative benefit of using multiple surrogates as opposed to a single one. Another aspect of the problem, discussed by Henderson *et al.* (2002), is the identification of longitudinal markers for survival. These authors focus on the use of longitudinal marker trajectories as individual-level surrogates for survival. Renard *et al.* (2002) used a joint model to explore the usefulness of prostate-specific antigen as a marker for prostate cancer.

Third, such joint models can be used when incomplete longitudinal data are collected. As stated in Section 3.3, whenever data are incomplete, one should a priori consider the joint distribution (3.2) of responses and missing

Missing Data in Clinical Studies G. Molenberghs and M.G. Kenward
© 2007 John Wiley & Sons, Ltd

data process. In this sense, selection models and pattern-mixture models are merely convenient ways to decompose this joint distribution. In a number of applications, it may be convenient to write this joint distribution in terms of latent variables, latent classes, or random effects. This leads to the so-called shared-parameter models (3.5). In principle, one can augment (3.2) with random effects

$$f(\boldsymbol{y}_i, \boldsymbol{r}_i, \boldsymbol{b}_i | X_i, W_i, Z_i, \boldsymbol{\theta}, \boldsymbol{\psi}, \boldsymbol{\xi}), \tag{17.1}$$

and then still consider the selection model factorization

$$f(\boldsymbol{y}_i, \boldsymbol{r}_i, \boldsymbol{b}_i | X_i, W_i, Z_i, \boldsymbol{\theta}, \boldsymbol{\psi})$$
$$= f(\boldsymbol{y}_i | X_i, \boldsymbol{b}_i, \boldsymbol{\theta}) f(\boldsymbol{r}_i | \boldsymbol{y}_i, \boldsymbol{b}_i, W_i, \boldsymbol{\psi}) f(\boldsymbol{b}_i | Z_i, \boldsymbol{\xi}) \tag{17.2}$$

and the PMM factorization

$$f(\boldsymbol{y}_i, \boldsymbol{r}_i, \boldsymbol{b}_i | X_i, W_i, Z_i, \boldsymbol{\theta}, \boldsymbol{\psi}, \boldsymbol{\xi})$$
$$= f(\boldsymbol{y}_i | \boldsymbol{r}_i, \boldsymbol{b}_i, X_i, \boldsymbol{\theta}) f(\boldsymbol{r}_i | \boldsymbol{b}_i, W_i, \boldsymbol{\psi}) f(\boldsymbol{b}_i | Z_i, \boldsymbol{\xi}). \tag{17.3}$$

The notation is the same as in Section 3.3, with in addition Z_i and $\boldsymbol{\xi}$ covariates and parameters, respectively, describing the random-effects distribution. Little (1995) refers to such decompositions as random-coefficient selection and pattern-mixture models, respectively.

Important early references to such models are Wu and Carroll (1988) and Wu and Bailey (1988, 1989). Wu and Carroll (1988) proposed such a model for what they termed informative right censoring. For a continuous response, Wu and Carroll suggested using a conventional Gaussian random-coefficient model combined with an appropriate model for to time to dropout, such as proportional hazards, logistic or probit regression. The combination of probit and Gaussian response allows explicit solution of the integral and was used in their application.

In a slightly different approach to modelling dropout time as a continuous variable in the latent variable setting, Schluchter (1992) and DeGruttola and Tu (1994) proposed joint multivariate Gaussian distributions for the latent variable(s) of the response process and a variable representing time to dropout. The correlation between these variables induces dependence between dropout and response. To permit more realistic distributions for dropout time, Schluchter proposes that dropout time itself should be some monotone transformation of the corresponding Gaussian variable. The use of a joint Gaussian representation does simplify computational problems associated with the likelihood. There are clear links here with the tobit model, and this is made explicit by Cowles *et al.* (1996) who use a number of correlated latent variables to represent various aspects of an individual's behaviour, such as compliance and attendance at scheduled visits. Models of this type handle non-monotone missingness quite conveniently. There are many ways in which such models can be extended and generalized.

An important simplification arises when Y_i and R_i are assumed independent, given the random effects. We then obtain shared-parameter decomposition (3.5) or, spelled out in full:

$$f(\boldsymbol{y}_i, \boldsymbol{r}_i, \boldsymbol{b}_i | X_i, W_i, Z_i, \boldsymbol{\theta}, \boldsymbol{\psi}, \boldsymbol{\xi})$$
$$= f(\boldsymbol{y}_i | X_i, \boldsymbol{b}_i, \boldsymbol{\theta}) f(\boldsymbol{r}_i | W_i, \boldsymbol{b}_i, \boldsymbol{\psi}) f(\boldsymbol{b}_i | Z_i, \boldsymbol{\xi}). \qquad (17.4)$$

This route was followed by Follmann and Wu (1995). Note that when $\boldsymbol{b}_i$ is assumed to be discrete, a latent-class or mixture model follows.

Rizopoulos *et al.* (2006) study the impact of random-effects misspecification in a shared-parameter model. Beunckens *et al.* (2006) combine continuous random effects with latent classes, leading to the simultaneous use of mixture and mixed-effects models ideas. This model is reported in Chapter 24.

It is natural to handle random-coefficient models, and in particular shared-parameter models, in a Bayesian framework. Examples in the missing value setting are provided by Best *et al.* (1996) and Carpenter *et al.* (2002).

18

Protective Estimation

18.1 INTRODUCTION

For multivariate Gaussian data, Brown (1990) constructed an estimator for the mean and covariance parameters of the joint normal distribution. He assumes that the missingness depends on the unobserved values, but not on the observed measurements, a particular and interesting type of MNAR. He called this estimator a *protective estimator*. Brown (1990) focused on an example where measurements are collected relatively far apart in time, such that the influence of a previous measurement on non-response might be deemed negligible. He allows for the presence of all possible response patterns, but each subject is measured at the first occasion. A key feature of this estimator is that there is no need to explicitly address the missing data mechanism, a very special MNAR version of ignorability, as it were.

Michiels and Molenberghs (1997) presented an analogous estimator for the repeated categorical case, still assuming each subject is observed at the first occasion, but with the important distinction that missingness is due to attrition, ruling out non-monotone patterns. Their protective estimator can be used in the selection and pattern-mixture framework. Estimation of measurement parameters is also possible, without explicitly modelling the dropout process. While Brown (1990) only gives necessary conditions for consistent solutions, Michiels and Molenberghs (1997) derive necessary and sufficient conditions for a unique solution in the interior of the parameter space and present an intuitive and appealing interpretation of these conditions. They present an algorithm consisting of the repeated calculation for a bivariate outcome, with the first one always observed and the second one possibly missing. This procedure circumvents the need to work with intractable systems of equations.

Missing Data in Clinical Studies   G. Molenberghs and M.G. Kenward
© 2007 John Wiley & Sons, Ltd

Lipsitz *et al.* (2004) returned to the Gaussian case, originally considered by Brown (1990), and extended it to the estimation of covariate effects in the marginal regression model. They made the further assumption that the missing data mechanism is conditionally independent of the regression covariate, given the outcome variable and the remaining covariates. A method of moments approach is used to obtain the protective estimator of the regression parameters, while jackknifing (Quenouille 1956) is employed to estimate the variance. The proposed method only requires the application of two separate ordinary least-squares regressions.

In Section 18.2 the protective estimator is introduced, and in Section 18.3 the analogous situation with repeated categorical measurements. The connection with direct likelihood estimation is given in Section 18.3.1, and a link with pseudo-likelihood estimation is established in Section 18.3.2. Section 18.3.3 is devoted to variance estimation. The precision estimates will be based on the delta method, the EM algorithm, and multiple imputation. The relative merits of these techniques are discussed and they are contrasted with the results from likelihood and pseudo-likelihood estimation. The method for categorical data is illustrated with two examples. The first, presented in Section 18.3.5, is the fluvoxamine trial. The second, a data set on presence or absence of colds, is analysed in Section 18.3.6.

Section 18.4 is devoted to the method proposed by Lipsitz *et al.* (2004). In Section 18.4.1 notation is presented, together with the complete data model and the observed data likelihood. In Section 18.4.2 the protective estimator for the linear regression parameters is developed. Finally, in Section 18.4.3, the proposed method is illustrated using the data on the persistence of maternal smoking from the six cities study (Ware *et al.* 1984).

18.2   BROWN'S PROTECTIVE ESTIMATOR FOR GAUSSIAN DATA

Brown (1990) introduced the *protective estimator* for normal data. He called it 'protective' because it retains its consistency over a wide range of non-random missing data mechanisms.

Let Y be an n-dimensional random variable, following a multivariate normal distribution. Let R be the usual vector of missingness indicators. As usual, Y_{ij} is the jth measure on the ith subject ($i = 1, \ldots, N$; $j = 1, \ldots, n$). The joint distribution of Y and R is factorized in a selection modelling manner (3.3). A *generalized censoring mechanism* is defined as

$$f(r_i|y_i) = \prod_{j=1}^{n} h_j(r_j|y_j),$$

where $h_j(\cdot)$, $j = 1, \ldots, n$, are functions bounded between 0 and 1, but without further restrictions. Under the generalized censoring mechanism, missingness on each outcome depends on the same variable only. Because one usually assumes the first measurement to be observed for every subject, it is natural to keep h_1 constant. The other h_j are left unspecified.

To obtain estimators for the unknown parameters in the model, Brown (1990) used statistics whose distributions do not depend on the mechanism and showed that this method leads to consistent estimators. We will exemplify the method for $n = 3$. Generalization to higher dimensions is straightforward.

The first two moments of Y_1 can be estimated independently from the missing data mechanism, because the first measurement is observed for all subjects. This leads to estimators for μ_1 and σ_{11}. Furthermore, the distributions of $Y_1|(y_2; R_2 = 1)$, $Y_1|(y_3; R_3 = 1)$, and $Y_1|(y_2, y_3; R_2 = 1, R_3 = 1)$ do not depend on the missing data mechanism. For example,

$$f(y_1|y_2; R_2 = 1) = \phi(y_1|y_2; \boldsymbol{\beta}),$$

where ϕ is the normal density and $\boldsymbol{\beta}$ are measurement parameters, that is, functions of $(\boldsymbol{\mu}, \Sigma)$. This implies the following statistics are independent of the mechanism: $\mu_1 - \sigma_{11}/\sigma_{22}\mu_2$, σ_{12}/σ_{22}, and $\sigma_{11.2} = \sigma_{11} - \sigma_{12}^2/\sigma_{22})$.

Under the mild assumption that neither σ_{12} nor σ_{13} equals zero, these statistics lead, using straightforward algebra, to $\mu_2, \sigma_{12}, \sigma_{22}, \mu_3, \sigma_{13}$, and σ_{33}. Furthermore, if one calculates the partial regression coefficients to predict Y_1,

$$\beta_{12.3} = \frac{\sigma_{12}\sigma_{33} - \sigma_{13}\sigma_{23}}{\sigma_{22}\sigma_{33} - \sigma_{23}^2},$$

$$\beta_{13.2} = \frac{-\sigma_{12}\sigma_{23} + \sigma_{13}\sigma_{22}}{\sigma_{22}\sigma_{33} - \sigma_{23}^2},$$

the only statistic not yet estimated is given by

$$\sigma_{23} = \begin{cases} -\sqrt{\dfrac{\beta_{13.2}\sigma_{12}\sigma_{33} - \beta_{12.3}\sigma_{13}\sigma_{22}}{\beta_{12.3}\sigma_{12} - \beta_{13.2}\sigma_{13}}} & \text{if } \rho_{12}^2 \neq \rho_{13}^2, \\[2em] \sqrt{\dfrac{\sigma_{12}\sigma_{33}}{\sigma_{13}}} & \text{if } \rho_{12}^2 = \rho_{13}^2 \neq 0 \text{ and } \beta_{12.3} = 0, \\[2em] \pm\sqrt{\sigma_{22}\sigma_{33}}\left(\sqrt{\dfrac{\sigma_{11}}{\sigma_{22}}\dfrac{\rho_{12}}{\beta_{12.3}}} - 1\right) & \text{if } \rho_{12} = \pm\rho_{13} \text{ and } \beta_{12.3} \neq 0. \end{cases}$$

The next step is to estimate all of these statistics. In the following, the superscripts indicate whether a measurement is observed (1), missing (0), or marginalized (.). Estimates for all the statistics we need are:

$$\widehat{\mu}_1 = \bar{Y}_1^{(1..)},$$

$$\widehat{\sigma}_{11} = s_{11}^{(1..)},$$

$$\widehat{\mu}_2 = \frac{\bar{Y}_1^{(1..)} - \bar{Y}_1^{(11.)}}{b_{12}^{(11.)}} + \bar{Y}_2^{(11.)},$$

$$\widehat{\sigma}_{22} = \frac{\widehat{\sigma}_{11} - s_{11.2}^{(11.)}}{(b_{12}^{(11.)})^2},$$

$$\widehat{\sigma}_{12} = b_{12}^{(11.)}\widehat{\sigma}_{22},$$

$$\widehat{\mu}_3 = \frac{\bar{Y}_1^{(1..)} - \bar{Y}_1^{(1.1)}}{b_{13}^{(1.1)}} + \bar{Y}_3^{(1.1)},$$

$$\widehat{\sigma}_{33} = \frac{\widehat{\sigma}_{11} - s_{11.3}^{(1.1)}}{(b_{13}^{(1.1)})^2},$$

$$\widehat{\sigma}_{13} = b_{13}^{(1.1)}\widehat{\sigma}_{33}.$$

We obtain $\widehat{\sigma}_{23}$ by minimizing a residual variance expression for $Y_1|y_2, y_3$ in terms of previously calculated estimates. Define

$$M_{1.23}(y_2, y_3; \sigma_{23}^*) = \widehat{\mu}_1 + \frac{\widehat{\sigma}_{12}\widehat{\sigma}_{33} - \widehat{\sigma}_{13}\sigma_{23}^*}{\widehat{\sigma}_{22}\widehat{\sigma}_{33} - (\sigma_{23}^*)^2}(y_2 - \widehat{\mu}_2) + \frac{\widehat{\sigma}_{13}\widehat{\sigma}_{22} - \widehat{\sigma}_{12}\sigma_{23}^*}{\widehat{\sigma}_{22}\widehat{\sigma}_{33} - (\sigma_{23}^*)^2}(y_3 - \widehat{\mu}_3).$$

Then, $\widehat{\sigma}_{23}$ is the value for σ_{23}^* minimizing

$$\sum_{s: r_{s1} = r_{s2} = r_{s3} = 1} \{y_{s1} - M_{1.23}(y_{s2}, y_{s3}; \sigma_{23}^*)\}^2.$$

Brown (1990) also gives necessary conditions to have consistent estimators:

$$\forall t : \rho_{1t} \neq 0 \text{ and } P(Y_t \text{ is observed}) > 0.$$

However, they are not sufficient.

A drawback of this method is that all missingness patterns (with the first variable observed) are needed to obtain the necessary estimates. Hence, in a study with dropout only, no complete solution exists for the protective estimator with normal data.

18.3   A PROTECTIVE ESTIMATOR FOR CATEGORICAL DATA

The class of protective estimators for repeated categorical data, introduced by Michiels and Molenberghs (1997), will be presented next. In contrast to the protective estimator for normal data (Section 18.2), in the case of categorical data we have to restrict to dropout to find unique estimates. The hypothetically complete data, organized in a contingency table, are written $Z_{d,k_1 \ldots k_n}^c$, with multinomial cell probabilities

$$\nu_{d,k_1 \ldots k_n}^c = P(D_i = d, Y_{i1} = k_1, \ldots, Y_{in} = k_n). \tag{18.1}$$

Here, D_i is the dropout indicator for subject i. Let r denote the number of levels the categorical outcomes Y_{ij} can take. We will use the following simplified notation for the selection model and the pattern-mixture model, respectively:

$$\nu^c_{d,k_1...k_n} = \mu^c_{k_1...k_n} \, \phi^c_{d|k_1...k_n},$$
$$\nu^c_{d,k_1...k_n} = \phi^c_d \, \mu^c_{k_1...k_n|d}. \tag{18.2}$$

Since we only observed the first d measures, the observed data are $Z_{d,k_1...k_d}$. So we can estimate the probabilities

$$\mu^c_{k_1...k_d|d} \tag{18.3}$$

directly from the data, as well as derived marginal and conditional probabilities. These probabilities are of a pattern-mixture nature and correspond to a 'partial classification' of model (18.2). The aim is to construct the cell probabilities $\mu^c_{k_1...k_n}$, when a selection model is thought appropriate, or $\mu^c_{k_1...k_n|d}$ for PMMs.

A key assumption for protective estimation is that dropout (possibly) depends on the unobserved outcome, but not on the (previously) observed outcomes. The method used to estimate the probabilities is based on statistics that are independent of the missing data mechanism. Factor the probability $\nu^c_{(D\geq d),k_1k_2...k_t}$ first as

$$\nu^c_{(D\geq d),k_1k_2...k_t} = \nu^c_{(D\geq d),k_2...k_t} \, \nu^c_{k_1|k_2...k_t;(D\geq d)} \tag{18.4}$$

and alternatively as

$$\begin{aligned}
\nu^c_{(D\geq d),k_1k_2...k_t} &= \mu^c_{k_1k_2...k_t} \, \phi^c_{(D\geq d)|k_1k_2...k_t} \\
&= \mu^c_{k_1k_2...k_t} \, \phi^c_{(D\geq d)|k_2...k_t} \\
&= \nu^c_{(D\geq d),k_2...k_t} \, \nu^c_{k_1|k_2...k_t},
\end{aligned} \tag{18.5}$$

where we assume, as Brown (1990) did, that the first variable is always observed, and hence dropout does not depend on its value. Equating (18.4) and (18.5) yields

$$\nu^c_{k_1|k_2...k_t;(D\geq d)} = \nu^c_{k_1|k_2...k_t}. \tag{18.6}$$

Choosing $t = d$, the left-hand side of (18.6) contains the probabilities directly observed through the patterns for which at least d measurements are available, written as $\mu_{k_1|k_2...k_d}$. The right-hand side contains the complete data measurement probabilities marginalized over all dropout patterns, that is, $\mu^c_{k_1|k_2...k_d}$, and hence (18.6) can be rewritten as $\mu^c_{k_1|k_2...k_d} = \mu_{k_1|k_2...k_d}$. This result simply means that the conditional probability of the first outcome, given the $d-1$ subsequent measures, can be estimated directly from the observed data.

We summarize the relevant quantities directly available from the data. First, table d yields $\mu^c_{k_1 \ldots k_d | d}$. Second, tables d to n provide the conditional probabilities

$$\mu^c_{k_1 | k_2 \ldots k_d}. \tag{18.7}$$

In particular, all tables contribute to $\mu^c_{k_1}$, whereas only the last table contributes to $\mu^c_{k_1 | k_2 \ldots k_T}$. The next step is the computation of $\mu^c_{k_1 \ldots k_d}$, for all d. Denote by $\mu_{k_1 \ldots k_d}$ the directly observed cell probabilities, estimated from tables d to T.

For $d = 1$, $\mu^c_{k_1}$ follows from the data. Consider first the construction of $\mu^c_{k_1 k_2}$. Recall that neither the observed $\mu_{k_1 k_2}$ nor the $\mu_{k_1 k_2 | d}$ for $d \geq 2$ are of direct use; they only contribute through (18.7) by estimating $\mu^c_{k_1 | k_2}$. Then, $\mu^c_{k_1 k_2}$ is determined by solving the system of equations

$$\sum_{k_2 = 1}^{r} \mu^c_{k_1 | k_2} \mu^c_{k_2} = \mu^c_{k_1}, \qquad k_1 = 1, \ldots r, \tag{18.8}$$

where $\mu^c_{k_1 | k_2}$ act as coefficients and $\mu^c_{k_2}$ as unknowns. Solving this system yields $\mu^c_{k_2}$, whereupon $\mu^c_{k_1 k_2}$ is obtained by a simple multiplication. Writing (18.8) as $M_{1|2} M_2 = M_1$, it clearly follows that a unique solution can be found if and only if the determinant of the matrix $M_{1|2}$ is non-zero. This is equivalent to $\det(M_{12}) = \det(\mu_{k_1 k_2}) \neq 0$. To obtain a valid solution, one has to guarantee that all components of M_2 are non-negative. Necessary and sufficient conditions are given in Theorem 18.1 below.

We can now proceed by induction. Suppose we have constructed all marginal probabilities up to order $d - 1$. We will then construct $\mu^c_{k_1 \ldots k_d}$. For a fixed multi-index $(k_2, \ldots, k_{d-1})$, consider the system of equations

$$\sum_{k_d = 1}^{r} \mu^c_{k_1 | k_2 \ldots k_d} \mu^c_{k_d | k_2 \ldots k_{d-1}} = \mu^c_{k_1 | k_2 \ldots k_{d-1}}, \qquad k_1 = 1, \ldots r. \tag{18.9}$$

Solving this system yields $\mu^c_{k_d | k_2 \ldots k_{d-1}}$ and hence $\mu^c_{k_1 k_d | k_2 \ldots k_{d-1}}$, resulting in

$$\mu^c_{k_1 k_2 \ldots k_{d-1} k_d} = \mu^c_{k_1 k_2 \ldots k_{d-1}} \frac{\mu^c_{k_1 k_d | k_2 \ldots k_{d-1}}}{\mu^c_{k_1 | k_2 \ldots k_{d-1}}}, \tag{18.10}$$

all quantities on the right-hand side being determined. Writing (18.9) as

$$M_{1|d}^{(k_2 \ldots k_{d-1})} M_d^{(k_2 \ldots k_{d-1})} = M_1^{(k_2 \ldots k_{d-1})}, \tag{18.11}$$

we obtain a family of systems of equations, one for each combination of occasions $(k_2, \ldots, k_{d-1})$. Each one of these is exactly of the form (18.8). We now state the conditions for a valid solution.

Theorem 18.1 *The system of equations (18.9) has a unique, valid (i.e., non-negative) solution if and only if:*

(i) $\det(\mu_{k_1 \ldots k_d}) \neq 0$, for $k_2, \ldots, k_{d-1}$ fixed;

(ii) the column vector $M_1^{(k_2 \ldots k_{d-1})} = (\mu_{k_1|k_2 \ldots k_{d-1}})_{k_1}$ is an element of the convex hull of the r column vectors, indexed by k_d, $((\mu_{k_1|k_d;k_2 \ldots k_{d-1}})_{k_1})$.

Note that the vectors $\{(\mu_{k_1|k_d;k_2 \ldots k_{d-1}})_{k_1}\}$ are the columns of $M_{1|d}^{(k_2 \ldots k_{d-1})}$. By requiring that this theorem holds for all $d = 2, \ldots, T$ and for all $1 \leq k_2, \ldots, k_{d-1} \leq r$, one ensures the existence of an overall solution.

Proof. Clearly, the matrix equation has a unique root if and only if $\det M_{1|d}^{(k_2 \ldots k_{d-1})} \neq 0$, where only k_1 and k_d are free indices. Whether or not this determinant is zero is not altered by multiplying each column of the matrix by $\mu_{k_d|k_1 \ldots k_{d-1}}$. Equivalently, one can construct the determinant of the two-way table, obtained from the observed probabilities $\mu_{k_1 \ldots k_d}$ by keeping $k_2, \ldots, k_{d-1}$ fixed.

We need to establish that the solution is non-negative if and only if the column on the right-hand side is an element of the convex hull of the columns of the matrix $M_{1|d}^{(k_2 \ldots k_{d-1})}$. However, the convex hull is formed by all elements for which there exists a linear combination of which all coefficients are in the unit interval and summing to 1, that is, a vector of probabilities. This completes the proof. $\square$

These conditions can be interpreted as follows. The model implies that the column distributions in both tables are the same, as indicated by (18.6). Therefore, the single column we observe on the right-hand side of (18.9) must be a convex linear combination of the set of column distributions we observe on the left-hand side. An interesting consequence is that a negative solution points to a violation of the assumptions: the data can contradict the model, even without applying a model checking procedure. A non-zero determinant is equivalent to a set of column distributions which is of full rank. We could call this condition the 'full association' condition. It is worth noting that in the case of binary outcomes ($r = 2$) these conditions reduce to: (1) the odds ratio of the table on the left-hand side is different from 1; (2) the (marginal) odds of the only column on the right-hand side lies in the interval bounded by the two (conditional) odds of the columns on the left-hand side. For the binary case, these conditions were given by Baker and Laird (1988, p. 67).

The algorithm presented here is not the only method for finding the cell probabilities. By requiring that the cell probabilities $\mu_{k_1 \ldots k_n}^c$ sum to 1 and have (18.7) as conditionals, one is able to construct a single system of r^n equations in r^n unknowns. Although appealing at first sight, the procedure advocated in this section has several important advantages. First, a potentially complex procedure is broken into a sequence of simple, identical procedures, for which the validity requirements are readily verified. No large matrices have to be inverted. If the method yields a non-valid solution, one can at least compute the estimator for a subset of the outcomes – for example, the first $t - 1$ outcomes, when the first problem occurs at variable t. By removing the 'problematic' variables, one can compute the estimator for a maximal subset.

18.3.1 Likelihood estimation

The protective estimator for two measurements can also be derived through likelihood estimation, by considering a saturated measurement model and a dropout model that only depends on the unobserved outcome, that is, the likelihood based on the factorization $\nu^c_{d,k_1 k_2} = \mu^c_{k_1 k_2} \, \phi^c_{d|k_2}$. This model saturates the degrees of freedom available in the data. Maximizing the likelihood

$$L \propto \prod_{k_1,k_2} (\mu^c_{k_1 k_2} \, \phi^c_{2|k_2})^{z_{2,k_1 k_2}} \prod_{k_1} (\mu^c_{k_1 1} \, \phi^c_{1|1} + \mu^c_{k_1 2} \, \phi^c_{1|2})^{z_{1,k_1}} \qquad (18.12)$$

yields the protective estimator, which is also equal to the estimator for the model $(Y_1 Y_2, Y_2 R)$ discussed in Baker and Laird (1988, their equation 2.1). The likelihood estimator is apparently attractive in allowing for flexible dependence on outcomes and covariates, but explicit and often untestable assumptions about the dropout process have to be made. The protective estimator leaves the dropout model unspecified and therefore uses fewer degrees of freedom.

An explicit solution to (18.12) can be derived:

$$\widehat{\mu}^c_{11} = \frac{z_{2,11}}{z_{+,++}} \left(\frac{(z_{1,1} + z_{2,11})z_{2,22} - (z_{1,2} + z_{2,21})z_{2,12}}{z_{2,11}z_{2,22} - z_{2,12}z_{2,21}} \right), \qquad (18.13)$$

$$\widehat{\mu}^c_{12} = \frac{z_{2,12}}{z_{+,++}} \left(\frac{(z_{1,2} + z_{2,22})z_{2,11} - (z_{1,1} + z_{2,12})z_{2,21}}{z_{2,11}z_{2,22} - z_{2,12}z_{2,21}} \right), \qquad (18.14)$$

$$\widehat{\mu}^c_{21} = \frac{z_{2,21}}{z_{+,++}} \left(\frac{(z_{1,1} + z_{2,11})z_{2,22} - (z_{1,2} + z_{2,21})z_{2,12}}{z_{2,11}z_{2,22} - z_{2,12}z_{2,21}} \right), \qquad (18.15)$$

$$\widehat{\mu}^c_{22} = \frac{z_{2,22}}{z_{+,++}} \left(\frac{(z_{1,2} + z_{2,22})z_{2,11} - (z_{1,1} + z_{2,12})z_{2,21}}{z_{2,11}z_{2,22} - z_{2,12}z_{2,21}} \right), \qquad (18.16)$$

$$\widehat{\phi}^c_{2|1} = \frac{z_{2,11}z_{2,22} - z_{2,12}z_{2,21}}{(z_{1,1} + z_{2,11})z_{2,22} - (z_{1,2} + z_{2,21})z_{2,12}}, \qquad (18.17)$$

$$\widehat{\phi}^c_{2|2} = \frac{z_{2,11}z_{2,22} - z_{2,12}z_{2,21}}{(z_{1,2} + z_{2,22})z_{2,11} - (z_{1,1} + z_{2,12})z_{2,21}}. \qquad (18.18)$$

Estimates (18.13)–(18.16) are identical to the protective estimator. Therefore, studying likelihood (18.12) can shed some light on situations where boundary restrictions are violated. Table 18.1 presents four artificial sets of data. The data in Table 18.1(a) satisfy the protective assumptions as the odds in the incomplete table are 1, well between 0.5 and 2. Table 18.1(b) presents data on the boundary, whereas the data in Table 18.1(c) violate the protective assumption. Finally, Table 18.1(d) is included to discuss model fit. Parameter estimates and standard errors are presented in the left-hand half of Table 18.2.

In all four cases, parameter estimates coincide with those found by the protective estimator (right-hand half of Table 18.2). For the data in Table 18.1(b) we estimate $\widehat{\phi}_{2|2} = 1.0$, implying that no observations from

Table 18.1 Four sets of artificial data. In each case a contingency table for the completers ($Y_1 = 1/2$, $Y_2 = 1/2$) and an additional contingency table for the dropouts ($Y_1 = 1/2$) is given.

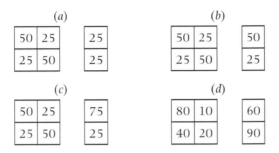

Table 18.2 Four sets of artificial data. Parameter estimates (standard errors). Methods of estimation are untransformed and transformed likelihood, and protective estimation with the delta method, the EM algorithm, and multiple imputation.

		Likelihood		Protective		
Data	Parameter	Untransformed	Transformed	Delta	EM	MI
(a)	μ_{11}	0.33 (0.05)	0.33 (0.05)	0.33 (0.06)	0.33 (0.05)	0.33 (0.05)
	μ_{12}	0.17 (0.04)	0.17 (0.04)	0.17 (0.04)	0.17 (0.05)	0.17 (0.04)
	μ_{21}	0.17 (0.04)	0.17 (0.04)	0.17 (0.04)	0.17 (0.04)	0.17 (0.04)
	μ_{22}	0.33 (0.05)	0.33 (0.05)	0.33 (0.06)	0.33 (0.05)	0.33 (0.05)
	$\phi_{2|1}$	0.75 (0.10)	0.75		0.75 (0.10)	
	$\phi_{2|2}$	0.75 (0.10)	0.75		0.75 (0.10)	
(b)	μ_{11}	0.44 (0.04)	0.44 (0.04)	0.44 (0.06)	0.44 (0.04)	0.43 (0.04)
	μ_{12}	0.11 (0.03)	0.11 (0.02)	0.11 (0.04)	0.11 (0.04)	0.12 (0.03)
	μ_{21}	0.22 (0.06)	0.22 (0.03)	0.22 (0.03)	0.22 (0.06)	0.21 (0.04)
	μ_{22}	0.22 (0.06)	0.22 (0.03)	0.22 (0.05)	0.22 (0.06)	0.24 (0.04)
	$\phi_{2|1}$	0.50 (0.07)	0.50		0.50 (0.07)	
	$\phi_{2|2}$	1.00 (0.23)	1.00		1.00 (0.23)	
(c)	μ_{11}	0.53 (0.04)	0.50 (0.03)	0.53 (0.05)	0.53 (0.04)	0.50 (0.03)
	μ_{12}	0.07 (0.03)	0.10 (0.02)	0.07 (0.05)	0.07 (0.03)	0.10 (0.02)
	μ_{21}	0.27 (0.07)	0.20 (0.02)	0.27 (0.02)	0.27 (0.07)	0.20 (0.03)
	μ_{22}	0.13 (0.07)	0.20 (0.02)	0.13 (0.03)	0.13 (0.07)	0.20 (0.03)
	$\phi_{2|1}$	0.38 (0.06)	0.43		0.38 (0.06)	
	$\phi_{2|2}$	1.50 (0.47)	1.00		1.50 (0.75)	
(d)	μ_{11}	0.33 (0.08)	0.33 (0.08)	0.33 (0.03)	0.33 (0.08)	0.33 (0.06)
	μ_{12}	0.17 (0.08)	0.17 (0.08)	0.17 (0.03)	0.17 (0.08)	0.17 (0.06)
	μ_{21}	0.17 (0.05)	0.17 (0.05)	0.17 (0.05)	0.17 (0.05)	0.17 (0.04)
	μ_{22}	0.33 (0.05)	0.33 (0.05)	0.33 (0.05)	0.33 (0.05)	0.33 (0.04)
	$\phi_{2|1}$	0.80 (0.19)	0.80		0.80 (0.19)	
	$\phi_{2|2}$	0.20 (0.06)	0.20		0.20 (0.06)	

the second column drop out. In the third example, the violation of the restrictions shows in the estimate for $\phi_{2|2}$. Note that the cell probabilities give no direct suggestion of parameter space violations. However, the probabilities predicted for the incomplete table are $\mu_{1,11} = 0.8333$, $\mu_{1,12} = -0.0833$, $\mu_{1,21} = 0.4167$, $\mu_{1,22} = -0.1667$. The latter probabilities are found with a pattern-mixture formulation of the protective estimator. The log-likelihood equals -423.94.

To avoid parameter space violations, one can reparameterize the probabilities as follows:

$$\mu^c_{k_1 k_2} = \exp[\alpha_1(k_1 - 1) + \alpha_2(k_2 - 1)$$
$$+ \alpha_3(k_1 - 1)(k_2 - 1) - A(\alpha_1, \alpha_2, \alpha_3)], \qquad (18.19)$$

where $A(\alpha_1, \alpha_2, \alpha_3)$ is a normalizing constant, and

$$\phi_{2|k_2} = \frac{\exp(\gamma_{k_2})}{1 + \exp(\gamma_{k_2})}. \qquad (18.20)$$

In this case, the parameters corresponding to the data in Table 18.1(b) are $\alpha_1 = 0.6932$, $\alpha_2 = 0$, $\alpha_3 = 1.3863$, $\gamma_1 = 0$, and γ_2 approaches infinity. The log-likelihood at maximum is -390.40, independent of whether the untransformed or transformed likelihoods are used.

Turning to Table 18.1(c) and again adopting parameterization (18.19) and (18.20), the log-likelihood at maximum becomes -424.66, obtained for parameters $\alpha_1 = 0.6932$, $\alpha_2 = 0$, $\alpha_3 = 1.6095$, $\gamma_1 = -0.2777$, while γ_2 approaches infinity. These values correspond to dropout probabilities $\phi_{2|1} = 0.4286$ and $\phi_{2|2} = 1.000$. This represents a slight decrease in the log-likelihood, but all estimated probabilities are valid. Corresponding marginal probabilities are given in the second column of Table 18.2. They are further divided over completers ($\nu^c_{2,11} = 0.2143$, $\nu^c_{2,12} = 0.1000$, $\nu^c_{2,21} = 0.0857$, $\nu^c_{2,22} = 0.2000$), and incomplete observations ($\nu^c_{1,11} = 0.2857$, $\nu^c_{1,12} = 0.0000$, $\nu^c_{1,21} = 0.1143$, and $\nu^c_{1,22} = 0.0000$). A boundary solution is obtained where all marginal probabilities are as observed, but the association as observed for the completers differs from the estimated association (consider, for example, the odds ratio). The differences in standard errors are discussed in Section 18.3.3.

Table 18.1(d) is generated by first assuming that $Z_{11} = Z_{22} = 100$ and $Z_{12} = Z_{21} = 50$ and also that $\phi_{2|1} = 0.8$ and $\phi_{2|2} = 0.2$. This implies that the table for the completers is as in Table 18.1(d), that the full data for the dropouts are $Z_{1,11} = 20$, $Z_{1,12} = 40$, $Z_{1,21} = 10$, $Z_{1,22} = 80$, and thus that the supplemental margin consists of the counts 60 and 90 as shown. Fitting a protective model to those data with all five methods yields exactly the same estimates. When these parameter estimates are used to construct fitted frequencies, then $Z_{1,jk}$ and $Z_{2,jk}(j, k = 1, 2)$ are recovered. The log-likelihood at maximum is -479.43.

As an alternative to maximizing likelihood (18.12), let us turn to the MAR likelihood

$$L \propto \prod_{k_1,k_2} (\mu^c_{k_1 k_2} \, \phi^c_{2|k_1})^{z_{2,k_1 k_2}} \prod_{k_1} (\mu^c_{k_1 1} \, \phi^c_{1|k_1} + \mu^c_{k_1 2} \, \phi^c_{1|k_1})^{z_{1,k_1}}$$

$$\propto \prod_{k_1,k_2} (\mu^c_{k_1 k_2})^{z_{2,k_1 k_2}} \prod_{k_1} (\mu^c_{k_1 +})^{z_{1,k_1}} \prod_{k_1} (\phi^c_{2|k_1})^{z_{2,k_1 +}} \prod_{k_1} (\phi^c_{1|k_1})^{z_{1,k_1 +}}.$$

Then, the fitted probabilities (with standard errors) are $\widehat{\mu}_{11} = 0.44 (0.03)$, $\widehat{\mu}_{12} = 0.06 (0.02)$, $\widehat{\mu}_{21} = 0.33 (0.04)$, and $\widehat{\mu}_{22} = 0.17 (0.03)$. The dropout probabilities are $\widehat{\phi}_{2|k_1=1} = 0.60 (0.04)$ and $\widehat{\phi}_{2|k_1=2} = 0.40 (0.04)$. While the table for the completers is recovered, the filled-in dropout table is estimated to be $\widehat{Z}_{1,11} = 53.33$, $\widehat{Z}_{1,12} = 6.67$, $\widehat{Z}_{1,21} = 60.00$, and $\widehat{Z}_{1,22} = 30.00$, entirely different from the true underlying structure. However, the value of the maximized log-likelihood is still -479.43. This points to a general problem with missing data: it is often impossible, or at least very difficult, to establish superiority of one dropout model over another, based on statistical considerations alone. Indeed, whereas the MAR and protective models both fit the observed data perfectly, they yield entirely different predictors for the underlying dropout table. Arguably, background and/or covariate information should be used to support the model builder's task. We return to this important issue in Chapter 19.

18.3.2 Pseudo-likelihood estimation

While generalizing the likelihood method of the previous section to more than two measurement occasions is not computationally straightforward, progress can be made by switching to pseudo-likelihood estimation (Arnold and Strauss 1991). Pseudo-likelihood has been used in the context of spatial data by Cressie (1991), for correlated binary data by le Cessie and Van Houwelingen (1994), and for clustered data by Geys *et al.* (1999), to name but a few.

Let us concentrate on three measurement occasions. The protective estimator first determines $\mu^c_{k_1 k_2}$ and then $\mu^c_{k_1 k_3 | k_2}$. Each of these steps can be handled by means of likelihood (18.12). This naturally leads to a new expression,

$$L^* \propto \prod_{k_1,k_2} (\mu^c_{k_1 k_2} \, \phi^c_{2|k_2})^{z_{k_1 k_2}} \prod_{k_1} \left(\sum_{k_2} \mu^c_{k_1 k_2} \, \phi^c_{1|k_2} \right)^{z_{k_1}}$$

$$\times \prod_{k_1,k_2,k_3} \left(\mu^c_{k_1 k_3 | k_2} \, \phi^{(k_2)c}_{2|k_3} \right)^{z_{k_1 k_3 | k_2}}$$

$$\times \prod_{k_1,k_2} \left(\sum_{k_3} \mu^c_{k_1 k_3 | k_2} \, \phi^{(k_2)c}_{1|k_3} \right)^{z_{k_1 | k_2}}. \tag{18.21}$$

All counts used in (18.21) are based on the maximal amount of information, except for z_{k_1}, which is calculated using the subjects being observed at the first time point only. This is clearly not a likelihood since the factors are incorrectly assumed to be independent.

While the point estimator is consistent, one has to be careful with estimating the precision (Arnold and Strauss 1988; Geys *et al.* 1999). In particular, let

$$\lambda = \left\{ \mu^c_{k_1 k_2}, \mu^c_{k_1 k_3 | k_2}, \phi^c_{1|k_2}, \phi^c_{2|k_2}, \phi^{(k_2)c}_{1|k_3}, \phi^{(k_2)c}_{2|k_3}; \text{for all } k_1, k_2, k_3 \right\}$$

and

$$\ell(\lambda) = \sum_{i=1}^{N} \ell_i(\lambda) = \ln(L^*(\lambda)),$$

where $\ell_i(\lambda)$ is the contribution of subject i to the log pseudo-likelihood and N is the total sample size. Then, $\sqrt{N}(\widehat{\lambda} - \lambda)$ converges in distribution to the normal distribution $N(\mathbf{0}, \mathbf{J}(\lambda)^{-1} \mathbf{K}(\lambda) \mathbf{J}(\lambda)^{-1})$ where

$$\mathbf{J}(\lambda) = E\left(\frac{\partial^2 l(\lambda)}{\partial \lambda \partial \lambda'} \right)$$

and

$$\mathbf{K}(\lambda) = \sum_{i=1}^{N} E\left(\frac{\partial l_i(\lambda)}{\partial \lambda} \left(\frac{\partial l_i(\lambda)}{\partial \lambda} \right)' \right).$$

This result is very close in spirit to the sandwich estimator, known from generalized estimating equations (Liang and Zeger 1986). It yields an asymptotic measure of precision for $\mu^c_{k_1 k_2}$ and $\mu^c_{k_1 k_3 | k_2}$ from which the precision for $\mu^c_{k_1 k_2 k_3}$ easily follows using a standard delta method argument. Precision for the dropout probabilities is also available. The method will be contrasted with different methods for variance calculation for the protective estimator, described in the next subsection.

18.3.3 Variance estimation

Whereas estimating the variance under MNAR is more involved than under MAR, we are further hampered by the fact that the dropout parameters are not estimated. Brown (1990) does not provide a way to estimate the variance of the parameters. We will discuss three procedures. The first is based on the delta method (Agresti 1990, 2002). The second uses EM-aided differentiation (Meilijson 1989). The final technique makes use of multiple imputation (Chapter 9). We will then revisit the artificial examples considered in Section 18.3.1.

Delta method

In the following, the superscripts c will be dropped from the probabilities. Write (18.11) as $M_{1|d}M_d = M_1$. As M_1 and $M_{1|d}$ are directly observed from the data, their covariance matrices are immediate. Let $V(\cdot)$ indicate the covariance function. First, M_1, the vector of probabilities μ_{k_1}, has multinomial covariance matrix

$$V(M_1) = \frac{1}{n_1}\{\mathrm{diag}(M_1) - M_1 M_1'\}, \tag{18.22}$$

n_1 indicating the sample size. In order to be able to work conveniently with the matrix $M_{1|d}$, a matrix of which the columns represent independent multinomial distributions, we introduce some extra notation. The components are $\mu_{k_1|k_d}$, while column k_d (corresponding to the k_dth conditional distribution) is denoted by $\mu_{.|k_d}$. The covariance matrix $V(M_{1|d})$ is block diagonal with blocks

$$V(M_{1|d})(k_d) = \frac{1}{n_{1|k_d}}\{(\mathrm{diag}(\mu_{.|k_d}) - \mu_{.|k_d}\mu_{.|k_d}'\}. \tag{18.23}$$

It is convenient to write the components of M_1 as $\mu_{k_1|0}$. The quantity $\mu_{.|0}$ is defined similarly. Then (18.23) encompasses (18.22) by letting $k_d = 0, 1, \ldots, r$. Thus, k_d will be allowed to assume the value 0 also, which should be read as 'unconditional'. From these covariance matrices and the observation that $M_d = M_{1|d}^{-1}M_1$, the covariance $V(M_d)$ is obtained by applying the delta method. Note that M_d is a vector-valued function, of which the arguments are a non-redundant set of components of M_1 and $M_{1|d}$. The redundancies are given by the following identities:

$$g_{k_d} = \sum_{k_1=1}^{r} \mu_{k_1|k_d} - 1 = 0, \quad k_d = 0, 1, \ldots, r. \tag{18.24}$$

A possible non-redundant set is given by the first $r - 1$ components of each probability vector. Let us denote these sets by $\widetilde{M}_1$ and $\widetilde{M}_{1|d}$, with similar notation for the vectors $\widetilde{\mu}_{.|k_d}$. Grouping the vectors $\widetilde{\mu}_{.|k_d}$ into a vector T and the remaining $\mu_{r|k_d}$ into Y, we can express the total derivative of M_d with respect to T as

$$\frac{dM_d}{dT} = \frac{\partial M_d}{\partial T} - \frac{\partial M_d}{\partial Y}\left(\frac{\partial G}{\partial Y}\right)^{-1}\frac{\partial G}{\partial T},$$

where G is the set of functions described by (18.24). It follows immediately that

$$\frac{\partial G}{\partial Y} = I_{r+1},$$

$$\frac{\partial G}{\partial T} = I_{r+1} \otimes 1_{1,r-1},$$

$$\frac{\partial M_d}{\partial M_1} = M_{1|d}^{-1},$$

$$\frac{\partial M_d}{\partial \mu_{k_1|k_d}} = -M_{1|d}^{-1} E_{k_1 k_d} M_d, \quad k_1, k_d = 1, \ldots, r,$$

where $E_{k_1 k_d}$ is a zero matrix, except for a single 1 in entry (k_1, k_d). Using these expressions, we obtain

$$\Phi = \frac{dM_d}{d\boldsymbol{T}} = (\Phi_1, -M_{1|d}^{-1}\Phi_2),$$

where Φ_1 is an $r \times (r-1)$ matrix of which the columns are $\xi_{.|k_d} - \xi_{.|r}$ ($k_d = 1, \ldots, r-1$), $\xi_{.|k_d}$ are the columns of $M_{1|d}^{-1}$, and $\Phi_2 = (\Phi_{21}, \ldots, \Phi_{2r})$ with

$$\Phi_{2k_d} = \begin{pmatrix} \mu_{k_d} I_{r-1} \\ -\mu_{k_d} \mathbf{1}_{1,r-1} \end{pmatrix}.$$

Finally, $V(M_d) = \Phi W \Phi'$, with

$$W = \mathrm{cov}(\boldsymbol{T}) = \left(\begin{array}{c|c} V(\widetilde{M}_1) & V_{1,1|d} \\ \hline V'_{1,1|d} & V(\widetilde{M}_{1|d}) \end{array} \right).$$

The matrix $V(\widetilde{M}_1)$ is found from $V(M_1)$ by omitting the last row and column. Replacing $\mu_{.|k_d}$ by $\widetilde{\mu}_{.|k_d}$ in (18.23) yields $V(\widetilde{M}_{1|d})$. Finally, $V_{1,1|d}$ describes the covariance function of M_1 and $M_{1|d}$. A typical element is

$$\mathrm{cov}(\mu_{k_1}, \mu_{k'_1|k_d}) = \frac{1}{n_{12}} \mu_{k'_1|k_d} (\delta_{k_1 k'_1} - \mu_{k_1}),$$

$k_1, k'_1 = 1, \ldots, r-1; k_d = 1, \ldots, r$, with n_{12} the number of subjects, observed at both occasions.

With similar computations, the covariance matrix of M_{1d} (with this matrix appropriately vectorized) is found to be

$$V(\mathrm{vec}(M_{1d})) = \Phi_3 V(\widetilde{\mu}_{.|k_d}) \Phi'_3 + \mathrm{bdiag}_{k_d=1}^r \{ \Phi_{2k_d} V(\widetilde{\mu}_{.|k_d}) \Phi'_{2k_d} \},$$

with Φ_3 given by

$$\Phi_3 = \begin{pmatrix} \mu_{.|1} & & & \\ & \mu_{.|2} & & \\ & & \ddots & \\ & & & \mu_{.|r-1} \\ -\mu_{.|r} & \cdots & & -\mu_{.|r} \end{pmatrix},$$

and where 'bdiag' denotes a block diagonal matrix with blocks given by the indexed argument.

Probabilities of the form $\mu^c_{k_1\ldots k_d}$ can be written as a product of probabilities that have been determined:

$$\mu^c_{k_1\ldots k_d} = \mu^c_{k_1 k_d | k_2 \ldots k_{d-1}} \prod_{t=2}^{d-1} \mu^c_{k_t | k_2 \ldots k_{t-1}}. \tag{18.25}$$

Deriving a variance estimator from this expression is straightforward. One only has to take into account that in each matrix (set of probabilities) a sum constraint applies. This fact needs to be discounted in computing the derivatives.

EM-aided differentiation

The computations based on the delta method are somewhat involved because of the fact that a linear system of equations needs to be solved. We will show that a computational scheme based on the EM algorithm (Chapter 8) is useful to circumvent this step. The price to pay is that, although the dropout parameters are not necessary for estimating the model parameters, they are required for variance estimation. Suppose we wish to estimate $\mu^c_{k_1 k_d | k_2 \ldots k_{d-1}}$. Without loss of generality, we will describe the algorithm for $\mu_{k_1 k_2}$ (setting $d = 2$ and dropping the superscript). Information is based on two tables: those observed at both occasions, summarized in table $Z_{2,k_1 k_2}$ and those observed at the first occasion only, Z_{1,k_1}.

Choosing starting values $\mu^{(0)}_{k_1 k_2}$, one iterates between the E step and the M step until convergence. The E step first calculates probabilities $\mu^{(t)}_{k_1 | k_2}$, given $\mu^{(t)}_{k_1 k_2}$. Together with the probabilities μ_{1,k_1}, directly computed from the incomplete table Z_{1,k_1}, the probabilities $\mu^{(t)}_{1,k_1 k_2}$ are found by solving

$$\sum_{k_2=1}^{r} \mu^{(t)}_{k_1 | k_2} \mu^{(t)}_{1,k_2} = \mu_{1,k_1}, \tag{18.26}$$

and hence $\mu^{(t)}_{1,k_1 k_2} = \mu^{(t)}_{1,k_2} \mu^{(t)}_{k_1 | k_2}$. From these probabilities and the observed data Z_{1,k_1} the expected counts in the completed table $Z^{(t)}_{1,k_1 k_2}$ are readily found. Note that the dropout probabilities are implicitly determined since

$$\phi_{2|k_1 k_2} = \phi_{2|k_2} = \frac{\mu_{2,k_1 k_2}}{\mu_{k_1 k_2}}.$$

The M step merely sums over both tables $Z^{(t)}_{k_1 k_2} = Z^{(t)}_{1,k_1 k_2} + Z_{2,k_1 k_2}$ and determines an update for the probabilities:

$$\mu^{(t+1)}_{k_1 k_2} = \frac{Z^{(t)}_{k_1 k_2}}{Z_{++}}. \tag{18.27}$$

Observe the strong connection with the likelihood approach since (18.27) maximizes the complete data log-likelihood

$$\ell^{(t)} = \sum_{k_1,k_2} Z^{(t)}_{k_1 k_2} \ln(\mu^{(t+1)}_{k_1 k_2}). \qquad (18.28)$$

An important advantage of this technique is that log-likelihood (18.28) can be replaced by another one, such as the independence log-likelihood, thereby opening up the possibility of modelling the effect of predictor variables. This is feasible without distorting the protective restrictions as they are used only in the E step.

To calculate the variance, we will use the method proposed by Meilijson (1989). Suppose we define $\boldsymbol{\beta}$ to be a non-redundant set of $\mu_{k_1 k_2}$. In the E step the only probabilities used are $\mu_{1.k_1}$ and $\mu_{1.k_1 k_2}(\boldsymbol{\beta}_i)$. The former are fixed, the latter change as they depend on the small perturbations of the parameter vector. This implies that the dropout probabilities are implicitly changed, whereas they are a formal part of the parameter vector, and should remain fixed. A simple solution is to compute the dropout probabilities and consider them as a formal part of the parameter vector,

$$\phi_{2|k_2} = \frac{Z_{2,k_1 k_2}}{Z_{k_1 k_2}}, \qquad (18.29)$$

with the complete data cell counts evaluated at the maximum. The right-hand side of (18.29) is independent of k_1 due to the protective assumption.

The corresponding E step will be based on $\mu_{1.k_1}(\boldsymbol{\beta}_i)$ and $\mu_{2.k_1 k_2}(\boldsymbol{\beta}_i)$, and hence the correct information matrix is obtained. There is another reason for the use of the $\boldsymbol{\phi}$ parameters. Because the covariance between the $\boldsymbol{\mu}$ and the $\boldsymbol{\phi}$ parameters is generally non-zero, unless one assumes MAR, the correct covariance matrix is obtained only if it is based on the full information for both $\boldsymbol{\mu}$ and $\boldsymbol{\phi}$.

In conclusion, the EM algorithm is a simple method to compute parameter estimates and their variances, but there are two caveats. First, the estimates can easily be determined using the methods of Section 18.3, making the technique redundant for parameter estimation. Second, for variance estimation, estimation of dropout probabilities is required, thereby weakening the advantage of protective estimation. An important advantage of the method is that it can be used to calculate a variance estimator for general n-dimensional outcome vectors. To this end, the EM computations can be used to replace the variance computations for all $r \times r$ tables occurring, whereupon a delta method argument is applied to combine these variances into a variance for the multivariate cell probabilities.

Multiple imputation

We present an approach based on multiple imputation (Chapter 9) for the special case of two measurements, and then generalize it to n-dimensional contingency tables. Interest lies in estimating the parameter vector $\boldsymbol{\beta}$, containing a non-redundant subset of $\mu^c_{k_1 k_2}$. The set of easily estimable parameters $\boldsymbol{\gamma}$ includes μ_{1,k_1} and the conditional probabilities $\mu_{k_1|k_2}$ determined from $\mu_{2,k_1 k_2}$.

Using a normal posterior distribution for $\boldsymbol{\theta}$, the algorithm for 'filling in' the data is as follows:

1. Draw $\boldsymbol{\gamma}^*$ from the posterior distribution of $\boldsymbol{\gamma}$. This yields $\mu^*_{k_1|k_2}$ and μ^*_{1,k_1}, which are easily transformed to $\mu^*_{1,k_1 k_2}$ using the algorithm of Section 18.3.
2. Draw $Z^*_{1,k_1 k_2}$ from $f(Z_{1,k_1 k_2}|Z_{1,k_1},\boldsymbol{\gamma}^*)$. This is easily realized using a uniform random generator.
3. Calculate the estimate of the parameter of interest, and its estimated variance, using the completed data:

$$\widehat{\mu}_{k_1 k_2} = \frac{Z^*_{1,k_1 k_2} + Z_{2,k_1 k_2}}{Z_{+,++}},$$

$$U = \widehat{\mathrm{var}}(\widehat{\boldsymbol{\beta}}) = \frac{1}{Z_{+,++}}\left(\mathrm{diag}(\widehat{\boldsymbol{\mu}}) - \widehat{\boldsymbol{\mu}}\widehat{\boldsymbol{\mu}}'\right).$$

Repeating these three steps M times, and combining the results as in Section 9.2, the parameters and variances of interest are found.

The method described above can easily be generalized to n-dimensional contingency tables. One obvious method is to use multiple imputation to estimate the variance of each two-way table occurring in the computational method outlined in Section 18.3, and to combine the variance estimators into an estimator for the n-dimensional table using, for example, the delta method (similar to the extension suggested in previous section). Another is to use multiple imputation to complete all partial tables into n-dimensional contingency tables.

Although some of the draws may yield negative $\mu^*_{1,k_1 k_2}$, this does not imply that the procedure breaks down. It merely means that the corresponding table $Z^*_{1,k_1 k_2}$ will contain structural zeros. Further, a variance estimate is obtained without having to estimate the dropout probabilities, which is closer in spirit to protective estimation than the EM algorithm. This reduction in the number of parameters to be estimated may result in a more efficient variance estimator. Assuming that $\boldsymbol{\gamma}$ is normally distributed is only an approximation, which may result in small-sample bias.

18.3.4 Analysis of artificial data

To illustrate the use of the three protective (variance) estimation procedures, consider the artificial data of Table 18.1. Parameter estimates and standard errors are shown in Table 18.2. In all four cases, the EM-based estimator coincides exactly with the likelihood estimator. A disadvantage is that again negative probabilities are found. Two solutions to this problem can be proposed. First, one can use a different (parameterization of the) likelihood in the M step. Second, one can enforce restrictions in the E step. When the conditions of Theorem 18.3.1 are not satisfied, the probabilities found from (18.26) are invalid and have to be replaced by the appropriate boundary solution. Applying this technique to Table 18.1(c) yields exactly the same solution as found with the transformed likelihood. It has been omitted from Table 18.2. A further disadvantage is that the dropout probabilities need to be estimated.

Although the delta method does not require the dropout probabilities, it also suffers from parameter space violations. Moreover, the delta method is known to be somewhat inefficient, although reasonable agreement is observed for Table 18.1(a) and the method turns out to be superior for Table 18.1(d). For Table 18.1(b) caution should be used because parameters lie on the boundary, and for Table 18.1(c) parameter estimates are not even meaningful.

For Table 18.1(a), multiple imputation (based on 5000 samples) yields the same result as both the direct likelihood and EM methods. Although the procedure is more time-consuming, we obtain the correct answer without having to estimate the dropout probabilities. With Table 18.1(b) small differences are seen. The effect of these is that parameters move slightly away from the boundary. Indeed, the direction in which the MI parameters move is the same as seen for Table 18.1(c). In the latter case, the MI estimator yields different results than seen with other methods, but they coincide with the transformed likelihood parameters (and with the EM parameters when a valid solution in the E step is ensured). In other words, using multiple imputation automatically ensures valid parameters, whereas other methods require some additional work such as finding a solution on the boundary, which is quite involved when the number of categories r is large. The standard errors differ between the two methods, but also the standard errors between both likelihood procedures differ, owing to the fact that one of the dropout parameters with the transformed likelihood equals infinity, and asymptotic properties should be interpreted with great care. For Table 18.1(d) the MI standard errors are slightly smaller than the likelihood-based standard errors. In conclusion, multiple imputation seems to be a recommendable technique, not only for variance estimation, but also to estimate the parameters.

18.3.5   Analysis of the fluvoxamine trial

The fluvoxamine data were introduced in Section 2.6 and then analysed in Sections 12.6, 15.4.2, 15.5.1, and 16.8. We used the observations at times 2, 3, and 4, leading to the data of Table 18.3.

Table 18.4 gives the cell probability estimators and estimates of the standard errors under MAR with all three protective estimators, with pseudo-likelihood

Table 18.3 Fluvoxamine trial. Dichotomized side-effect and therapeutic effect outcomes at occasions 2, 3, and 4.

Cell	Side effect	Therapeutic effect
000	94	11
001	6	1
010	4	0
011	8	2
100	31	46
101	5	3
110	26	52
111	68	127
00*	5	1
01*	2	0
10*	3	2
11*	16	23
0**	9	4
1**	22	27
Total	299	299

and for the subset of completers. Both side effects and therapeutic effect are analysed. Let us discuss the results for side effects first.

Clearly the three protective estimation strategies yield (virtually) the same results, apart from very large standard errors found with both the delta method and with the EM algorithm for cells 110 and 111, because the information for cells 110 and 111 is largely the same as they are imputed from the same cells (11* and 1**). No violations of the boundary restrictions were encountered. The results obtained using pseudo-likelihood are very close to the delta and EM results. Point estimates coincide, and standard errors are very similar. Once again, MI seems to yield more precise standard errors because there is no need to sacrifice information to the estimation of dropout parameters. To assess model fit, a deviance statistic was computed. To obtain a saturated model, one needs to consider a different probability table for each of the three observed patterns. The deviance is 11.23 for the protective estimator and 9.40 for the MAR model, on 4 degrees of freedom in each case. Assuming a χ^2 distribution, p-values are 0.024 and 0.052, respectively, pointing to a similar (lack of) fit for both models.

An alternative strategy consists of estimating both the measurement parameters and the dropout model, using the model proposed by Molenberghs *et al.* (1997; see Section 15.4 above), and using likelihood-based estimation. Describing the dropout probability, given the outcomes, by a logistic regression, where the linear predictor describes the effect of both the previous and the current (possibly unobserved) outcome, we have

$$\text{logit}(\phi_{d|k_{d-1}k_d}) = \beta_0 + \beta_{d-1}k_{d-1} + \beta_d k_d.$$

Table 18.4 Fluvoxamine trial. Estimated cell probabilities (standard errors). All quantities were multiplied by 1000. Each cell gives the outcomes at the three times considered. Six methods were used: likelihood estimation once for the completers only, and once assuming MAR; protective estimation using the delta method, the EM algorithm and multiple imputation to calculate standard errors; and finally pseudo-likelihood using the protective assumption.

	Likelihood		Protective			
Cell	Completers	MAR	Delta	EM	MI	Pseudo-likelihood
Side effects						
000	388 (31)	355 (28)	342 (33)	342 (34)	343 (30)	342 (34)
001	25 (10)	23 (91)	31 (15)	31 (21)	30 (13)	31 (21)
010	17 (8)	17 (81)	18 (29)	18 (27)	19 (9)	18 (27)
011	33 (11)	34 (111)	37 (25)	37 (29)	36 (12)	37 (28)
100	128 (21)	129 (21)	113 (20)	113 (21)	115 (20)	113 (21)
101	21 (9)	21 (9)	26 (13)	26 (13)	24 (10)	26 (13)
110	107 (20)	117 (21)	115 (179)	115 (179)	129 (35)	115 (178)
111	281 (29)	305 (29)	318 (186)	318 (180)	305 (40)	318 (179)
Therapeutic effect						
000	45 (13)	51 (13)	44 (30)	48 (—)	50 (15)	46 (18)
001	4 (4)	5 (5)	12 (36)	9 (—)	7 (6)	15 (15)
010	0 (0)	0 (0)	0 (0)	0 (—)	0 (0)	2 (3)
011	8 (6)	9 (6)	7 (5)	7 (—)	7 (5)	11 (6)
100	190 (25)	177 (23)	184 (117)	200 (—)	205 (33)	187 (70)
101	12 (7)	12 (7)	37 (105)	22 (—)	17 (10)	35 (61)
110	215 (26)	217 (27)	265 (29)	265 (—)	254 (35)	168 (273)
111	525 (32)	531 (31)	449 (37)	449 (—)	461 (41)	536 (275)

Several models can be considered. These models are similar in spirit to (15.5). Parameter estimates (standard errors) for the marginal cell probabilities and for the dropout parameters are given in Table 18.5.

Several observations can be made. First, the overall deviances (corresponding to the likelihood of measurement and dropout processes simultaneously) convey a different message than the deviances of the dropout process. The overall deviances do not show a clear distinction between MAR and informative models. Although both terms in the informative model MNAR(2) are significant, the MAR model and the informative model MNAR(1), with dependence on the current outcome only, describe the data equally well. This seems to be due to the 'balance' which is achieved between dropout and measurement processes. Indeed, when the dropout model shows a better fit, achieved by including relevant parameters, the measurement model (with the same number of parameters) can afford to show a greater lack of fit. It clearly shows that the likelihood is very flat and similar likelihood values are obtained for conceptually very different models. This observation is in agreement with those made in Section 18.3.1 regarding the comparison of MAR and protective models for

Table 18.5 Fluvoxamine trial. Parametric models for the side-effects outcome. Likelihood-based estimation. Each cell gives the outcomes at the three measurement times considered. Measurement probabilities are multiplied by 1000.

Cell probabilities

	MCAR	MAR	MNAR(1)	MNAR(2)
000	355 (28)	355 (28)	346 (29)	331 (44)
001	23 (9)	23 (9)	25 (10)	29 (17)
010	17 (8)	17 (8)	17 (8)	18 (9)
011	34 (11)	34 (11)	40 (13)	50 (25)
100	129 (21)	125 (21)	115 (20)	99 (33)
101	21 (9)	21 (9)	22 (9)	22 (9)
110	117 (21)	117 (21)	108 (20)	99 (26)
111	305 (29)	305 (29)	327 (29)	353 (54)

Dropout model

Effect	Parameter	MCAR	MAR	MNAR(1)	MNAR(2)
Intercept	β_0	−2.19	−3.56	−4.33	−5.59 (0.34)
Current	β_d			1.35	2.71 (0.14)
Previous	β_{d-1}		0.86		−0.70 (0.38)
Deviance (overall)		618.16	613.86	613.69	613.55
Deviance (dropout)		184.98	180.67	174.33	160.08

Table 18.1(d). Second, when either the previous measurement only or the current observation only is included to describe the dropout process, the latter is the clear winner in terms of fitting the dropout process. However, in this latter case the current, possibly unobserved, outcome is used as a covariate in the dropout model and hence this model should be considered jointly with the measurement model, at which level the fit is comparable. The conclusion is that at least one outcome should be included in the dropout model. This has been observed before by Diggle and Kenward (1994) and Molenberghs *et al.* (1997). In Section 15.4.2 we found that dropout in the fluvoxamine trial mainly depends on the size of side effects, whereas a decrease in the therapeutic outcome seems to be responsible for dropout. From the deviances (p. 520) of the models in Table 18.4 one would infer that the previous measurement is the better candidate to describe dropout with respect to the side-effects outcome. The fitted cell probabilities reported in Tables 18.4 and 18.5 are of similar magnitude. In contrast to the examples in Section 18.3.1, the standard errors are smaller for likelihood estimation than for protective estimation.

Therapeutic effect is more complicated because one of the combinations (010) does not occur. EM and the delta method show slightly different estimates because the use of EM automatically enforces the boundary conditions.

No sensible precision estimates are obtained with the EM method. Multiple imputation yields similar results and automatically satisfies the conditions. Note that the delta estimator still yields a valid set of probabilities. But when the corresponding dropout probabilities are computed, a situation comparable to that in Table 18.1(c) occurs. For example, for the cross-classification of the first and third observations, given the second one equals 0, the counts are $Z_{00|0} = 11$, $Z_{01|0} = 1$, $Z_{10|0} = 46$, $Z_{11|0} = 3$, $Z_{0*|0} = 1$, $Z_{1*|0} = 2$, and hence violation of the restrictions might be due to chance. This means that the hypothetically complete table will have negative (but small) cell counts. Therefore, the delta method estimator can still be considered sensible. The zero cell counts lead to instability of the pseudo-likelihood estimator. A satisfactory solution is provided by applying a continuity correction, adding 0.5 to all cell counts. The results then differ slightly from those obtained with the delta method.

For therapeutic effect, Section 15.4.2 reported that MAR and MCAR fitted equally well, even though the fit was much improved by allowing for MNAR. In our analysis, the deviance for the MAR model is 5.57 on 4 degrees of freedom, which has to be contrasted with a deviance of 20.28 on 4 degrees of freedom for the protective estimator. Interpretation of these statistics should be done with caution, as the frequencies in some cells are very small and the estimator lies on the boundary.

18.3.6   Presence or absence of colds

Koch *et al.* (1992) looked at data on the presence or absence of colds recorded for 5554 subjects over three successive years. Covariates are sex (M/F) and the area of the residence of the subject (1/2). Considering the monotone sequences only, we have a subsample of 3112 subjects. Table 18.6 shows estimated cell probabilities for different strata. Apart from the entire set of data, we can also stratify by sex, by area, or by sex and area simultaneously. For all strata, we considered both an MAR and a protective model. All zeros in the table correspond to a boundary estimate and are not due to rounding. It is interesting to observe that a boundary solution for strata combined does not imply a boundary solution for the strata separately (e.g., all data versus stratified by area) and vice versa (e.g., area 1 versus area 1 stratified by sex).

Finally, EM and multiple imputation estimators are slightly different when applied to those tables in which boundary problems occur. As an example, we consider the estimates for the full set of data with EM: 23, 9, 6, 12, 11, 8, 9, and 22, respectively. These are much closer to the MAR solution, with the multiple imputation estimates even closer. This phenomenon is observed for all other tables as well. It means that the correction for parameter space violations is too extreme with the delta method estimator.

Table 18.6 Presence or absence of colds. Estimated cell probabilities (all quantities were multiplied by 100). Stratification for sex is indicated by male (M) and female (F); stratification for area is indicated by area 1 (1) and area 2 (2). A + indicates that the corresponding stratifying variable is not used.

	++	M+	F+	+1	+2	M1	M2	F1	F2
Protective estimators
111	23	20	29	21	26	15	21	24	32
112	9	7	10	9	11	9	11	11	11
121	0	3	0	3	6	7	7	8	4
122	18	16	17	15	11	11	10	10	12
211	11	13	10	11	11	11	13	10	9
212	8	7	8	10	6	12	6	10	7
221	0	5	0	4	12	12	14	11	11
222	31	30	27	29	17	24	19	18	16
MAR estimators
111	22	17	27	24	16	27	24	35	32
112	10	10	11	12	8	3	11	8	11
121	7	7	7	5	2	0	3	4	4
122	11	11	10	12	17	18	15	12	12
211	10	11	10	10	12	16	10	10	9
212	9	9	8	7	10	2	10	6	7
221	12	13	11	11	3	0	3	10	11
222	20	22	17	19	33	34	25	16	16

18.4 A PROTECTIVE ESTIMATOR FOR GAUSSIAN DATA

We return now to the Gaussian case and describe the method proposed by Lipsitz *et al.* (2004) allowing a protective estimate to be made of the effect of a covariate in a linear regression relationship. The method relies on the assumption that the outcome variable and the covariate of interest have an approximate bivariate normal distribution, conditional on the remaining covariates. In addition, it is assumed that the missing data mechanism is conditionally independent of this covariate, given the outcome variable and the remaining covariates. This could be termed the *protective* assumption. A method of moments approach is used to obtain the protective estimator of the regression parameters, and variance estimation is conducted using jackknife methods (Quenouille 1956).

18.4.1 Notation and maximum likelihood

Consider a linear regression model with N independent subjects $(i = 1, \ldots, n)$. Let Y_i denote the outcome variable for the ith subject and let $\boldsymbol{x}_i =$

$(x_{i1}, \ldots, x_{ip})'$ denote a $p \times 1$ vector of covariates. The primary interest is in estimation of the vector of regression coefficients $\boldsymbol{\beta}' = (\beta_0, \boldsymbol{\beta}')$ for the linear regression model

$$\mu_i = E(Y_i|\boldsymbol{x}_i, \boldsymbol{\beta}) = \beta_0 + \boldsymbol{x}_i'\boldsymbol{\beta}. \tag{18.30}$$

The error term is assumed to be $N(0, \sigma^2)$. Assume that, although the covariates are fully observed, Y_i is missing for a subset of the subjects. The missing data mechanism is allowed to be MNAR. Maximum likelihood estimation of $\boldsymbol{\beta}$ (and σ^2) requires specification of the conditional distribution of y_i given $\boldsymbol{x}_i$. As usual, the missing data indicator $R_i = 1$ (0) if Y_i is observed (missing). Under MNAR, Ibrahim and Lipsitz (1996) and Ibrahim *et al.* (1999) propose basing inferences on

$$f(y_i, r_i|\boldsymbol{x}_i, \boldsymbol{\alpha}, \boldsymbol{\beta}, \sigma^2) = f(y_i|\boldsymbol{x}_i, \boldsymbol{\beta}, \sigma^2)f(r_i|\boldsymbol{x}_i, y_i, \boldsymbol{\alpha}), \tag{18.31}$$

where $\boldsymbol{\alpha}$ parameterizes the missing data mechanism. For example, a logistic regression model could be specified for the Bernoulli random variable R_i given $(\boldsymbol{x}_i, y_i)$,

$$f(r_i|\boldsymbol{x}_i, y_i, \boldsymbol{\alpha}) = \pi_i^{r_i}(1 - \pi_i)^{(1-r_i)}, \tag{18.32}$$

where

$$\pi_i = \frac{\exp(\alpha_0 + \boldsymbol{\alpha}_1'\boldsymbol{x}_i + \alpha_2 y_i)}{1 + \exp(\alpha_0 + \boldsymbol{\alpha}_1'\boldsymbol{x}_i + \alpha_2 y_i)}, \tag{18.33}$$

where $\boldsymbol{\alpha} = (\boldsymbol{\alpha}_1', \alpha_2)'$. The likelihood contribution for a subject with Y_i unobserved equals

$$f(r_i|\boldsymbol{x}_i, \boldsymbol{\alpha}, \boldsymbol{\beta}, \sigma^2) = \int f(y_i|\boldsymbol{x}_i, \boldsymbol{\beta}, \sigma^2)f(r_i|\boldsymbol{x}_i, y_i, \boldsymbol{\alpha})dy_i,$$

the observed data log-likelihood is

$$\sum_{i=1}^{N} r_i \log[f(r_i, y_i|\boldsymbol{x}_i, \boldsymbol{\alpha}, \boldsymbol{\beta}, \sigma^2)] + (1 - r_i) \log[f(r_i|\boldsymbol{x}_i, \boldsymbol{\alpha}, \boldsymbol{\beta}, \sigma^2)], \tag{18.34}$$

and the maximum likelihood estimates follow from maximizing (18.34) over $(\boldsymbol{\alpha}, \boldsymbol{\beta}, \sigma^2)$. In the next subsection we describe the protective alternative proposed by Lipsitz *et al.* (2004).

18.4.2 Protective estimator

To develop the protective estimator we must assume that one of the covariates, x_{i1} say, has a normal distribution. We use the partition $x_i = (x_{i1}, x'_{i2})'$, and assume that $f(y_i, x_{i1} | x_{i2})$ has a bivariate normal distribution. The joint density is

$$\begin{pmatrix} Y_i \\ X_{i1} \end{pmatrix} \Bigg| x_{i2} \sim N\left[\begin{pmatrix} \theta_0 + \theta_1 x_{i2} \\ \gamma_0 + \gamma_1 x_{i2} \end{pmatrix}, \begin{pmatrix} \sigma_{11}^2 & \sigma_{12} \\ \sigma_{12} & \sigma_{22}^2 \end{pmatrix} \right]. \tag{18.35}$$

The regression model is given by

$$E(Y_i | x_i) = \theta_0 + \theta_1 x_{i2} + \frac{\sigma_{12}}{\sigma_{22}^2}(x_{i1} - \gamma_0 - \gamma_1 x_{i2})$$

$$= \left(\theta_0 - \frac{\sigma_{12}}{\sigma_{22}^2} \gamma_0 \right) + \frac{\sigma_{12}}{\sigma_{22}^2} x_{i1} + \left(\theta_1 - \frac{\sigma_{12}}{\sigma_{22}^2} \gamma_1 \right) x_{i2} \tag{18.36}$$

$$= \beta_0 + \beta_1 x_{i1} + \beta_2 x_{i2},$$

where

$$\beta_0 = \theta_0 - \frac{\sigma_{12}}{\sigma_{22}^2} \gamma_0, \tag{18.37}$$

$$\beta_1 = \frac{\sigma_{12}}{\sigma_{22}^2}, \tag{18.38}$$

$$\beta_2 = \theta_1 - \frac{\sigma_{12}}{\sigma_{22}^2} \gamma_1. \tag{18.39}$$

Further, the conditional variance is

$$\text{var}(Y_i | x_i) = \sigma_{11}^2 - \frac{\sigma_{12}}{\sigma_{22}^2}. \tag{18.40}$$

Rather than using the full joint distribution, the protective estimator uses the conditional distributions $f(x_{i1} | x_{i2})$ and $f(x_{i1} | y_i, x_{i2})$ to estimate the parameters $(\theta_0, \theta_1, \gamma_0, \gamma_1, \sigma_{11}^2, \sigma_{12}, \sigma_{22}^2)$, which is done, through (18.37)–(18.39). Since x_{i1} and x_{i2} are both fully observed, it is straightforward to estimate the parameters $(\gamma_0, \gamma_1, \sigma_{22}^2)$ from $f(x_{i1} | x_{i2})$, using all observations. Indeed, from (18.35), the conditional mean of X_{i1} given x_{i2} is

$$E(X_{i1} | x_{i2}, \gamma) = \gamma_0 + \gamma_1 x_{i2}, \tag{18.41}$$

with conditional variance

$$\text{var}(X_{i1} | x_{i2}) = \sigma_{22}^2. \tag{18.42}$$

Hence, ordinary least squares can be used for these parameters.

However, since y_i is only partially observed, it is not straightforward to estimate the remaining parameters $(\theta_0, \boldsymbol{\theta}_1, \sigma_{11}^2, \sigma_{12})$ from $f(x_{i1}|y_i, \boldsymbol{x}_{i2})$ unless additional assumptions are made. Write

$$f(x_{i1}|y_i, \boldsymbol{x}_{i2}, R_i = 1) = \frac{f(x_{i1}|y_i, \boldsymbol{x}_{i2}) \cdot P(R_i = 1|x_{i1}, y_i, \boldsymbol{x}_{i2})}{P(R_i = 1|y_i, \boldsymbol{x}_{i2})}. \tag{18.43}$$

Making the *protective assumption*

$$P(R_i = 1|x_{i1}, y_i, \boldsymbol{x}_{i2}) = P(R_i = 1|y_i, \boldsymbol{x}_{i2}), \tag{18.44}$$

(18.43) reduces to

$$f(x_{i1}|y_i, \boldsymbol{x}_{i2}, R_i = 1) = f(x_{i1}|y_i, \boldsymbol{x}_{i2}). \tag{18.45}$$

Result (18.45) implies that the complete cases ($R_i = 1$) can be used to consistently estimate the parameters of the conditional distribution of X_{i1} given $(y_i, \boldsymbol{x}_{i2})$. In particular,

$$E(X_{i1}|\boldsymbol{x}_{i2}, y_i, R_i = 1, \boldsymbol{\gamma}, \boldsymbol{\theta}) = E(X_{i1}|\boldsymbol{x}_{i2}, y_i, \boldsymbol{\gamma}, \boldsymbol{\theta}).$$

Using (18.35), the conditional mean of X_{i1} given $(\boldsymbol{x}_{i2}, y_i)$, is

$$E(X_{i1}|\boldsymbol{x}_{i2}, y_i, \boldsymbol{\gamma}, \boldsymbol{\theta}) = (\gamma_0 + \boldsymbol{\gamma}_1 \boldsymbol{x}_{i2}) + \frac{\sigma_{12}}{\sigma_{11}^2}(y_i - \theta_0 - \boldsymbol{\theta}_1 \boldsymbol{x}_{i2})$$

$$= \phi_0 + \boldsymbol{\phi}_1 \boldsymbol{x}_{i2} + \phi_2 y_i, \tag{18.46}$$

where

$$\phi_0 = \gamma_0 - \frac{\sigma_{12}}{\sigma_{11}^2}\theta_0 = \gamma_0 - \phi_2 \theta_0,$$

$$\boldsymbol{\phi}_1 = \boldsymbol{\gamma}_1 - \frac{\sigma_{12}}{\sigma_{11}^2}\boldsymbol{\theta}_1 = \boldsymbol{\gamma}_1 - \phi_2 \boldsymbol{\theta}_1,$$

$$\phi_2 = \frac{\sigma_{12}}{\sigma_{11}^2}.$$

The conditional variance is given by

$$\text{var}(X_{i1}|\boldsymbol{x}_{i2}, y_i) = \sigma_{22}^2 - \frac{\sigma_{12}^2}{\sigma_{11}^2}. \tag{18.47}$$

The parameters $[\phi_0, \boldsymbol{\phi}_1, \phi_2, \text{var}(X_{i1}|\boldsymbol{x}_{i2}, y_i)]$ can now be estimated, based on the complete cases, via ordinary least-squares regression with outcome variable X_{i1} and covariates $(\boldsymbol{x}_{i2}, y_i)$. These, in turn, give rise to a sequence of estimates

$$\widehat{\theta}_0 = (\widehat{\gamma}_0 - \widehat{\phi}_0)/\widehat{\phi}_2,$$

$$\widehat{\theta}_1 = (\widehat{\gamma}_1 - \widehat{\phi}_1)/\widehat{\phi}_2,$$

$$\widehat{\sigma}_{12} = \frac{\widehat{\sigma}_{22}^2 - \widehat{\mathrm{var}}(X_{i1}|\boldsymbol{x}_{i2}, y_i)}{\widehat{\phi}_2},$$

$$\widehat{\sigma}_{11}^2 = \frac{\widehat{\sigma}_{12}}{\widehat{\phi}_2} = \frac{\widehat{\sigma}_{22}^2 - \widehat{\mathrm{var}}(X_{i1}|\boldsymbol{x}_{i2}, y_i)}{\widehat{\phi}_1^2}.$$

Finally, the protective estimator of $\boldsymbol{\beta} = (\beta_0, \beta_1, \boldsymbol{\beta}_2')'$ is given by

$$\widehat{\beta}_0 = \widehat{\theta}_0 - \frac{\widehat{\sigma}_{12}}{\widehat{\sigma}_{22}^2}\widehat{\gamma}_0,$$

$$\widehat{\beta}_1 = \frac{\widehat{\sigma}_{12}}{\widehat{\sigma}_{22}^2},$$

$$\widehat{\beta}_2 = \widehat{\theta}_1 - \frac{\widehat{\sigma}_{12}}{\widehat{\sigma}_{22}^2}\widehat{\gamma}_1.$$

Lipsitz *et al.* (2004) established the consistency and asymptotic normality of $\widehat{\boldsymbol{\beta}}$. The covariance matrix can be consistently estimated using the delta method or the jackknife (Quenouille 1956). Because $\boldsymbol{\beta}$ is a complicated function of $(\theta_0, \theta_1, \gamma_0, \gamma_1, \sigma_{11}^2, \sigma_{12}, \sigma_{22}^2)$, the jackknife method may be more attractive. An expression for this variance estimator is

$$\widehat{\mathrm{var}}(\widehat{\boldsymbol{\beta}}) = \frac{n-1}{n}\sum_{i=1}^{n}(\widehat{\boldsymbol{\beta}}_{-i} - \widehat{\boldsymbol{\beta}})(\widehat{\boldsymbol{\beta}}_{-i} - \widehat{\boldsymbol{\beta}})', \qquad (18.48)$$

where $\widehat{\boldsymbol{\beta}}_{-i}$ is the estimate of $\boldsymbol{\beta}$ obtained by deleting the data for the *i*th subject.

Lipsitz *et al.* (2004) report on a simulation study set up to compare the protective estimator with maximum likelihood as well as with the conventional complete case estimator.

18.4.3 The six cities study

In this subsection we illustrate the protective regression estimator using data on the persistence of maternal smoking from the six cities study. We consider a subsample concerned with the health effects of air pollution (Ware *et al.* 1984). The outcome variable of interest is a measure of the mother's smoking (in cigarettes per day) when her child is 10 years old. It is of interest to determine how changes in the mother's smoking behaviour (from the previous year) are related to her child's wheeze status at age 9 (yes or no) and the city of residence (there are two participating cities). Preliminary analyses have shown that the square-root transformation of the maternal smoking variable is approximately normal. As a result, it is of interest to estimate the parameters in the linear regression of the outcome (square root of maternal smoking when child is aged 10, S_{i2}) on the prior measure of maternal smoking (square root of maternal smoking when child is aged 9, S_{i1}), the child's wheeze status at age 9, and the city of residence. Notably, 208 (or 35%) of the 574 subjects have missing outcome data. With such a large amount of missing data, a complete case analysis would potentially be biased and inefficient at the same time. Data for 30 randomly selected subjects are shown in Table 18.7.

Table 18.7 Six cities study. Data on 30 randomly selected subjects. Maternal smoking is expressed in number of cigarettes.

Subject	City	Child wheeze, age 9	Maternal smoking age 9	Maternal smoking age 10
1	1	no	0	—
2	1	no	1	—
3	1	yes	10	—
4	0	no	13	—
5	0	yes	15	—
6	0	no	20	—
7	1	yes	20	—
8	0	no	30	—
9	0	yes	35	—
10	0	yes	≥ 40	—
11	1	no	≥ 40	—
12	0	no	0	0
13	0	yes	0	0
14	1	no	0	0
15	1	yes	0	0
16	0	no	12	0
17	0	no	4	3
18	0	no	10	6
19	0	no	1	7
20	1	no	10	10
21	0	yes	20	10
22	1	no	20	10
23	0	no	20	20
24	0	yes	20	20
25	0	no	30	20
26	1	no	20	21
27	1	no	35	25
28	0	yes	≥ 40	30
29	1	yes	≥ 40	30
30	1	yes	2	≥ 40

The important variables are S_{i1}, S_{i2},

$$W_i = \begin{cases} 1 & \text{if child wheezed at age 9,} \\ 0 & \text{if child did not wheeze at age 9,} \end{cases}$$

and C_i, which takes values 0 and 1 to distinguish between the participating cities. The regression model

$$E(S_{i2}|C_i, W_i, S_{i1}) = \beta_0 + \beta_1 S_i + \beta_2 C_i + \beta_2 W_i \qquad (18.49)$$

is of interest, and the missing data model takes the form

$$\text{logit}(\pi_i) = \alpha_0 + \alpha_1 S_{i2} + \alpha_2 S_{i1} + \alpha_3 W_i + \alpha_3 C_i, \qquad (18.50)$$

where $\pi_i = P(R_i = 1|S_{i2}, S_{i1}, W_i, C_i, \boldsymbol{\alpha})$. Table 18.8 displays the maximum likelihood estimates of $\boldsymbol{\alpha}$. With due caution, we might conclude that there is some evidence in favour of MNAR. If we accept this model at face value, we can conclude that missingness in the outcome appears to be significantly related to the outcome S_{i2}, the city of residence ($p < 0.0001$), and marginally related to wheeze.

To use protective estimation we assume that $f(S_{i2}, S_{i1}|W_i, C_i)$ is bivariate normal. Since the probability of missingness in (18.50) does not appear to be related to S_{i1}, and the marginal distributions of S_{i2} and S_{i1} each appear to be approximately normal in the preliminary analyses, the two assumptions required for the protective estimator to be consistent appear to hold. We note, however, that because of the inherent sensitivities in fitting MNAR models, ordinarily it will not be possible to determine whether the missingness probabilities are conditionally independent of x_{i1}. In general, the assumption must often be made on subject-matter grounds.

Table 18.9 provides the estimates of β obtained from maximum likelihood, protective estimation and complete case analysis. All three approaches yield very similar estimates of the intercept, and the effects of S_{i1} and wheeze. Nevertheless, for the latter, the CC estimate is negative, whereas the other two

Table 18.8 Six cities study. Maximum likelihood estimates (standard errors) and p-values for logistic regression for the missing data model, $P(R_i = 1|y_i, \boldsymbol{x}_i)$.

Effect	Estimate (s.e.)	p-value
Intercept	2.359 (0.260)	< 0.0001
S_{i2}	−0.405 (0.075)	< 0.0001
S_{i1}	−0.016 (0.051)	0.758
Wheeze	−0.382 (0.229)	0.096
City	−1.521 (0.210)	< 0.0001

Table 18.9 Six cities study. Estimates (s.e.) and p-values for linear regression model for $E(Y_i|\boldsymbol{x}_i)$. Estimation methods are complete case analysis (CC), maximum likelihood (ML), and protective estimation (PR).

Effect	Method	Estimate (s.e.)	p-value
Intercept	CC	0.892 (0.162)	< 0.0001
	ML	1.169 (0.156)	< 0.0001
	PR	1.045 (0.286)	< 0.0001
S_{i1}	CC	0.294 (0.047)	< 0.0001
	ML	0.301 (0.042)	< 0.0001
	PR	0.416 (0.086)	< 0.0001
Wheeze	CC	−0.045 (0.245)	0.853
	ML	0.075 (0.222)	0.736
	PR	0.083 (0.556)	0.881
City	CC	−0.025 (0.221)	0.910
	ML	0.460 (0.199)	0.021
	PR	0.424 (0.495)	0.392

estimates are positive. However, we note that the estimate of the city effect is similar for maximum likelihood and the protective estimate, but discernibly different from the CC estimate. The maximum likelihood estimator appears to be the most efficient, and most notably so for estimation of the city effect, in which the protective estimate is estimated to be only 16% as efficient as the maximum likelihood estimate. Thus, even though the maximum likelihood and the protective estimates of the city effect are quite similar, the larger sampling variability of the protective estimate yields a non-significant p-value.

18.5   CONCLUDING REMARKS

In this chapter we have reviewed so-called protective estimation, both for the Gaussian and the categorical case. Broadly speaking, such estimators apply when missingness on a particular measurement is allowed to depend on that very measurement, but on no other measurements. Brown (1990), Michiels and Molenberghs (1997), and Lipsitz *et al.* (2004) have shown that under such assumptions the missing data mechanism does not have to be modelled to estimate measurement model parameters. In a sense, this result is related to ignorability, in spite of the MNAR nature of such mechanisms. Both ignorable and protective estimators are valid under a class of missingness mechanisms, rather than under a single one. This opens up the possibility of sensitivity analysis. Both Michiels and Molenberghs (1997) and Lipsitz *et al.* (2004) established a connection with full likelihood estimation, the former authors also with pseudo-likelihood. For precision estimation, such methods as the delta method, the EM algorithm, multiple imputation, and jackknifing can be used.

Part V
Sensitivity Analysis

19

MNAR, MAR, and the Nature of Sensitivity

19.1   INTRODUCTION

Over the last decade a variety of models to analyse incomplete multivariate and longitudinal data have been proposed, many of which allow for the missingness mechanism to be MNAR. Several of these models have been reviewed and illustrated earlier in Chapters 15–17.

The fundamental problems implied by such models, to which we refer as sensitivity to unverifiable modelling assumptions, have, in turn, sparked off various strands of research in what is now termed *sensitivity analysis*. The nature of sensitivity originates from the fact that an MNAR model is not fully verifiable from the data, rendering the formal distinction between MNAR and random missingness (MAR), where only covariates and observed outcomes influence missingness, hard or even impossible, unless one is prepared to accept the posited MNAR model in an unquestioning way. In this introductory chapter to the sensitivity analysis part of this book, we show that the formal data-based distinction between MAR and MNAR is not possible, in the sense that each MNAR model fit to a set of observed data can be reproduced exactly by an MAR counterpart. Of course, such a pair of models will produce different predictions of the unobserved outcomes, given the observed ones.

Such a position is in contrast to the view that one can test for an MNAR mechanism using the data under analysis. Such tests, comparing MAR and MNAR mechanisms, can of course be constructed using conventional statistical methodology as done, for example, by Diggle and Kenward (1994) and discussed in Section 15.2 of this volume. We again remind the reader that such tests are conditional upon the alternative model holding, which can only be assessed as far as it fits the *observed* data, not the *unobserved*.

Missing Data in Clinical Studies   G. Molenberghs and M.G. Kenward
© 2007 John Wiley & Sons, Ltd

In Section 19.2 we show formally that for every MNAR model an MAR counterpart can be constructed that has exactly the same fit to the observed data, in the sense that it produces exactly the same predictions to the observed data (e.g., fitted counts in an incomplete contingency table) as the original MNAR model, and depending on exactly the same parameter vector. In Section 19.3 the specific case of incomplete contingency tables is studied. In Section 19.4 we apply the ideas developed to data from the Slovenian public opinion survey, introduced in Section 2.10 and analysed previously by Rubin *et al.* (1995) and Molenberghs *et al.* (2001a). The fact that models with different implications at the complete data level might produce exactly the same fit has, of course, important implications for model selection and assessment. Some of these are discussed in Section 19.5. Jansen *et al.* (2006b) have shown that such tests are also subject to theoretical concerns, and these are presented in Section 19.6.

19.2   EVERY MNAR MODEL HAS AN MAR BODYGUARD

In this section, we will show that for every MNAR model fitted to a set of data, there is an MAR counterpart providing exactly the same fit. The following steps are involved: (1) an MNAR model is fitted to the data; (2) the fitted model is reformulated in a PMM form; (3) the density or distribution of the unobserved measurements given the observed ones, and given a particular response pattern, is replaced by its MAR counterpart; (4) it is established that such an MAR counterpart exists and is unique. Throughout this section, we will suppress covariates $\mathbf{x}_i$ from the notation, while allowing them to be present.

In the first step, an MNAR model is fitted to the observed set of data. Suppose, for example, that the model is written in selection model format. Then the observed data likelihood is

$$L = \prod_i \int f(\mathbf{y}_i^o, \mathbf{y}_i^m | \boldsymbol{\theta}) f(\mathbf{r}_i | \mathbf{y}_i^o, \mathbf{y}_i^m, \boldsymbol{\psi}) d\mathbf{y}_i^m. \tag{19.1}$$

Similar expressions hold for pattern-mixture and shared-parameter models. Denoting the resulting parameter estimates by $\widehat{\boldsymbol{\theta}}$ and $\widehat{\boldsymbol{\psi}}$ respectively, the fit to the hypothetical full data is

$$f(\mathbf{y}_i^o, \mathbf{y}_i^m, \mathbf{r}_i | \widehat{\boldsymbol{\theta}}, \widehat{\boldsymbol{\psi}}) = f(\mathbf{y}_i^o, \mathbf{y}_i^m | \widehat{\boldsymbol{\theta}}) f(\mathbf{r}_i | \mathbf{y}_i^o, \mathbf{y}_i^m, \widehat{\boldsymbol{\psi}}). \tag{19.2}$$

For the second step, the full density (19.2) can be re-expressed in PMM form as

$$f(\mathbf{y}_i^o, \mathbf{y}_i^m | \mathbf{r}_i, \widehat{\boldsymbol{\theta}}, \widehat{\boldsymbol{\psi}}) f(\mathbf{r}_i | \widehat{\boldsymbol{\theta}}, \widehat{\boldsymbol{\psi}})$$
$$= f(\mathbf{y}_i^o | \mathbf{r}_i, \widehat{\boldsymbol{\theta}}, \widehat{\boldsymbol{\psi}}) f(\mathbf{r}_i | \widehat{\boldsymbol{\theta}}, \widehat{\boldsymbol{\psi}}) f(\mathbf{y}_i^m | \mathbf{y}_i^o, \mathbf{r}_i, \widehat{\boldsymbol{\theta}}, \widehat{\boldsymbol{\psi}}). \tag{19.3}$$

A similar reformulation can be considered for a shared-parameter model. In a PMM setting, the model will have been expressed in this form to begin with. Note that, in line with PMM theory, the final term on the right-hand side of (19.3), $f(\boldsymbol{y}_i^m|\boldsymbol{y}_i^o, d_i, \widehat{\boldsymbol{\theta}}, \widehat{\boldsymbol{\psi}})$, is not identified from the observed data. In this case, it is determined solely from modelling assumptions. Within the PMM framework, identifying restrictions have to be considered (Section 16.5 above; Little 1994a; Molenberghs *et al.* 1998b; Kenward *et al.* 2003).

In the third step this factor is replaced by the appropriate MAR counterpart. For this we need the following lemma, which defines MAR within the PMM framework.

Lemma 19.1 *In the PMM framework, the missing data mechanism is MAR if and only if*

from marginal density $f(Y)$; can be estimated from complete cases

$$f(\boldsymbol{y}_i^m|\boldsymbol{y}_i^o, \boldsymbol{r}_i, \boldsymbol{\theta}) = f(\boldsymbol{y}_i^m|\boldsymbol{y}_i^o, \boldsymbol{\theta}).$$

This means that, in a given pattern, the conditional distribution of the unobserved components given the observed ones equals the corresponding distribution marginalized over the patterns. The proof, after Molenberghs *et al.* (1998b) is as follows:

Proof. Suppressing parameters and covariates from the notation, the decomposition of the full data density, in both selection model and PMM fashion, whereby MAR is applied to the selection model version, produces

$$f(\boldsymbol{y}_i^o, \boldsymbol{y}_i^m)f(\boldsymbol{r}_i|\boldsymbol{y}_i^o) = f(\boldsymbol{y}_i^o, \boldsymbol{y}_i^m|\boldsymbol{r}_i)f(\boldsymbol{r}_i). \tag{19.4}$$

Further factoring the right-hand side and moving the second factor on the left to the right as well gives

$$f(\boldsymbol{y}_i^o, \boldsymbol{y}_i^m) = f(\boldsymbol{y}_i^m|\boldsymbol{y}_i^o, \boldsymbol{r}_i)\frac{f(\boldsymbol{y}_i^o|\boldsymbol{r}_i)f(\boldsymbol{r}_i)}{f(\boldsymbol{r}_i|\boldsymbol{y}_i^o)}$$

$$= f(\boldsymbol{y}_i^m|\boldsymbol{y}_i^o, \boldsymbol{r}_i)\frac{f(\boldsymbol{y}_i^o, \boldsymbol{r}_i)}{f(\boldsymbol{r}_i|\boldsymbol{y}_i^o)}$$

$$f(\boldsymbol{y}_i^m|\boldsymbol{y}_i^o)f(\boldsymbol{y}_i^o) = f(\boldsymbol{y}_i^m|\boldsymbol{y}_i^o, \boldsymbol{r}_i)f(\boldsymbol{y}_i^o),$$

and hence

$$f(\boldsymbol{y}_i^m|\boldsymbol{y}_i^o) = f(\boldsymbol{y}_i^m|\boldsymbol{y}_i^o, \boldsymbol{r}_i).$$

This concludes the proof. $\square$

Using Lemma 19.1, it is clear that $f(\boldsymbol{y}_i^m|\boldsymbol{y}_i^o, \boldsymbol{r}_i, \widehat{\boldsymbol{\theta}}, \widehat{\boldsymbol{\psi}})$ needs to be replaced by

$$h(\boldsymbol{y}_i^m|\boldsymbol{y}_i^o, \boldsymbol{r}_i) = h(\boldsymbol{y}_i^m|\boldsymbol{y}_i^o) = f(\boldsymbol{y}_i^m|\boldsymbol{y}_i^o, \widehat{\boldsymbol{\theta}}, \widehat{\boldsymbol{\psi}}), \tag{19.5}$$

where the $h(\cdot)$ notation is used for shorthand purposes. Note that the density in (19.5) follows from the selection model-type marginal density of the complete data vector. Sometimes, therefore, it may be more convenient to replace the notation $\boldsymbol{y}_i^o$ and $\boldsymbol{y}_i^m$ by one that explicitly indicates which components under consideration are observed and missing in pattern $\boldsymbol{r}_i$:

$$h(\boldsymbol{y}_i^m|\boldsymbol{y}_i^o,\boldsymbol{r}_i) = h(\boldsymbol{y}_i^m|\boldsymbol{y}_i^o) = f[(y_{ij})_{\underset{r_{ij}}{r_j=0}}|(y_{ij})_{\underset{r_{ij}}{r_j=1}},\widehat{\boldsymbol{\theta}},\widehat{\boldsymbol{\psi}}]. \qquad (19.6)$$

Thus, (19.6) provides a unique way of extending the model fit to the observed data, within the MAR family. To show formally that the fit remains the same, we consider the observed data likelihood based on (19.1) and (19.3):

$$L = \prod_i \int f(\boldsymbol{y}_i^o,\boldsymbol{y}_i^m|\boldsymbol{\theta})f(\boldsymbol{r}_i|\boldsymbol{y}_i^o,\boldsymbol{y}_i^m,\boldsymbol{\psi})d\boldsymbol{y}_i^m$$

$$= \prod_i \int f(\boldsymbol{y}_i^o|\boldsymbol{r}_i,\boldsymbol{\theta},\boldsymbol{\psi})f(\boldsymbol{r}_i|\boldsymbol{\theta},\boldsymbol{\psi})f(\boldsymbol{y}_i^m|\boldsymbol{y}_i^o,\boldsymbol{r}_i,\boldsymbol{\theta},\boldsymbol{\psi})d\boldsymbol{y}_i^m$$

$$= \prod_i f(\boldsymbol{y}_i^o|\boldsymbol{r}_i,\boldsymbol{\theta},\boldsymbol{\psi})f(\boldsymbol{r}_i|\boldsymbol{\theta},\boldsymbol{\psi})$$

$$= \prod_i \int f(\boldsymbol{y}_i^o|\boldsymbol{r}_i,\boldsymbol{\theta},\boldsymbol{\psi})f(\boldsymbol{r}_i|\boldsymbol{\theta},\boldsymbol{\psi})h(\boldsymbol{y}_i^m|\boldsymbol{y}_i^o)d\boldsymbol{y}_i^m.$$

The above results justify the following theorem:

Theorem 19.2 *Every fit to the observed data, obtained from fitting an MNAR model to a set of incomplete data, is exactly reproducible from an MAR model.*

The key computational consequence is the need to obtain $h(\boldsymbol{y}_i^m|\boldsymbol{y}_i^o)$ in (19.5) or (19.6). This means that, for each pattern, the conditional density of the unobserved measurements given the observed ones needs to be extracted from the marginal distribution of the complete set of measurements. ACMV restrictions (Sections 3.6 and 16.5) provide a practical computational scheme. Recall that ACMV states:

$$\forall t \geq 2, \forall s < t:$$

$$f(y_{it}|y_{i1},\ldots,y_{i,t-1},d_i = s) = f(y_{it}|y_{i1},\ldots,y_{i,t-1},d_i \geq t). \qquad (19.7)$$

In words, the density of a missing measurement, conditional on the measurement history, is determined from the corresponding density over all patterns for which all of these measurements are observed. For example, the density of the third measurement in a sequence, given the first and second ones, in patterns with only one or two measurements taken, is determined from the corresponding density over all patterns with three or more measurements. Thijs *et al.* (2002) and Verbeke and Molenberghs (2000, p. 347) derived a practical computational method for the factors in (19.7):

$$f(y_{it}|y_{i1},\ldots,y_{i,t-1},d_i=s)$$

$$=\frac{\sum_{d=s}^{n}\alpha_d f_d(y_{i1},\ldots,y_{is})}{\sum_{d=s}^{n}\alpha_d f_d(y_{i1},\ldots,y_{i,s-1})}$$

$$=\sum_{d=s}^{n}\left(\frac{\alpha_d f_d(y_{i1},\ldots,y_{i,s-1})}{\sum_{d=s}^{n_i}\alpha_d f_d(y_{i1},\ldots,y_{i,s-1})}\right)f_d(y_s|y_{i1},\ldots,y_{i,s-1}). \qquad (19.8)$$

Here, α_d is the probability of belonging to pattern d. Details can be found in Section 16.5.

The above identifications for the monotone case are useful when an MNAR pattern-mixture model has been fitted to begin with, since then the identifications under MAR can be calculated from the pattern-specific marginal distributions. When a selection model has been fitted in the initial step, $f(y_{i1},\ldots,y_{in_i}|\widehat{\boldsymbol{\theta}})$ has been estimated, from which all conditional distributions needed in (19.6) can be derived. When the initial model is an MNAR PMM model and the missing data patterns are non-monotone, then it is necessary to first rewrite the PMM in selection model form, and derive the required conditional distributions from the resultant selection-based measurement model. This essentially comes down to calculating a weighted average of the pattern-specific measurement models. In some cases, such as for contingency tables, this step can be done in an alternative way by fitting a saturated MAR selection model to the fit obtained from the PMM model.

We will illustrate and contrast the monotone and non-monotone cases using a bivariate and trivariate outcome with dropout on the one hand and a bivariate non-monotone outcome on the other hand. While the theorem applies to both the monotone and non-monotone settings we will see that only for the former do relatively simple and intuitively appealing expressions arise. In the next section we study the aforementioned general contingency table setting to which a PMM has been fitted.

19.2.1 A bivariate outcome with dropout

Dropping covariates, parameters, and the subject index i from notation, the selection model–PMM equivalence for the case of two outcomes, the first of which is always observed but the second one partially missing, is given by:

$$f(y_1,y_2)\widetilde{g}(d=2|y_1,y_2)=f_2(y_1,y_2)\widetilde{\alpha}(d=2),$$

$$f(y_1,y_2)\widetilde{g}(d=1|y_1,y_2)=f_1(y_1,y_2)\widetilde{\alpha}(d=1).$$

This is the setting considered by Glynn *et al.* (1986). For more details on their perceived paradox, see Section 16.3. Here, $\widetilde{g}(\cdot)$ is used for the selection model dropout model, with $\widetilde{\alpha}(\cdot)$ denoting the PMM probabilities of belonging to one of the patterns. Because $\widetilde{\alpha}(d = 1) + \widetilde{\alpha}(d = 2) = 1$ and a similar result holds for the $\widetilde{g}(\cdot)$ functions, it is convenient to write:

$$f(y_1, y_2)g(y_1, y_2) = f_2(y_1, y_2)\alpha, \qquad (19.9)$$

$$f(y_1, y_2)[1 - g(y_1, y_2)] = f_1(y_1, y_2)[1 - \alpha]. \qquad (19.10)$$

Assuming MCAR, it is clear that $\alpha = g(y_1, y_2)$, producing, without any difficulty,

$$f(y_1, y_2) = f_2(y_1, y_2) = f_1(y_1, y_2). \qquad (19.11)$$

Under MAR, $g(y_1, y_2) = g(y_1)$ and hence (19.9) produces

$$f(y_1)f(y_2|y_1)g(y_1) = f_2(y_1)f_2(y_2|y_1)\alpha.$$

Upon reordering, we find that

$$\frac{f(y_1)g(y_1)}{f_2(y_1)\alpha} = \frac{f_2(y_2|y_1)}{f(y_2|y_1)}. \qquad (19.12)$$

The same arguments can be applied to (19.10), from which we derive:

$$f(y_2|y_1) = f_2(y_2|y_1) = f_1(y_2|y_1). \qquad (19.13)$$

Note that (19.13) is strictly weaker than (19.11). The last term in (19.13) is not identified in itself, and hence, it needs to be set equal to its counterpart from the completers which, in turn, is equal to the marginal distribution. This is in agreement with (19.6) as well as with the specific identifications applicable in the monotone and hence the ACMV setting.

19.2.2   A trivariate outcome with dropout

Identification (19.13) does not involve mixtures. This is no longer true when there are three or more outcomes. The equations corresponding to (19.9) and (19.10), applied to the MAR case, are:

$$f(y_1, y_2, y_3)g_0 = f_0(y_1, y_2, y_3)\alpha_0, \qquad (19.14)$$

$$f(y_1, y_2, y_3)g_1(y_1) = f_1(y_1, y_2, y_3)\alpha_1, \qquad (19.15)$$

$$f(y_1, y_2, y_3)g_2(y_1, y_2) = f_2(y_1, y_2, y_3)\alpha_2, \qquad (19.16)$$

$$f(y_1, y_2, y_3)g_3(y_1, y_2) = f_3(y_1, y_2, y_3)\alpha_3. \qquad (19.17)$$

We have chosen to include pattern 0, the one without follow-up measurements, as well, and will return to it. We could write $g_3(\cdot)$ as a function of y_3 as well, but because the sum of the $g_d(\cdot)$ equals one, it is clear that $g_3(\cdot)$ ought to be independent of y_3. With arguments similar to those developed in the case of two measurements, we can rewrite (19.17) as

$$\frac{f(y_1,y_2)}{f_3(y_1,y_2)} \cdot \frac{g_3(y_1,y_2)}{\alpha_3} = \frac{f_3(y_3|y_1,y_2)}{f(y_3|y_1,y_2)}.$$

Exactly the same argument can be made based on (19.16), and hence

$$f_3(y_3|y_1,y_2) = f(y_3|y_1,y_2) = f_2(y_3|y_1,y_2). \tag{19.18}$$

The first factor identifies the second, and hence also the third. Starting from (19.15), we obtain

$$f_1(y_2,y_3|y_1) = f(y_2,y_3|y_1),$$

which produces two separate identities,

$$f_1(y_2|y_1) = f(y_2|y_1), \tag{19.19}$$

$$f_1(y_3|y_1,y_2) = f(y_3|y_1,y_2) = f_3(y_3|y_1,y_2) = f_2(y_3|y_1,y_2). \tag{19.20}$$

For (19.20), identity (19.18) has been used as well. The density $f(y_2|y_1)$, needed in (19.19), is determined from the general ACMV result (19.8):

$$f(y_2|y_1) = \frac{\alpha_2 f_2(y_2|y_1) + \alpha_3 f_3(y_2|y_1)}{\alpha_2 + \alpha_3}.$$

Finally, turning attention to (19.14), it is clear that $g_0 = \alpha_0$ and hence also $f_0(y_1,y_2,y_3) = f(y_1,y_2,y_3)$. From the latter density, only $f(y_1)$ has not yet been determined, but this one follows again directly from the general ACMV result:

$$f(y_1) = \frac{\alpha_1 f_1(y_1) + \alpha_2 f_2(y_1) + \alpha_3 f_3(y_1)}{\alpha_1 + \alpha_2 + \alpha_3}.$$

In summary, the MAR identifications needed follow directly from both the PMM and the selection model formulations of the model.

19.2.3 A bivariate outcome with non-monotone missingness

The counterparts to (19.9)–(19.10) and (19.14)–(19.17) for a bivariate outcome with non-monotone missingness are

$$f(y_1,y_2)g_{00}(y_1,y_2) = f_{00}(y_1,y_2)\alpha_{00}, \tag{19.21}$$

$$f(y_1,y_2)g_{10}(y_1,y_2) = f_{10}(y_1,y_2)\alpha_{10}, \tag{19.22}$$

$$f(y_1,y_2)g_{01}(y_1,y_2) = f_{01}(y_1,y_2)\alpha_{01}, \tag{19.23}$$

$$f(y_1,y_2)g_{11}(y_1,y_2) = f_{11}(y_1,y_2)\alpha_{11}. \tag{19.24}$$

Clearly, under MCAR, the $g_{r_1 r_2}(\cdot)$ functions do not depend on the outcomes and hence $f_{r_1 r_2}(y_1, y_2) = f(y_1, y_2)$ for all four patterns. For the MAR case, (19.21)–(19.24) simplify to

$$f(y_1, y_2) g_{00} = f_{00}(y_1, y_2) \alpha_{00}, \tag{19.25}$$

$$f(y_1, y_2) g_{10}(y_1) = f_{10}(y_1, y_2) \alpha_{10}, \tag{19.26}$$

$$f(y_1, y_2) g_{01}(y_2) = f_{01}(y_1, y_2) \alpha_{01}, \tag{19.27}$$

$$f(y_1, y_2) g_{11}(y_1, y_2) = f_{11}(y_1, y_2) \alpha_{11}. \tag{19.28}$$

Observe that there are four identifications across the $g_{r_1 r_2}(y_1, y_2)$ functions:

$$g_{00} + g_{10}(y_1) + g_{01}(y_2) + g_{11}(y_1, y_2) = 1,$$

for each (y_1, y_2). Also $\sum_{r_1, r_2} \alpha_{r_1, r_2} = 1$. Applying the usual algebra to (19.25)–(19.28), we obtain three identifications for the unobservable densities:

$$f_{00}(y_1, y_2) = f(y_1, y_2), \tag{19.29}$$

$$f_{10}(y_2 | y_1) = f(y_2 | y_1), \tag{19.30}$$

$$f_{01}(y_1 | y_2) = f(y_1 | y_2). \tag{19.31}$$

19.3 THE GENERAL CASE OF INCOMPLETE CONTINGENCY TABLES

In Sections 19.2.1–19.2.3 we derived general identification schemes for an MAR extension of a fitted model to a binary or trivariate outcome with dropout, as well as to a bivariate outcome with non-monotone missingness. Whereas the monotone cases provide explicit expressions in terms of the pattern-specific densities, (19.29)–(19.31) provide an identification only in terms of the marginal probability. This in itself is not a problem, since the marginal density is always available, either directly when a selection model is fitted, or through marginalization when a PMM or a shared-parameter model is fitted.

In the specific case of contingency tables, further progress can be made since we can show a saturated MAR model is always available for any incomplete contingency table setting. This implies that one can start from the fit of an MNAR model to the observed data and then extend it, using this result, to MAR. We will present the general result and then discuss its precise implications for practical applications.

Assume that we have a $\prod_{k=1}^{n} c_k$ contingency table with supplemental margins. The table of completers is indexed by $r = 1 = (1, \ldots, 1)$. A particular incomplete table is indexed by an $r \neq 1$. The full set of tables can, but need not, be present. The number of cells is

$$\#\text{cells} = \sum_r \prod_{k=1}^n c_k^{r_k}. \tag{19.32}$$

Denote the measurement model probabilities by $p_j = p_{j_1 \ldots j_n}$ for $j_k = 1, \ldots, c_k$ and $k = 1, \ldots, n$. Clearly, these probabilities sum to one. The missingness probabilities, assuming MAR, are

$$p(r|j) = \begin{cases} p(r|j_k \text{ with } r_k = 1) & \text{if } r \neq 1, \\ 1 - \sum_{r \neq 1} p(r|j) & \text{if } r = 1. \end{cases} \tag{19.33}$$

Summing over r implies summing over those patterns for which actual observations are available. The number of parameters in the saturated model is

$$\#\text{parameters} = \left(\prod_{k=1}^n c_k - 1 \right) + \sum_{r \neq 1} \prod_{k=1}^n c_k^{r_k}. \tag{19.34}$$

The first term in (19.34) is for the measurement model, the second is for the missingness model. Clearly, the number of parameters equals one less than the number of cells, establishing the claim. The situation where covariates are present is covered automatically, merely by considering one extra dimension in the contingency table, $j = 0$ say, with c_0 referring to the total number of covariate levels in the set of data.

We will now study the implications for the simple but important settings studied in Sections 19.2.1 and 19.2.3.

19.3.1   A bivariate contingency table with dropout

In Section 19.2.1 identifications were derived for the bivariate case with monotone missingness. For contingency tables, these can be also be derived by further fitting the saturated MAR model, described in the previous section, to the fit obtained from the original MNAR model. Denote the counts obtained from the fit of the original model by $z_{2,jk}$ and $z_{1,j}$, for the completers and dropouts, respectively. Denote the measurement model probabilities by p_{jk} and the dropout probabilities by q_j. Then, due to ignorability, the likelihood factors into two components:

$$\ell_1 = \sum_{j,k} z_{2,jk} \ln p_{jk} + \sum_j z_{1,j} \ln p_{j+} - \lambda \left(\sum_{j,k} p_{jk} - 1 \right), \tag{19.35}$$

$$\ell_2 = \sum_{j,k} z_{2,jk} \ln q_j + \sum_j z_{1,j} \ln(1 - q_j). \tag{19.36}$$

$$0 = z_{2,jk} / p_{jk} + z_{1,j} / p_{j+} - \lambda$$

$$0 = z_{2,jk} / q_j - z_{1,j} / (1 - q_j)$$

$$0 = p_{++} - \lambda$$

We have used an undetermined Lagrange multiplier λ to incorporate the sum constraint on the marginal probabilities. Solving the score equations for (19.35) and (19.36) produces

$0 = z_{2,j+} \cdot p_{j+} + z_{\cdot,j} p_{j+} - \lambda p_{j+}^2$

$0 = z_{2,j+}(1 - q_j) - z_{1,j} q_j$

$0 = p_{++} - 1$

and $\quad z_{2,++} + z_{1,+} = n$

$$\widehat{p}_{jk} = \frac{1}{n} z_{2,jk} \left(\frac{z_{2,j+} + z_{1,j}}{z_{2,j+}} \right), \tag{19.37}$$

$$\widehat{q}_j = \frac{z_{2,j+}}{z_{2,j+} + z_{1,j}}, \tag{19.38}$$

where n is the total sample size. Combining parameter estimates leads to the new, MAR-based, fitted counts:

$$\widehat{z_{2,jk}} = n\widehat{p}_{jk}\widehat{q}_j = z_{2,jk}, \tag{19.39}$$

$$\widehat{z_{1,jk}} = n\widehat{p}_{jk}(1 - \widehat{q}_j) = z_{1,j}\frac{z_{2,jk}}{z_{2,j+}}, \tag{19.40}$$

$$\widehat{z_{1,j+}} = z_{1,j+}. \tag{19.41}$$

From (19.39) and (19.41) it is clear that the fit in terms of the observed data has not changed. The expansion of the incomplete data so that they are complete is described by (19.40). Equations (19.39) and (19.40) can be used to produce the MAR counterpart to the original model, without any additional calculations. This is not as simple in the non-monotone case, as we now demonstrate.

19.3.2 A bivariate contingency table with non-monotone missingness

The counterparts to (19.35)–(19.36) for this case are

$$\ell_1 = \sum_{j,k} z_{11,jk} \ln p_{jk} + \sum_{j} z_{10,j} \ln p_{j+} + \sum_{k} z_{01,k} \ln p_{+k}$$

$$+ z_{00} \ln p_{++} - \lambda \left(\sum_{j,k} p_{jk} - 1 \right), \tag{19.42}$$

$$\ell_2 = \sum_{j,k} z_{11,jk} \ln(1 - q_{10,j} - q_{01,k} - q_{00}) + \sum_{j} z_{10,j} \ln q_{10,j}$$

$$+ \sum_{k} z_{01,k} \ln q_{01,k} + z_{00} \ln q_{00}. \tag{19.43}$$

The notation has been modified in accordance with the design. The q quantities correspond to the $g(\cdot)$ model in Section 19.2.3.

While $p_{++} = 1$ and hence z_{00} does not contribute information to the measurement probabilities, it does add to the estimation of the missingness model.

Deriving the score equations from (19.42) and (19.43) is straightforward but, in contrast to the previous section, no closed form exists. Chen and Fienberg (1974) derived an iterative scheme for the probabilities p_{jk}, based on setting the expected sufficient statistics equal to their *complete data* counterparts:

$$np_{jk} = z_{11,jk} + z_{10,j}\frac{p_{jk}}{p_{j+}} + z_{01,k}\frac{p_{jk}}{p_{\mid k}} + z_{00}\frac{p_{jk}}{p_{++}}$$

(with $p_{++} = 1$) and hence

$$(n - z_{00})p_{jk} = z_{11,jk} + z_{10,j}\frac{p_{jk}}{p_{j+}} + z_{01,k}\frac{p_{jk}}{p_{+k}}. \tag{19.44}$$

The same equation is obtained from the first derivative of (19.42). Chen and Fienberg's iterative scheme results from initiating the process with a set of starting values for the p_{jk}, for example from the completers, and then evaluating the right-hand side of (19.44). Equating it to the left-hand side provides an update for the parameters. The process is repeated until convergence.

While there are no closed-form counterparts to (19.37) and (19.38), the expressions equivalent to (19.39)–(19.41) are

$$\widehat{z_{11,jk}} = z_{11,jk}, \tag{19.45}$$

$$\widehat{z_{10,jk}} = z_{10,j}\frac{p_{jk}}{p_{j+}}, \tag{19.46}$$

$$\widehat{z_{01,jk}} = z_{01,k}\frac{p_{jk}}{p_{+k}}, \tag{19.47}$$

$$\widehat{z_{00,jk}} = z_{00}p_{jk}. \tag{19.48}$$

However, there is an important difference between (19.39)–(19.41) on the one hand and (19.45)–(19.48) on the other. In the monotone case, the expressions on the right-hand side are in terms of the counts z only, whereas here the marginal probabilities p_{jk} intervene, which have to be determined from a numerical fit.

19.4   THE SLOVENIAN PUBLIC OPINION SURVEY

The practical use of the results in the previous section is illustrated now on data from the Slovenian public opinion survey. Molenberghs *et al.* (2001a) reanalysed these data and used them as motivation to introduce their so-called *intervals of ignorance*, a formal way of incorporating uncertainty stemming from incompleteness into the analysis of incomplete contingency tables. For this they used the convenient model family proposed by Baker *et al.* (1992) and introduced in a somewhat modified and expanded form in Section 15.5 above. In Section 19.4.1 the original formulation will be introduced. In Section 19.4.2 the original analyses, conducted by Rubin *et al.* (1995) and Molenberghs *et al.* (2001a) will be reviewed, followed by application of the BRD models in Section 19.4.3.

19.4.1   The BRD models

Baker *et al.* (1992) proposed the original form of the models presented in Section 15.5, also in terms of the four-way classification of both outcomes, together with their respective missingness indicators:

$$
\nu_{10,jk} = \nu_{11,jk}\beta_{jk},
$$
$$
\nu_{01,jk} = \nu_{11,jk}\alpha_{jk}, \qquad\qquad (19.49)
$$
$$
\nu_{00,jk} = \nu_{11,jk}\alpha_{jk}\beta_{jk}\gamma,
$$

with

$$
\alpha_{jk} = \frac{\phi_{01|jk}}{\phi_{11|jk}}, \qquad \beta_{jk} = \frac{\phi_{10|jk}}{\phi_{11|jk}}, \qquad \gamma = \frac{\phi_{11|jk}\phi_{00|jk}}{\phi_{10|jk}\phi_{01|jk}}.
$$

The α (β) parameters describe missingness in the independence (attendance) question, and γ captures the interaction between them. The subscripts are missing from γ since Baker *et al.* (1992) showed that this quantity is independent of j and k in every identifiable model. These authors considered nine models, based on setting α_{jk} and β_{jk} constant in one or more indices:

$$
\begin{array}{lll}
\text{BRD1}: (\alpha, \beta) & \text{BRD4}: (\alpha, \beta_k) & \text{BRD7}: (\alpha_k, \beta_k) \\
\text{BRD2}: (\alpha, \beta_j) & \text{BRD5}: (\alpha_j, \beta) & \text{BRD8}: (\alpha_j, \beta_k) \\
\text{BRD3}: (\alpha_k, \beta) & \text{BRD6}: (\alpha_j, \beta_j) & \text{BRD9}: (\alpha_k, \beta_j).
\end{array}
$$

Interpretation is straightforward. For example, BRD1 is MCAR, and in BRD4 missingness in the first variable is constant, while missingness in the second variable depends on its value. BRD6–BRD9 saturate the observed data degrees of freedom, while the lower-numbered ones do not, leaving room for a non-trivial model fit to the observed data.

19.4.2   Initial analysis

We first review a number of analyses previously done on these data, primarily by Rubin *et al.* (1995) and Molenberghs *et al.* (2001a), and then illustrate the ideas laid out in earlier sections. We will concentrate on the independence and attendance outcomes, that is, collapsing Table 2.12.

Rubin *et al.* (1995) conducted several analyses of the data. Their main emphasis was on determining the proportion θ of the population that would attend the plebiscite and vote for independence. The three other combinations of these two binary outcomes would be treated as voting 'no'. Their estimates are reproduced in Table 19.1, which also shows the proportion ν of 'no' via non-attendance (i.e., the proportion of the population who would not attend the plebiscite). The conservative method is to use the ratio of the (yes, yes) answers to the (attendance, independence) pair and the total sample, that is, $1439/2074 = 0.694$. This is the most pessimistic scenario. At the opposite end of the spectrum, we can add to their analysis the most optimistic estimate that replaces the numerator by all who are not a definite 'no':

$$\frac{1439 + 159 + 144 + 136}{2074} = \frac{1878}{2074} = 0.905.$$

These figures are obtained by first collapsing over the secession variable and then summing the counts of the (yes, yes), (yes, *), (*, yes) and (*, *) categories. Both estimates together yield the interval

$$\theta \in [0.694, 0.905]. \tag{19.50}$$

The corresponding interval for ν (no through non-attendance) is

$$\nu \in [0.031, 0.192]. \tag{19.51}$$

The complete case estimate for θ is based on the subjects answering all three questions,

$$\widehat{\theta} = \frac{1191 + 158}{1454} = 0.928,$$

Table 19.1 Slovenian public opinion survey. Estimates of the proportion θ attending the plebiscite and voting for independence, as presented in Rubin *et al.* (1995) and Molenberghs *et al.* (2001a).

Estimation method	Voting in favour of independence $\widehat{\theta}$	Noes via non-attendance $\widehat{\nu}$
Pessimistic–optimistic bounds	[0.694, 0.905]	[0.031, 0.192]
Complete cases	0.928	0.020
Available cases	0.929	0.021
MAR (2 questions)	0.892	0.042
MAR (3 questions)	0.883	0.043
~~MAR~~ MNAR	0.782	0.122
Plebiscite	0.885	0.065

and the available case estimate is based on the subjects answering the two questions of interest here,

$$\widehat{\theta} = \frac{1191 + 158 + 90}{1549} = 0.929.$$

It is noteworthy that both estimates fall outside the pessimistic–optimistic interval and should be disregarded, since these seemingly straightforward estimators do not take into account the decision to treat absences as noes and thus discard available information.

Rubin *et al.* (1995) considered two MAR models, the first based on the two questions of direct interest only, the second using all three, yielding $\widehat{\theta} = 0.892$ and $\widehat{\theta} = 0.883$, respectively. Finally, they considered a single MNAR model, based on the assumption that missingness on a question depends on the answer to that question but not on the other questions. They argued that this is a plausible assumption. The corresponding estimator is $\widehat{\theta} = 0.782$.

Figure 19.1 shows the relative position of the estimates of Rubin *et al.* In summary, we see that: (1) the available case and complete case estimates are outside the pessimistic–optimistic range (19.50) (indicated by vertical bars); (2) both MAR estimates are very close to and the MNAR estimate is very far from the 'truth', which is the proportion who voted yes at the actual plebiscite, $\theta = 0.885$. Based on these findings, and those from other carefully designed surveys, the authors conclude that the MAR assumption can be plausible, when there is limited non-response and good covariate information. While we agree with the closeness of the MAR analyses in this case, it is of course unclear whether MAR will always be the preferred non-response mechanism. In addition, we aim to place the MAR analysis within a whole family of non-ignorable models, in order to shed additional light on these data, as will be done next.

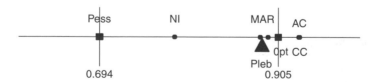

Figure 19.1 The Slovenian public opinion survey. Relative position for the estimates of proportion of yes votes, based on the models considered in Rubin *et al.* (1995). The vertical lines indicate the non-parametric pessimistic–optimistic bounds. (Pess, pessimistic boundary; Opt, optimistic boundary; MAR, Rubin *et al.*'s MAR model; NI, Rubin *et al.*'s MNAR model; AC, available cases; CC, complete cases; Pleb, plebiscite outcome.)

19.4.3   BRD analysis

Molenberghs *et al.* (2001a) fitted all nine BRD models to the Slovenian public opinion survey and presented a summary table. There was a small computational error that has been corrected. The corrected results are presented in Table 19.2. BRD1 produces $\widehat{\theta} = 0.892$, exactly the same as the first MAR estimate obtained by Rubin *et al.* (1995). This does not come as a surprise, since both models assume MAR and use information from the two main questions. A graphical representation of the original analyses (Section 19.4.2) and the BRD models combined is given in Figure 19.2.

The connection between MNAR models and their associated MAR bodyguards can be illustrated easily by means of four models from the BRD family. We select models BRD1, BRD2, BRD7, and BRD9. Model BRD1 assumes missingness to be MCAR. All others are of the MNAR type. Model BRD2 has seven free parameters, and hence does not saturate the observed data degrees of freedom, whereas models BRD7 and BRD9 do saturate the eight data degrees of freedom. The collapsed data, together with the model fits, are displayed in Tables 19.3

Table 19.2 Slovenian public opinion survey. Analysis restricted to the independence and attendance questions. Summaries for each of the models BRD1–BRD9 are presented.

Model	Structure	d.f.	Log-likelihood	$\widehat{\theta}$	Confidence interval	$\widehat{\theta}_{MAR}$
BRD1	(α, β)	6	−2495.29	0.892	[0.878; 0.906]	0.8920
BRD2	(α, β_j)	7	−2467.43	0.884	[0.869; 0.900]	0.8915
BRD3	(α_k, β)	7	−2463.10	0.881	[0.866; 0.897]	0.8915
BRD4	(α, β_k)	7	−2467.43	0.765	[0.674; 0.856]	0.8915
BRD5	(α_j, β)	7	−2463.10	0.844	[0.806; 0.882]	0.8915
BRD6	(α_j, β_j)	8	−2431.06	0.819	[0.788; 0.849]	0.8919
BRD7	(α_k, β_k)	8	−2431.06	0.764	[0.697; 0.832]	0.8919
BRD8	(α_j, β_k)	8	−2431.06	0.741	[0.657; 0.826]	0.8919
BRD9	(α_k, β_j)	8	−2431.06	0.867	[0.851; 0.884]	0.8919

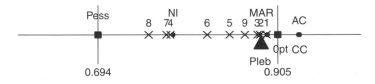

Figure 19.2 Slovenian public opinion survey. Relative position for the estimates of proportion of yes votes, based on the models considered in Rubin *et al.* (1995) and on the Baker *et al.* (1992) models. The vertical lines indicate the non-parametric pessimistic–optimistic bounds. (Letter symbols as in Figure 19.1; numbers refer to BRD models.)

Table 19.3 Slovenian public opinion survey. Analysis restricted to the independence and attendance questions. The observed data are shown, as well as the fit of models BRD1, BRD2, BRD7, and BRD9, and their MAR counterparts, to the observed data.

Observed data and
fit of BRD7, BRD7(MAR), BRD9, and BRD9(MAR) to incomplete data

1439	78	159
16	16	32

144	54	136

Fit of BRD1 and BRD1(MAR) to incomplete data

1381.6	101.7	182.9
24.2	41.4	8.1

179.7	18.3	136.0

Fit of BRD2 and BRD2(MAR) to incomplete data

1402.2	108.9	159.0
15.6	22.3	32.0

181.2	16.8	136.0

and 19.4. Each of the four models is paired with its MAR counterpart. For each pairing, Tables 19.3 and 19.4 also show the fit to the observed and the hypothetical complete data. The fits of models BRD7, BRD9, and their MAR counterparts coincide with the observed data. As the theory states, every MNAR model and its MAR counterpart will produce exactly the same fit to the observed data, which is therefore also seen for BRD1 and BRD2. However, while models BRD1 and BRD1(MAR) coincide in their fit to the hypothetical complete data, this is not the case for the other three models. The reason is clear: since model BRD1 belongs to the MAR family from the start, its counterpart BRD1(MAR) will not produce any difference, but merely copies the fit of BRD1 to the unobserved data, given the observed ones. Finally, while BRD7 and BRD9 produce a different fit to the complete data, BRD7(MAR) and BRD9(MAR) coincide. This is because the fits of BRD7 and BRD9 coincide with respect to their fit to the observed data and, because they are saturated, coincide with the observed data as such. This fit is the sole basis for the models' MAR extensions. It is noteworthy that, while BRD7, BRD9, and BRD7(MAR)≡BRD9(MAR) all saturate the observed data degrees of freedom, their complete data fits are dramatically different.

We return now to the implications of our results for the primary estimand θ, the proportion of people voting yes by simultaneously being in favour of independence and deciding to take part in the vote. Rubin *et al.* (1995) considered, apart from simple models such as complete case analysis ($\widehat{\theta} = 0.928$) and available case analysis ($\widehat{\theta} = 0.929$), both ignorable models ($\widehat{\theta} = 0.892$

Table 19.4 Slovenian public opinion survey. Analysis restricted to the independence and attendance questions. The fit of models BRD1, BRD2, BRD7, and BRD9, and their MAR counterparts, to the hypothetical complete data is shown.

Fit of BRD1 and BRD1(MAR) to complete data

1381.6	101.7	170.4	12.5	176.6	13.0	121.3	9.0
24.2	41.4	3.0	5.1	3.1	5.3	2.1	3.6

Fit of BRD2 to complete data

1402.2	108.9	147.5	11.5	179.2	13.9	105.0	8.2
15.6	22.3	13.2	18.8	2.0	2.9	9.4	13.4

Fit of BRD2(MAR) to complete data

1402.2	108.9	147.7	11.3	177.9	12.5	121.2	9.3
15.6	22.3	13.3	18.7	3.3	4.3	2.3	3.2

Fit of BRD7 to complete data

1439	78	3.2	155.8	142.4	44.8	0.4	112.5
16	16	0.0	32.0	1.6	9.2	0.0	23.1

Fit of BRD9 to complete data

1439	78	150.8	8.2	142.4	44.8	66.8	21.0
16	16	16.0	16.0	1.6	9.2	7.1	41.1

Fit of BRD7(MAR) and BRD9(MAR) to complete data

1439	78	148.1	10.9	141.5	38.4	121.3	9.0
16	18	11.8	20.2	2.5	15.6	2.1	3.6

when based on the two main questions and $\widehat{\theta} = 0.883$ when using the secession question as an auxiliary variable) and a MNAR one ($\widehat{\theta} = 0.782$). Since the value of the plebiscite was $\theta_{\text{pleb}} = 0.885$, an important benchmark obtained four weeks after the survey, they concluded that the MAR-based estimate was preferable. Molenberghs *et al.* (2001a) supplemented these analysis with a so-called pessimistic–optimistic interval, obtained from replacing the incomplete data with no and yes, respectively, and obtained $\theta \in [0.694, 0.904]$. Further, they considered all nine BRD models, producing a range for θ from 0.741 to 0.892.

We now consider the model fit of all nine BRD models. Conducting likelihood ratio tests for BRD1 versus the ones with seven parameters, and then in turn for BRD2–BRD5 versus the saturated ones, suggests the lower-numbered models should not be considered further. In particular, this seems to imply that the MAR-based value 0.892 is also inappropriate. However, recomputing the MAR value from each of the models BRD1(MAR)–BRD9(MAR), as displayed in the last column of Table 19.2, it is clear that this value is remarkably stable. Obviously, since models BRD6(MAR)–BRD9(MAR) are exactly the same, the corresponding probabilities $\widehat{\theta}_{\text{MAR}}$ are exactly equal too. Even though BRD2(MAR)–BRD5(MAR) are different, in this case, the probability of being in favour of independence and attending the plebiscite is constant across all four models. This is a coincidence, since all three other cell probabilities are different, but only slightly so. For example, the probability of being in favour of independence combined with not attending ranges over 0.066–0.0685 across these four models.

We have made the following two-stage use of models BRD6(MAR)–BRD9(MAR). First, in a conventional way, the fully saturated model is selected as the only adequate description of the observed data. Second, these models are transformed into their MAR counterpart, from which inferences are drawn. As such, the MAR counterpart provides a useful supplement to the original set of models BRD6–BRD9 and one further, important scenario to model the incomplete data. In principle, the same exercise could be conducted if the additional secession variable were used.

19.5   IMPLICATIONS FOR FORMAL AND INFORMAL MODEL SELECTION

Model selection and assessment are a well-established component of statistical analysis. This has been the case for univariate data settings, but methods for multivariate, longitudinal, clustered, and otherwise correlated data follow suit.

There are several strands of intuition surrounding model selection and assessment. First, it is researchers' common understanding that 'observed $\simeq$ expected' in a very broad sense. This is usually understood to imply that observed and fitted profiles ought to be sufficiently similar, or similarly observed and fitted counts in contingency tables, and so on. Second, in a likelihood-based context, deviances and related information criteria are considered useful and practical tools for model assessment. Third, saturated models are uniquely defined and at the top of the model hierarchy. For contingency tables, such a saturated model is one which exactly reproduces the observed counts. Fourth, for the special case of samples from univariate or multivariate normal distributions, the estimators for the mean vector and the variance–covariance matrix are independent, both in a small-sample as well as in an asymptotic sense. Fifth, in the same situation, the least-squares and maximum likelihood estimators are identical as far as mean parameters are concerned, and asymptotically equal for covariance parameters.

It is very important to realize that the five points of intuition are based on our experience with well-balanced designs and complete sets of data. We have already seen a number of counterexamples. For example, the analysis of the incomplete version of the orthodontic growth data set in Section 5.3 and the ensuing discussion in Section 5.4 showed that 'observed $\simeq$ expected' does not need to hold. This is graphically illustrated in Figures 5.2 (model 1) and 5.3. In Table 5.4 we noticed that the maximum likelihood based estimates differ from the ordinary least-squares estimates (MANOVA and ANOVA for each time point). A more formal derivation of these results was given in Section 4.4. For the bivariate normal case, the frequentist (or moments) estimator (4.17) is strictly different from the likelihood-based estimator (4.19). Analogous results were derived for the contingency table case in Section 4.4.2, where expressions (4.22) and (4.23) can be usefully juxtaposed.

At the same time, (4.19) clearly establishes that the estimators for mean and variance in a normal setting are *not* independent, owing to the presence of $\widehat{\beta}_1$.

The nature of the problem is that, when fitting models to incomplete data, we have to manage two aspects rather than one, as represented schematically in Figure 19.3. The contrast between data and model can be expressed at both a complete and at an incomplete data level. Ideally, we would want to consider the situation depicted in Figure 19.3(b), where the comparison is fully made at the complete level. Of course, the complete data are, by definition, beyond reach, and there is a real danger in settling for the situation in Figure 19.3(c). This would happen, for example, if we were to conclude that the fit of model 1, shown in Figure 5.2, is poor. Such a conclusion would ignore the fact that the model fit is at the complete data level, accounting for 16 boys and 11 girls at the age of 10, whereas the data only represent the remaining 11 boys and 7 girls at the age of 10.

Thus, a fair model assessment should be confined to the situations laid out in Figures 19.3(b) and 19.3(d) only. We will start out with the simpler (d) and then return to (b).

Assessing how well model 1 fits the incomplete version of the growth data can be done by comparing the observed means at the age of 10 to the values predicted by the model. This implies we have to confine model fit to those children actually observed at the age of 10. However, it is clear from the form of estimator (4.19) that the model perfectly predicts the observed data points. Clearly, this quick assessment makes use of normality and the fact that the model is saturated. This cannot always be done, a point to which we will return.

Turning to the analysis of the Slovenian public opinion survey, the principle behind Figure 19.3(d) would lead to the conclusion that models BRD7, BRD7(MAR), BRD9, and BRD9(MAR9) fit the observed data perfectly, as can be seen in Table 19.3 (top). The same conclusion would apply to BRD6, BRD8, and their MAR counterparts, since they too saturate the observed data degrees of freedom, as can be seen from Table 19.3.

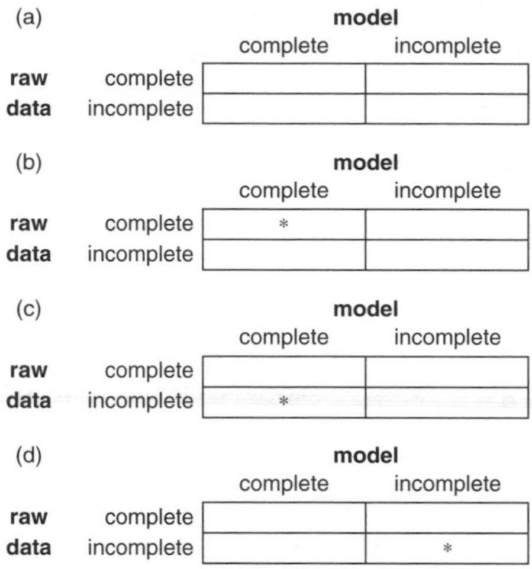

Figure 19.3 Model assessment when data are incomplete. (a) Two dimensions in model (assessment) exercise when data are incomplete. (b) Ideal situation. (c) Dangerous situation, bound to happen in practice. (d) Comparison of data and model at coarsened, observable level.

However, Table 19.4 illustrates the fact that these models are different at the complete data level. To be precise, BRD6–BRD9 each lead to different predictions of the underlying complete tables. These four MNAR models are different as well from their MAR counterparts, but BRD6(MAR)–BRD9(MAR) is only one single model. These observations have ramifications for inferences on, for example, the proportion voting in favour of independence, $\widehat{\theta}$ and $\widehat{\theta}_{MAR}$, a quantity estimated in the range $[0.74, 0.89]$ across these five models. Thus, while we can conclude these models fit the observed data perfectly, we can never be sure about the fit to the hypotetical complete data, a point to which we return in chapters to come, in particular in Chapter 21.

While it is relatively easy to check the fit of the model to the observed contingency table, we have observed that this is slightly more awkward for continuous data, as illustrated by the orthodontic growth data. Gelman *et al.* (2005) proposed a method fitting into the situation depicted in Figure 19.3(b). The essence of the approach is as follows. First, a model is fitted to the observed data. Second, using the model, the data are completed M times, for example, using multiple imputation (Chapter 9). From the data sets thus completed characteristics are computed (e.g., means or standard deviations) or plotted (e.g., average profiles). This allows for a straightforward comparison between model and data at the complete data level.

While the method is elegant, one has to be careful about the realm of the conclusion. This is best seen using the Slovenian public opinion survey. Applying the method to BRD7, for example, would tell us the model is a perfect fit. What it means, though, is that the fit to the *incomplete* data is perfect. This still leaves us in the dark as to the plausibility of the story told by the model about the fit to the complete data since exactly the same story would apply to BRD6, BRDD8, BRD9, and the MAR bodyguard of these models.

In summary, there are two important aspects in selection and assessment when data are incomplete. First, the model needs to fit the *observed* data sufficiently well. This aspect alone is already more involved than in the complete/balanced case. Second, sensitivity analysis is necessary to assess to what extent the conclusions drawn are dependent on the explicit or implicit assumptions a model makes about the conditional behaviour of the incomplete data given the observed, because such assumptions usually have an impact on the inferences of interest.

19.6 BEHAVIOUR OF THE LIKELIHOOD RATIO TEST FOR MAR VERSUS MNAR

In the previous section we have seen that, in a well-defined sense, that it is not possible to distinguish between MAR and MNAR using the incomplete data. This may be seem contradictory given that a test for MAR versus MNAR can be conducted within, say, the model proposed by Diggle and Kenward (1994; see Section 15.2 above). However, the difference is that there we have the narrow choice between a single posited MNAR model and one predefined MAR-type simplification. Thus, one might be tempted to conclude that such a test is acceptable, given that one is prepared to believe the alternative model is the correct description of the truth, something that can never be verified but perhaps is backed up by enough scientific and empirical evidence. Even given this, there remain a number of problems associated with the statistical behaviour – that is, likelihood ratio tests for such hypotheses – as will be illustrated in this section, which based on work by Jansen *et al.* (2006b).

We report on a simulation study designed to examine the finite-sample behaviour of the likelihood ratio test (LRT) for testing MAR versus MNAR within the selection model framework of Diggle and Kenward (1994). For comparison we also consider the test for MCAR versus MAR. The behaviour of a parametric and a semi-parametric bootstrap approach in this context is also investigated.

It follows from standard theory that the LRT for MCAR versus MAR has the usual asymptotic χ_1^2 distribution, but the test for MNAR versus MAR is a non-standard situation. Rotnitzky *et al.* (2000) have shown that for a similar but simpler setting the limiting distribution is a χ^2 mixture with characteristics governed by the singularity properties of the information matrix. The score equation associated with the MNAR parameter ψ_2 apparently generates a quasi-linear dependence structure in the system of score equations. When reducing the model to an MAR/MCAR model, this dependency disappears.

Moreover, they have shown that convergence to this limiting distribution is extremely slow.

Similar theoretical considerations show that the same phenomena hold for the model of Diggle and Kenward (1994). The slow convergence also raises the question whether, even if known, an asymptotic distribution is of any practical use. Thus, it is of interest to examine the finite-sample properties of the LRT in this setting and to investigate whether a bootstrap simulated null distribution, known to be a (slightly) better approximation in several classical settings, could be a useful alternative to χ^2-based distributions.

The simulation settings are as follows. The measurement model takes the general linear mixed model form

$$\boldsymbol{y}_i \sim N(X_i\boldsymbol{\beta}, V_i) \tag{19.52}$$

$(i = 1, \ldots, N)$ in which $\boldsymbol{\beta}$ is a vector of regression coefficients (or fixed effects), and where the marginal variance–covariance matrix is decomposed in the typical mixed model fashion: $V_i = Z_i G Z_i' + \Sigma_i$ for matrices G and Σ_i. The parameters in $\boldsymbol{\beta}$, G, and Σ_i are assembled into $\boldsymbol{\theta}$.

We set $N = 200$, $n_i = 3$, $X_i = 1$ (intercept only), mean vector $\beta = (2, 0, -2)'$ and compound symmetric covariance structure with common variance equal to 8 and common covariance equal to 6; the missingness model given by

$$\text{logit}\,[P(D_i = j | D_i \geqslant j, \boldsymbol{y}_i)] = \psi_0 + \psi_1 y_{i,j-1} + \psi_2 y_{ij}. \tag{19.53}$$

Consider the following hypotheses: (1) $\psi_1 = 0$ in (19.53) with $\psi_2 = 0$ (MCAR versus MAR); (2) $\psi_2 = 0$ in (19.53) with $\psi_1 \neq 0$ (MAR versus MNAR). When not set to zero, we took $\psi_0 = -2$, $\psi_1 = 1$, $\psi_2 = 2$.

19.6.1   Simulated null distributions

Figure 19.4, based on 800 samples generated under each of the two null hypotheses, shows the simulated null distribution of the LRT. As expected, the simulated null distribution deviates in a more pronounced way from the χ_1^2 distribution when going from hypothesis 1 to hypothesis 2. The p-value of the Kolmogorov–Smirnov goodness-of-fit test is 0.0548 for hypothesis 1 and less than 0.00001 for hypothesis 2. The mean and variance are 0.94 and 1.75 respectively under hypothesis 1, and 2.54 and 8.11 under Hypothesis 2, clearly showing an increase in the values of the LRT. This is also confirmed by the 10%, 5%, and 1% quantiles as shown on the bottom lines of Tables 19.5 and 19.6. Whereas the theoretical results of Rotnitzky *et al.* (2000) indicate that in this setting the asymptotic distribution is stochastically smaller than a

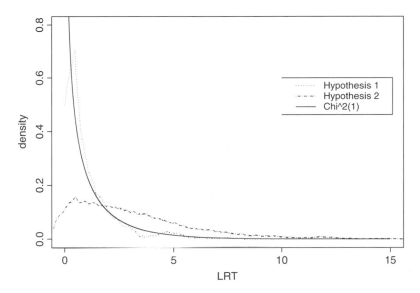

Figure 19.4 Simulation study. Kernel density plots of the simulated null distribution based on 800 samples, under each hypothesis $i = 1, 2$, together with the density of the χ_1^2 distribution.

χ_1^2 distribution, that is, a mixture with a χ_0^2, the simulated null distribution is stochastically larger. It is plausible that the slow rate of convergence is causing this opposite behaviour. Experimentation with larger sample sizes did not substantially change this result.

This small simulation experiment clearly shows that the use of the χ_1^2 distribution, which holds in standard situations, is not appropriate in the settings studied here. An alternative approach is needed, and in the next section we describe two bootstrap approaches proposed by Jansen *et al.* (2006b) and consider the extent to which their use leads to a resolution of the problem.

19.6.2 Performance of bootstrap approaches

Jansen *et al.* (2006b) proposed a parametric and a semi-parametric bootstrap LRT. If the asymptotic null distribution does not depend on unknown parameters, the bootstrap is expected to exhibit a smaller order of magnitude for the error level (Efron 1979; Efron and Tibshirani 1998; Davison and Hinkley 1997). Beran (1988) showed that the bootstrap LRT automatically accomplishes the Bartlett adjustment, at least in a standard setting.

Parametric bootstrap

Given the data, a parametric bootstrap procedure for testing hypothesis 1 or 2 in Diggle and Kenward's selection model can be implemented using the following four-step algorithm:

1. Fit the initial data under the null and the alternative hypothesis, resulting in $(\widehat{\boldsymbol{\theta}}_{H_0}, \widehat{\boldsymbol{\psi}}_{H_0})$ and $(\widehat{\boldsymbol{\theta}}_{H_1}, \widehat{\boldsymbol{\psi}}_{H_1})$ respectively, where $\boldsymbol{\theta}$ denotes the parameter vector for the measurement part and $\boldsymbol{\psi}$ for the missingness part; compute the LRT for the hypotheses under consideration.
2. Generate a 'bootstrap sample' from the selection model, reflecting the null hypothesis by using the estimates $(\widehat{\boldsymbol{\theta}}_{H_1}, \widehat{\boldsymbol{\psi}}_{H_0})$.
3. Compute the LRT test for the bootstrap sample.
4. Repeat steps 2 and 3 B times and determine the bootstrap p-value as the proportion of bootstrap LRT values larger than its value for the original data from the first step.

Alternatively, step 2 could be based on the estimates $(\widehat{\boldsymbol{\theta}}_{H_0}, \widehat{\boldsymbol{\psi}}_{H_0})$. But some exploratory simulations showed that both choices resulted in essentially the same p-values. Instead of a p-value, one can also compute critical points of the bootstrap approximate null distribution (10%, 5%, and 1% quantiles) in step 4 (Tables 19.5 and 19.6).

The parametric bootstrap depends heavily on the quality of the estimates $(\widehat{\boldsymbol{\theta}}_{H_1}, \widehat{\boldsymbol{\psi}}_{H_0})$. When the initial data are generated under the alternative, one would expect uncertainty in these to adversely affect the performance of the procedure, especially for hypothesis 2. This would lead to the generation of bootstrap data in the second step, which would obey the null constraint but which would be substantially different from the initial data in many other respects. A semi-parametric model based on resampling and less dependent on the estimates from the initial sample might perform better.

Semi-parametric bootstrap

Given the data, a semi-parametric bootstrap procedure for testing hypothesis 1 or 2 in the selection model can be implemented using the following algorithm:

1. Fit the models to the initial data under the null and the alternative hypotheses resulting in $(\widehat{\boldsymbol{\theta}}_{H_0}, \widehat{\boldsymbol{\psi}}_{H_0})$ and $(\widehat{\boldsymbol{\theta}}_{H_1}, \widehat{\boldsymbol{\psi}}_{H_1})$ respectively; compute the LRT for the hypothesis under consideration.
2. Impute the missing data, conditionally on the observed outcomes at the previous occasion, and based on the probability model for the measurement part (19.52) using the estimate $\widehat{\boldsymbol{\theta}}_{H_1}$ (this is a parametric part).
3. Draw (complete) observations from the augmented data set (resulting from step 2), with replacement, yielding a new sample of the same size N (this resampling is the non-parametric part).
4. Observations at time $t \geq 2$ are deleted with a probability according the logistic dropout model (19.53) using the estimate $\widehat{\boldsymbol{\psi}}_{H_0}$ (thus reflecting the

null hypothesis; this is again a parametric part); this is the final bootstrap sample.

5. Compute the LRT test for the bootstrap sample.
6. Repeat steps 2–5 B times and determine the bootstrap p-value as the proportion of bootstrap LRT values larger than its value from the initial data from the first step.

For more details about similar semi-parametric bootstrap implementations in other settings, see Davison and Hinkley (1997).

For hypothesis $i\,(i = 1, 2)$, two initial data sets were generated under three scenarios.

Scenario 1. All N observations generated under hypothesis i.
Scenario 2. All N observations generated under the alternative: $\psi_1 = 1$ for $i = 1$, $\psi_2 = 2$ for $i = 2$.
Scenario 3. Ten observations generated under hypothesis i and 190 observations under the corresponding alternative.

For each hypothesis i, for each scenario j and for each initial data set, $B = 400$ bootstrap samples were generated and bootstrap LRT values were computed. The results (p-values and quantiles) for these 18 combinations are shown in Tables 19.5 and 19.6.

Table 19.5 Simulation study. Hypothesis 1. Critical points based on the parametric and semi-parametric bootstrap procedure (400 bootstrap runs) for two initial data sets. Lower lines show the critical points of the simulated null distribution based on 800 samples, together with those of the χ_1^2 distribution.

Scenario	Bootstrap method	Quantiles			p-value
		0.10	0.05	0.01	
1	Parametric	3.04	4.17	6.12	0.7556
		2.53	3.35	6.76	0.3566
	Semi-parametric	2.96	3.83	6.22	0.7890
		2.46	4.16	6.60	0.3616
2	Parametric	2.55	3.39	6.36	< 0.0025
		2.83	3.68	7.02	< 0.0025
	Semi-parametric	2.41	3.39	6.49	< 0.0025
		2.68	3.68	6.37	< 0.0025
3	Parametric	2.35	3.72	7.91	0.9352
		3.00	3.93	6.48	< 0.0025
	Semi-parametric	2.83	4.13	8.00	0.6085
		2.70	4.40	6.49	< 0.0025
	Simulated H_0	2.23	3.27	6.04	
	χ_1^2 distribution	2.71	3.84	6.63	

Table 19.6 Simulation study. Hypothesis 2. Critical points based on the parametric and semi-parametric bootstrap procedure (400 bootstrap runs) for two initial data sets. Lower lines show the critical points of the simulated null distribution based on 800 samples, together with those of the χ_1^2 distribution.

Scenario	Bootstrap method	Quantiles			
		0.10	0.05	0.01	p-value
1	Parametric	38.71	42.68	46.21	0.1870
		9.62	12.25	19.77	1.0000
	Semi-parametric	4.86	6.74	10.48	0.0998
		7.40	9.35	14.47	0.2743
2	Parametric	22.07	24.84	30.32	0.0349
		9.36	11.39	14.04	0.0025
	Semi-parametric	12.35	15.63	20.88	0.0050
		17.05	19.75	27.56	0.0224
3	Parametric	8.17	10.09	15.02	0.0175
		15.46	17.85	24.38	0.9351
	Semi-parametric	15.68	19.11	25.58	0.1397
		8.11	10.46	13.55	0.6085
	Simulated H_0	6.44	9.17	12.10	
	χ_1^2 distribution	2.71	3.84	6.63	

Fitting the selection model, obtaining the maximum likelihood estimates and computing the LRT is a non-trivial iterative computing exercise, and so does not lend itself to extensive simulation studies. A full simulation study based on, for example, 100 initial samples was computationally not feasible. The 'optmum' procedure in Gauss 3.2.32 was used. The optimization method used the Broyden–Fletcher–Goldfarb–Shanno procedure to obtain starting values for the Newton–Raphson procedure, and it took about one week to obtain the results for one of the 18 combinations. Nevertheless we would argue that the limited results obtained do reveal the main characteristics of the performance of both bootstrap procedures.

For hypothesis 1, Table 19.5 shows that, for all scenarios, the χ_1^2 approximation and the bootstrap approximation to the null distribution are consistent and in line with our expectations. Note that the results for the two initial data sets under scenario 3 are not in agreement: one clearly rejects the hypothesis and the other clearly does not. Since only 5% of the initial data are generated under the alternative, a less clear rejection pattern is to be expected here.

The results in Table 19.6 globally show that for testing MAR versus MNAR (hypothesis 2), the bootstrap is unable to approximate the true null distribution and, in particular, the behaviour of the parametric bootstrap is unstable and inconsistent. The semi-parametric version seems to perform a little better, especially for scenario 1. As the bootstrap is also an asymptotic method, it suffers from the same slow convergence as the χ^2-type distributions.

19.7 CONCLUDING REMARKS

In Section 19.2 we have shown that every MNAR model, fitted to a set of incomplete data, can be replaced by an MAR version which produces exactly the same fit to the observed data. There are, in particular, two important implications of this. First, unless one puts a priori belief in the posited MNAR model, it is not possible to use the fit of an MNAR model for or against MAR. Second, the full flexibility of the MNAR modelling framework can be used to ensure that a model fits well to the observed data, but then the MAR version can be used for the actual data analysis, as an additional sensitivity analysis tool.

A reanalysis of the Slovenian public opinion survey data has shown that, while a set of MNAR models produces a widely varying range of conclusions about the proportion of people who are jointly in favour of independence and plan to attend the plebiscite, the corresponding MAR models produce a very narrow range of estimates, which in addition all lie close to the outcome of the plebiscite.

The determination of the MAR version of an MNAR model is straightforward in the case of dropout, since the ACMV restrictions, established by Molenberghs *et al.* (1998b) and translated into a computational scheme by Thijs *et al.* (2002), provide a convenient algorithm. In the case of non-monotone missingness, the marginal density of the outcomes is needed. This is straightforward when the model fitted is of the selection model type. When a PMM is fitted, the marginal density follows from a weighted sum over the pattern-specific measurement models.

While the result of Theorem 19.2 is general, we have focused on selection model and PMM formulations. It is worth re-emphasizing that the shared-parameter model also falls within this framework. In this case, the likelihood is expressed as

$$L = \prod_i \int f(\boldsymbol{y}_i^o, \boldsymbol{y}_i^m | \boldsymbol{\theta}, \boldsymbol{b}_i) f(\boldsymbol{r}_i | \boldsymbol{\psi}, \boldsymbol{b}_i) d\boldsymbol{y}_i^m, \qquad (19.54)$$

with $\boldsymbol{b}_i$ the shared parameter often taking the form of random effects. To apply our result, $f(\boldsymbol{y}_i^o, \boldsymbol{y}_i^m | \widehat{\boldsymbol{\theta}}, \boldsymbol{b}_i)$ needs to be integrated over the shared parameter. The model as a whole needs to be used to produce the fit to the observed data, and then (19.6) is used to extend the observed data fit to complete data MAR version.

Turning to the test for MAR versus the alternative of MNAR in, say, the Diggle and Kenward (1994) model, Section 19.6 has underscored that this is a non-regular problem and hence the behaviour of the likelihood ratio statistic is not standard. The information on the parameter ψ_2 in (19.53), available in the data, is very scarce and interwoven with other features of the measurement and dropout model. This translates mathematically into dependent systems of estimating equations and thus singularities in the corresponding information matrix. The rate of convergence to the asymptotic null distribution is extremely slow, implying that well-established bootstrap methods also appear to be deficient.

This implies that there is much less information available, even with increasing sample sizes, than one conventionally would expect. As a result of this, the ψ_2 parameter is more vulnerable than others for all sorts of deviations in the model, in particular to unusual profiles.

All the results in this chapter underscore the great sensitivity of inferences based on MNAR models, to posited and unverifiable model assumptions. As a consequence a primary (definitive) analysis should not be based on a single MNAR model. A further consequence is that *no* single analysis provides conclusions that are free of dependence in some way or other on untestable assumptions. This implies that any such analysis should be supported by carefully considered and contextually relevant sensitivity analysis, a view that is consistent with the position of the International Conference on Harmonization guidelines (1999). The rest of this part of this part of the book is therefore devoted to an exploration and demonstration of a variety of sensitivity analysis tools. It is intended that these should be of value to the practitioner, but the coverage should not be seen as complete. Research and development in the field of sensitivity analysis for incomplete data is very active and likely to remain that way for the foreseeable future.

20

Sensitivity Happens

20.1 INTRODUCTION

A key message from the previous chapter is that a model can be assessed in terms of its fit to the observed data, but not to the unobserved data, given the observed. This has implications not only for model fit, but also for inferences, as was seen in the analysis of the Slovenian public opinion survey. In particular, it was shown that every MNAR model has an MAR counterpart, producing exactly the same fit to the observed data, but potentially leading to different inferences. Together these point to the need for sensitivity analysis.

In a broad sense we can define a sensitivity analysis as one in which several statistical models are considered simultaneously and/or a statistical model is further scrutinized using specialized tools (such as diagnostic measures). This rather loose and very general definition encompasses a wide variety of useful approaches. The simplest procedure is to fit a selected number of (MNAR) models which are all deemed plausible or one in which a preferred (primary) analysis is supplemented by a number of modifications. The degree to which conclusions (inferences) are stable across such ranges provides an indication of the confidence that can be placed in them. In the missing data context modifications to a basic model can be constructed in different ways. One obvious strategy is to consider various dependencies of the missing data process on the outcomes and/or on covariates. One can choose to supplement an analysis within the selection framework, say, with one or several in the pattern-mixture framework which explicitly modify the future behaviour of the missing data given the observed. Alternatively, the distributional assumptions of the models can be altered.

Various forms of sensitivity analysis will be discussed in the remaining chapters in this part of the book. In this chapter, we will further illustrate

Missing Data in Clinical Studies   G. Molenberghs and M.G. Kenward
© 2007 John Wiley & Sons, Ltd

some issues that may occur when analysing incomplete data, in particular using models that allow for MNAR, such as the occurrence of non-unique, invalid, and boundary solutions. It is convenient to work within the reasonably straightforward framework of incomplete contingency tables, but similar illustrations would apply in different settings, too. This chapter is largely based on Molenberghs *et al.* (1999a).

In Section 20.2 a range of MNAR models is presented for an incomplete 2×2 contingency table with non-monotone missingness and fitted to a simple but illustrative set of data, introduced in Little (1993). This allows us to illustrate a variety of issues. In Section 20.3 we show that a given model can be identifiable for certain data configurations, but non-identifiable for others. In Section 20.4 we consider further analyses of the fluvoxamine trial.

20.2   A RANGE OF MNAR MODELS

Consider a two-way contingency table where a subset of subjects only has margins observed. Decompose the cell probabilities as $\mu_{jk}\phi_{r_1 r_2|jk}$, where $j, k = 1, 2$ index the categorical outcome levels and $r_1, r_2 = 0, 1$ index the response pattern (1 indicating observed). The Baker *et al.* (1992) models provide one route to the analysis of such data (Section 19.4.1). A further set of models are displayed in Table 20.1. A simple set of data, first introduced by Little (1993), is reproduced in Table 20.2. For these, pattern $(r_1, r_2) = (0, 0)$ is absent. The problem of non-response patterns for which there are no observations is a very common one and requires careful attention, a further motivation for the data in Table 20.2.

Assuming that the missing data mechanism is MCAR (model I in Table 20.1), the missingness probabilities reduce to $\phi_{r_1 r_2}$ $(r_1, r_2 = 0, 1)$. The cell probabilities μ_{jk} are the same under MCAR and MAR, while the missingness probabilities would differ between them.

One may assume that $\phi_{00} \equiv 0$ and hence drop it from the model. Alternatively, one can include this parameter and estimate it. It then follows that $\widehat{\phi}_{00} = 0$. Both approaches are equivalent in terms of model fit, but might lead to different inferences. Assuming ϕ_{00} is dropped, a set of non-redundant parameters is given by $(\mu_{11}, \mu_{12}, \mu_{21}, \phi_{11}, \phi_{10})'$. Parameter estimates and standard errors are presented in Table 20.3. The estimated complete data counts are shown in Table 20.4 (model I). The fourth pattern in this table corresponds to the subjects without a single measurement; the observed count corresponding to this pattern is zero. Observe that the standard errors for the μ parameters are slightly bigger than their complete data counterparts, reflecting the additional uncertainty.

Next, we will consider several non-random missingness processes. Confining attention to the three patterns observed, there are seven degrees of freedom in the data, suggesting that we can use at most four parameters for the

Table 20.1 Non-response models for binary two-way tables with supplemental margins.

I	$\phi_{11|jk} = p_1$
	$\phi_{10|jk} = p_2$
	$\phi_{01|jk} = p_3$
	$\phi_{00|jk} = 1 - p_1 - p_2 - p_3$
II	$\phi_{11|jk} = p_1(j,k)p_2(j,k)$
	$\phi_{10|jk} = p_1(j,k)[1 - p_2(j,k)]$
	$\phi_{01|jk} = [1 - p_1(j,k)]p_3(j,k)$
	$\phi_{00|jk} = [1 - p_1(j,k)][1 - p_3(j,k)]$
A	logit $p_1(j,k) = \alpha_1 + \alpha_J I(j=1) + \alpha_K I(k=1)$
	logit $p_2(j,k) = \alpha_2 + \alpha_J I(j=1) + \alpha_K I(k=1)$
	logit $p_3(j,k) = \alpha_3$
B	logit $p_1(j,k) = \alpha_1 + \alpha_J I(j=1)$
	logit $p_2(j,k) = \alpha_2 + \alpha_K I(k=1)$
	logit $p_3(j,k) = \alpha_3 + \alpha_K I(k=1)$
C	logit $p_1(j,k) = \alpha_1 + \alpha_J I(j=1) + \alpha_K I(k=1)$
	logit $p_2(j,k) = \alpha_2 + \alpha_J I(j=1) + \alpha_K I(k=1)$
	logit $p_3(j,k) = \alpha_3 + \alpha_J I(j=1) + \alpha_K I(k=1)$
D	logit $p_1(j,k) = \alpha_1$
	logit $p_2(j,k) = \alpha_2 + \alpha_J I(j=1)$
	logit $p_3(j,k) = \alpha_3 + \alpha_J I(j=1)$
E	logit $p_1(j,k) = \alpha_1$
	logit $p_2(j,k) = \alpha_2 + \alpha_K I(k=1)$
	logit $p_3(j,k) = \alpha_3 + \alpha_K I(k=1)$
F	logit $p_1(j,k) = \alpha_1$
	logit $p_2(j,k) = \alpha_2 + \alpha_{JK}[I(j=1) - I(k=1)]$
	logit $p_3(j,k) = \alpha_3 + \alpha_{JK}[I(j=1) - I(k=1)]$
G	logit $p_1(j,k) = \alpha_1$
	logit $p_2(j,k) = \alpha_2 + \alpha_{JK}[I(j=1) + I(k=1)]/2$
	logit $p_3(j,k) = \alpha_3 + \alpha_{JK}[I(j=1) + I(k=1)]/2$
III	$\phi_{11|jk} = p_1(j,k)p_2(j,k)$
	$\phi_{10|jk} = p_1(j,k)[1 - p_2(j,k)]$
	$\phi_{01|jk} = [1 - p_1(j,k)]p_2(j,k)$
	$\phi_{00|jk} = [1 - p_1(j,k)][1 - p_2(j,k)]$
A	logit $p_1(j,k) = \alpha_1 + \alpha_J I(j=1)$
	logit $p_2(j,k) = \alpha_2 + \alpha_K I(k=1)$
B	logit $p_1(j,k) = \alpha_0 + \alpha_1 I(j=1)$
	logit $p_2(j,k) = \alpha_0 + \alpha_2 I(k=1)$
C	logit $p_1(j,k) = \alpha_1$
	logit $p_2(j,k) = \alpha_2 + \alpha_J I(j=1)$
D	logit $p_1(j,k) = \alpha_1$
	logit $p_2(j,k) = \alpha_2 + \alpha_K I(k=1)$
IV	logit $\phi_{11|jk} = \alpha_1 + \alpha_J I(j=1) + \alpha_K I(k=1)$
	logit $\phi_{10|jk} = \alpha_2 + \alpha_J I(j=1) + \alpha_K I(k=1)$
	$\phi_{01|jk} = 1 - \phi_{11|jk} - \phi_{10|jk}$
	$\phi_{00|jk} = 0$

Table 20.2 The Little (1993) data. Two-way
contingency table with two supplemental margins.

100	50
75	75

30
60

28	60

missingness model, given the measurement model is left fully general. Family II in Table 20.1 belongs to the recursive models proposed by Fay (1986), where $p_1(j, k)$ is the probability of being observed at the first measurement occasion, given outcomes j and k, $p_2(j, k)$ is the probability of being observed at the second occasion, given outcomes j and k and given that a measurement was obtained at the first occasion, and $p_3(j, k)$ is the probability of being observed at the second occasion, given outcomes j and k and given that the measurement at the first occasion is missing. When missingness at one occasion does not depend on missingness at the other occasion, $p_2(j, k) \equiv p_3(j, k)$, and family III is obtained. In family II, similarly to family I, the fact that there are only three out of four patterns observed is taken into account by setting $p_3(j, k) = 1$. When family III is seriously considered for candidate models, one must explicitly address the observations with pattern (0,0). Below, we discuss families II and III in turn.

In model IIA, missingness is allowed to depend on the outcome at both measurements. The dependence is the same at both occasions, but the overall rate (compare intercepts α_1 and α_2) is allowed to differ. Parameter estimates are shown in Table 20.2. The model is saturated in the sense that the predicted and observed counts coincide and thus the likelihood ratio statistic $G^2 = 0$. The predicted probabilities for the hypothetical complete data all lie in the interior of the parameter space. Further, estimated complete data counts are all positive, as shown in Table 20.4. These add up to the observed counts in Table 20.2. These properties are desirable, but will not always obtain. Furthermore, they do not yield conclusive evidence for the plausibility of the model. We illustrate these points by changing the non-response model.

For model IIB, the probability of missingness in each outcome depends solely on its own values, and these probabilities are allowed to differ on the two measurement occasions. Keeping $p_3 \equiv 1$, the number of parameters in models IIA and IIB is the same. Model IIB clearly saturates the degrees of freedom and at the same time yields a non-zero deviance. This is also seen by inspecting the imputed cell counts (Table 20.4): expected counts for the first pattern are different from the observed ones, as are the relevant margins for the second and third patterns.

The zero cells in Table 20.4 are a consequence of high values found for the parameters α_J and α_K, which are diverging to infinity, implying that $p_1(1, k) = p_2(j, 1) = 1$, $\phi_{10}(j, 1) = \phi_{01}(1, k) = 0$. In other words, a boundary solution is found. Should the same model be fitted without constraints on the parameters, for example by directly modelling missingness probabilities, negative cell counts

Table 20.3 The Little (1993) Data. Parameter estimates (standard errors) for models fitted to the data in Table 20.2.

Parameter	I(MCAR)	IIA	IIB	IIIA	IV	IV(EM)
μ_{11}	0.280 (0.023)	0.263 (0.022)	0.209 (0.019)	0.236 (0.028)	0.362 (0.029)	0.312
μ_{12}	0.174 (0.021)	0.168 (0.022)	0.167 (0.017)	0.141 (0.026)	0.253 (0.031)	0.200
μ_{21}	0.239 (0.023)	0.231 (0.023)	0.216 (0.019)	0.243 (0.034)	0.181 (0.025)	0.227
μ_{22}	0.308 (0.024)	0.338 (0.025)	0.408 (0.023)	0.380 (0.035)	0.204 (0.031)	0.262
ϕ_{11}	0.628 (0.022)					
ϕ_{10}	0.188 (0.018)					
ϕ_{01}	0.184 (0.018)					
α_1		0.942 (0.152)	0.870 (0.127)	0.870 (0.127)	1.198 (0.376)	0.543
α_2		0.596 (0.165)	0.329 (0.138)	1.054 (0.374)	-1.059 (0.297)	-1.521
α_J		0.559 (0.264)	$+\infty(-)$	$+\infty(-)$	-1.546 (0.480)	-0.515
α_K		0.795 (0.219)	$+\infty(-)$	1.019 (1.245)	0.664 (0.144)	0.489
Odds ratio	2.071 (0.388)	2.295 (0.433)	2.367 (0.457)	2.621 (0.510)	1.613 (0.305)	1.809
Log-likelihood	-971.872	-958.674	-959.384	-986.506	-958.674	-960.747
Model d.f.	5	7	7	7	7	7

Table 20.4   The Little (1993) data. Complete data counts for models fitted to Table 20.2.

	(1,1)		(1,0)		(0,1)		(0,0)	
I(MCAR)	83.84	52.21	25.15	15.66	24.59	15.31	0	0
	71.62	92.33	21.49	27.70	21.00	27.08	0	0
IIA	100.00	50.00	14.24	15.76	11.51	14.66	0	0
	75.00	75.00	18.67	41.33	16.49	45.34	0	0
IIB	100.00	46.51	0.00	33.49	0.00	0.00	0	0
	72.58	79.89	0.00	57.52	30.42	57.58	0	0
IIIA	100.00	50.00	12.58	17.42	0.00	0.00	0.00	0.00
	72.58	95.13	9.13	33.15	30.42	39.87	3.82	13.89
IV	100.00	50.00	21.69	8.31	51.22	62.50	0	0
	75.00	75.00	34.87	25.13	−23.22	−2.50	0	0
IV(EM)	100.00	50.00	21.13	8.87	28.00	36.23	0	0
	75.00	75.00	33.57	26.43	0.00	23.77	0	0

would be predicted. This phenomenon can be seen as evidence against the model, a point also raised by Baker *et al.* (1992).

Since model IIB saturates the degrees of freedom and yet yields a non-zero deviance, the question arises as to whether the model can be extended. Going one step further, one might include *two* additional parameters in the model, by extending model IIB to

$$\text{logit} p_1(j, k) = \alpha_1 + \alpha_{j1} I(j = 1) + \alpha_{K1} I(k = 1),$$

$$\text{logit} p_2(j, k) = \alpha_2 + \alpha_{j2} I(j = 1) + \alpha_{K2} I(k = 1).$$

This model is clearly overparameterized. For different starting values, the maximization routine will lead to different solutions. The range of solutions thus obtained will reproduce the observed data counts exactly. Of course, the corresponding information matrix is singular.

Family III will always assign mass to all four patterns. Thus, it differs from the previous families in that the zero count in pattern (0,0) has to be treated as a sampling zero. Model IIIA is similar in spirit to model IIB, but family III assumes missingness at both occasions to be independent. Complete data cell counts are displayed in Table 20.4. Clearly, the fit of model IIIA is inferior to that of model IIB. This can be seen by calculating the deviance, but also by considering the prediction for the observed data counts. Note that this model predicts non-zero counts for pattern (0,0), in spite of the zero count observed for this pattern. Furthermore, model IIIA shows a boundary solution as well, albeit in one table only. This indicates that the assumption of independence is unrealistic.

The difference in fit between models IIB and IIIA is expected from the difference in the observed data log-likelihoods. However, the log-likelihoods for models IIA and IIB are fairly close, but the predicted complete data cell counts are very different. This fact points towards a general problem with MNAR mechanisms. One could decompose the full data distribution into two parts: that for the observed counts; and that for the observations over the missing cells, given their observed margin. Models IIA and IIB are in good agreement on the first part, but very different on the second (a reasonably balanced fit for IIA versus a boundary IIB solution). This follows from the fact that missingness in model IIA depends on a combination of influences of both measurements, while in IIB missingness in a given outcome depends on its own realization only. These are indeed radically different assumptions. Some criticism can be directed to model IIA: parameter identification is borrowed from equating the J and K effects at both times. Given the difference in interpretation of p_1 (unconditional) and p_2 (conditional on the status of the first outcome), this may well be a questionable assumption.

Arbitrariness in distributing the observed counts over the missing cells is illustrated further by considering the somewhat peculiar model IV, which is a special case of the model considered by Baker (1994). Parameter estimates are shown in Table 20.3. This model saturates the degrees of freedom and has a deviance of $G^2 = 0$, properties shared with model IIA. However, the imputed cell counts are very different: the non-response model does not constrain the probabilities to lie in the unit interval, and negative cell counts, as opposed to a boundary solution, are obtained under unconstrained maximum likelihood estimation. Although models IIA and IV describe the *observed* data equally well (see also Chapter 19), there are large differences between both, exhibited by the (non-allowable) imputed values for the complete cell counts (Table 20.4). The negative counts are not to be considered the true maximum likelihood estimates, which would be found by constraining the counts to be non-negative. Use of the EM algorithm (Chapter 8) provides one route for overcoming this problem. This solution is also displayed in Table 20.3, while the counts are given in Table 20.4 (IV-EM). The fit for the completers does not change and the fit for the second pattern is very similar. However, the complete counts for the third pattern are drastically different. The model is saturated in terms of degrees of freedom, but the deviance is now positive. Baker *et al.* (1992) argue that, particularly in large samples, a negative solution (and its corresponding boundary solution) can be viewed as evidence against the model and hence it is not necessary to compute boundary solutions. Apart from these problems, another point of criticism for model IV is that the missingness model treats the third pattern entirely differently from the others: whereas the effect on the first and second patterns is linear on the logit scale, the effect on the third is highly non-linear, and not constrained to be non-negative. Arguably, one has to think harder about formulating a missingness model such that (1) undesirable asymmetries are avoided and (2) non-negative solutions are ensured (with the possibility of having a boundary solution).

The fact that the predicted complete data counts can change dramatically with the non-response mechanism does not imply that all quantities of interest will change accordingly. It was noted for the models considered by Baker *et al.* (1992) that the odds ratio in the 2×2 table, collapsed over all response patterns, is very stable and in fact, for many models, equal to the one in the completers' table. Thus, it is interesting to compute the marginal odds ratio. Estimates for this quantity (and standard errors, obtained with the delta method), have been calculated and are displayed in Table 20.3. Knowing that the odds ratio for the completers' table equals 2.000 (0.476), it is clear that the estimates for the models fitted are reasonably close, although the one for model IV, obtained by the Newton–Raphson method, is on the opposite side of the value for the completers than the other models. The value obtained for the boundary solution is again closer to the completers' value.

20.3   IDENTIFIABILITY PROBLEMS

When MNAR models are used, it is important also to be aware of the potential occurrence of parameter redundancy. Even if the degrees of freedom are not saturated, the MLE may be obtained on a proper subset of the parameter space. We will illustrate this point using a simple example, displayed in Table 20.5. Observe that the row and column classifications are independent (Baker 1995b).

Suppose that we adopt model IIIB of Table 20.1, with the additional constraint $\alpha_J = \alpha_K$. This model implies that the probabilities of non-response at each occasion are equal but independent, and influenced by the *current* observation only. The data are exactly reproduced by $\mu_{jk} = 0.25$ $(j, k = 1, 2)$ and $\alpha_1 = \alpha_J = \alpha_K = 0$. The corresponding log-likelihood is -3327.11. All 16 complete data counts are 100. However, there are multiple maxima, each one yielding a perfect fit, but different predicted complete data counts. We explore this issue analytically. Write $\beta_1 = p_1(1, k) = p_2(j, 1)$ and $\beta_2 = p_1(2, k) = p_2(j, 2)$. The likelihood equations are easily derived in the spirit of Baker *et al.* (1992), using Birch's (1963) theorem adapted to incomplete data. Algebraic manipulation leads to a one-parameter family of solutions to likelihood equations. Choosing $\mu_{11} = \mu$, $\mu_{12} = \mu_{21} = \sqrt{\mu} - \mu$ and $\mu_{22} = (1 - \sqrt{\mu})^2$ yields $\beta_1 = 1/(4\sqrt{\mu})$, and $\beta_2 = 1/[4(1 - \sqrt{\mu})]$, which is valid provided $\mu \in [0.0625, 0.5625]$. An overview of the ranges for the other parameters is given in Table 20.6. Scanning the entire range can usefully be seen as a sensitivity analysis. This route has been explored before by Nordheim (1984), Philips (1993), and in logistic regression by Vach and Blettner (1995). Some parameters exhibit a range too wide to draw useful conclusions, such as the concordant cells μ_{11} and μ_{22}, the missingness

Table 20.5   Two-way contingency table with three supplemental margins.

100 100		200		200 200		400
100 100		200				

Table 20.6 Data from Table 20.5. Ranges for the parameters of the model.

Parameter	Minimum	Maximum
μ_{11}	0.0625	0.5625
μ_{12}	0.1875	0.2500
μ_{22}	0.0625	0.5625
β_1	0.3333	1.0000
β_2	0.3333	1.0000
μ_{1+}	0.2500	0.7500
μ_{+1}	0.2500	0.7500
ψ	1.0000	1.0000

parameters and the marginal probabilities. However, for the discordant cells $\mu_{12} = \mu_{21}$ the range [0.1875, 0.2500] is relatively narrow, and the odds ratio

$$\psi = \frac{\mu_{11}\mu_{22}}{\mu_{12}\mu_{21}} = 1,$$

since the entire family consists of independence models.

The complete data probabilities, expressed as functions of $\mu = \mu_{11}$, are displayed in Table 20.7. It is interesting to consider these counts for the limiting cases $\mu = 0.0625 = 1/16$ and $\mu = 0.5625 = 9/16$ and for $\mu = 0.25$. The results are displayed in Table 20.8. Clearly, it is hard to draw meaningful conclusions about the complete data probabilities as the probability mass can be distributed freely over the unobserved margin (patterns 10 and 01), with an even more extreme behaviour for pattern 00.

This artificial data example illustrates parameter identifiability problems when an MNAR missingness model is assumed. If a single maximum is required, a different path ought to be followed. First, a different model could be chosen, for example assuming MAR. Second, one could ensure that more data are available, for example all measurements at baseline. If the unidentified model is thought reasonable, one can still perform a sensitivity analysis, hoping that some parameters of interest show a relatively narrow range, like the odds ratio in our example. Finally, prior knowledge about some of the parameters could be included, to distinguish between the members of a family of solutions.

Table 20.7 Data from Table 20.5. Complete data probabilities given $\mu = \mu_{11}$.

$\frac{1}{16}$	$\frac{1}{16}$	$\frac{4\sqrt{\mu}-1}{16}$	$\frac{3-4\sqrt{\mu}}{16}$	$\frac{4\sqrt{\mu}-1}{16}$	$\frac{4\sqrt{\mu}-1}{16}$	$\frac{16\mu-8\sqrt{\mu}+1}{16}$	$\frac{-16\mu+16\sqrt{\mu}-3}{16}$
$\frac{1}{16}$	$\frac{1}{16}$	$\frac{4\sqrt{\mu}-1}{16}$	$\frac{3-4\sqrt{\mu}}{16}$	$\frac{3-4\sqrt{\mu}}{16}$	$\frac{3-4\sqrt{\mu}}{16}$	$\frac{-16\mu+16\sqrt{\mu}-3}{16}$	$\frac{16\mu-24\sqrt{\mu}+9}{16}$

Table 20.8 Data from Table 20.5. Complete data probabilities for $\mu = 1/16$, $\mu = 4/16$, and $\mu = 9/16$.

$$\mu = \frac{1}{16} \quad \begin{bmatrix} \frac{1}{16} & \frac{1}{16} \\ \frac{1}{16} & \frac{1}{16} \end{bmatrix} \begin{bmatrix} 0 & \frac{2}{16} \\ 0 & \frac{2}{16} \end{bmatrix} \begin{bmatrix} 0 & 0 \\ \frac{2}{16} & \frac{2}{16} \end{bmatrix} \begin{bmatrix} 0 & 0 \\ 0 & \frac{4}{16} \end{bmatrix}$$

$$\mu = \frac{4}{16} \quad \begin{bmatrix} \frac{1}{16} & \frac{1}{16} \\ \frac{1}{16} & \frac{1}{16} \end{bmatrix} \begin{bmatrix} \frac{1}{16} & \frac{1}{16} \\ \frac{1}{16} & \frac{1}{16} \end{bmatrix} \begin{bmatrix} \frac{1}{16} & \frac{1}{16} \\ \frac{1}{16} & \frac{1}{16} \end{bmatrix} \begin{bmatrix} \frac{1}{16} & \frac{1}{16} \\ \frac{1}{16} & \frac{1}{16} \end{bmatrix}$$

$$\mu = \frac{9}{16} \quad \begin{bmatrix} \frac{1}{16} & \frac{1}{16} \\ \frac{1}{16} & \frac{1}{16} \end{bmatrix} \begin{bmatrix} \frac{2}{16} & 0 \\ \frac{2}{16} & 0 \end{bmatrix} \begin{bmatrix} \frac{2}{16} & \frac{2}{16} \\ 0 & 0 \end{bmatrix} \begin{bmatrix} \frac{4}{16} & 0 \\ 0 & 0 \end{bmatrix}$$

20.4   ANALYSIS OF THE FLUVOXAMINE TRIAL

In the previous sections, as well as in Chapter 19, it was argued that several models can look equally plausible if the fit of the model to the *observed* data is considered as the sole criterion, even though the implications for the complete (partly unobserved) data can be radically different. In this section we apply the ideas developed so far using artificial data, to the fluvoxamine trial, introduced in Section 2.6 and then analysed in Sections 12.6, 15.4.2, 15.5.1, 16.8, and 18.3.5. The advantage is that subject-matter knowledge can be introduced into the analysis.

We focus on the occurrence of side effects (no/yes) and the presence of therapeutic effect (no/yes) at the first and last visits. All four non-response patterns are considered. The data are shown in Tables 20.9(a) and 20.9(b), and agree with those of Table 12.7, but now the non-monotone pattern and the number of people without follow-up measurements are also considered. In addition, the effect of sex and age on side effects will be studied for completers and for patients who drop out (excluding two patients who are observed at the second occasion only, as well as 14 patients without measurements). The raw data, collapsed over age, are shown in Table 20.9(c). The slight discrepancy between the counts in Table 20.9(a) and the summed counts in Table 20.9(c) is due to missing baseline information for a few patients.

All the models listed in Table 20.1 (except for IV) have been fitted to both Tables 20.9(a) and 20.9(b). This means that a few models have been added (IID–G and IIIC–D). These models reflect a priori information: (1) the data are collected in a time-ordered fashion and hence missingness at the second occasion could possibly depend on the measurement at the first occasion, while

Table 20.9   Fluvoxamine trial. Dichotomized side-effect
and therapeutic effect outcomes, at the first and last visits.

(a) *Side effects*

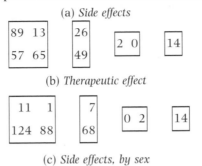

(b) *Therapeutic effect*

(c) *Side effects, by sex*

		Time 2	
	Completers		Dropouts
Time 1	1	2	*
Males			
1	34	6	10
2	12	19	23
Females			
1	55	7	15
2	44	42	26

the reverse is unlikely; (2) missingness at the second occasion is much more frequent than at the first occasion. Therefore, missingness at the first occasion could be considered purely accidental, while missingness at the second occasion is likely to be data-dependent. The parameter $p_1(j, k)$ is held constant in all the models. The family II models are considered more likely than the family III models a priori because, in a longitudinal study, missingness is often dominated by dropout, forcing dependence between non-response at the various occasions. This is reflected in the association in the marginal probabilities of falling in one of the four response patterns (0.71, 0.24, 0.0063, and 0.045 respectively, yielding an odds ratio of 21.1). We describe the models in terms of the effect of the measurements on missingness at the second occasion they assume. In models IIIC and IID, non-response depends on the outcome at the first occasion only; in models IIID and IIE it depends on the second occasion only; in model IIF it depends on the increment between both measurements; and in model IIG it depends on the average of both measurements.

We discuss the side effects first, the results for which are shown in Table 20.10. First, some models are not considered further since unconstrained maximization would yield negative expected complete data counts if a boundary solution is not imposed. This additional phrase is important because the presence

Table 20.10 Fluvoxamine trial. Model fit for side effects. (d.f., degrees of freedom; G^2, likelihood ratio test statistic.)

Model	d.f.	G^2	p-value	Marginal odds ratio
I	6	4.52	0.1044	7.80 (2.39)
IIA	8	0.00	—	5.07 (1.71)
IIC	8	0.00	—	5.07 (1.71)
IID	7	1.52	0.2176	7.84 (2.35)
IIE	7	0.96	0.3272	7.70 (2.14)
IIF	7	2.04	0.1532	7.26 (2.25)
IIG	7	1.32	0.2506	7.98 (2.34)
IIIB	5	70.04	< 0.0001	6.18 (2.04)
IIIC	6	27.88	< 0.0001	7.81 (2.34)
IIID	6	27.88	< 0.0001	7.81 (2.18)

of the sampling zero in pattern (0,1) implies that some models (including several that saturate the degrees of freedom) yield boundary solutions even with unconstrained maximization. Models not considered are IIB and IIIA. These two models are similar in that they all assume dropout depends only on the realization of the associated outcome. Among the remaining models, those belonging to family III are strongly rejected. This is anticipated from the dependence between non-response at both occasions. The other models would be acceptable if goodness of fit were the only criterion considered. This includes MCAR (models I). The best fit, among the non-saturated models, is given by IIE, but models IID and IIG are very similar in fit. These models assume constant non-response at the first occasion, and non-response at the second occasion that depends on either the first outcome or on the second outcome, or on the average of both. Inspecting the complete data counts of these models, it is reassuring that all yield similar conclusions (with a slightly inferior fit for MCAR). They are displayed in Table 20.11. Thus, the conclusion of our sensitivity analysis might be that missingness at the first occasion of side effects is constant, whereas missingness at the second occasion depends on the values of side effects themselves (whether measured at the first occasion, the second occasion, or both). Further, the association between both side-effect measures is very high, with an odds ratio around 7.8 (standard error around 2.2).

The results from the analysis of the therapeutic effect are shown in Table 20.12. The same models are excluded on the basis of boundary values. Again, the fit of family III models is very poor. Among the remaining non-saturated models, the only convincing fit is for IIE. In IIE, non-response at time 2 depends on the time 2 measurement. Model IIG would still be acceptable, but far less so than the others mentioned. Thus, the picture is much less clear than with side effects. Even for the marginal odds ratio, two of the saturated models show a relatively small value, while the others are higher. Of course,

Table 20.11 Fluvoxamine trial. Complete data counts for models fitted to side-effects data.

	(1,1)		(1,0)		(0,1)		(0,0)	
I(MCAR)	84.00	12.12	28.13	4.06	0.74	0.11	5.26	0.76
	60.21	67.67	20.16	22.66	0.53	0.60	3.77	4.23
IID	89.60	12.89	22.56	3.24	0.92	0.13	5.08	0.73
	57.12	64.41	23.11	26.06	0.44	0.49	3.86	4.35
IIE	89.69	13.12	17.55	7.84	0.95	0.07	4.79	1.05
	57.04	64.24	11.16	38.37	0.60	0.33	3.05	5.16
IIG	89.68	12.95	21.30	4.33	0.94	0.11	5.00	0.82
	57.06	64.35	19.07	30.26	0.48	0.44	3.59	4.62

Table 20.12 Fluvoxamine trial. Model fit for therapeutic effect.

Model	d.f.	G^2	p-value	Marginal odds ratio
I	6	5.08	0.0789	7.77 (6.44)
IIA	8	0.00	—	1.13 (0.49)
IIC	8	0.00	—	1.13 (0.49)
IID	7	3.62	0.0571	7.86 (6.39)
IIE	7	0.08	0.7773	8.25 (8.32)
IIF	7	4.74	0.0295	7.10 (5.31)
IIG	7	2.90	0.0886	8.20 (7.18)
IIIB	5	27.56	<0.0001	7.67 (5.98)
IIIC	6	29.84	<0.0001	7.81 (6.27)
IIID	6	29.94	<0.0001	8.25 (8.44)

this effect is less severe than it appears owing to the large standard errors. These are undoubtably influenced by the count of one in the completers' table.

Again, an inspection of the complete data counts sheds some light on these findings (Table 20.13). It turns out that both models IIC and IIE yield boundary solutions for pattern (1,0), while this need not be the case even for a saturated model. Indeed, several model parameter estimates tend to infinity. In addition, the way in which this pattern is filled in depends crucially on the model assumptions. In model IIC, all dropouts are assumed to have arisen in spite of a therapeutic effect at the second occasion. In model IIE, the situation is exactly reversed. The conclusions for pattern (0,0) are similar. Clearly, imputation in model IIC is driven by the zero count in the observed data of pattern (0,1). This feature is less desirable and model IIC should be discarded. Model IIE, on the other hand, is able to reverse the zero columns in patterns (1,0) and (0,1), through two parameters at infinity (α_2 and α_K, with opposite signs). Model IIG is similar to but less extreme than IIE, with some differences in pattern (0,0). Retaining the picture

Table 20.13 Fluvoxamine trial. Complete data counts for models fitted to therapeutic data.

	(1,1)		(1,0)		(0,1)		(0,0)	
IIC	11.00	1.00	0.00	7.00	0.00	0.11	0.00	4.96
	124.00	88.00	0.00	68.00	0.00	1.89	0.00	9.04
IIE	11.57	1.00	6.43	0.00	0.00	0.02	0.96	0.03
	123.43	88.00	68.57	0.00	0.00	1.98	10.27	2.73
IIG	10.42	0.98	7.17	0.38	0.06	0.01	0.89	0.07
	123.51	89.19	47.87	19.48	0.91	0.96	8.26	4.86

behind IIE and IIG, we might conclude that non-response at the second occasion is caused by a less favourable evolution and/or level of therapeutic effect.

From this model-building exercise it is clear that selecting a model solely on its basis of fit to the observed data is not sufficient when MNAR models are considered. First, models which produce boundary or invalid solutions should be treated with caution. Arguably, such models should be discarded. Second, one should question the plausibility of non-response mechanisms in terms of design information (e.g., time ordering of measurements) and subject-matter knowledge (e.g., prior knowledge about the directionality of treatment effect).

Next, we consider what can be gained from the incorporation of covariates. A marginal odds ratio model was fitted in which a logit link is assumed to relate the probability of outcome at each measurement occasion to covariates and the association between outcomes is modelled in terms of log odds ratios. The corresponding results are presented in Table 20.14.

Age has been selected as a predictor for the marginal measurement models. For both measurements, age increases the risk of side effects in the fitted model. Although association between both outcomes was allowed to depend on covariates, no evidence of such association was found and the log odds ratio was set constant. In the dropout model, sex was the only sufficiently significant predictor to be kept in the model. We consider four dropout models: MCAR; MAR; MNAR(1), where dropout depends on both measurements; and MNAR(2), where dropout depends only on the value of the second measurement, the so-called protective assumptions (see also Chapter 18). The most general dropout model retained assumes the form

$$\text{logit}(\phi_{ijk}) = \text{logit}(P(\text{non-dropout}|Y_1 = j, Y_2 = k, x_i))$$

$$= \alpha_0 + \alpha_1 I(j = 1) + \alpha_2 I(k = 1) + \alpha_3 x_i,$$

where x_i is the sex of subject i. From the MAR model we conclude that dropout chances increase for subjects with side effects at the first visits and are higher for men than for women.

Table 20.14   Fluvoxamine trial. Estimates (standard errors) for side effects (covariates).

Parameter	MCAR	MAR	MNAR(1)	MNAR(2)
Measurements model				
First time				
Intercept	0.640 (0.402)	0.640 (0.402)	0.642 (0.402)	0.639 (0.402)
Age effect	−0.022 (0.009)	−0.022 (0.009)	−0.022 (0.009)	−0.022 (0.009)
Second time				
Intercept	1.598 (0.489)	1.598 (0.489)	1.745 (0.597)	1.403 (0.489)
Age effect	−0.023 (0.011)	−0.023 (0.011)	−0.021 (0.011)	−0.025 (0.010)
Log odds ratio	1.955 (0.357)	1.955 (0.357)	1.808 (0.515)	1.935 (0.347)
Dropout model				
Intercept	0.766 (0.211)	1.085 (0.275)	0.951 (0.315)	1.382 (0.435)
1st measurement		−0.584 (0.284)	−0.963 (0.623)	
2nd measurement			1.237 (2.660)	−1.231 (0.627)
Sex effect	0.518 (0.275)	0.568 (0.277)	0.636 (0.294)	0.493 (0.289)
Log-likelihood	−480.485	−478.302	−478.149	−478.600
Model d.f.	7	8	9	8

Observe that the MAR model and the MNAR models lead to approximately the same fit. This is in line with our findings in Table 20.10. First, the association between both measurements is considerable, given a log odds ratio of about 2, found in all models. MAR and MNAR(2) both indicate a strong dependence of dropout on the level of side effect: the regression coefficients have the same sign. In conclusion, all three models show a strong dependence of dropout on the occurrence of side effects, irrespective of whether the first, the second, or both measurements are used, that is, the same conclusion as in the analysis without covariates.

20.5   CONCLUDING REMARKS

Incomplete *categorical* data are ideally suited to the illustration of the fundamental issues surrounding the use of non-random missingness models. First, models with an entirely different interpretation at the complete data level might exhibit the similar or the same deviance, or even saturate the observed data. Second, models saturating the degrees of freedom might yield a boundary solution and strictly positive deviance in both the complete data counts and in some of the parameter estimates. Without constraints built in to ensure non-negative solutions, some iterative algorithms can yield invalid solutions. Third, non-unique solutions can be obtained, in particular when the row and column variables are independent. When responses at different occasions are associated, but only weakly so, one should expect to see very flat likelihoods, unstable parameter estimates, and/or low precision. Some of these points have been documented by Little and Rubin (1987, Section 11.6), Park and Brown (1994), and Baker (1995b).

These phenomena underscore the fact that fitting a model to incomplete data necessarily encompasses a part that cannot be assessed from the observed data, a central point also of Chapter 19. In particular, whether or not a dropout model is acceptable cannot be determined solely by mechanical model-building exercises. Arbitrariness can be removed partly by careful consideration of the plausibility of a model. One should use as much context-derived information as possible. Prior knowledge can give an idea of which models are more plausible. Covariate information can be explicitly included in the model to increase the range of plausible models which can be fitted. Moreover, covariates can help explain the dependence between response mechanism and outcomes. Good non-response models in a longitudinal setting should make use of the temporal and/or association structure among the repeated measures.

21

Regions of Ignorance and Uncertainty

21.1 INTRODUCTION

We have seen repeatedly, especially in Chapters 19 and 20, that there are fundamentally untestable components of models for incomplete data that have the potential to seriously affect inferences. Thus, solely relying on a single model, whether of MCAR, MAR, or MNAR type, is not advisable, and the only reasonable way forward in the light of this is to use appropriate sensitivity analysis. A number of early references include Nordheim (1984), Little (1994b), Rubin (1994), Laird (1994), Vach and Blettner (1995), Fitzmaurice *et al.* (1995), Molenberghs *et al.* (1999a), Kenward (1998), and Kenward and Molenberghs (1999). Many of these are to be considered potentially useful but *ad hoc* approaches. Whereas such informal sensitivity analyses are an indispensable step in the analysis of incomplete longitudinal data, it is desirable to have more formal frameworks within which to develop such analyses. Such frameworks can be found in Scharfstein *et al.* (1999), Thijs *et al.* (2000), Verbeke *et al.* (2001b), Molenberghs *et al.* (2001a, 2001b), Kenward *et al.* (2001), Van Steen *et al.* (2001), and Jansen *et al.* (2006b).

One way forward, the topic of this chapter, is to acknowledge both the status of *imprecision* due to (finite) random sampling, as well as *ignorance* due to incompleteness. Molenberghs *et al.* (2001) and Kenward *et al.* (2001) combined both concepts into *uncertainty*.

Section 21.2 introduces a very simple yet illustrative example, concerned with HIV prevalence estimation in Kenyan women. Key concepts are introduced in Section 21.3. Conventional sensitivity analyses for monotone patterns (Section 21.4) and for non-monotone patterns (Section 21.5) are presented next. The general principles behind the sensitivity analysis approach of this

Missing Data in Clinical Studies   G. Molenberghs and M.G. Kenward
© 2007 John Wiley & Sons, Ltd

chapter are studied in Section 21.6. We then turn to the analysis of data from the fluvoxamine study in Section 21.7, followed by the analysis of a number of artificial yet insightful sets of data in Section 21.8. Then, in Section 21.9, we continue with the Slovenian public opinion survey. Finally, in Section 21.10, we briefly discuss the theoretical foundations behind the approach developed in this chapter, as set out in Vansteelandt *et al.* (2006).

21.2   PREVALENCE OF HIV IN KENYA

In the context of disease monitoring, HIV prevalence is to be estimated in a population of pregnant women in Kenya. To this end, $N = 787$ samples from Kenyan women were sampled, with the following results: known HIV+, r=52; known HIV−, $n - r = 699$; and (owing to test failure) unknown HIV status, $N - n = 36$. We deduce immediately that the number of HIV+ women lies within [52,88] out of 787, producing a *best–worst case interval* of [6.6,11.2]%. This example is extremely important from a public health point of view on the one hand, and provides the simplest setting for sensitivity analysis on the other hand. Furthermore, the best–worst case interval produces the simplest answer to the sensitivity analysis question. This idea has been used, for example, in the survey literature. While Cochran (1977) considered and subsequently rejected it on the grounds of overly wide intervals, we believe that in this particular example it does provide useful information and, more importantly, that it leads to a versatile starting point for more elaborate modelling, based on which the width of the intervals can be reduced further.

21.3   UNCERTAINTY AND SENSITIVITY

To fix ideas, we focus on monotone patterns first. Formally, these can be regarded as coming from two 2×2 tables, of which the probabilities are displayed in Table 21.1. In contrast, we only observe data corresponding to the probabilities as displayed in Table 21.2, where + indicates summation over the corresponding subscript.

A sample from Table 21.2 produces empirical proportions representing the corresponding πs with error. This results in so-called *imprecision*, which is usually captured by way of such quantities as standard errors and confidence intervals. In sufficiently regular problems, imprecision disappears as the sample size tends to infinity and the estimators are consistent. What remains is *ignorance*

Table 21.1   Theoretical distribution over completed cells for monotone patterns.

$\pi_{1,11}$	$\pi_{1,12}$		$\pi_{0,11}$	$\pi_{0,12}$
$\pi_{1,21}$	$\pi_{1,22}$		$\pi_{0,21}$	$\pi_{0,22}$

Table 21.2 Theoretical distribution over observed cells for monotone patterns.

$\pi_{1,11}$	$\pi_{1,12}$	$\pi_{0,1+}$
$\pi_{1,21}$	$\pi_{1,22}$	$\pi_{0,2+}$

regarding the redistribution of $\pi_{0,1+}$ and $\pi_{0,2+}$ over the second outcome value. In Table 21.2, there is constrained ignorance regarding the values of $\pi_{0,jk}$ ($j, k = 1, 2$) and hence regarding any derived parameter of scientific interest. For such a parameter, ψ say, a region of possible values which is consistent with Table 21.2 is called the region of ignorance. Analogously, an observed incomplete table leaves ignorance regarding the would-be observed complete table, which in turn leaves imprecision regarding the true complete probabilities. The region of estimators for ψ that is consistent with the observed data provides an estimated region of ignorance. We then conceive a $(1 - \alpha)100\%$ *region of uncertainty* as a larger region in the spirit of a confidence region, designed to capture the combined effects of imprecision and ignorance. It can be seen as a confidence region around the ignorance region. In Section 21.10 we briefly discuss its theoretical properties, such as convergence and coverage.

In standard statistical practice, ignorance is hidden in the consideration of a single identified model. In Sections 21.4 and 21.5 we first contrast several identified models for both the monotone and the non-monotone patterns of missingness, producing a conventional sensitivity analysis. When introducing more formal instruments, it is shown that a conventional assessment can be inadequate and even misleading.

21.4 MODELS FOR MONOTONE PATTERNS

Applying a selection model factorization (3.3) to Table 21.1, we get

$$\pi_{r,jk} = p_{jk}q_{r|jk},\qquad(21.1)$$

with handwritten annotations: *3 d.f.* and *1, ..., 4 d.f.*

where p_{jk} parameterizes the measurement process and $q_{r|jk}$ determines the non-response (or dropout) mechanism. In what follows we will leave p_{jk} unconstrained and consider various forms for $q_{r|jk}$, as listed in Table 21.3.

As a consequence of incompleteness, we can consider degrees of freedom both at the level of the observed data (Table 21.2), and in terms of the hypothetical complete data (Table 21.1). We refer to these as d.f.(obs) and d.f.(comp), respectively. It is important to realize that identification or saturation of a model is relative to the type of d.f. considered.

Model MNAR(0) is also termed 'protective' since its missing data mechanism satisfies the protective assumption, studied in Chapter 18. Model MNAR(II) is referred to as 'M_{sat}' since it has three measurement parameters and four dropout

Table 21.3 Dropout models corresponding to the setting of Table 21.1. The function $g(\cdot)$ refers to a link function, for example the logit link.

Model	$q_{r\mid jk}$	No. of parameters	Observed d.f.	Complete d.f.
1. MCAR	q_r	4	Non-saturated	Non-saturated
2. MAR	$q_{r\mid j}$	5	Saturated	Non-saturated
3. MNAR(0) (protective)	$q_{r\mid k}$	5	Saturated	Non-saturated
4. MNAR(I)	$g(q_{r\mid jk}) = \alpha + \beta_j + \gamma_k$	6	Overspecified	Non-saturated
5. MNAR(II) (M_{sat})	$g(q_{r\mid jk}) = \alpha + \beta_j + \gamma_k + \delta_{jk}$	7	Overspecified	Saturated

(handwritten annotations:)

$\alpha + \beta\, I(j=1) + \gamma\, I(k=1)$

$\alpha + \beta\, I(j=1) + \gamma\, I(k=1) + \delta \cdot I(j=1 \text{ and } k=1)$

parameters and therefore saturates d.f.(comp). However, there are only five observable degrees of freedom, rendering this model overspecified when fitted to the observed data.

To ensure a model is identifiable, one has to impose restrictions. Conventional restrictions result from assuming an MCAR or MAR model (models 1 and 2, respectively). Models 2 and 3 both saturate d.f.(obs) and hence are indistinguishable in terms of their fit to the observed data, although they will produce different complete data tables, in line with the issues discussed in Chapter 19. In model 4, dropout is allowed to depend on both measurements but not on their interaction. As a consequence, it overspecifies d.f.(obs) and underspecifies d.f.(comp).

We are dealing here with the simplest possible longitudinal setting, for which there are only a very small number of identifiable models. It is important to see how these observations carry over to settings where a much larger number of identifiable models can be constructed. A natural generalization which allows such an extended class of models is the non-monotone setting.

21.5   MODELS FOR NON-MONOTONE PATTERNS

We now consider the problem of modelling all the patterns in Table 21.4, an example of which will be encountered in Table 21.8. The discrepancy between d.f.(comp) = 15 and d.f.(obs) = 8 is larger. A natural class of models for this situation is the one proposed by Baker *et al.* (1992), presented in Section 19.4.1 above. The complete data and observed data cell probabilities for this setting are presented in Tables 21.4 and 21.5, respectively. The notation employed in the previous section is extended in an obvious way.

Table 21.4 Theoretical distribution over completed cells for non-monotone patterns.

$\pi_{11,11}$	$\pi_{11,12}$	$\pi_{10,11}$	$\pi_{10,12}$	$\pi_{01,11}$	$\pi_{01,12}$	$\pi_{00,11}$	$\pi_{00,12}$
$\pi_{11,21}$	$\pi_{11,22}$	$\pi_{10,21}$	$\pi_{10,22}$	$\pi_{01,21}$	$\pi_{01,22}$	$\pi_{00,21}$	$\pi_{00,22}$

Table 21.5 Theoretical distribution over observed cells for non-monotone patterns.

$\pi_{11,11}$	$\pi_{11,12}$		$\pi_{10,1+}$			
$\pi_{11,21}$	$\pi_{11,22}$		$\pi_{10,2+}$			

$$\pi_{01,+1} \quad \pi_{01,+2} \qquad \pi_{00,++}$$

21.6 FORMALIZING IGNORANCE AND UNCERTAINTY

As we have emphasized in Section 21.3, the adoption of a single identified model masks what we have termed ignorance. Examples are models 1–3 in Table 21.3 and models BRD1–9 (Section 19.4.1) of Section 21.5 for the monotone and non-monotone settings, respectively. Among these, a number of different models such as models 2 and 3 in the monotone case, and BRD6–9, typically saturate d.f.(obs). Naturally, these models cannot be distinguished in terms of their fit to the observed data alone, yet they can produce substantially different inferences, as exemplified in Section 19.4. A straightforward sensitivity analysis for the situations considered in Sections 21.4 and 21.5 uses a collection of such models. The resulting parameter ranges implied by the estimates of such models are *ad hoc* in nature and lack formal justification as a measure of ignorance. Therefore, we need to parameterize the set of models considered by means of one or more continuous parameters and then to consider all (or at least a range of) models along such a continuum, this as suggested by Nordheim (1984). Foster and Smith (1998) expand on this idea and, referring to Baker and Laird (1988) and to Rubin *et al.* (1995), suggest imposing a prior distribution on a range. While this is an obvious way to account for ignorance and still produce a single inference, these authors also note that the posterior density is, due to the lack of information, often a direct or indirect reproduction of the prior. Little (1994a) presents confidence intervals for a number of values along a range of sensitivity parameters. In this way, he combines ignorance and imprecision. Similar ideas are found in Little and Wang (1996).

Molenberghs *et al.* (2001a), Kenward *et al.* (2001), and Vansteelandt *et al.* (2006) formalized the idea of such ranges of models. A natural way to achieve this goal is to consider models that would be identified if the data were complete, and then fit them to the observed, incomplete data, thereby producing a range of estimates rather than a point estimate. Where such overspecified models have appeared in the literature (Catchpole and Morgan 1997), various strategies are used, such as applying constraints, to recover identifiability. In contrast, our goal is to use the non-identifiability to delineate the range of inferences consistent with the observed data, that is, to capture ignorance. Maximization of the likelihood function of the overspecified model is a natural approach.

We consider the simple setting of the data on HIV prevalence in Kenya, where r denotes the number of observed successes, $n - r$ the number of observed failures, and $N - n$ the number of unclassified subjects. Independent of the parameterization chosen, the observed data log-likelihood can be expressed in the form

$$\ell = r \ln \alpha + (n - r) \ln \beta + (N - n) \ln(1 - \alpha - \beta),$$

with α the probability of an observed success and β the probability of an observed failure. It is sometimes useful to denote $\gamma = 1 - \alpha - \beta$. We consider two models, of which the parameterization is given in Table 21.6. The first is identified, the second is overparameterized. Here, p is the probability of a success (whether observed or not), q_1 (q_2) is the probability of being observed given a success (failure), and λ is the odds of being observed for failures versus successes. For model I, the latter is assumed to be unity.

Denote the corresponding log-likelihoods by ℓ_I and ℓ_{II} respectively. In both cases,

$$\hat{\alpha} = \frac{r}{N}, \qquad \hat{\beta} = \frac{n - r}{N}.$$

Maximum likelihood estimates for p and q follow immediately under model I, either by observing that the moments (α, β) map one-to-one onto the pair (p, q) or by directly solving ℓ_I. The solutions are given in Table 21.6. The asymptotic variance–covariance matrix for p and q is block-diagonal with well-known elements $p(1 - p)/n$ and $q(1 - q)/N$. Observe that we now obtain only one solution, a strong argument in favour of the current model. The probability of HIV+ is $\hat{p} = 0.069$ (95% confidence interval [0.0511, 0.0874]) and the response probability is $\hat{q} = 0.954$.

Table 21.6 Two transformations of the observed data likelihood.

Model I (MAR)	Model II (MNAR, M_{sat})
Parameterization:	
$\alpha = pq$	$\alpha = pq_1$
$\beta = (1 - p)q$	$\beta = (1 - p)q_2$
$\gamma = 1 - q$	$\gamma = 1 - pq_1 - (1 - p)q_2$
	$q_1 = q$
	$q_2 = q\lambda$
Solution:	
$\hat{p} = \dfrac{\hat{\alpha}}{\hat{\alpha} + \hat{\beta}} = \dfrac{r}{n}$	$pq_1 = \dfrac{r}{N}$
$\hat{q} = \hat{\alpha} + \hat{\beta} = \dfrac{n}{N}$	$(1 - p)q_2 = \dfrac{n - r}{N}$
	$\dfrac{r}{q_1} + \dfrac{n - r}{q_2} = N$
	$p : \left[\dfrac{r}{N}, \dfrac{N - n + r}{N} \right]$

A similar standard derivation is not possible for model II, since the triplet (p, q_1, q_2) or, equivalently, the triplet (p, q, λ) is redundant. This follows directly from Catchpole and Morgan (1997) and Catchpole *et al.* (1998) whose theory shows that model II is rank-deficient and model I is of full rank. Since model I is a submodel of model II and saturates the observed data, so must every solution to ℓ_{II}, implying the relationships

$$pq_1 = \frac{r}{N}, \qquad (1-p)q_2 = \frac{n-r}{N}. \qquad (21.2)$$

Constraints (21.2) imply

$$\hat{p} = \frac{r}{Nq_1} = 1 - \frac{n-r}{Nq_2}$$

and hence

$$\frac{r}{q_1} + \frac{n-r}{q_2} = N. \qquad (21.3)$$

The requirement that $q_1, q_2 \le 1$ in (21.2) implies an allowable range for p:

$$p \in \left[\frac{r}{N}, \frac{N-n+r}{N} \right]. \qquad (21.4)$$

For the prevalence of HIV in Kenya example, the best–worst case range [0.066, 0.112] is recovered. Within this interval of ignorance, the MAR estimate obtained earlier is rather extreme, which is entirely due to the small proportion of HIV+ subjects. To account for the sampling uncertainty, the left estimate can be replaced by a 95% lower limit and the right estimate can be replaced by a 95% upper limit, yielding an interval of uncertainty [0.0479, 0.1291].

Such overspecification of the likelihood can be managed in a more general fashion by considering a minimal set of parameters η, conditional upon which the others, μ, are identified, where $\psi = (\eta, \mu)$ upon possible reordering. We term η the *sensitivity parameter* and μ the *estimable parameter*. Clearly, there will almost never be a unique choice for η and hence for μ. Each value of η will produce an estimate $\hat{\mu}(\eta)$. The union of these produces the estimated region of ignorance. A natural estimate of the region of uncertainty is the union of confidence regions for each $\hat{\mu}(\eta)$. For the HIV+ example, one could choose $\mu = (p, q_1)$ and $\eta = q_2$ or $\mu = (p, q)$ and $\eta = \lambda$. The latter choice motivates our inclusion of λ in Table 21.6 as a sensitivity parameter.

It is not always the case that the range for η will be an entire line or real space, and hence specific measures may be needed to ensure that η is within its allowable range. As the choice of sensitivity parameter is non-unique, a proper choice can greatly simplify the treatment. It will be seen in what follows that the choice of λ as in Table 21.6 is an efficient one from a computational point of view. In contrast, the choice $\theta = q_2 - q_1$ would lead to cumbersome computations and will not be pursued. Of course, what is understood by a proper choice will depend on the context. For example, the sensitivity parameter can be chosen from the nuisance parameters, rather than from the parameters of direct scientific interest. Whether the parameters of direct scientific interest can overlap with the sensitivity set or not is itself an issue (White and Goetghebeur 1998). For example, if the scientific question is a sensitivity analysis for treatment effect, then one should consider the implications of including the treatment effect parameters in the sensitivity set. There will be no direct estimate of imprecision available for the sensitivity parameter. Alternatively, if, given a certain choice of sensitivity parameter, the resulting profile likelihood has a simple form (analogous to the Box–Cox transformation, where conditioning on the transformation parameter produces essentially a normal likelihood), then such a parameter is an obvious candidate.

Given our choice of sensitivity parameter λ, simple algebra yields estimates for p and q (subscripted by λ to indicate dependence on the sensitivity parameter):

$$p_\lambda = \frac{\hat{\alpha}\lambda}{\hat{\beta} + \hat{\alpha}\lambda} = \frac{\lambda r}{n - r(1 - \lambda)}, \tag{21.5}$$

$$q_\lambda = \frac{\hat{\beta} + \hat{\alpha}\lambda}{\lambda} = \frac{n - r(1 - \lambda)}{N\lambda}. \tag{21.6}$$

Using the delta method, an asymptotic variance–covariance matrix of p_λ and q_λ is seen to be constructed from:

$$\widehat{\text{var}}(p_\lambda) = \frac{p_\lambda(1 - p_\lambda)}{N\lambda q_\lambda} \left\{ 1 + \frac{1 - \lambda}{\lambda}(1 - p_\lambda)[1 - p_\lambda q_\lambda(1 - \lambda)] \right\}, \tag{21.7}$$

$$\widehat{\text{cov}}(p_\lambda, q_\lambda) = -\frac{1}{N} p_\lambda(1 - p_\lambda)\frac{1 - \lambda}{\lambda} q_\lambda, \tag{21.8}$$

$$\widehat{\text{var}}(q_\lambda) = \frac{q_\lambda(1 - q_\lambda)}{N} \left\{ 1 + \frac{1 - p_\lambda}{1 - q_\lambda}\frac{1 - \lambda}{\lambda} \right\}.$$

Note that the parameter estimates are asymptotically correlated, except when $\lambda = 1$, that is, under the MAR assumption, or under boundary values ($p_\lambda = 0, 1$; $q_\lambda = 0$). This is in line with the ignorable nature of the MAR model.

We need to determine the set of allowable values for λ by requiring $0 \leq p_\lambda, q_\lambda, \lambda q_\lambda \leq 1$. These six inequalities reduce to

$$\lambda \in \left[\frac{n - r}{N - r}, \frac{N - (n - r)}{r} \right].$$

Clearly, $\lambda = 1$ is always valid. For the prevalence of HIV in Kenya example, the range equals $\lambda \in [0.951, 1.692]$.

Table 21.7 Prevalence of HIV in Kenya. Limiting cases for the sensitivity parameter analysis.

Estimator	λ	$\lambda = \frac{n-r}{N-r}$	$\lambda = 1$	$\lambda = \frac{N-(n-r)}{r}$
p_λ	$\frac{\lambda r}{n-r(1-\lambda)}$	$\frac{r}{N}$	$\frac{r}{n}$	$\frac{N-n+r}{N}$
q_λ	$\frac{n-r(1-\lambda)}{N\lambda}$	1	$\frac{n}{N}$	$\frac{r}{N-(n-r)}$
$q_\lambda\lambda$	$\frac{n-r(1-\lambda)}{N}$	$\frac{n-r}{N-r}$	$\frac{n}{N}$	1
$\frac{p_\lambda}{1-p_\lambda}$	$\lambda\frac{r}{n-r}$	$\frac{r}{N-r}$	$\frac{r}{n-r}$	$\frac{N-(n-r)}{n-r}$

Prevalence of HIV in Kenya

p_λ	$\frac{52\lambda}{699+52\lambda}$	0.066	0.069	0.112
q_λ	$\frac{699+52\lambda}{787\lambda}$	1.000	0.954	0.591
$q_\lambda\lambda$	$\frac{699+52\lambda}{787}$	0.951	0.954	1.000
$\frac{p_\lambda}{1-p_\lambda}$	0.074λ	0.071	0.074	0.126

Table 21.7 presents estimates for limiting cases. In particular, results for the HIV example are presented. The interval of ignorance for the success probability is thus seen to be as in (21.4). It is interesting to observe that the success odds estimator is linear in the sensitivity parameter; the resulting interval of ignorance equals

$$\text{odds}(p) : \left[\frac{r}{N-r}, \frac{N-n+r}{n-r}\right].$$

For the HIV case, the odds vary between 0.071 and 0.126.

For the success probability, the variance of p_λ is given by (21.7). For the success odds, we obtain

$$\widehat{\text{var}}(\text{odds}(p_\lambda)) = \frac{1}{N\lambda q_\lambda}\frac{p_\lambda}{1-p_\lambda}\left\{1 + \frac{1-\lambda}{\lambda}(1-p_\lambda)[1-p_\lambda q_\lambda(1-\lambda)]\right\},$$

and for the success logit

$$\widehat{\text{var}}(\text{logit}(p_\lambda)) = \frac{1}{N\lambda q_\lambda}\frac{1}{p_\lambda(1-p_\lambda)}\left\{1 + \frac{1-\lambda}{\lambda}(1-p_\lambda)[1-p_\lambda q_\lambda(1-\lambda)]\right\}.$$

For each λ, a confidence interval C_λ can be constructed for every point within the allowable range of λ. The union of the C_λ is the *interval of uncertainty*, for either p, its odds, or its logit.

Figure 21.1 represents intervals of ignorance and uncertainty for the prevalence of HIV in Kenya study. Note that the interval of ignorance (the inner

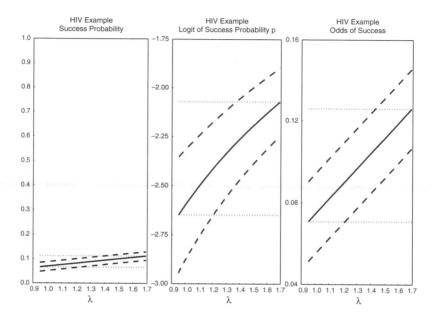

Figure 21.1 HIV prevalence study. Graphical representation of interval of ignorance and interval of uncertainty. The thick solid line represents the point estimates conditional on the sensitivity parameter; its extremes (which are projected on the vertical axis) provide the limits of the interval of ignorance. The thick dashed lines graph the lower and upper confidence limits, conditional on the sensitivity parameter. The extremes form the interval of uncertainty (projecting lines on the vertical axis not shown.)

interval, indicated by the projecting horizontal lines) is sufficiently narrow to be of practical use. The outer interval, formed by the lowest point of the lower and the highest point of the higher thick dashed lines, represents the interval of uncertainty. This is also sufficiently narrow from a practical viewpoint.

21.7 ANALYSIS OF THE FLUVOXAMINE TRIAL

These data were introduced in Section 2.6 and then analysed in Sections 12.6, 15.4.2, 15.5.1, 16.8, 18.3.5, and 20.4. We will focus on a dichotomized version (present/absent) of side effects at the first and the last visit. We use this simplification of the problem because the ideas conveyed here are sufficiently uncommon (although not complicated) to deserve the simplest setting that is sufficiently rich. In addition, a similar dichotomization of therapeutic effect (present/absent) will be considered. The non-monotone nature of the response variable ensures that there are enough 'missing' degrees of freedom to capture the full richness of the approach.

Table 21.8 Fluvoxamine trial. The first subtable contains the complete observations. Subjects with only the first outcome, only the last outcome, or no outcome at all reported are presented in the second, third, and fourth subtables, respectively.

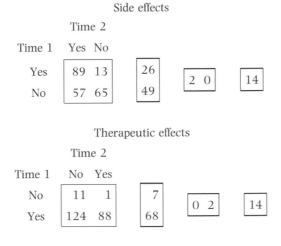

The relevant observed data are given in Table 21.8. There are two patients with a non-monotone pattern of follow-up, while 14 subjects have no follow-up data at all. This enables us to treat these data both from the monotone non-response or dropout perspective, as well as from the more complicated but more general non-monotone point of view.

In Section 21.7.1 we restrict attention to the identified models, whereas overspecified models are studied in Section 21.7.2.

21.7.1 Identified models

We consider the monotone patterns first. Table 21.9 shows the predicted complete tables for models 1, 2, and 3. The effect of ignorance is clearly seen by comparing the MAR and protective models: they provide a substantially different prediction for the partially observed table, while producing the same deviance. In addition, the protective model produces a boundary solution, or even an invalid solution if predicted proportions are not constrained to lie within the unit interval, for therapeutic effect.

We now interpret these results in terms of possible quantities of interest, for instance the first and second marginal probability of side effects and the odds ratio, capturing the association between both measurements (Table 21.10). Models 4 and 5 will be discussed in Section 21.7.2.

Both models 1 and 2 are ignorable and hence all measurement model quantities are independent of the choice between MAR and MCAR.

The quantities in Tables 21.9 and 21.10 differ in one important way. The former quantities are calculated conditionally on the dropout pattern, while the

Table 21.9 Fluvoxamine trial. Identifiable models fitted to the monotone patterns.

	(1,1)		(1,0)		Deviance
Side effects	83.7	12.2	28.0	4.1	495.8
Model 1 (MCAR)	59.9	68.3	20.0	22.9	
Side effects	89.0	13.0	22.7	3.3	494.4
Model 2 (MAR)	57.0	65.0	22.9	26.1	
Side effects	89.0	13.0	18.6	7.4	494.4
Model 3 (protective)	57.0	65.0	11.9	37.1	
Therapeutic effect	13.0	1.2	4.4	0.4	386.5
Model 1 (MCAR)	122.7	87.1	41.1	29.2	
Therapeutic effect	11.0	1.0	6.4	0.6	385.8
Model 2 (MAR)	124.0	88.0	39.8	28.2	
Therapeutic effect	11.0	1.0	7.1	−0.1	385.8
Model 3 (protective, unconstrained)	124.0	88.0	80.5	−12.5	
Therapeutic effect	11.6	1.0	6.4	0.0	385.8
Model 3 (protective, constrained)	123.4	88.0	68.5	0.0	

Table 21.10 Fluvoxamine trial. Marginal probabilities and (log) odds ratio for monotone patterns of side-effects data. (Models 1–3, point estimates and 95% confidence interval; models 4–5, interval of ignorance (II) and interval of uncertainty (IU). Models are defined in Section 21.4.)

Parameter		Model 1/2	Model 3	Model 4	Model 5
1st margin	II	0.43	0.43	0.43	0.43
	IU	[0.37, 0.48]	[0.37, 0.48]	[0.37, 0.48]	[0.37, 0.48]
2nd margin	II	0.64	0.59	[0.49, 0.74]	[0.49, 0.74]
	IU	[0.58, 0.70]	[0.53, 0.65]	[0.43, 0.79]	[0.43, 0.79]
Log odds ratio	II	2.06	2.06	[1.52, 2.08]	[0.41, 2.84]
	IU	[1.37, 2.74]	[1.39, 2.72]	[1.03, 2.76]	[0.0013, 2.84]
Odds ratio	II	7.81	7.81	[4.57, 7.98]	[1.50, 17.04]
	IU	[3.95, 15.44]	[4.00, 15.24]	[2.79, 15.74]	[1.0013, 32.89]

latter follow directly from the marginal measurement probabilities p_{jk}, which are common to all three models, while the dropout probabilities $q_{r|jk}$ depend on the model. As a consequence, while MAR and MCAR are equivalent for the quantities in Table 21.10, this does not carry over to the predicted cell counts in Table 21.9. Further, the stability of the estimates in Table 21.10 (at least for models 1–3) is in marked contrast to the variation among the predicted cell counts in Table 21.9. These considerations suggest that stability may be restricted to *certain* functions of parameters in *certain* sets of data.

Table 21.11 Fluvoxamine trial. Complete data counts for models fitted to side-effects data.

	(1,1)		(1,0)		(0,1)		(0,0)		(+,+)	
BRD1	84.00	12.12	28.13	4.06	0.74	0.11	5.26	0.76	118.13	17.05
	60.21	67.67	20.16	22.66	0.53	0.60	3.77	4.23	84.67	95.16
BRD2	89.42	12.89	22.73	3.27	0.80	0.12	4.24	0.61	117.19	16.89
	57.27	64.42	23.06	25.94	0.51	0.58	4.30	4.82	85.14	95.76
BRD3	83.67	12.22	28.02	4.09	1.17	0.00	8.16	0.00	121.01	16.31
	59.85	68.25	20.04	22.85	0.83	0.00	5.84	0.00	86.57	91.11
BRD4	89.42	12.89	18.58	7.42	0.80	0.12	3.47	1.39	112.27	21.82
	57.27	64.42	11.90	37.10	0.51	0.58	2.22	6.93	71.90	109.03
BRD7	89.00	13.00	18.58	7.42	1.22	0.00	8.53	0.00	117.33	20.42
	57.00	65.00	11.90	37.10	0.78	0.00	5.47	0.00	75.15	102.10
BRD9	89.00	13.00	22.69	3.31	1.22	0.00	6.97	0.00	119.87	16.31
	57.00	65.00	22.89	26.11	0.78	0.00	7.03	0.00	87.71	91.11

We now introduce the non-monotone patterns into the analysis. The fitted counts of the models with an interior solution are given in Table 21.11 and the marginal quantities of interest are displayed in Table 21.12. It is important to note that a subgroup of models produces invalid solutions without appropriate constraints.

Even though we are now looking at a larger class of models, the results are comparable with those obtained for the monotone patterns. Table 21.12 reveals that models BRD1–9 show little variation in the marginal probabilities and in the measure of association. Considered as an informal sensitivity analysis, this could be seen as evidence for the robustness of these measures. We will revisit this conclusion following a more formal sensitivity analysis and conclude that the above assertion can be seriously misleading.

21.7.2 Sensitivity analysis

We first consider the monotone patterns. In addition to the three identifiable models from Table 21.3, fitted in Section 21.4, we now fit overspecified models 4 and 5 to the same data. Results for these additional models are also given in Table 21.10.

For model 4 there is one sensitivity parameter, which we choose to be γ (measuring the extent of non-randomness). When $\gamma = 0$ the MAR model 2 is recovered. The value of γ which corresponds to $q_{r|jk} = q_{r|k}$ in Table 21.3 yields the protective model 3. Because there is only one sensitivity parameter, a graphical representation (Figure 21.2) is straightforward. For the monotone cases the first measurement is always recovered, so there no ignorance about the first marginal probability, and hence the interval of ignorance for this quantity is a point. This is not true for the other two quantities.

Table 21.12 Fluvoxamine trial. Model fit for side effects. (G^2, likelihood ratio test statistic for model fit, corresponding *p*-value, estimates and 95% confidence limits for marginal probabilities and marginal (log) odds ratio.) For model 10 (21.10), intervals of ignorance and uncertainty are presented instead.

Model	No. of parameter	G^2	p-value	Marginal probabilities		Odds ratio	
				First	Second	Original	Log
BRD1	6	4.5	0.104	0.43 [0.37, 0.49]	0.64 [0.58, 0.71]	7.80 [3.94, 15.42]	2.06 [1.37, 2.74]
BRD2	7	1.7	0.192	0.43 [0.37, 0.48]	0.64 [0.58, 0.70]	7.81 [3.95, 15.44]	2.06 [1.37, 2.74]
BRD3	7	2.8	0.097	0.44 [0.38, 0.49]	0.66 [0.60, 0.72]	7.81 [3.95, 15.44]	2.06 [1.37, 2.74]
BRD4	7	1.7	0.192	0.43 [0.37, 0.48]	0.58 [0.49, 0.68]	7.81 [3.95, 15.44]	2.06 [1.37, 2.74]
BRD7	8	0.0	—	0.44 [0.38, 0.49]	0.61 [0.53, 0.69]	7.81 [3.95, 15.44]	2.06 [1.37, 2.74]
BRD9	8	0.0	—	0.43 [0.38, 0.49]	0.66 [0.60, 0.72]	7.63 [3.86, 15.10]	2.03 [1.35, 2.71]
Model 10: II	9	0.0	—	[0.425, 0.429]	[0.47, 0.75]	[4.40, 7.96]	[1.48, 2.07]
Model 10: IU	9	0.0	—	[0.37, 0.49]	[0.41, 0.80]	[2.69, 15.69]	[0.99, 2.75]

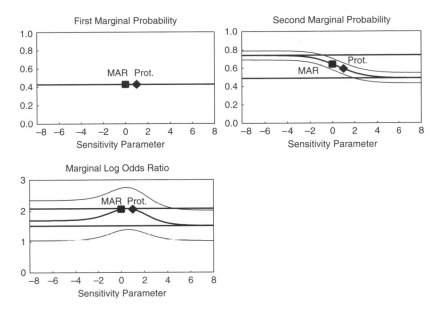

Figure 21.2 Fluvoxamine trial. Graphical representation of intervals of ignorance and intervals of uncertainty for the monotone patterns and for the side-effects outcome. The thick curves graph the point estimates conditional on the sensitivity parameter. The thick horizontal lines project the interval of ignorance on the vertical axes. The extremes of the thin lines correspond to the interval of uncertainty. The MAR and protective point estimates have been added.

Commonly, fitting a pair of identifiable models (e.g., models 2 and 3) is regarded as a sensitivity analysis. This example shows how misleading this can be. Both models differ by about 0.05 in the second marginal probability, but the interval of ignorance of model 4 shows the range is about 0.25! Similarly, models 2 and 3 yield virtually the same result for the odds ratio, but the interval of ignorance of model 4 shows that this proximity is fortuitous.

The impact of fitting an overspecified but, at the complete data level, non-saturated model is seen by contrasting model 4 with the fully saturated model 5. The sensitivity parameter for model 4 is γ_1 in Table 21.3; for model 5 the two sensitivity parameters are γ_1 and δ_{11} (all other γ and δ parameters need to be set to zero for classical identifiability purposes). As expected, both models coincide for the first marginal probability. It turns out that their respective intervals of ignorance and uncertainty for the second marginal probability exhibit considerable overlap. In contrast, the interval of ignorance for the log odds ratio is now about 5 times longer. For model 5 the lower limit of the interval of uncertainty is very close to zero, whereas under its model 4 counterpart there is clear evidence for a strong positive association between both outcomes.

By construction, the data do not provide evidence for choosing between models 4 and 5. Both are overspecified at the observed data level and both encompass models 2 and 3. Model 5 is saturated at the observed data level as well, and therefore the limits derived from it are not model-based. The reduced width of the intervals produced under model 4 follows from the unverifiable model assumption that the dropout probability depends on both outcomes through their main effects only and *not* on the interaction between both outcomes. If this assumption is deemed not plausible, it can easily be avoided by including an extra degree of freedom. However, in more complicated settings, such as when covariates are included or with continuous responses, assumptions are unavoidable in the interests of model parsimony.

Once we include the non-monotone patterns, any model within the BRD family (19.49), with nine or more parameters, is non-identifiable. To simplify the sensitivity analysis, we consider the equivalent parameterization (see also Section 15.5)

$$\pi_{r_1 r_1, jk} = p_{jk} \frac{\exp[\beta_{jk}^*(1 - r_2) + \alpha_{jk}^*(1 - r_1) + \gamma^*(1 - r_1)(1 - r_2)]}{1 + \exp(\beta_{jk}^*) + \exp(\alpha_{jk}^*) + \exp(\beta_{jk}^* + \alpha_{jk}^* + \gamma^*)}, \qquad (21.9)$$

which contains the marginal success probabilities p_{jk} and forces the missingness probabilities to obey their range restrictions.

While models BRD1–9 have shown stability in the estimates of the marginal parameters of interest (Section 21.5), it was revealed in Section 21.7.2, in the monotone context, that such a conclusion can be deceptive. To study this further, we consider an overspecified model, analogous to model 4 in Table 21.3. The choice can be motivated by observing that both BRD7 and BRD9 yield an interior solution and differ only in the β-model. Therefore, model 10 will be defined as (α_k, β_{jk}) with

$$\beta_{jk} = \beta_0 + \beta_j + \beta_k. \qquad (21.10)$$

Since one parameter is redundant, we propose to use β_k as the sensitivity parameter. While the interval of ignorance obtained in this way is acceptable, the interval of uncertainty shows aberrant behaviour (plot not shown) towards larger values of the sensitivity parameter, leading to very wide intervals of uncertainty. This problem is entirely due to the zero count in pattern $(0,1)$ (see Table 21.8), as can be seen by adding 0.5 to this zero count. The results are presented in Figure 21.3. The resulting intervals of ignorance and uncertainty are presented in Table 21.12, and they are very similar to the results for model 4, as displayed in Table 21.10. Because of the presence of the non-monotone patterns, there is a small but non-zero degree of ignorance in the first marginal probability as well, in contrast to the monotone setting. Once again, it is seen that fitting identifiable models only may be misleading because, for example, the log odds ratio shows much more variability than results from models BRD1–9.

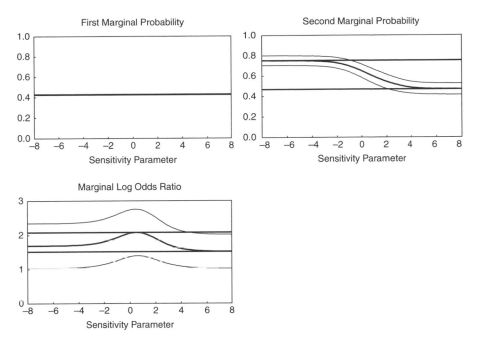

Figure 21.3 Fluvoxamine trial. Graphical representation of intervals of ignorance and intervals of uncertainty for the non-monotone patterns and the side-effects outcome. A value of 0.5 has been added to the zero count in pattern $(1, 0)$. The thick curves graph the point estimates conditional on the sensitivity parameter. The thick horizontal lines project the interval of ignorance on the vertical axes. The extremes of the thin lines correspond to the interval of uncertainty.

21.8 ARTIFICIAL EXAMPLES

To study the behaviour of the intervals of ignorance and uncertainty, we consider eight artificial sets of data, as presented in Table 21.13. The complete data counts are presented. It is easy to derive the observed data. For example, set (a) produces:

$$\begin{array}{|c|c|} \hline 200 & 100 \\ \hline 100 & 200 \\ \hline \end{array} \quad \begin{array}{|c|} \hline 300 \\ \hline 300 \\ \hline \end{array} \qquad \begin{array}{|c|c|} \hline 300 & 300 \\ \hline \end{array} \qquad \begin{array}{|c|} \hline 600 \\ \hline \end{array}$$

The eight sets are chosen to illustrate the impact of three factors. First, sets (a)–(d) are MCAR (BRD1), whereas (e)–(h) are MNAR (BRD9). Second, in sets (a), (b), (e), and (f), the proportions in the four response patterns are (25%,25%,25%,25%), whereas in the other sets this is (50%,20%,20%,10%). The parameters α and β in (21.9) were chosen to approximate these proportions. In (e)–(f) we set $\alpha_0 = 0$, $\alpha_1 = 0.75$, $\beta_0 = 0$, $\beta_1 = -1$, and in

Table 21.13 Artificial sets of data.

Set	(1,1)		(1,0)		(0,1)		(0,0)	
(a)	200	100	200	100	200	100	200	100
	100	200	100	200	100	200	100	200
(b)	2000	1000	2000	1000	2000	1000	2000	1000
	1000	2000	1000	2000	1000	2000	1000	2000
(c)	400	200	160	80	160	80	80	40
	200	400	80	160	80	160	40	80
(d)	4000	2000	1600	800	1600	800	800	400
	2000	4000	800	1600	800	1600	400	800
(e)	200	64	200	64	200	136	200	136
	146	188	54	69	146	397	54	146
(f)	2000	640	2000	640	2000	1360	2000	1360
	1460	1880	540	690	1460	3970	540	1460
(g)	417	154	254	94	80	94	49	58
	281	417	54	80	54	254	11	49
(h)	4170	1540	2540	940	800	940	490	580
	2810	4170	540	800	540	2540	110	490

(g)–(h) we set $\alpha_0 = -1.65$, $\alpha_1 = -0.5$, $\beta_0 = -05$, $\beta_1 = -1.65$. In both cases, $\gamma = 0$, although due to rounding this is only approximately true for the MNAR models. Third, the sample size in (b), (d), (f), and (h) is ten times that in (a), (c), (e), and (g).

The results of fitting overspecified model 10 to the artificial data are summarized in Table 21.14. There are three intervals. First, we present the non-parametric bounds on the probability of answering yes/yes, as was done in (19.50). Next, we present intervals of ignorance and intervals of uncertainty. Recall that the interval of ignorance reflects uncertainty due to missingness,

Table 21.14 Artificial sets of data. Estimates of the proportion θ (confidence interval) attending the plebiscite and voting for independence, based on the pessimistic–optimistic range and on overspecified model BRD10 (interval of ignorance and interval of uncertainty).

Set	Mechanism	Incompleteness	Sample	Pess–Opt	II	IU
(a)	MCAR	large	small	[0.083, 0.583]	[0.167, 0.417]	[0.140, 0.443]
(b)	MCAR	large	large	[0.083, 0.583]	[0.167, 0.417]	[0.161, 0.425]
(c)	MCAR	small	small	[0.167, 0.467]	[0.233, 0.383]	[0.215, 0.405]
(d)	MCAR	small	large	[0.167, 0.467]	[0.233, 0.383]	[0.228, 0.390]
(e)	MNAR	large	small	[0.083, 0.561]	[0.167, 0.429]	[0.148, 0.455]
(f)	MNAR	large	large	[0.083, 0.561]	[0.167, 0.429]	[0.161, 0.437]
(g)	MNAR	small	small	[0.174, 0.444]	[0.208, 0.402]	[0.191, 0.423]
(h)	MNAR	small	large	[0.174, 0.444]	[0.208, 0.402]	[0.203, 0.409]

while the interval of uncertainty combines both sources of uncertainty, that is, it also reflects sampling variability.

We can make several observations. First, the effect of the sample size is seen only in the interval of uncertainty: each pair of sets yields the same non-parametric bounds and the same interval of ignorance, but the even sets produce sharper intervals of uncertainty than the odd ones.

Second, the proportion of incompleteness is larger in sets (a), (b), (e), and (f), as opposed to (c), (d), (g), and (h), respectively. This is reflected in larger ignorance, that is, in larger non-parametric ranges and larger intervals of ignorance.

Third, comparing the non-parametric range and the interval of ignorance shows the consequences of the modelling strategy. The interval of ignorance is neither based on an identifiable model nor fully non-parametric. Rather, it has aspects of both by allowing overspecification, but in a controlled fashion. In this case, we chose to illustrate the potential by including one extra parameter (one sensitivity parameter), by means of model 10. Of course, in a real-life situation one has to reflect on the plausibility of such model assumptions. It then provides a compromise between the acknowledgement of ignorance due to incompleteness (abandoning a single point estimate), and practically useful lengths of the corresponding intervals (avoiding the non-parametric bounds).

Finally, there is a striking symmetry between the results for the MCAR models (a)–(d) and their MNAR counterparts (e)–(h). This implies that, other things being equal, the precise form of the MNAR mechanism seems to be less relevant. This feature distinguishes our sensitivity analysis from fitting a single identified model. Let us expand on this point. If we consider BRD1–9 for set (a), then all models produce $\hat{\theta} = 0.333$, the 'true' value. This follows from the fact that all the models are extensions of the MCAR model (BRD1), which fits the data exactly. However, model 10 intrinsically includes deviations from MCAR by considering a whole range for the sensitivity parameter. In contrast, if we fit BRD1–9 to set (e), then we obtain

BRD1:	0.317	BRD4:	0.426	BRD7:	0.426
BRD2:	0.342	BRD5:	0.167	BRD8:	0.193
BRD3:	0.321	BRD6:	0.167	BRD9:	0.333

In other words, BRD1–9 span a wide variety of estimates. This also holds for the subset BRD6–9 of the saturated models. These almost reproduce the entire interval of ignorance. Thus, the formal sensitivity analysis, removes the *ad hoc* nature of intervals, computed from fitting a number of identified models. In this case, we have shown that intervals can be anything from a single point to almost the entire interval of ignorance.

21.9   THE SLOVENIAN PUBLIC OPINION SURVEY

We now turn to the Slovenian public opinion survey data, introduced in Section 2.10. An overview of simple and more complex analyses on these data was presented in Section 19.4.

The estimated intervals of ignorance and intervals of uncertainty are shown in Table 21.15, while a graphical representation of the yes votes is given in Figure 21.4. A representation for the proportion of noes via non-attendance is

Table 21.15 Slovenian public opinion survey. Parameter estimates (confidence interval) of the proportion θ (confidence interval) attending the plebiscite and of the proportion v of noes via non-attendance, following from fitting the Baker *et al.* (1992) models. BRD1–BRD9 are identifiable, while models 10–12 are overspecified.

Model	d.f.	Log-likelihood	$\hat{\theta}$	$\hat{v}$
BRD1	6	−2495.29	0.892 [0.878, 0.906]	0.042 [0.032, 0.052]
BRD2	7	−2467.43	0.884 [0.869, 0.900]	0.047 [0.036, 0.058]
BRD3	7	−2463.10	0.881 [0.866, 0.897]	0.045 [0.034, 0.056]
BRD4	7	−2467.43	0.765 [0.674, 0.856]	0.047 [0.036, 0.058]
BRD5	7	−2463.10	0.844 [0.806, 0.882]	0.110 [0.071, 0.150]
BRD6	8	−2431.06	0.819 [0.788, 0.849]	0.137 [0.107, 0.168]
BRD7	8	−2431.06	0.764 [0.697, 0.832]	0.047 [0.035, 0.059]
BRD8	8	−2431.06	0.741 [0.657, 0.826]	0.137 [0.105, 0.169]
BRD9	8	−2431.06	0.867 [0.851, 0.884]	0.059 [0.045, 0.074]
Model 10(II)	9	−2431.06	[0.762, 0.893]	[0.037, 0.044]
Model 10(IU)	9	−2431.06	[0.744, 0.907]	[0.029, 0.055]
Model 11(II)	9	−2431.06	[0.766, 0.883]	[0.032, 0.193]
Model 11(IU)	9	−2431.06	[0.715, 0.920]	[−0.037, 0.242]
Model 12(II)	10	−2431.06	[0.694, 0.905]	[0.032, 0.193]

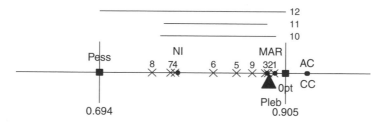

Figure 21.4 Slovenian public opinion survey. Relative position for the estimates of proportion of yes votes, based on the models considered in Rubin *et al.* (1995), and on the BRD models. The vertical lines indicate the non-parametric pessimistic–optimistic bounds. (Pess, pessimistic boundary; Opt, optimistic boundary; MAR, Rubin *et al.*'s MAR model; NI, Rubin *et al.*'s MNAR model; AC, available cases; CC, complete cases; Pleb, plebiscite outcome. Numbers refer to the BRD models. Intervals of ignorance (models 10–12) are represented by horizontal bars.)

given in Figure 21.5. Apart from the overspecified model 10, defined by (21.10), we consider another, analogous overspecified model with one extra parameter. This model 11 takes the form (α_{jk}, β_j) and uses

$$\alpha_{jk} = \alpha_0 + \alpha_j + \alpha_k, \qquad (21.11)$$

an additive decomposition of the missingness parameter on the attendance question. Furthermore, we define model 12, $(\alpha_{jk}, \beta_{jk})$, as a combination of both (21.10) and (21.11).

We first consider the proportion θ of yes votes. Model 10 shows an interval of ignorance which is very close to [0.741, 0.892], the range produced by the models BRD1–BRD9, while model 11 is somewhat sharper and just fails to cover the plebiscite value. However, it should be noted that the corresponding intervals of uncertainty contain the true value.

Interestingly, Model 12 virtually coincides with the non-parametric range (19.50), even though it does not saturate the complete data degrees of freedom. To do so, not two but in fact seven sensitivity parameters would have to be included. Thus, it appears that a relatively simple sensitivity analysis is sufficient to increase the insight in the information provided by the incomplete data about the proportion of valid YES votes. This simplicity may not hold in all cases, as will be illustrated next.

We now turn to ν, the proportion of noes via non-attendance. In some aspects, a similar picture holds in the sense that model 10 just fails to cover the plebiscite value, while models 11 and 12 produce intervals of ignorance which virtually coincide with the non-parametric range. A major difference between θ and ν is that in the first case the MAR models of Rubin *et al.* (1995) are very close to the plebiscite value, while in the second case the MAR models are relatively far from it. This and related issues were discussed in Section 19.4. The plebiscite value of the proportion of noes via non-attendance is best reproduced by BRD9. Thus, a specific model, such as MAR, can be acceptable for one estimand but not necessarily for another.

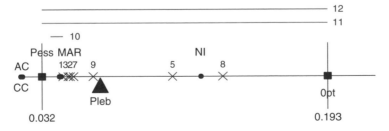

Figure 21.5 Slovenian public opinion survey. Relative position for the estimates of proportion of no votes via non-attendance, based on the models considered in Rubin *et al.* (1995), and on the BRD models. The vertical lines indicate the non-parametric pessimistic–optimistic bounds. (For key to symbols, see Figure 21.4.)

We can enhance our insight by studying the *pair* (θ, ν). For this it is useful to plot the region of ignorance for both θ and ν. Since models 10 and 11 are based on a single sensitivity parameter, the regions of ignorance are one-dimensional curves, while a two-dimensional planar region is obtained for model 12. A graphical sketch is given in Figure 21.6. The left- and right-hand panels contain the same information. The left-hand panel is useful for answering the substantive questions. The conclusion we reach from it is that, even when ignorance is taken into account, a convincing majority will vote for independence and only a very small proportion will provide a no vote through non-attendance. The right-hand panel focuses on the region of ignorance to provide a clearer picture of its main features. This figure combines the univariate intervals from Figures 21.4 and 21.5. Models 10 and 11 are represented by curves. In order to obtain a representation for model 12, points of the sensitivity parameter are sampled from a bivariate uniform distribution. For each of those pairs, the model is fitted and the corresponding $(\hat{\theta}, \hat{\nu})$ determined. These points are then plotted. A black square marks the plebiscite values for both quantities. The MAR analysis is represented by a bullet. It is clear that the plebiscite

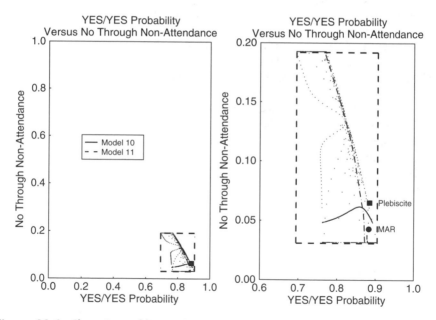

Figure 21.6 Slovenian public opinion survey. Graphical representation of regions of ignorance. Proportion of yes votes versus proportion of noes via non-attendance. The interval of ignorance is the envelope of the points so obtained. Models 10 (solid line), 11 (dashed line), and 12 (sampled points). The optimistic–pessimistic bounds are reproduced by means of the dashed box. The left-hand panel gives an absolute impression of ignorance in the unit square. The right-hand panel focuses on the relative position of the models by zooming in on the relevant region.

result is *on the boundary* of the range produced by model 12, while it is not on the boundary of the optimistic–pessimistic range (represented by means of a dashed box). Thus, while the univariate intervals of ignorance clearly include the plebiscite value, this is less true for the bivariate region, indicating that it enhances our understanding. Note that a saturated model would incorporate five extra sensitivity parameters! Such an extended analysis would extend the region of ignorance in the direction of the optimistic–pessimistic box, thereby relaxing the boundary location of the plebiscite value.

21.10   SOME THEORETICAL CONSIDERATIONS

The introduction of regions (intervals) of ignorance and uncertainty cannot be done without revisiting such concepts as (weak and strong) convergence, bias, and asymptotic normality because the population quantities themselves have to be reconsidered: when data are incomplete these can be expressed as regions (intervals) rather than scalars. Vansteelandt *et al.* (2006) redefine these quantities and provide an illustration based on the data on prevalence of HIV in Kenya. In particular, these authors define a desirable set of properties for a 'point' estimator when region of ignorance ideas are applied. At the same time, they establish a logical framework for regions (intervals) of uncertainty.

21.11   CONCLUDING REMARKS

In this chapter we have defined the concept of *ignorance* and combined it with the familiar idea of statistical imprecision, producing a measure of *uncertainty*. As an extension of the concept of confidence, uncertainty is expressed as an interval for scalar unknowns (parameters) and a region for vectors, which reduce to conventional confidence intervals regions when it is assumed that there is no ignorance about the statistical model underlying the data. The construction of the intervals of uncertainty in the examples is seen to convey useful information about the problems concerned, providing insights not previously appreciated.

We have introduced three paths to sensitivity analysis. The first one is to look at the bounds produced by the most pessimistic and most optimistic scenarios. In the case of the Slovenian plebiscite, we learn that even the most pessimistic scenario translates into a clear majority in favour of independence. Second, a range of plausible models can be considered, such as those proposed by Baker *et al.* (1992). Here, their range is qualitatively similar to that obtained by the bounds, but enables further distinction between (a) well-fitting and poorly fitting models and (b) model formulations (dropout mechanisms) that are deemed plausible, in contrast to models where the dropout mechanism is not tenable on substantive grounds. This is necessarily subjective, but with incomplete data subjectivity should be controlled rather than avoided. Third, plausible but overspecified models can be considered. More overspecification will yield models that produce intervals of ignorance closer to the bounds, whereas models that are too parsimonious or not plausible may miss the 'true' value. The strategies presented here enable the consideration of *classes* of models, and the amount of parsimony can be controlled.

Of course, a sensitivity analysis can be conducted within different frameworks, and there are times where the setting will determine which framework is the more appropriate one (e.g., Bayesian or frequentist), in conjunction with technical and computational considerations. Draper (1995) has considered ways of dealing with model uncertainty in the very natural Bayesian framework.

We can approach the calculation of the interval of ignorance in several ways, but we have seen that a (possibly) overspecified model and associated likelihood are the more natural concepts to use. We have focused on the use of a sensitivity parameter in order to determine the set of maxima of this saturated likelihood. A formal study of the method and its properties can be found in Vansteelandt *et al.* (2006).

22

Local and Global Influence Methods

22.1 INTRODUCTION

The conclusions from models for incomplete longitudinal data are sensitive to model-based assumptions which cannot be checked from the data under analysis. Even if the multivariate normal model were the obvious choice of preference to describe the measurement process *if the data were complete*, then the analysis of the actually observed, incomplete version would be, in addition, subject to further untestable modelling assumptions (Jansen *et al.* 2006b). The growing body of modelling tools for selection models (Heckman 1976; Diggle and Kenward 1994) requires the understanding of such sensitivities (Glynn *et al.* 1986), as well as tools to deal with it (Draper 1995; Vach and Blettner 1995; Copas and Li 1997).

The sensitivity of MNAR selection models was illustrated by Verbeke and Molenberghs (2000, Chapter 17) who showed that, in the context of an onychomycosis study, excluding a small amount of measurement error drastically changes the likelihood ratio test statistics for the MAR null hypothesis. Kenward (1998) revisited the analysis of the mastitis data performed by Diggle and Kenward (1994). In this study, the milk yields of 107 cows were to be recorded for two consecutive years. While data were complete in the first year, 27 measurements were missing in year 2 because these cows developed mastitis which seriously affected their milk yield. While in the initial paper there was some evidence for MNAR, Kenward (1998) showed that removing two anomalous profiles from the 107 completely removed this evidence. Kenward also showed that changing the conditional distribution of the year 2 yield, given the year 1 yield, from a normal to a heavy-tailed *t* led to a similar conclusion.

Missing Data in Clinical Studies   G. Molenberghs and M.G. Kenward
© 2007 John Wiley & Sons, Ltd

Several authors have advocated using local influence tools (Verbeke *et al.* 2001b; Thijs *et al.* 2000; Molenberghs *et al.* 2001b; Van Steen *et al.* 2001; Jansen *et al.* 2006b) for sensitivity analysis purposes. In particular, Molenberghs *et al.* (2001b) revisited the mastitis example. They were able to identify the same two cows also found by Kenward (1998), in addition to another one. However, it is noteworthy that all three are cows with *complete* information, even though local influence methods were originally intended to identify subjects with other than MAR mechanisms of missingness. Thus, an important question concerns the combined nature of the data and model that leads to apparent evidence for a MNAR process. Jansen *et al.* (2006b) showed that a number of aspects, but not necessarily the (outlying) nature of the missingness mechanism in one or a few subjects, may be responsible for an apparent MNAR mechanism. Their work is reviewed in the next chapter.

Local and global influence methods for Gaussian outcomes are described in Section 22.2, and applied to the mastitis data in Section 22.3. A brief overview of alternative local influence based methods is provided in Section 22.4. A second application, concerned with milk protein contents in dairy cattle, is presented in Section 22.5. The final application in the Gaussian setting, in Section 22.6, is to the depression trials. Thereafter we turn to the categorical data setting. Influence methods for ordinal data are discussed in Section 22.7 and methods for binary data in Section 22.9. Both methods are illustrated by means of the fluvoxamine trial. Section 22.8 treats the outcome as ordinal, whereas a binary version is studied in Section 22.10.

22.2   GAUSSIAN OUTCOMES

Verbeke *et al.* (2001b), Thijs *et al.* (2000), and Molenberghs *et al.* (2001b) investigated the sensitivity of estimation of quantities of interest, such as treatment effect, growth parameters, and dropout model parameters, with respect to the dropout model assumptions. For this, they considered the following perturbed version of dropout model (15.3):

$$\text{logit}(g(\mathbf{h}_{ij}, y_{ij})) = \text{logit}\left[P(D_i = j | D_i \geqslant j, \mathbf{y}_i)\right] = \mathbf{h}'_{ij}\boldsymbol{\psi} + \omega_i y_{ij}, \qquad (22.1)$$

where the ω_i are local, individual-specific perturbations around a null model. These should not be confused with subject-specific parameters. Our null model will be the MAR model, corresponding to setting $\omega_i = 0$ in (15.3). Thus, the ω_i are perturbations that will be used only to derive influence measures (Cook 1986).

Using this set-up, one can study the impact on key model features, induced by small perturbations in the direction, or at least seemingly in the direction, of MNAR. This can be done by constructing local influence measures (Cook 1986). When small perturbations in a specific ω_i lead to relatively large differences in the model parameters, this suggests that the subject is likely to contribute in particular way to key conclusions. For example, if such a subject drove the model towards MNAR, then the conditional expectations of the unobserved measurements, given the observed ones, might deviate substantially from those under an MAR mechanism (Kenward 1998). Such an observation is also important for our approach since then the impact on dropout model parameters extends to all functions that include these dropout parameters. One such function is the conditional expectation of the unobserved measurements given the corresponding dropout pattern: $E(\boldsymbol{y}_i^m|\boldsymbol{y}_i^o, D_i, \boldsymbol{\theta}, \boldsymbol{\psi})$. As a consequence, the corresponding measurement model parameters will be affected as well.

Some caution is needed when interpreting local influence. Even though we may be tempted to conclude that an influential subject drops out non-randomly, this conclusion is misguided since we are not aiming to detect (groups of) subjects that drop out non-randomly but rather subjects that have a considerable impact on the dropout and measurement model parameters. An important observation is that a subject that drives the conclusions towards MNAR may be doing so not only because its true data-generating mechanism is of an MNAR type, but also for a wide variety of other reasons, such as an unusual mean profile or autocorrelation structure (Jansen *et al.* 2006b; see also Chapter 23 below). Similarly, it is possible that subjects, deviating from the bulk of the data because they are generated under MNAR, go undetected by this technique. Thus, subjects identified in a local influence analysis should be assessed carefully for their precise impact on the conclusions.

We start by reviewing the key concepts of local influence (Cook 1986). We denote the log-likelihood function corresponding to (22.1) by $\ell(\boldsymbol{\gamma}|\boldsymbol{\omega}) = \sum_{i=1}^{N} \ell_i(\boldsymbol{\gamma}|\omega_i)$, in which $\ell_i(\boldsymbol{\gamma}|\omega_i)$ is the contribution of the ith individual to the log-likelihood, and where $\boldsymbol{\gamma} = (\boldsymbol{\theta}, \boldsymbol{\psi})$ is the s-dimensional vector grouping the parameters of the measurement model and the dropout model, not including the $N \times 1$ vector $\boldsymbol{\omega} = (\omega_1, \omega_2, \ldots, \omega_N)'$ of weights defining the perturbation of the MAR model. It is assumed that $\boldsymbol{\omega}$ belongs to an open subset Ω of $\mathbb{R}^N$. For $\boldsymbol{\omega}$ equal to $\boldsymbol{\omega}_0 = (0, 0, \ldots, 0)'$, $\ell(\boldsymbol{\gamma}|\boldsymbol{\omega}_0)$ is the log-likelihood function which corresponds to an MAR dropout model.

Let $\widehat{\boldsymbol{\gamma}}$ be the maximum likelihood estimator for $\boldsymbol{\gamma}$, obtained by maximizing $\ell(\boldsymbol{\gamma}|\boldsymbol{\omega}_0)$, and let $\widehat{\boldsymbol{\gamma}}_{\boldsymbol{\omega}}$ denote the maximum likelihood estimator for $\boldsymbol{\gamma}$ under $\ell(\boldsymbol{\gamma}|\boldsymbol{\omega})$. In the local influence approach $\widehat{\boldsymbol{\gamma}}_{\boldsymbol{\omega}}$ is compared to $\widehat{\boldsymbol{\gamma}}$. Sufficiently different estimates suggest that the estimation procedure is sensitive to such perturbations. Cook (1986) proposed measuring the distance between $\widehat{\boldsymbol{\gamma}}_{\boldsymbol{\omega}}$ and $\widehat{\boldsymbol{\gamma}}$ by the so-called likelihood displacement, defined by $LD(\boldsymbol{\omega}) = 2[\ell(\widehat{\boldsymbol{\gamma}}|\boldsymbol{\omega}_0) - \ell(\widehat{\boldsymbol{\gamma}}_{\boldsymbol{\omega}}|\boldsymbol{\omega})]$. This takes into account the variability of $\widehat{\boldsymbol{\gamma}}$. Indeed, $LD(\boldsymbol{\omega})$ will be large if $\ell(\boldsymbol{\gamma}|\boldsymbol{\omega}_0)$ is strongly curved at $\widehat{\boldsymbol{\gamma}}$, which means that $\boldsymbol{\gamma}$ is estimated with high precision, and small otherwise. Therefore, a graph of $LD(\boldsymbol{\omega})$ versus $\boldsymbol{\omega}$ contains essential information on the influence of perturbations. It is useful to view this graph as the geometric surface formed by the values of the $(N+1)$-dimensional vector $\boldsymbol{\xi}(\boldsymbol{\omega}) = [\boldsymbol{\omega}', LD(\boldsymbol{\omega})]'$ as $\boldsymbol{\omega}$ varies throughout Ω. Since this *influence graph* can only be constructed when $N = 2$, Cook (1986) proposed looking at local influence, that is, at the normal curvatures C_h of $\xi(\omega)$ in ω_0, in the direction of some N-dimensional vector h of unit length. Let Δ_i be the s-dimensional vector defined by

$$\Delta_i = \frac{\partial^2 \ell_i(\gamma|\omega_i)}{\partial \omega_i \partial \gamma}\bigg|_{\gamma=\hat{\gamma}, \omega_i=0} \tag{22.2}$$

and define Δ as the $(s \times N)$ matrix with Δ_i as its ith column. Further, let $\ddot{L}$ denote the $(s \times s)$ matrix of second-order derivatives of $\ell(\gamma|\omega_0)$ with respect to γ, also evaluated at $\gamma = \hat{\gamma}$. Cook (1986) showed that C_h can be calculated as $C_h = 2|h'\Delta'\ddot{L}^{-1}\Delta h|$. Obviously, C_h can be calculated for any direction h. One obvious choice is the vector h_i containing one in the ith position and zeros elsewhere, corresponding to the perturbation of the ith weight only. This reflects the impact of allowing the ith subject to drop out non-randomly, while the others can only drop out at random. The corresponding local influence measure, denoted by C_i, then becomes $C_i = 2|\Delta_i'\ddot{L}^{-1}\Delta_i|$. Another important direction is h_{max} of maximal normal curvature C_{max}. This shows how the MAR model should be perturbed to obtain the largest local changes in the likelihood displacement. C_{max} is the largest eigenvalue of $-2\Delta'\ddot{L}^{-1}\Delta$ and h_{max} is the corresponding eigenvector. When a subset γ_1 of $\gamma = (\gamma_1', \gamma_2')'$ is of special interest, a similar approach can be used, replacing the log-likelihood by the profile log-likelihood for γ_1, and the methods discussed above for the full parameter vector directly carry over (Lesaffre and Verbeke 1998).

22.2.1 Application to the Diggle–Kenward model

Here we focus on the linear mixed model, combined with (15.3), as in Section 15.2. Using the $g(\cdot)$ factor notation, the dropout mechanism is described by

$$f(d_i|\boldsymbol{y}_i, \boldsymbol{\psi}) = \begin{cases} \prod_{j=2}^{n_i}[1 - g(\boldsymbol{h}_{ij}, y_{ij})] & \text{if completer } (d_i = n_i + 1), \\ \prod_{j=2}^{d-1}[1 - g(\boldsymbol{h}_{ij}, y_{ij})]g(\boldsymbol{h}_{id}, y_{id}) & \text{if dropout } (d_i = d \le n_i), \end{cases}$$

The log-likelihood contribution for a complete sequence is then

$$\ell_{i\omega} = \ln f(\boldsymbol{y}_i) + \ln f(d_i|\boldsymbol{y}_i, \boldsymbol{\psi}),$$

where the parameter dependencies are suppressed for ease of notation. The density $f(\boldsymbol{y}_i)$ is multivariate normal, following from the linear mixed model. The contribution from an incomplete sequence is more complicated. Its log-likelihood term is

$$\ell_{i\omega} = \ln f(y_{i1}, \dots, y_{i,d-1}) + \sum_{j=2}^{d-1} \ln[1 - g(\boldsymbol{h}_{ij}, y_{ij})] + \ln \int f(y_{id}|y_{i1}, \dots, y_{i,d-1})g(\boldsymbol{h}_{id}, y_{id})dy_{id}.$$

Further details can be found in Verbeke *et al.* (2001b). We need expressions for Δ and $\ddot{L}$. Straightforward derivation shows that the columns Δ_i of Δ are given by

$$\left. \frac{\partial^2 \ell_{i\omega}}{\partial \boldsymbol{\theta} \partial \omega_i} \right|_{\omega_i=0} = \mathbf{0}, \tag{22.3}$$

$$\left. \frac{\partial^2 \ell_{i\omega}}{\partial \boldsymbol{\psi} \partial \omega_i} \right|_{\omega_i=0} = -\sum_{j=2}^{n_i} \boldsymbol{h}_{ij} y_{ij} g(\boldsymbol{h}_{ij})[1 - g(\boldsymbol{h}_{ij})], \tag{22.4}$$

for complete sequences (no dropout) and by

$$\left. \frac{\partial^2 \ell_{i\omega}}{\partial \boldsymbol{\theta} \partial \omega_i} \right|_{\omega_i=0} = [1 - g(\boldsymbol{h}_{id})] \frac{\partial \lambda(y_{id}|\boldsymbol{h}_{id})}{\partial \boldsymbol{\theta}}, \tag{22.5}$$

$$\left. \frac{\partial^2 \ell_{i\omega}}{\partial \boldsymbol{\psi} \partial \omega_i} \right|_{\omega_i=0} = -\sum_{j=2}^{d-1} \boldsymbol{h}_{ij} y_{ij} g(\boldsymbol{h}_{ij})[1 - g(\boldsymbol{h}_{ij})]$$
$$- \boldsymbol{h}_{id} \lambda(y_{id}|\boldsymbol{h}_{id}) g(\boldsymbol{h}_{id})[1 - g(\boldsymbol{h}_{id})], \tag{22.6}$$

for incomplete sequences. All the above expressions are evaluated at $\widehat{\boldsymbol{\gamma}}$, and $g(\boldsymbol{h}_{ij}) = g(\boldsymbol{h}_{ij}, y_{ij})|_{\omega_i=0}$ is the MAR version of the dropout model. In (22.5), we make use of the conditional mean

$$\lambda(y_{id}|\boldsymbol{h}_{id}) = \lambda(y_{id}) + V_{i,21} V_{i,11}^{-1} [\boldsymbol{h}_{id} - \lambda(\boldsymbol{h}_{id})]. \tag{22.7}$$

The variance matrices follow from partitioning the responses as $(y_{i1}, \ldots, y_{i,d-1}|y_{id})'$.

The derivatives of (22.7) with respect to the measurement model parameters are

$$\frac{\partial \lambda(y_{id}|\boldsymbol{h}_{id})}{\partial \boldsymbol{\beta}} = \boldsymbol{x}_{id} - V_{i,21} V_{i,11}^{-1} X_{i,(d-1)},$$

$$\frac{\partial \lambda(y_{id}|\boldsymbol{h}_{id})}{\partial \boldsymbol{\alpha}} = \left[\frac{\partial V_{i,21}}{\partial \boldsymbol{\alpha}} - V_{i,21} V_{i,11}^{-1} \frac{\partial V_{i,11}}{\partial \boldsymbol{\alpha}} \right] V_{i,11}^{-1} [\boldsymbol{h}_{id} - \lambda(\boldsymbol{h}_{id})],$$

where $\boldsymbol{x}'_{id}$ is the dth row of X_i, $X_{i,(d-1)}$ indicates the first $d-1$ rows X_i, and $\boldsymbol{\alpha}$ indicates the subvector of covariance parameters within the vector $\boldsymbol{\theta}$.

In practice, the parameter $\boldsymbol{\theta}$ in the measurement model is often of primary interest. Since $\ddot{L}$ is block-diagonal with blocks $\ddot{L}(\boldsymbol{\theta})$ and $\ddot{L}(\boldsymbol{\psi})$, we have that for any unit vector $\boldsymbol{h}$, $C_{\boldsymbol{h}}$ equals $C_{\boldsymbol{h}}(\boldsymbol{\theta}) + C_{\boldsymbol{h}}(\boldsymbol{\psi})$, with

$$C_{\boldsymbol{h}}(\boldsymbol{\theta}) = -2\boldsymbol{h}' \left[\left. \frac{\partial^2 \ell_{i\omega}}{\partial \boldsymbol{\theta} \partial \omega_i} \right|_{\omega_i=0} \right]' \ddot{L}^{-1}(\boldsymbol{\theta}) \left[\left. \frac{\partial^2 \ell_{i\omega}}{\partial \boldsymbol{\theta} \partial \omega_i} \right|_{\omega_i=0} \right] \boldsymbol{h} \tag{22.8}$$

$$C_{\boldsymbol{h}}(\boldsymbol{\psi}) = -2\boldsymbol{h}' \left[\left. \frac{\partial^2 \ell_{i\omega}}{\partial \boldsymbol{\psi} \partial \omega_i} \right|_{\omega_i=0} \right]' \ddot{L}^{-1}(\boldsymbol{\psi}) \left[\left. \frac{\partial^2 \ell_{i\omega}}{\partial \boldsymbol{\psi} \partial \omega_i} \right|_{\omega_i=0} \right] \boldsymbol{h}, \tag{22.9}$$

evaluated at $\gamma = \widehat{\gamma}$. It now immediately follows from (22.3) and (22.5) that *direct* influence on θ only arises from those measurement occasions at which dropout occurs. In particular, from (22.5) it is clear that the corresponding contribution is large only if (1) the dropout probability was small but the subject disappeared nevertheless and (2) the conditional mean 'strongly depends' on the parameter of interest. This implies that complete sequences cannot be influential in the strict sense ($C_i(\theta) = 0$) and that incomplete sequences only contribute, in a direct fashion, at the actual dropout time. However, we make an important distinction between direct and indirect influence. It was shown that complete sequences can have an impact by changing the conditional expectation of the unobserved measurements given the observed ones *and given the dropout mechanism*. Thus, a complete observation which has a strong impact on the *dropout model parameters* can still drastically change the measurement model parameters and functions thereof.

Expressions (22.8)–(22.9) can be simplified further in specific cases. For example, Verbeke *et al.* (2001b) considered the compound symmetry setting for which they were able to split the overall influence into the approximate sum of three components, describing the mean model parameter β, the variance components σ^2 and τ^2, and the dropout model parameters ψ, respectively:

$$C_i^{\mathrm{ap}}(\beta) = 2[1 - g(\mathbf{h}_{id})]^2 (\xi_{id}\mathbf{x}_{id} + (1 - \xi_{id})\boldsymbol{\rho}_{id})'$$

$$\times \sigma^2 \left[\sum_{i=1}^{N} \left(\xi_{id} X'_{i(d-1)} X_{i(d-1)} + (1 - \xi_{id}) R'_{i(d-1)} R_{i(d-1)} \right) \right]^{-1}$$

$$\times (\xi_{id}\mathbf{x}_{id} + (1 - \xi_{id})\boldsymbol{\rho}_{id}), \tag{22.10}$$

$$C_i^{\mathrm{ap}}(\sigma^2, \tau^2) = 2[1 - g(\mathbf{h}_{id})]^2 \xi_{id}^2 (1 - \xi_{id})^2 [\widetilde{\mathbf{h}_{id} - \lambda(\mathbf{h}_{id})}]^2$$

$$\times \left(-1, \frac{1}{\tau^2} \right) \ddot{L}^{-1}(\sigma^2, \tau^2) \begin{pmatrix} -1 \\ 1 \\ \frac{1}{\tau^2} \end{pmatrix}, \tag{22.11}$$

$$C_i(\psi) = 2 \left(\sum_{j=2}^{d} \mathbf{h}_{ij} y_{ij} v_{ij} \right)' \left(\sum_{i=1}^{N} \sum_{j=2}^{d} v_{ij} \mathbf{h}_{ij} \mathbf{h}'_{ij} \right)^{-1}$$

$$\times \left(\sum_{j=2}^{d} \mathbf{h}_{ij} y_{ij} v_{ij} \right), \tag{22.12}$$

where $R_{i,d-1} = X_{i(d-1)} - \mathbf{1}_{d-1}\widetilde{X_{i(d-1)}}$, $\widetilde{X_{i(d-1)}} = \frac{1}{d-1}\mathbf{1}'_{d-1}X_{i(d-1)}$,

$$[\widetilde{\mathbf{h}_{id} - \lambda(\mathbf{h}_{id})}] = \frac{1}{d-1}\mathbf{1}'_{d-1}[\mathbf{h}_{id} - \lambda(\mathbf{h}_{id})],$$

$$\ddot{L}(\sigma^2, \tau^2) = \sum_{i=1}^{N} \frac{d-1}{2(\sigma^2 + (d-1)\tau^2)^2}$$
$$\times \begin{pmatrix} \sigma^2 + (d-1)\tau^2 - \tau^2 2\sigma^2 + (d-1)\tau^2 & 1 \\ 1 & d-1 \end{pmatrix},$$

$d = n_i$ for a complete case and where y_{id} needs to be replaced with

$$\lambda(y_{id}|\mathbf{h}_{id}) = \lambda(y_{id}) + (1 - \xi_{id})[\widetilde{\mathbf{h}_{id} - \lambda(\mathbf{h}_{id})}]$$

for incomplete sequences. Furthermore, v_{ij} equals $g(h_{ij})[1 - g(h_{ij})]$, which is the variance of the estimated dropout probability under MAR.

22.2.2 The special case of three measurements

In this section, we consider the special but insightful case of three measurement occasions, using the three-dimensional version of the linear mixed model (Section 7.3), where V_i follows a heterogeneous first-order autoregressive structure:

$$V_i = .5 \begin{pmatrix} \sigma_1^2 & \rho\sigma_1\sigma_2 & \rho^2\sigma_1\sigma_3 \\ \rho\sigma_1\sigma_2 & \sigma_2^2 & \rho\sigma_2\sigma_3 \\ \rho^2\sigma_1\sigma_3 & \rho\sigma_2\sigma_3 & \sigma_3^2 \end{pmatrix}.$$

Furthermore, we assume the following specific version of dropout model (22.1):

$$\text{logit}\,[P(D_i = j|D_i \geq j, \mathbf{y}_i)] = \psi_0 + \psi_1 y_{i,j-1} + \psi_2 y_{ij}. \tag{22.13}$$

As there are three measurements (Y_{i1}, Y_{i2}, Y_{i3}), three different situations can arise: (1) all three measurements are available (a completer); (2) only the first two measurements are available and the subject drops out after the second time point; or (3) only the first measurement is available, which means the subject drops out after the first measurement. In the first case, the components of the columns $\boldsymbol{\Delta}_i$ of $\boldsymbol{\Delta}$ are given by (22.3) and (22.4), and using (22.13) one obtains

$$g(\mathbf{h}_{ij}) = g(\mathbf{h}_{ij}, y_{ij})|_{\omega_i=0} = \frac{\exp(\psi_0 + \psi_1 y_{i,j-1})}{1 + \exp(\psi_0 + \psi_1 y_{i,j-1})}.$$

In the case of dropout, the components of the columns $\boldsymbol{\Delta}_i$ of $\boldsymbol{\Delta}$ are given by (22.5) and (22.6), which means we need $V_{i,11}$, $V_{i,21}$, and their derivatives with respect to the four variance components σ_1, σ_2, σ_3, and ρ.

Now, to get expressions for $\mathbf{h}_{id}$, $\lambda(y_{id})$, $\lambda(\mathbf{h}_{id})$, $V_{i,11}$, $V_{i,21}$, and their derivatives, we distinguish between dropout after the first measurement $(d = 2)$ and dropout after the second $(d = 3)$.

When $d = 2$, we have $\boldsymbol{h}_{id} = y_{i1}$, and since the mean of the measurement model is $X_i\boldsymbol{\beta}$, $\lambda(y_{id})$ equals the second value of $X_i\boldsymbol{\beta}$, whereas $\lambda(\boldsymbol{h}_{id})$ equals the first value of $X_i\boldsymbol{\beta}$. Further, $V_{i,11} = \sigma_1^2$, and $V_{i,21} = \rho\sigma_1\sigma_2$, and thus the derivatives are

$$\frac{\partial V_{i,11}}{\partial\sigma_1} = 2\sigma_1, \quad \frac{\partial V_{i,11}}{\partial\sigma_2} = \frac{\partial V_{i,11}}{\partial\sigma_3} = \frac{\partial V_{i,11}}{\partial\rho} = 0,$$

$$\frac{\partial V_{i,21}}{\partial\sigma_1} = \rho\sigma_2, \quad \frac{\partial V_{i,21}}{\partial\sigma_2} = \rho\sigma_1,$$

$$\frac{\partial V_{i,21}}{\partial\sigma_3} = 0, \quad \frac{\partial V_{i,21}}{\partial\rho} = \sigma_1\sigma_2.$$

Next, for the case $d = 3$, we have $\boldsymbol{h}_{id} = (y_{i1}, y_{i2})'$, $\lambda(y_{id})$ equals the third value of $X_i\boldsymbol{\beta}$, whereas $\lambda(\boldsymbol{h}_{id})$ is the vector of the first and second values of $X_i\boldsymbol{\beta}$. Furthermore,

$$V_{i,11} = \begin{pmatrix} \sigma_1^2 & \rho\sigma_1\sigma_2 \\ \rho\sigma_1\sigma_2 & \sigma_2^2 \end{pmatrix} \quad \text{and} \quad V_{i,21} = \begin{pmatrix} \rho^2\sigma_1\sigma_3 & \rho\sigma_2\sigma_3 \end{pmatrix},$$

and thus the derivatives are written as

$$\frac{\partial V_{i,11}}{\partial\sigma_1} = \begin{pmatrix} 2\sigma_1 & \rho\sigma_2 \\ \rho\sigma_2 & 0 \end{pmatrix}, \quad \frac{\partial V_{i,11}}{\partial\sigma_2} = \begin{pmatrix} 0 & \rho\sigma_1 \\ \rho\sigma_1 & 2\sigma_2 \end{pmatrix},$$

$$\frac{\partial V_{i,11}}{\partial\sigma_3} = \begin{pmatrix} 0 & 0 \\ 0 & 0 \end{pmatrix}, \quad \frac{\partial V_{i,11}}{\partial\rho} = \begin{pmatrix} 0 & \sigma_1\sigma_2 \\ \sigma_1\sigma_2 & 0 \end{pmatrix},$$

$$\frac{\partial V_{i,21}}{\partial\sigma_1} = \begin{pmatrix} \rho^2\sigma_3 & 0 \end{pmatrix}, \quad \frac{\partial V_{i,21}}{\partial\sigma_2} = \begin{pmatrix} 0 & \rho\sigma_3 \end{pmatrix},$$

$$\frac{\partial V_{i,21}}{\partial\sigma_3} = \begin{pmatrix} \rho^2\sigma_1 & \rho\sigma_2 \end{pmatrix}, \quad \frac{\partial V_{i,21}}{\partial\rho} = \begin{pmatrix} 2\rho\sigma_1\sigma_3 & \sigma_2\sigma_3 \end{pmatrix}.$$

Using all of this information, we can easily derive expressions (22.5) and (22.6), that is, the components of the columns $\boldsymbol{\Delta}_i$ of $\boldsymbol{\Delta}$.

We will calculate the following normal curvatures in the direction of the unit vector $\boldsymbol{h}_i$ containing one in the ith position and zero elsewhere: C_i, $C_i(\boldsymbol{\beta})$, $C_i(\boldsymbol{\alpha})$, $C_i(\boldsymbol{\theta})$, and $C_{\boldsymbol{h}}(\boldsymbol{\psi})$, as well as the normal curvature in the direction of $\boldsymbol{h}_{\max}$ of maximal normal curvature $C_{\max}$.

22.3 MASTITIS IN DAIRY CATTLE

The Mastitis data were introduced in Section 2.4. Diggle and Kenward (1994) and Kenward (1998) performed several analyses of these data. These are reviewed in Section 22.3.1. Local influence ideas are applied in Section 22.3.2.

22.3.1 Informal sensitivity analysis

In Diggle and Kenward (1994) a separate mean for each group defined by the year of first lactation and a common time effect was considered, together with an unstructured 2×2 covariance matrix. The dropout model included both Y_{i1} and Y_{i2} and was reparameterized in terms of the size variable $(Y_{i1} + Y_{i2})/2$ and the increment $Y_{i2} - Y_{i1}$. It turned out that the increment was important, in contrast to a relatively small contribution of the size. If this model were deemed to be plausible, MAR would be rejected on the basis of a likelihood ratio test statistic of $G^2 = 5.11$ on 1 degree of freedom.

Kenward (1998) carried out what we term a data-driven sensitivity analysis. He started from the original model in Diggle and Kenward (1994), albeit with a common intercept, since there was no evidence for a dependence on first lactation year. The right-hand panel of Figure 2.2 shows that there are two cows, nos 4 and 5, with unusually large increments. He conjectured that this might mean that these animals were ill during the first lactation year, producing an unusually low yield, whereas a normal yield was obtained during the second year. He then fitted t distributions to Y_{i2} given $Y_{i1} = y_{i1}$. Not surprisingly, his finding was that the heavier the tails of the t distribution, the better the outliers were accommodated. As a result, the difference in fit between the random and non-random dropout models vanished ($G^2 = 1.08$ for a t_2 distribution). Alternatively, removing these two cows and refitting the normal model shows complete lack of evidence for nonrandom dropout ($G^2 = 0.08$). The latter procedure is similar to a global influence analysis by means of deleting two observations. Parameter estimates and standard errors for random and non-random dropout, under several deletion schemes, are reproduced in Table 22.1. It is clear that the influence on the measurement model parameters is small in the random dropout case, although the gap on the time effect β_d between the random and non-random dropout models is reduced when cows4 and cows5 are removed.

We now look in more detail at these informal but insightful forms of sensitivity analysis. A simple bivariate Gaussian linear model is used to represent the marginal milk yield in the 2 years (i.e., the yield that would be, or was, observed in the absence of mastitis):

$$\begin{pmatrix} Y_1 \\ Y_2 \end{pmatrix} = N \left[\begin{pmatrix} \mu \\ \mu + \Delta \end{pmatrix}, \begin{pmatrix} \sigma_1^2 & \rho\sigma_1\sigma_2 \\ \rho\sigma_1\sigma_2 & \sigma_2^2 \end{pmatrix} \right].$$

Note that the parameter Δ represents the change in average yield between the 2 years. The probability of mastitis is assumed to follow the logistic regression model:

$$P(\text{dropout}) = \frac{e^{\psi_0 + \psi_1 y_1 + \psi_2 y_2}}{1 + e^{\psi_0 + \psi_1 y_1 + \psi_2 y_2}}. \tag{22.14}$$

Table 22.1 Mastitis in dairy cattle. Maximum likelihood estimates (standard errors) of random and non-random dropout models, under several deletion schemes.

Random dropout

Parameter	All	(53, 54, 66, 69)	(4, 5)	(66)	(4, 5, 66)
Measurement model					
β_0	5.77 (0.09)	5.69 (0.09)	5.81 (0.08)	5.75 (0.09)	5.80 (0.09)
β_d	0.72 (0.11)	0.70 (0.11)	0.64 (0.09)	0.68 (0.10)	0.60 (0.08)
σ_1^2	0.87 (0.12)	0.76 (0.11)	0.77 (0.11)	0.86 (0.12)	0.76 (0.11)
σ_2^2	1.30 (0.20)	1.08 (0.17)	1.30 (0.20)	1.10 (0.17)	1.09 (0.17)
ρ	0.58 (0.07)	0.45 (0.08)	0.72 (0.05)	0.57 (0.07)	0.73 (0.05)
Dropout model					
ψ_0	−2.65 (1.45)	−3.69 (1.63)	−2.34 (1.51)	−2.77 (1.47)	−2.48 (1.54)
ψ_1	0.27 (0.25)	0.46 (0.28)	0.22 (0.25)	0.29 (0.24)	0.24 (0.26)
$\omega = \psi_2$	0	0	0	0	0
−2 log-likelihood	280.02	246.64	237.94	264.73	220.23

Non-random dropout

Parameter	All	(53, 54, 66, 69)	(4, 5)	(66)	(4, 5, 66)
Measurement model					
β_0	5.77 (0.09)	5.69 (0.09)	5.81 (0.08)	5.75 (0.09)	5.80 (0.09)
β_d	0.33 (0.14)	0.35 (0.14)	0.40 (0.18)	0.34 (0.14)	0.63 (0.29)
σ_1^2	0.87 (0.12)	0.76 (0.11)	0.77 (0.11)	0.86 (0.12)	0.76 (0.11)
σ_2^2	1.61 (0.29)	1.29 (0.25)	1.39 (0.25)	1.34 (0.25)	1.10 (0.20)
ρ	0.48 (0.09)	0.42 (0.10)	0.67 (0.06)	0.48 (0.09)	0.73 (0.05)
Dropout model					
ψ_0	0.37 (2.33)	−0.37 (2.65)	−0.77 (2.04)	0.45 (2.35)	−2.77 (3.52)
ψ_1	2.25 (0.77)	2.11 (0.76)	1.61 (1.13)	2.06 (0.76)	0.07 (1.82)
$\omega = \psi_2$	−2.54 (0.83)	−2.22 (0.86)	−1.66 (1.29)	−2.33 (0.86)	0.20 (2.09)
−2 log-likelihood	274.91	243.21	237.86	261.15	220.23
G^2 for MNAR	5.11	3.43	0.08	3.57	0.005

The combined response/dropout model was fitted to the milk yields by maximum likelihood using a generic function maximization routine. In addition, the MAR model ($\psi_2 = 0$) was fitted. The latter is equivalent to fitting separately the Gaussian linear model for the milk yields and logistic regression model for the occurrence of mastitis. These fits produced the parameter estimates as displayed in the 'all' column of Table 22.1, standard errors and minimized value of twice the negative log-likelihood.

Using the likelihoods to compare the fit of the two models, we get a difference $G^2 = 5.11$. The corresponding tail probability from χ_1^2 is 0.02. This test essentially examines the contribution of ψ_2 to the fit of the model. Using the Wald statistic for the same purpose gives a statistic of $(-2.53)^2/0.83 = 9.35$, with corresponding χ_1^2 probability of 0.002. The discrepancy between the results of the two tests suggests that the asymptotic approximations on which these are based are not very accurate in this setting and the standard error probably underestimates the true variability of the estimate of ψ_2. Indeed, we showed in

Section 19.6 that such tests do not have the usual properties of likelihood ratio and Wald tests in regular problems. Nevertheless, there is a suggestion from the change in likelihood that ψ_2 is making a real contribution to the fit of the model. The dropout model estimated from the MNAR setting is as follows:

$$\text{logit}[P(\text{mastitis})] = 0.37 + 2.25y_1 - 2.54y_2. \tag{22.15}$$

Some insight into this fitted model can be obtained by rewriting it in terms of the milk yield totals $(Y_1 + Y_2)$ and increments $(Y_2 - Y_1)$:

$$\text{logit}[P(\text{mastitis})] = 0.37 - 0.145(y_1 + y_2) - 2.395(y_2 - y_1). \tag{22.16}$$

The probability of mastitis increases with larger negative increments; that is, those animals who showed (or would have shown) a greater decrease in yield over the 2 years have a higher probability of getting mastitis. The other differences in parameter estimates between the two models are consistent with this: the MNAR dropout model predicts a smaller average increment in yield (Δ), with larger second-year variance and smaller correlation caused by greater negative imputed differences between yields.

To get further insight into these two fitted models, we now take a closer look at the raw data and the predictive behaviour of the Gaussian MNAR model. Under an MNAR model, the predicted, or imputed, value of a missing observation is given by the ratio of expectations

$$\widehat{\boldsymbol{y}}_m = \frac{E_{Y_m|Y_o}[\boldsymbol{y}_m P(\boldsymbol{r} \mid \boldsymbol{y}_o, \boldsymbol{y}_m)]}{E_{Y_m|Y_o}[P(\boldsymbol{r} \mid \boldsymbol{y}_o, \boldsymbol{y}_m)]}. \tag{22.17}$$

Recall that the fitted dropout model (22.15) implies that the probability of mastitis increases with decreasing values of the increment $Y_2 - Y_1$. We therefore plot the 27 imputed values of this quantity together with the 80 observed increments against the first year yield Y_1. This plot is shown in Figure 22.1, in which the imputed values are indicated with triangles and the observed values with crosses. Note how the imputed values are almost linear in Y_1: this is a well-known property of the ratio (22.17) within this range of observations. The imputed values are all negative, in contrast to the observed increments, which are nearly all positive. With animals of this age, one would normally expect an increase in yield between the two years. The dropout model is imposing highly atypical behaviour on these animals and this corresponds to the statistical significance of the MNAR component of the model (ψ_2) but, of course, necessitates further scrutiny.

Another feature of this plot is the pair of outlying observed points circled in the top left-hand corner. These two animals have the lowest and third lowest yields in the first year, but moderately large yields in the second, leading to the largest positive increments. In a well-husbanded dairy herd, one would expect approximately Gaussian joint milk yields, and these two then represent outliers.

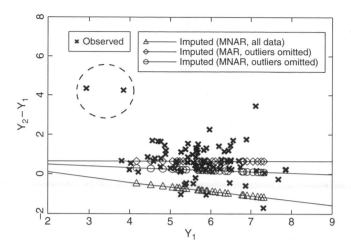

Figure 22.1 Mastitis in dairy cattle. Plot of observed and imputed year 2 − year 1 yield differences against year 1 yield. Two outlying points are circled.

It is likely that there is some anomaly, possibly illness, leading to their relatively low yields in the first year. One can conjecture that these two animals are the cause of the structure identified by the Gaussian MNAR model. Under the joint Gaussian assumption, the MNAR model essentially 'fills in' the missing data to produce a complete Gaussian distribution. To counterbalance the effect of these two extreme positive increments, the dropout model predicts negative increments for the mastitic cows, leading to the results observed. As a check on this conjecture, we omit these two animals from the data set and refit the MAR and MNAR Gaussian models. The resulting estimates are presented in the '(4,5)' column of Table 22.1.

The deviance is minimal and the MNAR model now shows no improvement in fit over MAR. The estimates of the dropout parameters, although still moderately large in an absolute sense, are of the same size as their standard errors which, as mentioned earlier, are probably underestimates. In the absence of the two anomalous animals, the structure identified earlier in terms of the MNAR dropout model no longer exists. The increments imputed by the fitted model are also plotted in Figure 22.1, indicated by circles. Although still lying in the lower region of the observed increments, these are now all positive and lie close to the increments imputed by the MAR model (diamonds). Thus, we have a plausible representation of the data in terms of joint Gaussian milk yields, two pairs of outlying yields and no requirement for an MNAR dropout process.

The two key assumptions underlying the outcome-based MNAR model are, first, the form chosen for the relationship between dropout probability and response and, second, the distribution of the response or, more precisely, the conditional distribution of the possibly unobserved response given the observed response. In the current setting for the first assumption, if there is dependence of mastitis occurrence on yield, experience with logistic regression tells us that the exact form of the link function in this relationship is unlikely to be critical. In terms of sensitivity, we therefore consider the second assumption, the distribution of the response.

All the data from the first year are available, and a normal probability plot of these (Figure 22.2), does not show great departures from the Gaussian assumption. Leaving this distribution unchanged, we therefore examine the effect of changing the conditional distribution of Y_2 given Y_1. One simple and obvious choice is to consider a heavy-tailed distribution, and for this we use the translated and scaled t_m distribution with density

$$f(y_2 \mid y_1) = \left\{ \sigma \sqrt{m} B(1/2, m/2) \right\}^{-1} \left\{ 1 + \frac{1}{m} \left(\frac{y_2 - \mu_{2\mid1}}{\sigma} \right)^2 \right\}^{-(m+1)/2},$$

where

$$\mu_{2\mid1} = \mu + \Delta + \frac{\rho \sigma_2 (y_1 - \mu)}{\sigma_1}$$

is the conditional mean of $Y_2 \mid y_1$. The corresponding conditional variance is

$$\frac{m}{m-2} \sigma^2.$$

Relevant parameter estimates from the fits of both MAR and MNAR models are presented in Table 22.2 for three values of m: 2, 10, and 25. Smaller values of m correspond to greater kurtosis and, as m becomes large, the model approaches

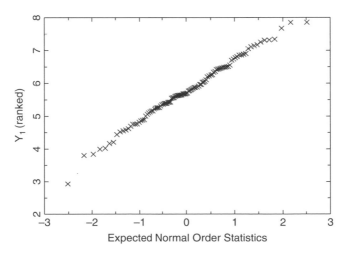

Figure 22.2 Mastitis in dairy cattle. Normal probability plot of the year 1 milk yields.

Table 22.2 Mastitis in dairy cattle. Details of the fit of MAR and MNAR dropout models, assuming a t_m distribution for the conditional distribution of Y_2 given Y_1. Maximum likelihood estimates (standard errors) are shown.

t d.f.	Parameter	MAR	MNAR
25	Δ	0.69 (0.10)	0.35 (0.13)
	ψ_1	0.27 (0.24)	2.11 (0.78)
	ψ_2		−2.33 (0.88)
−2 log-likelihood		275.54	271.77
10	Δ	0.67 (0.09)	0.38 (0.14)
	ψ_1	0.27 (0.24)	1.84 (0.82)
	ψ_2		−1.96 (0.95)
−2 log-likelihood		271.22	269.12
2	Δ	0.61 (0.08)	0.54 (0.11)
	ψ_1	0.27 (0.24)	0.80 (0.66)
	ψ_2		−0.65 (0.73)
−2 log-likelihood		267.87	266.79

the Gaussian one used in the previous section. It can be seen from the results for the MNAR model in Table 22.2 that as the kurtosis increases the estimate of ψ_2 decreases. Also, the maximized likelihoods of the MAR and MNAR models converge. With 10 and 2 degrees of freedom, there is no evidence at all to support the inclusion of ψ_2 in the model; that is, the MAR model provides as good a description of the observed data as the MNAR, in contrast to the Gaussian-based conclusions. Further, as m decreases, the estimated yearly increment in milk yield Δ from the MNAR model increases to the value estimated under the MAR model. In most applications of selection models, it will be quantities of this type that will be of prime interest, and it is clearly seen in this example how the dropout model can have a crucial influence on the estimate of this. Comparing the values of the deviance from the t-based model with those from the original Gaussian model, we also see that the former with $m = 10$ or 2 produces a slightly better fit, although no meaning can be attached to the statistical significance of the difference in these likelihood values.

The results observed here are consistent with those from the deletion analysis. The two outlying pairs of measurements identified earlier are not inconsistent with the heavy-tailed t distribution; so no 'filling in' would be required and hence no evidence for non-randomness in the dropout process under the second model. In conclusion, if we consider the data with outliers included, we have two models that effectively fit the observed data equally well. The first assumes a joint Gaussian distribution for the responses and a MNAR dropout model. The second assumes a Gaussian distribution for the first observation and a conditional t_m distribution (with small m) for the second given the first, with no requirement for a MNAR dropout component. Each provides a different explanation for what has been observed, with quite a different biological interpretation. In likelihood terms, the second model fits a little better than the first but, as has been stressed repeatedly in this book, a key feature of such dropout models is that the distinction between them should not be based on the observed data likelihood alone. As we have shown in Chapter 19, it is always possible to specify models with identical maximized observed data likelihoods that differ with respect to the unobserved data and dropout mechanism, and such models can have very different implications for the underlying mechanism generating the data. Finally, the most plausible explanation for the observed data is that the pairs of milk yields have joint Gaussian distributions, with no need for an MNAR dropout component, and that two animals are associated with anomalous pairs of yields.

22.3.2 Local influence approach

In the previous subsection, the sensitivity to distributional assumptions of conclusions concerning the randomness of the dropout process has been established in the context of the mastitis data. Such sensitivity has led some to conclude that such modelling should be avoided. We have argued that this conclusion is too strong. First, repeated measures tend to be incomplete and therefore consideration of the dropout process is simply unavoidable. Second, if a non-random dropout component is added to a model and the maximized likelihood changes appreciably, then some real structure in the data has been identified that is not encompassed by the original model. The MNAR analysis may tell us about inadequacies of the original model rather than the adequacy of the MNAR model. It is the interpretation of the identified structure that cannot be made unequivocally from the data under analysis. The mastitis data clearly illustrate this: using external information on the distribution of the response, a plausible explanation of the structure so identified *might* be made in terms of the outlying responses from two animals. However, it should also be noted that absence of structure in the data associated with an MNAR process does not imply that an MNAR process is not operating: different models with similar maximized likelihoods (i.e., with similar plausibility with respect to the observed data) may have completely different implications for the dropout process and the unobserved data. These points together suggest that the appropriate role of such modelling is as a component of a sensitivity analysis; we return to these issues later in Chapter 23.

The analysis of the previous section is characterized by its basis within substantive knowledge about the data. In this section, we will apply the local influence technique to the mastitis data, and see how the results compare with those found in Section 22.3.1. We suggest that here a combination of methodology and substantive insight will be the most fruitful approach.

Applying the local influence method to the mastitis data produces Figure 22.3, which suggests that there are four influential animals: 53, 54,

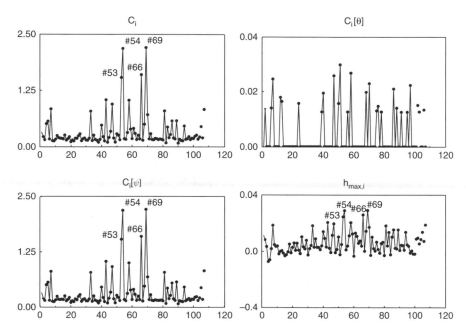

Figure 22.3 Mastitis in dairy cattle. Index plots of C_i, $C_i(\theta)$, $C_i(\psi)$, and of the components of the direction $\boldsymbol{h}_{max}$ of maximal curvature, when the dropout model is parameterized in terms of Y_{i1} and Y_{i2}.

66, and 69. The most striking feature of this analysis is that 4 and 5 are *not* recovered (see also Figure 2.2). It is interesting to consider an analysis with these four cows removed. Details are given in Table 22.1. In contrast to the consequences of removing 4 and 5, the influence on the likelihood ratio test is rather small: $G^2 = 3.43$ instead of the original 5.11. The influence on the measurement model parameters under both random and non-random dropout is small.

It is very important to realize that one should not expect agreement between deletion and our local influence analysis. The latter focuses on the sensitivity of the results with respect to the assumed dropout model; more specifically, on how the results change when the MAR model is extended in the direction of non-random dropout. In particular, all animals singled out so far are complete and hence $C_i(\boldsymbol{\theta}) \equiv 0$, placing all influence on $C_i(\boldsymbol{\psi})$ and $\boldsymbol{h}_{max,i}$. A comparison between local influence and deletion is given in Section 22.5.

Greater insight can also be obtained by studying the approximation for $C_i(\boldsymbol{\psi})$, derived by Verbeke *et al.* (2001b):

$$C_i(\boldsymbol{\psi}) \simeq 2(V_i y_{i2}^2) \left\{ V_i \boldsymbol{h}'_i \left(\sum_{i=1}^{N} V_i \boldsymbol{h}_i \boldsymbol{h}'_i \right)^{-1} \boldsymbol{h}_i \right\}, \qquad (22.18)$$

where the factor in braces equals the hat-matrix diagonal and $V_i = g(y_{i1})[1 - g(y_{i1})]$. For a dropout, y_{i2} has to be replaced by its conditional expectation. The contribution for animal i is made up of three factors. The first factor, V_i, is small for extreme dropout probabilities. The animals that have a very high probability of either remaining or leaving the study are less influential. Cows 4 and 5 have dropout probabilities equal to 0.13 and 0.17, respectively. The 107 cows in the study span the dropout probability interval [0.13, 0.37]. Thus, this component rather deflates the influence of 4 and 5. Second, (22.18) contains a leverage factor in braces. Third, an animal is relatively more influential when both milk yields are high. We now need to question whether this is plausible or relevant. Since both measurements are positively correlated, measurements with both milk yields high or low will not be unusual. In Section 22.3.1, we observed that cows 4 and 5 are unusual on the basis of their *increment*. This is in line with several other applications of similar dropout models (Diggle and Kenward 1994; Molenberghs *et al.* 1997) where it was found that a strong incremental component pointed to genuine non-randomness. In contrast, if correlations among succeeding measurements are not low, the size variable can often be replaced by just the history and hence the corresponding model is very close to random dropout.

Even though a dropout model expressed in terms of the outcomes themselves is equivalent to a model in the first variable Y_{i1} and the increment $Y_{i2} - Y_{i1}$, termed the incremental variables representation, we will show that they lead to different perturbation schemes of the form (22.1). At first, this feature can be seen as both an advantage and a disadvantage. The fact that reparameterizations of the linear predictor of the dropout model lead to different perturbation schemes requires careful reflection based on substantive knowledge in order to guide the analysis, such as the considerations on the incremental variable made earlier.

We will present the results of the incremental analysis and then offer further comments on the rationale behind this particular transformation. From the diagnostic plots in Figure 22.4, it is obvious that we recover three influential animals: 4, 5, and 66. Although Kenward (1998) did not consider 66 to be influential, it does appear to be somewhat distant from the bulk of the data (Figure 2.2). The main difference between both types is that the first two were plausibly ill during year 1, and this is not necessarily so for 66. An additional feature is that in all cases both $C_i(\psi)$ and $\mathbf{h}_{\max}$ show the same influential animals. In addition, $\mathbf{h}_{\max}$ suggests that the influence for cow 66 is different than for the others. It could be conjectured that the latter one pulls the coefficient ω in a different direction. The other values are all relatively small. This could indicate that for the remaining 104 animals, MAR is plausible, whereas a deviation in the direction of the incremental variable, *with differing signs*, appears to be necessary for animals 4, 5, and 66. At this point, a comparison between $\mathbf{h}_{\max}$ for the direct variable and incremental analyses is useful. Since the contributions h_i sum to 1, these two plots are directly comparable. There is no pronounced

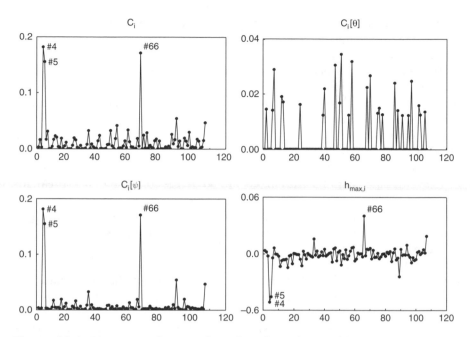

Figure 22.4 Mastitis in dairy cattle. Index plots of C_i, $C_i(\theta)$, $C_i(\psi)$, and of the components of the direction $\boldsymbol{h}_{\max}$ of maximal curvature, when the dropout model is parameterized in terms of Y_{i1} and $Y_{i2} - Y_{i1}$.

influence indication in the direct variables case and perhaps only random noise is seen. A more formal way to distinguish between signal and noise needs to be developed.

In Figure 22.5 we have decomposed (22.18) into its three components: the variance of the dropout probability V_i, the incremental variable $Y_{i2} - Y_{i1}$, which is replaced by its predicted value for a dropout, and the hat-matrix diagonal. In agreement with the preceding discussion, the influence clearly stems from an unusually large increment, which overcomes the fact that V_i actually downplays the influence because Y_{41} and Y_{51} are comparatively small, and dropout increases with the milk yield in the first year. Furthermore, a better interpretation can be made for the difference in sign of $h_{\max,4}$ and $h_{\max,5}$ versus $h_{\max,66}$.

We have noted already that animals 4 and 5 have relatively small dropout probabilities. In contrast, the dropout probability of 66 is large within the observed range [0.13, 0.37]. As the increment is large for these animals, changing the perturbation ω_i can have a large impact on the other dropout parameters ψ_0 and ψ_1. In order to avoid having the effects of the change for cows 4 and 5 cancel with the effect of 66, the corresponding signs need to be reversed. Such a change implies either that all three dropout probabilities move toward the centre of the range or are pulled away from it. (Note

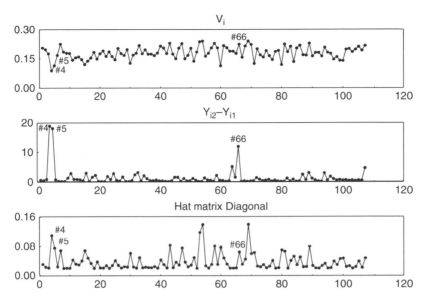

Figure 22.5 Mastitis in dairy cattle. Index plots of the three components of $C_i(\psi)$ when the dropout model is parameterized in terms of Y_{i1} and $Y_{i2} - Y_{i1}$.

that $-\boldsymbol{h}_{\max}$ is another normalized eigenvector corresponding to the largest eigenvalue.)

In the informal approach, extra analyses were carried out with cows 4 and 5 removed. The resulting likelihood ratio statistic reduces to $G^2 = 0.08$. When only cow 66 is removed, the likelihood ratio for non-random dropout is $G^2 = 3.57$, very similar to the one when 53, 54, 66, and 69 were removed. Removing all three (4, 5, and 66) results in $G^2 = 0.005$, indicating the complete disappearance of all evidence for non-random dropout. Details are given in Table 22.1.

We now explore the reasons why the transformation of direct outcomes to increments is useful. We have noted already that the associated perturbation schemes (22.1) are different. An important device in this respect is the equality

$$\psi_0 + \psi_1 y_{i1} + \psi_2 y_{i2} = \psi_0 + (\psi_1 + \psi_2) y_{i1} + \psi_2 (y_{i2} - y_{i1}). \qquad (22.19)$$

Equation (22.19) shows that the direct variables model can be used to assess the influence on the random dropout parameter ψ_1, whereas the equivalent statement for the incremental model is the random dropout parameter $\psi_1 + \psi_2$. Not only is this a different parameter, it is also estimated with higher precision. One often observes that $\widehat{\psi}_1$ and $\widehat{\psi}_2$ exhibit a similar variance and (strongly) negative correlation, in which case the linear combination with smallest variance is approximately in the direction of the sum $\psi_1 + \psi_2$. When the correlation is positive, the difference direction $\psi_1 - \psi_2$ is obtained instead.

Let us assess this in the case where all 107 observations are included. The estimated covariance matrix is

$$\begin{pmatrix} 0.59 & -0.54 \\ & 0.70 \end{pmatrix},$$

with correlation -0.84. The variance of $\widehat{\psi}_1 + \widehat{\psi}_2$, on the other hand, is estimated to be 0.21. In this case, the direction of minimal variance is along the direction (0.74, 0.67), which is indeed close to the sum direction. When all three influential subjects are removed, the estimated covariance matrix becomes

$$\begin{pmatrix} 3.31 & -3.77 \\ & 4.37 \end{pmatrix},$$

with correlation -0.9897. Removing only cows 4 and 5 yields an intermediate situation for which the results are not shown. The variance of the sum is 0.15, which is a further reduction and still close to the direction of minimal variance. These considerations reinforce the claim that an incremental analysis is strongly advantageous. It might therefore be interesting to routinely construct a plot such as in Figure 2.2 or Figure 22.1, with even longer measurement sequences. On the other hand, transforming the dropout model to a size variable $(Y_{i1} + Y_{i2})/2$ will worsen the problem since a poorly estimated parameter associated with Y_{i1} will result.

Finally, observe that a transformation of the dropout model to a size and incremental variable at the same time for the model with all three influential subjects removed gives a variance of the size and increment variables of 0.15 and 15.22, respectively. In other words, there is no evidence for an incremental effect, confirming that MAR is plausible.

Although local and global influence are, strictly speaking, not equivalent, it is useful to see how the global influence on $\boldsymbol{\theta}$ can be linked to the behaviour of $C_i(\boldsymbol{\psi})$. We observed earlier that all locally influential animals are completers and hence $C_i(\boldsymbol{\theta}) \equiv 0$. Yet, removing cows 4, 5, and 66 shows some effect on the discrepancy between the random dropout (MAR) and non-random dropout (MNAR) estimates of the time effect β_d. In particular, MAR and MNAR estimates with all three subjects removed are virtually identical (0.60 and 0.63, respectively). Let us do a small thought experiment. Since these animals are influential in $C_i(\boldsymbol{\psi})$, the MAR model could be improved by including incremental terms for these three. Such a model would still imply random dropout. In contrast, allowing a dependence on the increment in *all* subjects will influence $E(Y_{i2}|y_{i1}, \text{dropout})$ for all incomplete observations; hence, the measurement model parameters under MNAR will change. In conclusion, this provides a way to assess the *indirect* influence of the dropout mechanism on the measurement model parameters through local influence methods. In the milk yield data set, this influence is likely to be due to the fact that an exceptional increment which is caused by a different mechanism, perhaps a diseased animal during the first year, is nevertheless treated on an equal footing with the other observations within the dropout model. Such an investigation cannot be done with the case-deletion method because it is not possible to disentangle the various sources of influence.

In conclusion, it is found that an incremental variable representation of the dropout mechanism has advantages over a direct variable representation. Contrasting our local influence approach with a case-deletion scheme as applied in Kenward (1998), it is argued that the former approach is advantageous since it allows one to assess direct and indirect influences on the dropout and measurement model parameters, stemming from perturbing the random dropout model in the direction of non-random dropout. In contrast, a case-deletion scheme does not allow one to disentangle the various sources of influence.

22.4 ALTERNATIVE LOCAL INFLUENCE APPROACHES

The perturbation scheme used throughout this chapter has several elegant properties. The perturbation is around the MAR mechanism, which is often deemed a sensible starting point for an analysis. Additional calculations are limited and free of numerical integration. Influence decomposes into measurement and dropout parts, the first of which is zero in the case of a complete observation. Finally, if the special case of compound symmetry is assumed, the measurement part can approximately be written in interpretable components for the fixed-effects and variance component parts.

However, it is worthwhile considering alternative schemes as well. Most of the developments presented here can be adapted to such alternatives, although not all schemes will preserve the remarkable computational convenience. Also, interpretation of the influence expressions in an alternative scheme will require additional work.

Apart from MAR, MCAR may also considered a useful assumption in some settings. It is then natural to consider departures from the MCAR model, rather than from the MAR model. This would change (22.1) to

$$\text{logit}(g(\mathbf{h}_{ij}, y_{ij})) = \text{logit}\left[P(D_i = j | D_i \geq j, \mathbf{y}_i)\right]$$
$$= \mathbf{h}_{ij}\boldsymbol{\psi} + \omega_{i1}y_{i,j-1} + \omega_{i2}y_{ij}, \tag{22.20}$$

with an obvious change in the definition of $\mathbf{h}_{ij}$. In this way, the perturbation parameter becomes a two-component vector $\boldsymbol{\omega}_i = (\omega_{i1}, \omega_{i2})$. As a consequence, the ith subject produces a pair (h_{i1}, h_{i2}), which is a normalized vector, and hence the main interest lies in its direction. Also, $C_{\mathbf{h}} = C_i$ is the local influence on $\widehat{\boldsymbol{\gamma}}$ of allowing the ith subject to drop out randomly or non-randomly. Figure 22.6 shows the result of this procedure, applied to the mastitis data. Pairs (h_{i1}, h_{i2}) are plotted. The main diagonal corresponds to the size direction, whereas the other diagonal represents the purely incremental direction. Circles are used to indicate

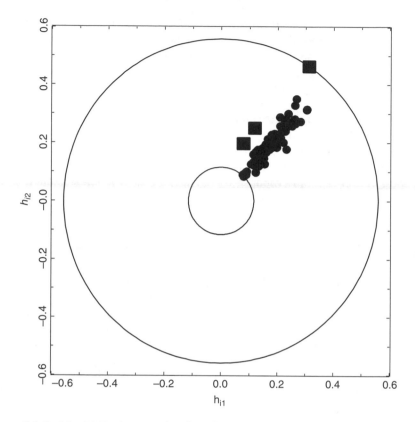

Figure 22.6 Mastitis in dairy cattle. Plot of C_i in the direction of $\mathbf{h}_i$.

the minimal and maximal distances to the origin. Finally, squares are used for animals 4, 5, and 66. Most animals lie in the *size direction*, but it is noticeable that 4, 5, and 66 tend toward the non-random direction. Furthermore, in this case, no excessively large C_i are seen.

Another extension would result from the observation that the choice of the incremental analysis in Section 22.3.2 may seem rather arbitrary, although motivated by substantive insight. Hence, it would be desirable to have a more automatic, data-driven selection of a direction. One way of doing this is to consider

$$\text{logit}(g(\mathbf{h}_{ij}, y_{ij})) = \text{logit}\left[P(D_i = j | D_i \geq j, \boldsymbol{y}_i)\right]$$
$$= \mathbf{h}_{ij}\boldsymbol{\psi} + \omega_i(\sin \theta y_{i,j-1} + \cos \theta y_{ij}). \qquad (22.21)$$

Now, it is possible to apply (22.21) for a selected number of angles θ, to range through a fine grid covering the entire circle, or to consider θ as another influence parameter. In the latter case, θ becomes subject-specific and the pair (ω_i, θ_i) is essentially a reparameterization of the pair $\boldsymbol{\omega}_i = (\omega_{i1}, \omega_{i2})$ in (22.21).

In a completely different local influence approach one would modify the general form (3.15) as follows:

$$f(\boldsymbol{y}_i^o, \boldsymbol{r}_i | \boldsymbol{\theta}, \boldsymbol{\psi}, \omega_i) = \int f(\boldsymbol{y}_i^o, \boldsymbol{y}_i^m | X_i \boldsymbol{\theta}) f(\boldsymbol{r}_i | \boldsymbol{y}_i^o, \boldsymbol{y}_i^m, W_i, \boldsymbol{\psi})^{\omega_i} d\boldsymbol{y}_i^m. \qquad (22.22)$$

Now, if $\omega_i = 0$, then the missing data process is considered random and only the measurement process is considered. If $\omega_i = 1$, the posited, potentially non-random, model is considered. Other values of ω_i correspond to partial case weighting.

22.5 THE MILK PROTEIN CONTENT TRIAL

Diggle (1990) and Diggle and Kenward (1994) analysed data taken from Verbyla and Cullis (1990), who, in turn, had obtained the data from a workshop at Adelaide University in 1989. The data consist of assayed protein content of milk samples taken weekly for 19 weeks from 79 Australian cows. The cows entered the experiment after calving and were randomly allocated to one of three diets: barley (25 animals), mixed barley and lupins (27), and lupins alone (27). The time profiles for all 79 cows are plotted in Figure 22.7. All cows remained on study during the first 14 weeks, following which the sample

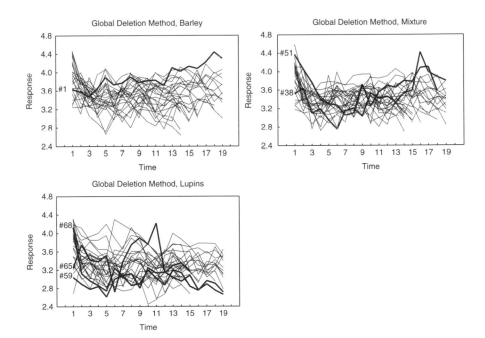

Figure 22.7 Milk protein content trial. Individual profiles, with globally influential subjects highlighted. Dropout modelled from week 15.

Table 22.3 Milk protein content trial. Dropout pattern and number of cows for each arm.

	Diet		
Dropout week	**Barley**	**Mixed**	**Lupins**
15	6	7	7
16	2	3	4
17	2	1	1
18			
19	2	2	1
Completers	13	14	14
Total	25	27	27

reduced to 59, 50, 46, 46, and 41, respectively, due to dropout. This means that dropout is as high as 48% by the end of the study. Table 22.3 shows the dropout pattern and the number of cows for each arm.

The primary objective of the milk protein experiment was to describe the effects of diet on the mean response profile of milk protein content over time. Previous analyses of the same data are reported by Diggle (1990, Chapter 5), Verbyla and Cullis (1990), Diggle *et al.* (1994), and Diggle and Kenward (1994), under different assumptions and with different modelling of the dropout process. Diggle (1990) assumed random dropout, whereas Diggle and Kenward (1994) concluded that dropout was non-random, based on their selection model. Once more, we supplement such an analysis with sensitivity analysis tools.

In addition to the usual problems with this type of model, serious doubts were raised about even the appropriateness of the 'dropout' concept in this study. In fact, unknown to the authors of the original papers, the animals did not drop out at all, but rather five cohorts started at different times. Interestingly, this was only revealed by Cullis (1994), the supplier of the data, in the light of the apparent non-random dropout identified by Diggle and Kenward (1994). Cullis knew from nature of the trial that non-random dropout was highly implausible, and an alternative reason lay behind the structure identified in the MNAR analysis. It was the search for this that led Cullis to uncover the actual cohort structure, which did imply that there were issues both with the original MAR analysis of Diggle (1990) and the later MNAR analysis. This illustrates well the point made in Section 22.3.2 that apparent evidence for an MNAR structure may indicate genuine lack of fit of a posited MAR model, but the interpretation of the identified structure as evidence of MNAR dropout cannot be made unequivocally without additional assumptions. In this case external information (which should have been present from the start) indicated that such an interpretation was quite wrong.

The initial, incomplete, description of the trial that produced these data is the main cause for so many conflicting issues related to their analysis. For this reason also it is a good candidate for sensitivity analysis. Modelling will be based upon the linear mixed-effects model with serial correlation, such as in (7.7). In Section 22.5.1 we examine the validity of the conclusions made in Diggle and Kenward (1994) by incorporating subject-matter information into the method of analysis, which was not available to the original authors. As dropout was due to design, the method of analysis should reflect this. We will investigate two approaches. The first approach involves restructuring the data set and then analysing the resulting data set using a selection modelling framework, whereas the second method involves fitting pattern-mixture models taking the missingness pattern into account. Both analyses consider the sequences as *unbalanced in length* rather than a formal instance of dropout. Local and global influence diagnostics are presented in Section 22.5.2.

22.5.1   Informal sensitivity analysis

The following is based on the most complete information that is now available about the trial. Several matched paddocks are randomly assigned to either of three diets: barley, lupins, or a mixture of the two. The experiment starts as the first cow experiences calving. As the first 5 weeks have passed, all 79 cows have entered their randomly assigned, randomly cultivated paddock. By week 19, all paddocks appear to approach the point of exhausting their food availability (in a synchronous fashion) and the experiment is terminated for all animals simultaneously.

Previously published analyses of these data wrongly assumed a fixed date for entry into the trial, and the crucial issue for these was how the dropout process should be accommodated. However, once we know that entry into the study was at random time points (i.e., after calving) and that the experiment was terminated at a fixed time, it is appropriate to take this time as the reference point. Given this, an attractive approach to the analysis is to reverse the time axis and to analyse the data in reverse, starting from the final reference time. Given the true structure of the trial, we find a partial solution to the problem because dropout has been replaced by ragged entry. Indeed, a crucial simplification now arises. Because entry into the trial depends solely on calving and gestation, it can be considered to be totally independent of the unobserved responses.

A problem with the alignment lies in the fact that virtually all cows showed a very steep decrease in milk protein content immediately after calving, lasting until the third week into the experiment. This behaviour could be due to a special hormone regulation of milk composition following calving, which lasts only for a few weeks. Such a process is most likely totally independent of diet and, probably, can also be observed in the absence of food, at the expense of the animal's natural reserves. Since entry is now ragged, the process is spread and influences the mean response level during the first 8 weeks. Of course, one might construct an appropriate model for the first 3 weeks with a separate model specification, by analogy with the one used in Diggle and Kenward (1994). Instead, we prefer to ignore the first 3 weeks, analogously in spirit to the approach taken in Verbyla and Cullis (1990). Hence, we have time series of length 16, with some observations missing at the beginning. Figure 22.8 displays the data manipulations for five selected cows. In Figure 22.8(a) the raw profiles are shown. In Figure 22.8(b) the plots are right aligned. Figure 22.8(c) illustrates the protein content levels for the five cows with the first three observations deleted, and Figure 22.8(d) presents these profiles when time is reversed.

To explore the patterns after transformation, we have plotted the newly obtained mean profiles. Figures 22.9(a) and 22.9(b) display the mean profiles before and after the transformation, respectively. Notice that the mean profiles have become parallel in Figure 22.9(b). To address the issue of correlation, we shall compare the corresponding two variograms (Verbeke and Molenberghs 2000; Diggle *et al.* 2002). The two graphs shown in Figure 22.10 are very similar, although slight differences can be noted in the estimated process variance, which is slightly lower after transformation. Complete decay of serial correlation appears to happen between time lags 9 and 10 in both variograms.

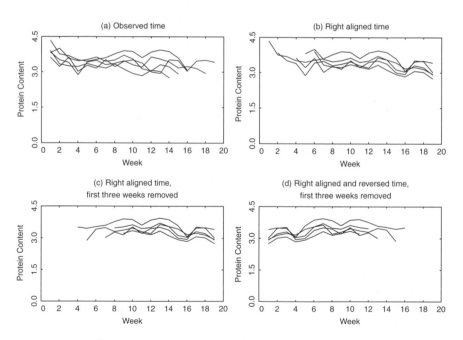

Figure 22.8 Milk protein content trial. Data manipulations on five selected cows: (a) raw profiles; (b) right aligned profiles; (c) deletion of the first three observations; (d) profiles with time reversal.

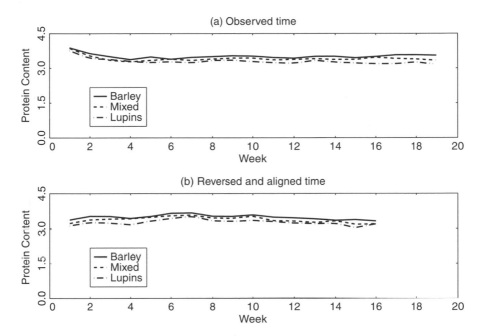

Figure 22.9   Milk protein content trial. Mean response profiles (a) on the original data and (b) after alignment and reversal.

There is virtually no evidence for random effects as the serial correlation levels off towards the process variance.

Table 22.4 presents maximum likelihood estimates for the original data, similar to the analysis by Diggle and Kenward (1994). The corresponding parameters after alignment and reversal are 3.45 (s.e. 0.06) for the barley group, with differences for the lupins and mixed groups estimated to be −0.21 (s.e. 0.08) and −0.12 (s.e. 0.08), respectively. The variance parameters roughly retain their relative magnitude, although even more weight is given to the serial process (90% of the total variance).

The analysis using aligned and reversed data shows little difference if compared to the original analysis by Diggle and Kenward (1994). It would be interesting to acquire knowledge about what mechanisms determined the systematic increase and decrease observed for the three parallel profiles illustrated in Figure 22.9(b). It is difficult to envisage that the parallelism of the profiles and their systematic peaks and troughs shown in Figure 22.8(b) is due entirely to chance. Indeed, many of the previous analyses debated the influence on variability for those factors common to the paddocks cultivated with the three different diets, such as meteorological factors, not reported by the experimenter. These factors may account for a large amount of variability in the data. Hence, the data exploration performed in this analysis may be

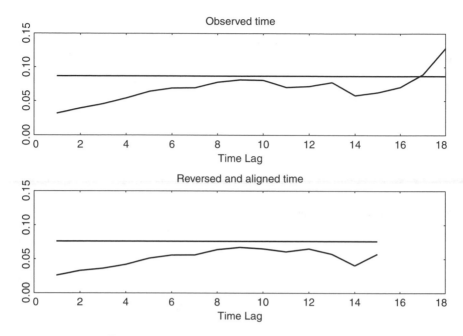

Figure 22.10 Milk protein content trial. Variogram for the original data and after alignment and reversal.

Table 22.4 Milk protein content trial. Maximum likelihood estimates (standard errors) of random and nonrandom dropout models. Dropout starts from week 15 onward.

Effect	Parameter	MAR	MNAR
Measurement model			
Barley	μ_1	4.147 (0.053)	4.152 (0.053)
Mixed	μ_2	4.046 (0.052)	4.050 (0.052)
Lupins	μ_3	3.935 (0.052)	3.941 (0.052)
Time effect	β	−0.226 (0.015)	−0.224 (0.015)
Random intercept variance	d	−0.001 (0.010)	0.002 (0.009)
Measurement error variance	σ^2	0.024 (0.002)	0.025 (0.002)
Serial variance	τ^2	0.073 (0.012)	0.067 (0.011)
Serial correlation	ρ	0.152 (0.037)	0.163 (0.039)
Dropout model			
Intercept	ψ_0	17.870 (3.147)	15.642 (3.535)
Previous measurement	ψ_1	−6.024 (0.998)	−10.722 (2.015)
Current measurement	ψ_2		5.176 (1.487)
−2 log-likelihood		51.844	37.257

shown to be a useful tool in gaining insight about the response process. For example, we note that after transformation, the inexplicable trend towards an increase in milk protein content, as the paddocks approach exhaustion, has in fact vanished or even reverted to a possible decrease. This was also confirmed in the stratified analysis where the protein level content tended to decrease prior to termination of the experiment (see Figure 22.11).

An alternative method of analysis is based on the premise that the protein content levels form distinct homogeneous subgroups for cows based on their cohort pattern. This leads very naturally to pattern-mixture models (Chapter 16). Marginal regression parameters are now made to depend on pattern. In its general form, the fixed-effects as well as the covariance parameters are allowed to vary unconstrained according to the dropout pattern. Alternatively, simplifications can be sought. For example, diet effect can vary linearly with pattern or can be pattern-independent. In the latter case, this effect becomes marginal. When the diet effect is pattern-dependent, an extra calculation is necessary to obtain the marginal diet effect. Details can be found in Section 16.6.2: specifically, the marginal effect can be computed as in (16.15), whereas the delta method variance expression is given by (16.16).

Denoting the parameter for diet effect $\ell = 1, 2$ (difference with respect to the barley group) in pattern $t = 1, 2, 3$ by $\beta_{\ell t}$ and letting π_t be the proportion of cows in pattern t, then the matrix A in (16.18) assumes the form

$$A = \frac{\partial(\beta_1, \beta_2)}{\partial(\beta_{11}, \beta_{12}, \beta_{13}, \beta_{21}, \beta_{22}, \beta_{23}, \pi_1, \pi_2, \pi_3)}$$
$$= \begin{pmatrix} \pi_1 & \pi_2 & \pi_3 & 0 & 0 & 0 & \beta_{11} & \beta_{12} & \beta_{13} \\ 0 & 0 & 0 & \pi_1 & \pi_2 & \pi_3 & \beta_{21} & \beta_{22} & \beta_{23} \end{pmatrix}.$$

Note that the simple multinomial model for the dropout probabilities could be extended when additional information concerning the dropout mechanism. For example, if covariates are known or believed to influence dropout, the simple multinomial model can be replaced by logistic regression or time-to-event methods (Hogan and Laird 1997).

Recall that Table 22.3 presents the dropout pattern by time in each of the three diet groups. As few dropouts occurred in weeks 16, 17, and 19, these three dropout patterns were collapsed into a single pattern. Thus, three patterns remain with 20, 18, and 41 cows, respectively. The model-fitting results are presented in Table 22.5. The most complex model for the mean structure assumes a separate mean for each diet by time by dropout pattern combination. As the variogram indicated no random effects, the covariance matrix was taken as first-order autoregressive with a residual variance term $\sigma_{jk} = \sigma^2 \rho^{|j-k|}$. Also the variance–covariance parameters are allowed to vary according to the dropout pattern. This model is equivalent to including time and diet as covariates in the model and stratifying for dropout pattern, and it provides a starting point for

Table 22.5 Milk protein content trial. Model fit summary for pattern-mixture models. (Ref., reference model for likelihood ratio test; AR(1) refers to first-order auto-regressive serial structure; meas refers to measurement error.)

	Mean	Covariance	No. of parameters	-2ℓ	Ref.	G^2	d.f.	p
1	Full interaction	AR1(t), meas(t)	162	−474.93				
2	Full interaction	AR1(t), meas	160	−470.79	1	4.44	2	0.111
3	Full interaction	AR(1), meas	156	−428.26	2	42.23	4	<0.001
4	Two-way interactions	AR1(t), meas	100	−439.96	2	30.53	50	0.987
5	Diet, time, pattern, diet×time, diet×pattern	AR1(t), meas	70	−202.40	4	237.56	30	<0.001
6	Diet, time, pattern, diet×time, time × pattern	AR1(t), meas	96	−430.55	4	9.41	4	0.052
7	Diet, time, pattern, diet × pattern, time × pattern	AR1(t), meas	64	−404.04	4	35.92	36	0.472
8	Time, pattern, time × pattern	AR1(t), meas	58	−378.22	7	25.82	6	<0.001
					6	52.33	38	0.061
9	Time, diet(time)	AR(1), meas	60					
10	Time, diet	AR(1), meas	24					

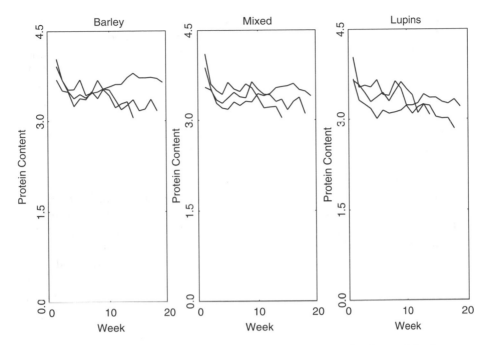

Figure 22.11 Milk protein content trial. Mean response level by diet and by dropout pattern.

model simplification through backward selection. We refer to the description of Strategy 2b in Section 16.4. The protein content levels over time are presented by pattern and diet in Figure 22.11. Note that the protein content profiles appear to vary considerably according to missingness pattern and time. Additionally, Diggle and Kenward (1994) suggested an increase in protein content level towards the end of the experiment. This observation is not consistent for the three plots in Figure 22.11. In fact, there is a tendency for a decrease in all diet by pattern subgroups prior to dropout.

To simplify the covariance structure presented in model 1, model 2 assumes the residual covariance parameter is equal in the three patterns. The likelihood ratio test indicates that model 2 compares favourably with model 1, suggesting a common residual variance (measurement error component) parameter (2 for the three groups; see Table 22.5 for details). However, comparing model 3 with model 2, we reject a common variance–covariance structure in the three groups.

Next, we investigate the mean structure. In model 4, the three-way interaction among pattern, time, and diet is removed. This simplified model is acceptable when contrasted with model 2, based on $p = 0.987$. Models 5, 6, and 7 are fitted to investigate the pairwise interaction terms. Comparing models 5 and 4 suggests a strong interaction between dropout pattern and time. Model 6 results in a borderline decrease in goodness of fit ($p = 0.052$). From Table 22.5, we observe that model 7 is a plausible simplification of model 4. Moreover, there is an apparent lack of fit for model 8, which includes only one interaction term, time by pattern, when compared to model 7. In conclusion, among the models presented, model 7 is the preferred one to summarize the data, as it is the simplest model consistent with the data. However, model 6 should be given some attention as well. By analogy with Diggle and Kenward (1994), we attempted to include time as a separate linear factor for the first 3 weeks and the subsequent 16 weeks. These models did not improve the fit (results not shown).

Recall that the objective of the experiment was to assess the influence of diet on protein content level. With selection models, the corresponding null hypothesis of no effect can be tested using, for example, the standard F tests on 2 numerator degrees of freedom as provided by the SAS procedure MIXED or similar software. In the pattern-mixture framework, such a standard test can be used only if the treatment effects do not interact with pattern. Otherwise, the marginal treatment (diet) effect has to be determined as in (16.15) and the delta method can be used to test the hypothesis of no effect. In model 6 the diet effect is independent of pattern, and the reverse holds for model 7. Reparameterizing model 6 by including the diet effect and diet-by-time interaction as one effect in the model provides us with an appropriate F test for the three diet profiles. The F test rejects the null hypothesis of no diet effect ($F = 1.57$ on 38 numerator degrees of freedom, $p = 0.015$). In the corresponding selection model, model 9, we remove all the terms from model 6 which include pattern. In that case, the F test is *not* significant ($F = 1.26$ on 38 numerator degrees of freedom, $p = 0.133$). The difference in the tests may be explained by the variance parameters which were larger in the selection model in the absence of stratification for pattern, thereby effectively diluting the strength of the difference. Additionally, the standard errors for the estimates of the fixed effects were slightly smaller in the pattern-mixture model. This is not surprising, as in the model fitting we found that the means and variance parameters were dependent on pattern. Thus, stratifying for pattern results in more homogeneous subgroups of cows, reducing the variance within each group and subsequently providing more precise estimates for the diet effect.

Using model 7, we test the global null hypothesis of no diet effect in any of the patterns. This analysis can be seen as a stratified analysis where a diet effect is estimated separately within each pattern. This model results in a significant F test for the diet effect ($F = 6.05$, on 6 numerator degrees of freedom, $p < 0.001$). Alternatively, we can consider the pooled estimate for the diet effect, provided by equation (16.15), and calculate the test statistic using the delta method. This test also indicates a significant diet effect ($F = 17.82$ on 2 numerator degrees of freedom, $p < 0.001$), as does the corresponding selection model, model 10 ($F = 8.51$ on 2 numerator degrees of freedom, $p < 0.001$).

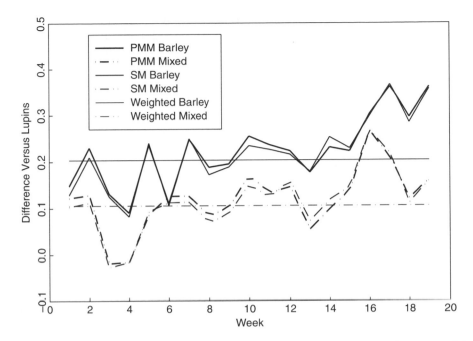

Figure 22.12 Milk protein content trial. Diet effect over time for the selection model (SM), the corresponding pattern-mixture model (PMM), and the estimate obtained after weighting the PMM contributions (weighted).

Figure 22.12 presents the diet by time parameter estimates for selection model 10, for the corresponding pattern-mixture model 7 and the weighted average estimates used in the delta method. The estimates for the selection model and the pattern-mixture model appear to differ only slightly. Since the model building within both families is done separately, this is a very reassuring sensitivity analysis outcome.

In conclusion, including pattern in the model improves the model fit significantly. In particular, the time-by-pattern and diet-by-pattern interactions are maintained in model 7, which is considered to be the most parsimonious model consistent with the data (Figure 22.11). In addition, the covariance parameters are also dependent on the missingness pattern. Dividing cows into more homogeneous groups based on their missingness patterns reduces the unexplained variation in the data and subsequently provides more precise parameter estimates.

This example and, in particular, the absence of genuine dropout illustrate once more that care has to be taken when analysing longitudinal outcomes with a non-rectangular structure.

The analyses discussed here provide an alternative to those obtained by Diggle and Kenward (1994), which it should be recalled relied on incomplete information about the actual conduct of the trial, but the conclusions are still fairly consistent. Rather, they convey the message that the use of sensitivity analysis should become standard practice when dropout occurs. We strongly stress the importance of careful data verification to be undertaken prior to any statistical analysis.

Our analysis of the correlation structure appears to agree with the general conclusions retained in the Diggle and Kenward (1994) analysis. Particularly, it is interesting to notice the absence of random effects. To explain the absence of random effects, we may assume that there were additional eligibility criteria for the trial (e.g., a specific breed of cow), which made random effects even more unlikely.

22.5.2 Formal sensitivity analysis

We now consider the more formal local and global influence analysis methods. Local influence was introduced in Section 22.2. For a global influence or case-deletion analysis we proceed as follows.

The best-known perturbation schemes are based on case deletion (Cook and Weisberg 1982; Chatterjee and Hadi 1988), in which the effect of completely removing cases from the analysis is studied. They were introduced by Cook (1977, 1979) for the linear regression context. Denote the likelihood function, corresponding to a linear mixed measurement model and dropout model (22.1), by

$$\ell(\boldsymbol{\gamma}) = \sum_{i=1}^{N} \ell_i(\boldsymbol{\gamma}), \tag{22.23}$$

in which $\ell_i(\boldsymbol{\gamma})$ is the contribution of the ith individual to the log-likelihood and where $\boldsymbol{\gamma} = (\boldsymbol{\theta}, \boldsymbol{\psi}, \omega)$ is the s-dimensional vector, grouping the parameters of the measurement model and the dropout model. Further, we denote by

$$\ell_{(-i)}(\boldsymbol{\gamma}) \tag{22.24}$$

the log-likelihood function where the contribution of the ith subject has been removed. Cook's distances (CD) are based on measuring the discrepancy between either the maximized likelihoods (22.23) and (22.24) or between (subsets of) the estimated parameter vectors $\widehat{\boldsymbol{\gamma}}$ and $\widehat{\boldsymbol{\gamma}}_{(-i)}$, with obvious notation. We consider both

$$\mathrm{CD}_{1i} = 2(\widehat{\ell} - \widehat{\ell}_{(-i)}) \tag{22.25}$$

and

$$\mathrm{CD}_2(\boldsymbol{\gamma}) = 2\,(\widehat{\boldsymbol{\gamma}} - \widehat{\boldsymbol{\gamma}}_{(-i)})'\ddot{L}^{-1}(\widehat{\boldsymbol{\gamma}} - \widehat{\boldsymbol{\gamma}}_{(-i)}). \tag{22.26}$$

Formulation (22.26) easily allows us to consider the global influence in a subvector of γ, such as the dropout parameters ψ, or the non-random parameter ω. This will be indicated using notation of the form $CD_{2i}(\psi)$, $CD_{2i}(\omega)$, and so forth.

Recall that Diggle and Kenward (1994) considered a linear mixed model where the mean model includes separate intercepts for the barley, mixed, and lupins groups, and a common time effect which is linear during the first 3 weeks and constant thereafter. The covariance structure is described by a random intercept, an exponential serial process, and measurement error. The dropout model includes dependence on the previous and current, possibly unobserved, measurements. Since dropout only happens from week 15 onwards, Diggle and Kenward (1994) chose to set the dropout probability for earlier occasions equal to zero. Thereafter, they allowed separate intercepts for each time point, but common dependencies on previous and current measurements. We will now introduce two models which use the same measurement model as Diggle and Kenward (1994) but different dropout models.

A first dropout model is closely related to that of Diggle and Kenward (1994), who defined occasion-specific intercepts ψ_{0k} ($k = 15, 16, 17, 19$), assumed slopes common, and set the dropout probability equal to zero at other occasions. We also model dropout from week 15 onwards, but we will keep the intercepts constant for occasions 15 to 19. Specifically, our first model contains three parameters (intercept ψ_0, dependence on the previous measurement ψ_1, and dependence on the current measurement ψ_2).

Parameter estimates for this model under both MAR and MNAR are listed in Table 22.4. The fitted model is qualitatively equivalent to the model used by Diggle and Kenward (1994), who concluded overwhelming evidence for non-random dropout (likelihood ratio statistic 13.9). In line with these results, we can also decide in favour of a nonrandom process (likelihood ratio statistic 14.59).

In our second dropout model, we allow dropout starting from the second week. Specifically, this model contains three parameters (intercept ψ_0, dependence on the previous measurement ψ_1, and dependence on the current measurement ψ_2) which are assumed constant throughout the whole 19-week period. The fit of this model is given in Table 22.6. A striking difference with the previous analysis is that the MAR assumption is borderline not rejected (likelihood ratio statistic 3.63). Apparently, this is a major source of sensitivity, to be explored further. As results from theory, the measurement model parameters do not change under the MAR model, compared to those displayed in Table 22.4. The measurement model obtained under MNAR has changed only slightly.

Which of the two analyses is to be preferred is debatable and depends on substantive rather than statistical considerations. The first analysis accounts for the *post hoc* observation that no dropout occurred prior to week 15. However, there is a (perhaps small) chance of the experiment terminating in a

Table 22.6 Milk protein content trial. Maximum likelihood estimates (standard errors) of random and nonrandom dropout models. Dropout starts from week 1 onwards.

Effect	Parameter	MAR	MNAR
Measurement model			
Barley	μ_1	4.147 (0.053)	4.152 (0.053)
Mixed	μ_2	4.046 (0.052)	4.050 (0.052)
Lupins	μ_3	3.935 (0.052)	3.941 (0.052)
Time effect	β	−0.226 (0.015)	−0.224 (0.015)
Random intercept variance	d	−0.001 (0.010)	0.002 (0.009)
Measurement error variance	σ^2	0.024 (0.002)	0.025 (0.002)
Serial variance	τ^2	0.073 (0.012)	0.067 (0.011)
Serial correlation	ρ	0.152 (0.037)	0.163 (0.040)
Dropout model			
Intercept	ψ_0	10.483 (2.010)	6.477 (2.867)
Previous measurement	ψ_1	−4.326 (0.651)	−5.917 (1.069)
Current measurement	ψ_2		2.732 (1.396)
−2 log-likelihood		194.316	190.691

particular field with less than 15 weeks of measurements, and our second model acknowledges this possibility. It is clear that there is an enormous sensitivity of the results due to this model choice and, therefore, an assessment of influence seems appropriate. In general, though, it may be questionable that the dropout model parameters remain constant over an extended period of time. Not only can the rate change over time, but also the dominant causes and the magnitude of their effect can change.

Global influence

Global influence results are shown in Figures 22.7, 22.13 and 22.14. They are based on fitting an MNAR model, with each of the cows deleted in turn. The Cook's distances for the first and second models are shown in Figure 22.13 and 22.14, respectively. The individual curves with influential subjects highlighted are plotted in Figure 22.7, where subject 38 should not be highlighted for the second model.

There is very little difference in some of the Cook's distance plots when Figures 22.13 and 22.14 are compared. Specifically, CD_{1i}, $CD_{2i}(\gamma)$, and $CD_{2i}(\theta)$ are virtually identical. The three others are similar in the sense that there is some overlap in the subjects indicated as peaks, but with varying magnitudes. Subject 38 is influential on the dropout measures $CD_{2,38}(\psi, \omega)$, $CD_{2,38}(\psi)$, and $CD_{2,38}(\omega)$. This is not surprising since this subject 38 is rather low in the middle portion of the measurement sequence, but very high from week 15 onwards. Therefore, this sequence is picked up in the second analysis only. By looking at a plot with the evolution of the parameters separately during the deletion process (not shown here), we can conclude that subject 38 has some impact on the serial correlation parameter while subject 65 is rather influential for the

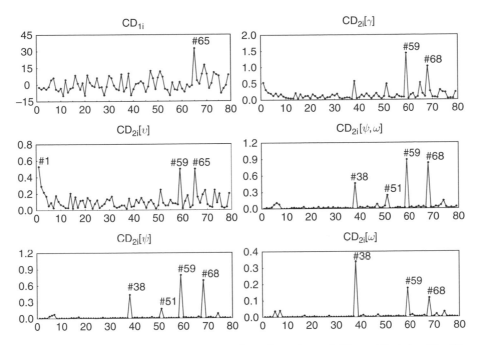

Figure 22.13 Milk protein content trial. Index plots of CD_{1i}, $CD_{2i}(\gamma)$, $CD_{2i}(\theta)$, $CD_{2i}(\psi, \omega)$, $CD_{2i}(\psi)$, and $CD_{2i}(\omega)$. Dropout modelled from week 15.

measurement error. In view of the fairly smooth deviation from a straight line of the former and the abrupt peaks in the latter, this is not a surprise.

Based on our second model, all forms of $CD_{2i}(\cdot)$, whether based on the entire parameter vector γ, the dropout parameters (ψ_0, ψ_1, ω), or subsets of the latter, indicate that subjects 51, 59, and 68 are influential. In contrast, CD_{1i}, which is based directly on the likelihood, does not reveal these subjects, but rather subject 65 stands out. Thus, although the former three subjects have a substantial impact on the parameter estimates, they do not change the likelihood in a noticeable fashion. From a plot of the dropout parameter estimates for each deleted case (not shown here), it is very clear that upward peaks in $\widehat{\psi}_{0(-i)}$ for subjects 51 and 59 are compensated with downward peaks in $\widehat{\omega}_{(-i)}$. An explanation for this phenomenon can be found in the variance–covariance matrix of the dropout parameters (correlations shown in the lower triangle):

$$\begin{pmatrix} 8.22 & 0.43 & -2.85 \\ (0.14) & 1.14 & -1.18 \\ (-0.71) & (-0.79) & 1.94 \end{pmatrix}.$$

From a principal components analysis, it follows that more than 90% of the variation is captured in the linear combination $0.93\psi_0 - 0.37\omega$. Hence, there is

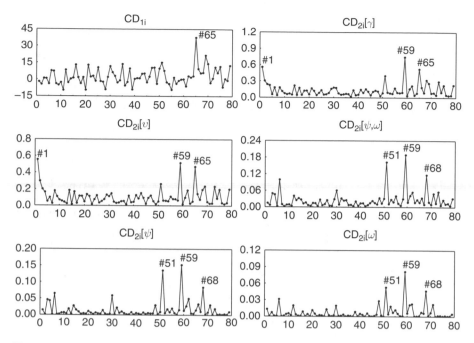

Figure 22.14 Milk protein content trial. Index plots of CD_{1i}, $CD_{2i}(\gamma)$, $CD_{2i}(\theta)$, $CD_{2i}(\psi, \omega)$, $CD_{2i}(\psi)$, and $CD_{2i}(\omega)$. Dropout modelled from week 1.

mass transfer between these two parameters, of course with sign reversal, little impact on the likelihood value, and little effect on the MAR parameter ψ_1. Note that a similar plot for the measurement model parameters can be constructed (not shown).

Let us now turn to the subjects which are globally influential. A first and common reason for those subjects to show up is the fact that they all have a rather strange profile. Remember that the overall trend is sloping downwards during the first 3 weeks and constant thereafter. Subject 65 appears with large $CD_{65,1}$ and large $CD_2(\theta)$. The reason for this can be found in the fact that its profile shows extremely low and high peaks. Subjects 51, 59, and 68, on the other hand, only show large values for $CD_2(\psi, \omega)$, $CD_2(\psi)$, $CD_2(\omega)$. This means that these subjects are influential for the dropout parameters. For subject 51, this can be explained by the fact that it drops out in spite of the rather large profile. Subjects 59 and 68, on the contrary, stay in the experiment even though they both have rather low profiles.

Local influence

Local influence plots and individual profiles, with the influential subjects highlighted, for the first model for raw and incremental data, respectively, are depicted in Figures 22.15–22.18. Corresponding graphs for our second model

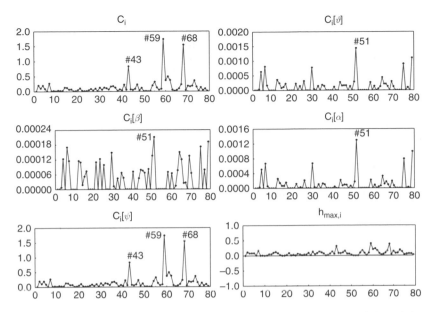

Figure 22.15 Milk protein content trial. Index plots of C_i, $C_i(\boldsymbol{\theta})$, $C_i(\boldsymbol{\beta})$, $C_i(\boldsymbol{\alpha})$, and $C_i(\boldsymbol{\psi})$, and of the components of the direction $\boldsymbol{h}_{\max}$ of maximal curvature. Dropout modelled from week 15.

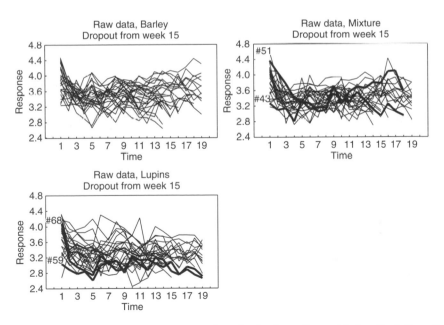

Figure 22.16 Milk protein content trial. Individual profiles, with locally influential subjects highlighted. Dropout modelled from week 15.

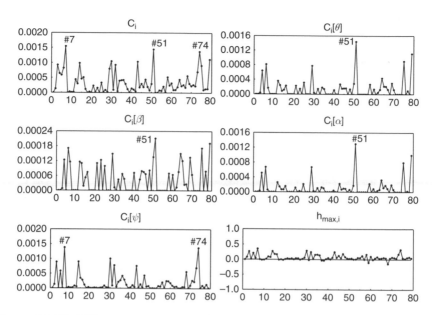

Figure 22.17 Milk protein content trial. Index plots of C_i, $C_i(\theta)$, $C_i(\beta)$, $C_i(\alpha)$, and $C_i(\psi)$, and of the components of the direction $\mathbf{h}_{\max}$ of maximal curvature. Dropout modelled from week 15. Incremental analysis.

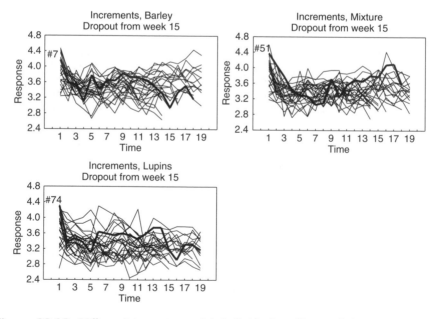

Figure 22.18 Milk protein content trial. Individual profiles, with locally influential subjects highlighted. Dropout modelled from week 15. Incremental analysis.

are shown in Figures 22.19–22.22. It is more convenient to discuss results of the second model up front and then compare them to the first model.

Observe that the plots for C_i and $C_i(\boldsymbol{\psi})$ are virtually identical. This is due to the relative magnitudes of the $\boldsymbol{\psi}$ and $\boldsymbol{\theta}$ components. Profiles 51, 59, and 66–68 are highlighted in Figure 22.20. A good feel for when $C_i(\boldsymbol{\psi})$ is large is obtained by approximating $h_{ij}y_{ij}v_{ij}$ by

$$F(y) = y^2 g(1-g), \qquad (22.27)$$

which is based on the assumption that previous and current measurements are approximately equal. Indeed, for ψ_0 and ψ_1 as in Table 22.6, the maximum is obtained for $y = 2.51$, exactly as seen in the influential profiles, which are all in the lupins group (Figure 22.20). Further, note that there is some agreement between the locally and globally influential subjects, although there is no compelling need for the two approaches to be identical (subject 51 appears in different influential components in the two approaches). Indeed, although global influence lumps together all sources of influence, our local influence approach is designed to detect subjects which, due to several causes, tend to have a strong impact on ω and therefore on the conclusion about the nature of the dropout mechanism.

Observe that one factor in (22.27) is the square of the response. This is a direct consequence of our parameterization of the dropout process, the logit of which

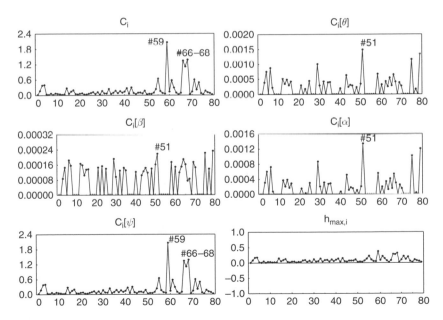

Figure 22.19 Milk protein content trial. Index plots of C_i, $C_i(\boldsymbol{\theta})$, $C_i(\boldsymbol{\beta})$, $C_i(\boldsymbol{\alpha})$, and $C_i(\boldsymbol{\psi})$, and of the components of the direction $\boldsymbol{h}_{\max}$ of maximal curvature. Dropout modelled from week 1.

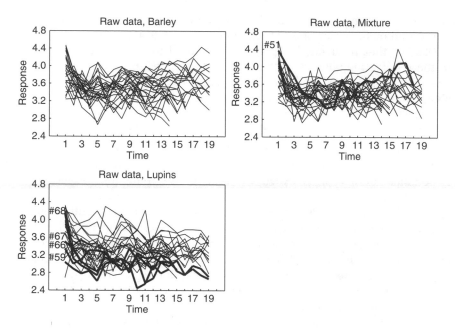

Figure 22.20 Milk protein content trial. Individual profiles, with locally influential subjects highlighted. Dropout modelled from week 1.

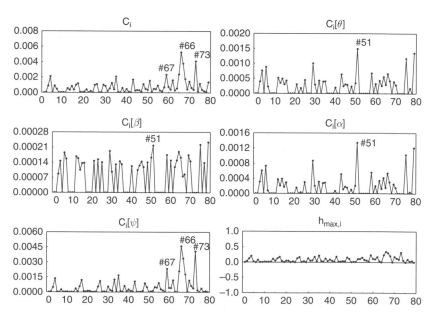

Figure 22.21 Milk protein content trial. Index plots of C_i, $C_i(\theta)$, $C_i(\beta)$, $C_i(\alpha)$, and $C_i(\psi)$, and of the components of the direction $\boldsymbol{h}_{\max}$ of maximal curvature. Dropout modelled from week 1. Incremental analysis.

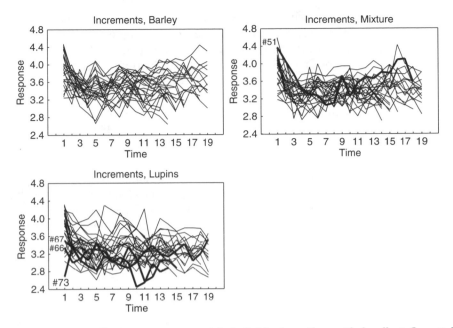

Figure 22.22 Milk protein content trial. Individual profiles, with locally influential subjects highlighted. Dropout modelled from week 1. Incremental analysis.

is in terms of the previous and current outcomes, to which no transformation is applied. As was argued in the mastitis case (p. 700), since two subsequent measurements are usually positively correlated, it is not unusual for both of them to be high. It is therefore wise to reparameterize the dropout model (22.1) in terms of the *increment*; that is, y_{ij} is replaced by $y_{ij} - y_{i,j-1}$. This is related to the approach of Diggle and Kenward (1994), who reparameterized their dropout model in terms of the increment just introduced and the size (the average of both measurements). Even though a dropout model in the outcomes themselves, termed the direct variables model, is equivalent to a model in the first variable Y_{i1} and the increment $Y_{i2} - Y_{i1}$, termed the incremental variable representation, it was shown that they lead to different perturbation schemes of the form (22.1). Indeed, from equality (22.19) or, more generally, from

$$\psi_0 + \psi_1 y_{i,j-1} + \psi_2 y_{ij} = \lambda_0 + \lambda_1 y_{i,j-1} + \lambda_2 (y_{ij} - y_{i,j-1}), \qquad (22.28)$$

it follows that $\psi_0 = \lambda_0$ and $\psi_1 = \lambda_1 - \lambda_2$. Thus, local influence is now focusing on a different set of parameters and one should not expect it to give the same answer. Therefore, it is crucial to guide the parameterization by careful substantive knowledge. In a sense, dependence on the increment is most dramatic since, at the time of dropout, there is no information about the increment, whereas size can be assessed reasonably well from $Y_{i,j-1}$, especially if the correlation is sufficiently high. The results of this analysis are presented in Figure 22.21 and the most influential profiles are highlighted in Figure 22.22. A slightly different but overlapping set of profiles is responsible for the influence now. The most important feature is that the influence is very minor. The components of the direction of maximal curvature h_{max} show virtually no peaks.

Finally, we compare both models. The direct variable results found in Figure 22.15 agree fairly well with those in Figure 22.19, the differences being the absence of subjects 66 and 67 and the appearance of subject 43. The latter profile is extremely low at the end of the period, where dropout is modelled, and therefore yields a large value for (22.27). For subjects 66 and 67, there is a logical explanation for their disappearance. These profiles are very low during the first part of the experimental period, in spite of which they do not drop out. However, during the latter part, their profile is still low *and* they drop out, which is totally plausible behaviour and, hence, their influence is marked in the second but not in this analysis.

For the incremental analysis there is a larger discrepancy between both models, as one can observe by comparing Figure 22.17 to Figure 22.21. While the direction of maximal curvature still shows no unusual subjects, C_i shows somewhat different subjects to be influential. Specifically, subjects 7, 51, and 74 are highly influential for the first model, whereas subjects 51 (again), 66, 67, and 73 are the ones detected with the second model. Although the cutoff is rather arbitrary, it is noteworthy that subject 51 appears in both C_i and $C_i(\boldsymbol{\theta})$ for the first model, indicating that the measurement model influence $C_i(\boldsymbol{\theta})$ is of the same order of magnitude as the dropout model influence $C_i(\boldsymbol{\psi})$, which is in contrast to the other analysis. Both subjects 7 and 74 are *on average* not particularly low profiles, but they are among the lowest ones during the last month of the experiment and, although there are some others with the same feature, these two have a low overall level, but a *high* increment, which is very unusual.

Overview

Table 22.7 summarizes the subjects which are found to be influential in the various analyses. Although it can be argued that the various influence analyses serve different purposes, it is of some importance to distinguish between those subjects who are influential overall and others which turn up in one or a few analyses. Cow 51 is highlighted in all six analyses and cows 59 and 68 show up four times, all others being seen three times or less. Clearly, cow 51 shows up unambiguously in the global influence plots and it yields the highest $C_i(\boldsymbol{\theta})$, $C_i(\boldsymbol{\beta})$, and $C_i(\boldsymbol{\alpha})$ values in the local influence analysis, even though one might argue that in some local influence plots it is closely followed by slightly lower peaks. Inspecting its profile more closely, we conclude that it deviates from the typical profile in a number of ways. First, it is among the highest profiles during the period of initial drop, whereafter it is fairly low during the first half of the period, followed by a period of almost linear increase until the

Table 22.7 Milk protein content trial. Summary of influential subjects.

Subject	Drop from week 15			Drop from week 1		
		Local			Local	
	Global	Raw	Incremental	Global	Raw	Incremental
1	*			*		
7			*			
38	*					
43		*				
51	*	*	*	*	*	*
59	*	*		*	*	
65	*			*		
66					*	*
67					*	*
68	*	*		*	*	
73						*
74			*			

end of the study. The other two, 59 and 68, are, on average, the lowest profiles, not only within their group, but overall.

Whereas global influence, as stated earlier, starts from deleting one subject completely, local influence only changes the dropout process for one subject from random dropout to non-random dropout. Because of the completely different approach, there is no need for both methods to yield similar results, although by looking at the influential subjects for all cases studied above, we notice some overlap.

Substantial differences are seen between the two models we formulated. The first one models dropout from week 15 onwards. The second allows dropout during the complete 19-week period. When dropout is based on the last 5 weeks, the model-fitting results are, as expected, very close to those of Diggle and Kenward (1994), with a highly significant indication for MNAR. When the dropout model is based on the entire period, there is little evidence for non-random dropout. Moreover, influential subjects in the two approaches are entirely different. Both analyses concentrate on behaviour in the period during which dropout is modelled. The latter indicates that the choice of period to which dropout applies is crucial.

In addition, we compared the direct variable analysis with an incremental one, where dropout depends on the difference between the current and previous measurements. In line with our analysis of the mastitis data set (Section 22.3.2), each analysis leads to different influential subjects, indicating that one should carefully discuss which analysis is preferable. Although both model formulations in (22.28) are equivalent, they lead to a different influence analysis, simply because the parameters at which the influence is targeted are different. Which one is chosen may depend on substantive considerations, as well as on the observation made by Molenberghs *et al.* (2001b) that the parameter $Y_{i,j-1}$ is the most efficiently calculated in the incremental model, provided $\widehat{\psi}_1$ and $\widehat{\psi}_2$ are negatively correlated. The latter condition is satisfied in many longitudinal applications, as already noted by Diggle and Kenward (1994).

22.6   ANALYSIS OF THE DEPRESSION TRIALS

The data from the depression trials, introduced in Section 2.5 and then examined in Chapter 6 and Sections 7.6 and 24.6, are analysed under MCAR, MAR, and MNAR assumptions, respectively. The six post-baseline visits correspond to the measurements taken at weeks 1, 2, 3, 5, 7, and 9. All six time points will be included in the analysis, regardless of the three-dimensional illustration (for the sake of clarity) in the previous section. In the measurement model (7.4) we include an intercept, and assume as fixed effects the following covariates: treatment, time, time^2, and the interactions of treatment with time and time^2. Random effects are modelled as part of the within-subject error correlations, with the covariance structure being of the heterogeneous first-order autoregressive type. Further, dropout model (22.13) is considered. Apart from the explicit MCAR, MAR, and MNAR versions of this model, we will also conduct an ignorable analysis (i.e., an analysis based on the measurement model only, ignoring the dropout model). The results for the measurement model parameters have to coincide, on theoretical grounds, with those of the MCAR and MAR analyses. In Table 22.8, parameter estimates and standard errors are listed for the four analyses, as well as the estimate of the treatment difference at the endpoint (week 9), which was the primary objective of the study, together with its *p*-value. The coincidence of MCAR, MAR, and ignorable measurement parameter estimates is observed, except for very small numerical differences. The *p*-value of the difference at the endpoint does not change much, being significant in all four cases.

As we have seen several times above, for the MNAR analysis, the estimates of the ψ_1 and ψ_2 parameters are approximately equally large, but with different sign. Recall that the cause of this is associated with two adjacent measurements being positively correlated. Rewriting the fitted dropout model in terms of the increment,

$$\text{logit}\left[P(D_i = j | D_i \geqslant j, \boldsymbol{y}_i)\right] = -2.46 + 0.03 y_{i,j-1} - 0.08(y_{ij} - y_{i,j-1}),$$

suggests that the probability of dropout increases with larger negative increments; that is, those patients who showed or would have shown a greater decrease in $HAMD_{17}$ score from the previous visit are more likely to drop out, given that the decrease from baseline at the previous visit is not large. In other

Table 22.8 Depression trials. Parameter estimates (standard errors) assuming ignorabilty, as well as explicitly modelling the missing data mechanism under MCAR, MAR, and MNAR assumptions, for all data. All subjects.

Effect	Parameter	Ignorable	MCAR	MAR	MNAR
Mean parameters					
Intercept	β_0	6.93 (1.49)	6.93 (1.48)	6.93 (1.48)	6.99 (1.48)
Baseline	β_1	-0.37 (0.07)	-0.37 (0.07)	-0.37 (0.07)	-0.37 (0.07)
Treatment	β_2	-0.34 (0.66)	-0.34 (0.65)	-0.34 (0.65)	-0.35 (0.67)
Time	β_3	-2.40 (0.29)	-2.40 (0.29)	-2.40 (0.29)	-2.49 (0.31)
Time^2	β_4	0.14 (0.03)	0.14 (0.03)	0.14 (0.03)	0.15 (0.03)
Time × treatment	β_5	0.59 (0.40)	0.59 (0.40)	0.59 (0.40)	0.60 (0.41)
Time^2 × treatment	β_6	-0.03 (0.04)	-0.03 (0.04)	-0.03 (0.04)	-0.04 (0.04)
Variance parameters					
Standard deviation (time 1)	σ_1	4.05	4.02 (0.17)	4.02 (0.17)	4.01 (0.17)
Standard deviation (time 2)	σ_2	5.29	5.27 (0.24)	5.27 (0.24)	5.25 (0.24)
Standard deviation (time 3)	σ_3	5.96	5.94 (0.27)	5.94 (0.27)	5.92 (0.27)
Standard deviation (time 4)	σ_4	6.52	6.49 (0.29)	6.49 (0.29)	6.55 (0.30)
Standard deviation (time 5)	σ_5	6.24	6.21 (0.28)	6.21 (0.28)	6.18 (0.27)
Standard deviation (time 6)	σ_6	6.33	6.29 (0.30)	6.29 (0.30)	6.26 (0.29)
Correlation	ρ	0.73	0.72 (0.02)	0.72 (0.02)	0.72 (0.02)
Missing data model					
Intercept	ψ_0		-2.46 (0.11)	-2.21 (0.14)	-2.46 (0.27)
Previous	ψ_1			-0.05 (0.02)	0.11 (0.05)
Current	ψ_2				-0.08 (0.06)
-2 log-likelihood			7949.4	7943.1	7941.6
Difference at endpoint (*p*-value)		2.20 (0.0179)	2.19 (0.0176)	2.19 (0.0176)	2.18 (0.0177)

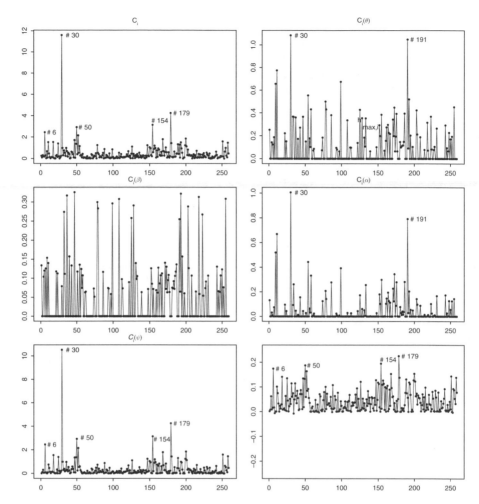

Figure 22.23 Depression trials. Index plots of C_i, $C_i(\boldsymbol{\theta})$, $C_i(\boldsymbol{\alpha})$, $C_i(\boldsymbol{\beta})$, $C_i(\boldsymbol{\psi})$ and of the components of the direction $\boldsymbol{h}_{\mathrm{max},i}$ of maximal curvature.

words, patients with a large improvement compared with the previous visit, a sudden shift in profile, are more likely to drop out.

We now switch to local influence. Figure 22.23 displays overall C_i and influences for subvectors $\boldsymbol{\theta}$, $\boldsymbol{\beta}$, $\boldsymbol{\alpha}$, and $\boldsymbol{\psi}$. In addition, the direction $\boldsymbol{h}_{\mathrm{max}}$, corresponding to maximal local influence, is given. The main emphasis should be put on the relative magnitudes. It is observed that patients 6, 30, 50, 154, and 179 have larger C_i values compared to other patients, which means they can be considered influential. Among these, patient 30 clearly shows the largest C_i. Virtually the same picture holds for $C_i(\boldsymbol{\psi})$. The large influence of patient 30 is caused by the patient achieving the biggest reduction in $HAMD_{17}$ score in the new drug group at week 1. Based on the dropout model under the MAR assumption, the dropout probability at week 2 for this subject was very small but the subject dropped out nevertheless. Hence the subject had a large influence on θ from (22.5). For the same reason, the values of h_{ij} and $\lambda_{ij|h_{ij}}$ are large in (22.6), resulting in a large value of $C_i(\boldsymbol{\psi})$. Since patients 6, 50, 154, and 179 are completers, all their influence affects $\boldsymbol{\beta}$. It immediately follows from (22.3) and (22.5) that direct influence on θ only arises from those measurement occasions at which dropout occurs. Their relatively large influence on ψ is due to two facts. First, their profiles are relatively higher in magnitude than others, and hence y_{ij} and h_{ij} in (22.4) are large. Second, since all of these patients are completers, (22.3) contains a maximal number of large terms. Turning attention to the influence on the measurement model, we see that for $C_i(\boldsymbol{\beta})$ there are no relatively high peaks, whereas $C_i(\boldsymbol{\alpha})$ again reveals a considerable peak for patients 30 and 191. Note that patient 191 does not have a high peak for the overall C_i. This is due to the fact that the scale for $C_i(\boldsymbol{\alpha})$ is relatively small, comparing to the overall C_i. Nevertheless, these patients can still be considered influential. The relatively large influence of patient 191 is due to the large residual $h_{id} - \lambda(h_{id})$. This can be explained by the fact that the observed change in $HAMD_{17}$ score from baseline at visit 5 was zero, which is distant from the group mean at that time point. Finally, the direction of maximum curvature does not really highlight any influential patients, although the four influential completers seem to have the highest values.

In Figure 22.24, the individual profiles of the influential observations are highlighted. Let us now take a closer look at these cases. Patients 30 and 191 dropped out of the study, whereas the others completed the 9 weeks. In many previous analyses, the influential subjects were completers, making this application important in its own right. Furthermore, patients 30 and 154 belong to the new drug group, while patients 6, 50, 179, and 191 were on placebo.

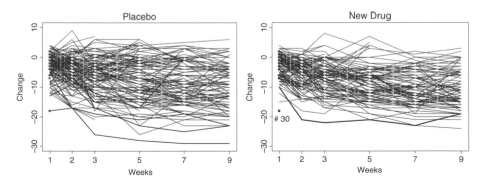

Figure 22.24 Depression trials. Individual profiles for both treatment arms, with influential subjects highlighted.

As we can see from Figure 22.24, patient 30 dropped out after the first post-baseline measurement occasion. This patient achieved the largest change in $HAMD_{17}$ at week 1, with a score going down from 24 at baseline to 6 at week 1. The second incomplete influential subject, patient 191, dropped out at the second last measurement occasion, resulting in five observed measurements. It is clear from Figure 22.24 that this patient's $HAMD_{17}$ was decreasing up to the fourth measurement occasion, meaning s/he was improving. However, at the last observed measurement occasion, his/her value became 0 again, so his/her $HAMD_{17}$ score was again the same as the one at baseline, indicating a marked worsening from the previous visit. Finally, all the other influential patients had a big improvement within the first three weeks, which remained more or less constant afterwards.

It is interesting to consider an analysis without these influential observations. Therefore, we apply the selection model to three subsets of the data. For the first subset, patient 30 was removed, as this is overall the most influential one. For the second, patients 30 and 191, who seemed to be influencing the measurement model the most, were removed. Finally, for the third, all six influential patients mentioned above were removed. The results from these analyses are summarized in Tables 22.9 and 22.10. We compare the results of the MAR and MNAR analyses.

The largest C_i is observed for patient 30. This patient's relatively large influence is caused by a large improvement, that is, big drop in $HAMD_{17}$ score, just before dropout. By removing patient 30, the estimate of ψ_1 changes from 0.11 to 0.12. Formulating the dropout model in terms of the increment $y_{ij} - y_{i,j-1}$ and the previous measurement $y_{i,j-1}$, the coefficient for the increments does not change, while the coefficient for $y_{i,j-1}$ increases from 0.03 to 0.04. Since the coefficient for the current measurement y_{ij} does not change by removing patient 30, there is not much influence on the likelihood ratio test for MAR against MNAR: $G^2 = 1.3$ compared to $G^2 = 1.5$. The parameter for the main treatment effect decreases, as well as the difference between the new drug and placebo at week 9, resulting in a slightly increased p-value. This holds for both MAR and MNAR. This can be explained by the patient's big improvement before dropout, and membership of the new drug group.

Removing patients 30 and 191 changes the parameter for the interaction between time and treatment under MAR from 0.59 to 0.64. The estimate for $time^2$-by-treatment interaction also changes slightly from -0.04 to -0.03. The change in these estimates is due to the unusual individual profile for patient 191. Observe in Figure 22.24 that the $HAMD_{17}$ score decreases during the first four post-baseline visits and suddenly goes back to the level at baseline at visit 5. Figure 22.25 shows the fitted mean profiles of the change in $HAMD_{17}$, both for placebo and the new drug group, for all subjects and for the subset with patients 30 and 191 removed. We used the mean baseline value to calculate the mean values. For the new drug group, the coefficients for time and $time^2$ remain the same for all subjects and for the subset, the two mean profiles are

Table 22.9 Depression trials. Parameter estimates (standard errors) assuming ignorability, as well as explicitly modelling the missing data mechanism under MCAR/MAR assumptions, after removing subjects 30 (set 1), 30 and 191 (set 2), and 6, 30, 50, 154, 179, and 191 (set 3).

Effect	Parameter	Set 1	Set 2	Set 3
Mean parameters				
Intercept	β_0	6.74 (1.46)	6.70 (1.46)	5.41 (1.41)
Baseline	β_1	−0.35 (0.07)	−0.35 (0.07)	−0.29 (0.07)
Treatment	β_2	−0.47 (0.65)	−0.51 (0.64)	−0.40 (0.63)
Time	β_3	−2.41 (0.30)	−2.40 (0.29)	−2.36 (0.29)
Time^2	β_4	0.14 (0.03)	0.14 (0.03)	0.14 (0.03)
Time × treatment	β_5	0.60 (0.40)	0.64 (0.40)	0.65 (0.39)
Time^2 × treatment	β_6	−0.03 (0.04)	−0.04 (0.04)	−0.04 (0.04)
Variance parameters				
Standard deviation (time 1)	σ_1	3.93 (0.17)	3.95 (0.17)	3.76 (0.16)
Standard deviation (time 1)	σ_1	5.23 (0.23)	5.25 (0.24)	5.05 (0.23)
Standard deviation (time 1)	σ_1	5.91 (0.26)	5.93 (0.27)	5.71 (0.26)
Standard deviation (time 1)	σ_1	6.46 (0.29)	6.41 (0.28)	6.25 (0.28)
Standard deviation (time 1)	σ_1	6.19 (0.27)	6.15 (0.27)	5.95 (0.27)
Standard deviation (time 1)	σ_1	6.27 (0.29)	6.26 (0.29)	6.09 (0.29)
Correlation	ρ	0.72 (0.02)	0.72 (0.02)	0.71 (0.02)
Missing data model				
Intercept	ψ_0	−2.20 (0.14)	−2.22 (0.14)	−2.23 (0.15)
Previous	ψ_1	−0.05 (0.02)	0.05 (0.02)	0.05 (0.02)
−2 log-likelihood		7919.8	7875.2	7701.6
Difference at endpoint (*p*-value)		2.15 (0.0197)	2.07 (0.0241)	2.40 (0.0082)

parallel and the difference between the fitted mean profile of all subjects and the subset excluding patients 30 and 191 is relatively small. In the placebo group, the mean profile becomes steeper by removing the two patients. The estimate for treatment effect falls from −0.35 to −0.51, mainly due to the big improvement on patient 30. Overall, the difference at endpoint decreases from 2.19 to 2.07, and the *p*-value for this difference increases from 0.0176 to 0.0241. A similar pattern is seen for the MNAR analysis.

It is noted that removing patients 30 and 191 leads to a small impact on the likelihood ratio test for MAR against MNAR. The value of G^2 changes from 1.5 to 2.07. This is partially due to a weaker incremental component in the dropout model. The coefficient for the increments $y_{ij} - y_{i,j-1}$ changes from −0.08 to −0.07, and the coefficient of the previous measurement increases from 0.03 to 0.04.

To better understand the influence of this patient, his/her demographic information was investigated. This patient was in his/her first major depressive disorder (MDD) episode, when s/he was enrolled. The patient dropped out of the

Table 22.10 The Depression Trials. Parameter estimates (standard errors) assuming ignorability, as well as explicitly modelling the missing data mechanism under MNAR assumptions, after removing subjects 30 (set 1), 30 and 191 (set 2), and 6, 30, 50, 154, 179, and 191 (set 3).

Effect	Parameter	Set 1	Set 2	Set 3
Mean parameters				
Intercept	β_0	6.79 (1.44)	6.75 (1.46)	5.47 (1.41)
Baseline	β_1	−0.35 (0.07)	−0.35 (0.07)	−0.29 (0.07)
Treatment	β_2	−0.47 (0.64)	−0.51 (0.66)	−0.40 (0.64)
Time	β_3	−2.50 (0.30)	−2.49 (0.30)	−2.45 (0.30)
Time^2	β_4	0.15 (0.03)	0.15 (0.03)	0.14 (0.03)
Time × treatment	β_5	0.61 (0.40)	0.64 (0.40)	0.65 (0.40)
Time^2 × treatment	β_6	−0.04 (0.04)	−0.04 (0.04)	−0.04 (0.04)
Variance parameters				
Standard deviation (time 1)	σ_1	3.92 (0.17)	3.94 (0.17)	3.75 (0.16)
Standard deviation (time 1)	σ_1	5.19 (0.23)	5.22 (0.23)	5.02 (0.23)
Standard deviation (time 1)	σ_1	5.88 (0.26)	5.90 (0.26)	5.69 (0.26)
Standard deviation (time 1)	σ_1	6.51 (0.30)	6.46 (0.29)	6.31 (0.29)
Standard deviation (time 1)	σ_1	6.15 (0.27)	6.11 (0.27)	5.92 (0.26)
Standard deviation (time 1)	σ_1	6.24 (0.29)	6.23 (0.29)	6.07 (0.29)
correlation	ρ	0.72 (0.02)	0.72 (0.02)	0.70 (0.02)
Missing data model				
intercept	ψ_0	−2.43 (0.27)	−2.44 (0.27)	−2.47 (0.28)
previous	ψ_1	0.12 (0.06)	0.11 (0.05)	0.11 (0.06)
current	ψ_2	−0.08 (0.06)	−0.07 (0.06)	−0.08 (0.06)
−2 log-likelihood		7918.5	7873.9	7700.2
Difference at endpoint (*p*-value)		2.14 (0.0198)	2.07 (0.0237)	2.39 (0.0083)

study after week 1, based on his/her own decision, and claimed that the symptoms of depression were caused by high carbon monoxide levels in his/her house. Given this information, it is unlikely such a patient provides meaningful information regarding the risks and benefits of the investigational treatment, and it is probably best to consider the merits of the drug after excluding this observation.

And while excluding this patient had little effect on interpretations of the treatment effect in this well-powered confirmatory clinical trial, which is very useful information in and of itself, it is also useful to consider the benefits of sensitivity analyses in a proof of concept setting where the sample sizes are much smaller. For example, if there had been only 40 subjects per arm, excluding this one subject would have had a much bigger impact. Knowing how strongly results depend on one or a few subjects, or on specific assumptions, could potentially improve decisions on whether to continue or discontinue development of an intervention.

Finally, we perform the same analyses on the third subset with patients 6, 30, 50, 154, 179, and 191 removed. Again, we observe for the MAR analysis that the parameter for the interaction between time and treatment changes to 0.65,

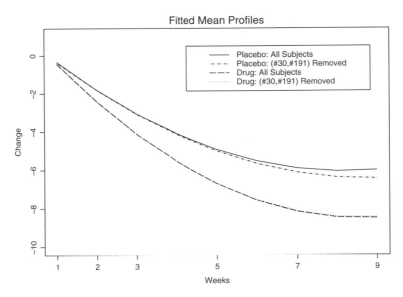

Figure 22.25 Depression trials. Fitted mean profiles, both for placebo group and treatment group, for all subjects and for the subset resulting from removing subjects 30 and 191. Mean baseline value is used to calculate the means.

mainly due to the unusual profile of patient 191. There is an increase of 0.31 in the difference between the new drug and placebo at the endpoint. Also, the p-value for this difference decreases from 0.0176 to 0.0082. A similar pattern is found for the MNAR analysis. This change in difference at the endpoint could be due to the fact that the profiles for patients 6, 50, and 179 are relatively low in the placebo group. The estimates of the parameters in the dropout model do not change much, and the deviance for MAR against MNAR is nearly the same.

Clearly, sensitivity analysis and local influence tools are useful for the analyses of incomplete clinical trial data. A careful study of influential subjects, combined with knowing how the results of primary interest change by removing such subjects and by altering assumptions regarding missing data, can lead to a better understanding of the nature of clinical trial data. Sensitivity analyses can also help develop an appropriate level of confidence in the originally proposed primary analysis and help develop alternative analyses in which more confidence can be placed by the researchers.

22.7 A LOCAL INFLUENCE APPROACH FOR ORDINAL DATA WITH DROPOUT

Incomplete longitudinal ordinal data can be modelled using a simple logistic regression formulation for the dropout process and using a multivariate Dale model for the response (Molenberghs and Lesaffre 1994, 1999; Molenberghs *et al.* 1997), as described in Section 15.4. To explore the sensitivity of this selection model for repeated ordinal outcomes, Van Steen *et al.* (2001) considered a local influence approach. The expressions derived take the form (22.8) and (22.9), as in the Gaussian case, where now the appropriate likelihood is used.

22.8   ANALYSIS OF THE FLUVOXAMINE DATA

Van Steen *et al.* (2001) applied the local influence ideas of the previous section to the fluvoxamine study introduced in Section 2.6 and then analysed in Sections 12.6, 15.4.2, 15.5.1, 16.8, 18.3.5, 20.4, and 21.7.

To investigate the sensitivity of inferences reported with respect to modelling assumptions for the dropout process, the overall C_i, influences $C_i(\boldsymbol{\theta})$ and $C_i(\boldsymbol{\psi})$ for the measurement parameters and dropout parameters, as well as $\boldsymbol{h}_{\max}$ of maximal curvature are displayed in Figure 22.26. Note that the largest C_i are observed for patients 34 and 252 (both having side effects surpassing the therapeutic effect at visit 1 and visit 2), followed by patients 182, 64, 122, 28, 108, 287, 232, 112, and 245, all of whom yield the worst score on side effects at visit 1 and drop out at visit 2. We pay special attention to patient 239, showing side effects interfering significantly with functionality at visit 1, after which dropout occurs.

In addition, Figure 22.26 shows some evidence of the fact that influence on measurement model parameters can theoretically only arise from those measurement occasions at which dropout occurs, a fact already observed by Verbeke *et al.* (2001b). Nevertheless, it should be noted that influence on the measurement model parameters can also arise from complete observations. Indeed, when small perturbations in a specific ω_i lead to relatively large differences in the model parameters, the subject's impact on dropout parameters indirectly influences all functions that include these dropout parameters. An example of such a function is the conditional mean of an unobserved measurement, given the observed measurements and given the fact that the patient belongs to a certain dropout pattern. As a consequence, the corresponding measurement model parameters will *indirectly* be affected as well (Verbeke *et al.* 2001b).

Influential completers occur in the index plots of C_i, $C_i(\boldsymbol{\psi})$, and of the components of the direction $\boldsymbol{h}_{\max}$ of maximal curvature, but are absent in the index plot of $C_i(\boldsymbol{\theta})$. Focusing on $C_i(\boldsymbol{\theta})$, Figure 22.26 reveals the highest peaks for patients 239 and 128. It appears that the influence of allowing subject 239 to drop out non-randomly is best visible on the measurement model parameters. Patient 128 has an incomplete sequence, with a relatively mild score for side effects (side effects not interfering with functionality). Hence, the relatively large value for $C_i(\boldsymbol{\theta})$ is somewhat unusual, especially because other index plots do not show evidence of any influential effect, not even globally. One could

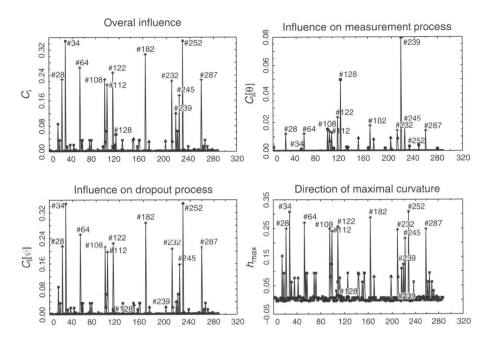

Figure 22.26 Fluvoxamine trial. Index plots of C_i, $C_i(\boldsymbol{\theta})$, $C_i(\boldsymbol{\psi})$, and of the components of the direction $\boldsymbol{h}_{\max}$ of maximal curvature. The x-axis merely contains sequential indicators. Relevant patient IDs have been added to the plot. Stars indicate completers (patients with observed responses at visit 1 and visit 2). Circles, squares, triangles, and plus signs indicate subjects with side-effects scores at visit 1 of 1,2,3, and 4, respectively. Patients with a non-monotone dropout pattern are discarded.

ask the question whether other, unmeasured factors could have caused this phenomenon.

Before addressing this question, we turn attention to $C_i(\boldsymbol{\psi})$ and $\boldsymbol{h}_{\max}$. To avoid confusion, observe that the scale is different from that of $C_i(\boldsymbol{\theta})$. The most influential patients appear to be the same as for the overall C_i (34, 252 and 182, 64, 122, 28, 108, 287, 232, 112, 245). The same patients are also shown in the index plot for $\boldsymbol{h}_{\max}$.

Observe that in all plots, 'layers' of influential cases may be distinguished. The higher the layers, the more they seem to be associated with particular response levels. For instance, in Figure 22.26, patients 34 and 252 give rise to components of $\boldsymbol{h}_{\max}$ that are larger than 0.3. Patients 182, 64, 122, 28, 108, 287, 232, 112 and 245 (corresponding to the influential patients in the previous paragraph) refer to $\boldsymbol{h}_{\max}$ components that are all smaller than 0.3 but larger than 0.2. The layer formation is not clear though, and, recalling the particular behaviour of patient 128, one is led to believe that another distorting factor is involved, blurring the picture. Therefore, we investigate the effect of covariates on the ability to interpret influence plots.

For this purpose, we consider two additional models. The first includes sex as the only covariate in the measurement model, the second uses age as the only covariate. These models perform worse than the model including both age and sex, augmented with duration and severity, but they are merely intended for illustrative purposes. The resulting influence plots are enlightening. Figure 22.27 shows the index plots when age is included as the only covariate, while Figure 22.28 displays the corresponding pictures when sex is the only source of covariate information. In both cases, much smaller values are obtained for $C_i(\boldsymbol{\theta})$. The high peaks for patients 239 and 128 have disappeared. Patients 122, 245, and 182 also show up in Figure 22.27 with the highest peaks for $C_i(\boldsymbol{\theta})$, although hard to distinguish from the peaks for patients 287, 232, 28, 108, 64, and 112. The variability observed in $C_i(\boldsymbol{\theta})$ values also appears in Figure 22.28. However, in this case, it seems to be caused by the fact that patients 108, 182, 287, and 232 have $C_i(\boldsymbol{\theta})$ equal to about 0.0116 compared to approximately 0.0097 for patients 28, 245, 64, 122, and 112. This layer effect may be explained by the binary character of sex as opposed to age, the latter of which entered the model as a continuous variable. Also note that

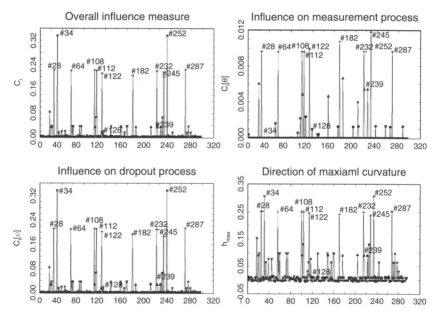

Figure 22.27 Fluvoxamine trial. Index plots of C_i, $C_i(\boldsymbol{\theta})$, $C_i(\boldsymbol{\psi})$, and of the components of the direction $\boldsymbol{h}_{\max}$ of maximal curvature, where age is considered as the sole covariate in the Dale model. The x-axis contains sequential indicators. Stars indicate completers. Circles, squares, triangles, and plus signs indicate subjects with side-effects scores at visit 1 of 1, 2, 3, and 4, respectively.

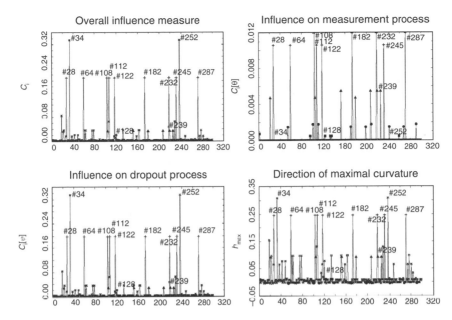

Figure 22.28 Fluvoxamine trial. Index plots of C_i, $C_i(\theta)$, $C_i(\psi)$, and of the components of the direction h_{max} of maximal curvature, where sex is considered as the only covariate in the Dale model. The x-axis contains sequential indicators. Stars indicate completers. Circles, squares, triangles, and plus signs indicate non-completers with side-effects scores at visit 1 of 1, 2, 3, and 4, respectively.

patients 108, 182, 287, and 232 are all male, whereas patients 28, 245, 64, 122, and 112 are all female. All these patients drop out at visit 2 and showed side effects surpassing therapeutic effect at visit 1. In Figures 22.27 and 22.28 the same patient group (i.e., patients 34, 252, 287, 108, 28, 112, 64, 232, 122, 182, and 245) is distinguished as globally influential, with highest C_i values for 34 and 252. The layering effect is again the most explicit when sex is considered as only the covariate (Figure 22.28). Influential patients for $C_i(\psi)$ and h_{max} appear to be the same as before, where sex and age were both considered in the pool of covariates, with the exception of subject 239 whose corresponding component in h_{max} is now less than 0.1000. The distribution over potential values becomes more discrete when age is considered to be the only covariate in the multivariate Dale model. Changing age for sex causes the distribution to be even more discrete and therefore the layer effect more explicit.

In an attempt to improve insight into the driving forces present in the data set, which may explain possible deviations from a random-dropout process, we exclude patients 34 and 252 from the data set and apply the same measurement model as before, including the covariates age, sex, duration, and severity.

Provided MAR is the correct alternative hypothesis and provided the parametric form for the MAR process is correct (again, no covariates were included), there seems to be even less evidence for MAR; the likelihood ratio test statistic comparing MCAR with MAR equals $G^2 = 0.94$, based on 1 degree of freedom ($p = 0.333$). Note that now borderline evidence for MNAR is observed, since a comparison between the non-random and random dropout models generates a likelihood ratio test statistic of $G^2 = 3.74$ with 1 degree of freedom ($p = 0.053$). Hence, the suggested local influence approach bridges the gap between the random and the non-random models: some of the mechanisms that cannot be explained by the random model and are captured by the non-random model, the latter resting on untestable assumptions, can be attributed to the observations for patients 34 and 252.

Repeating the previous analysis on a reduced data set, where patient 239 is excluded instead of patients 34 and 252, we find no evidence for MAR against MCAR ($G^2 = 0.01$, $p = 0.913$). After investigating the likelihood ratio test statistic for comparing the non-random with the random dropout model ($G^2 = 2.13$, $p = 0.145$), we may conclude that the MCAR assumption is fairly plausible. It is not surprising that conclusions remain similar. Indeed, although patient 239 appeared to be most influential patient with respect to the measurement model parameters, it should be noted that (i) the value for $C_i(\boldsymbol{\theta})$ is 'only' 0.079 (further investigation is required to define some critical value above which $C_i(\boldsymbol{\theta})$ can be said to be statistically significantly large) and that (ii) patient 239 did not appear to be influential overall.

22.9   A LOCAL INFLUENCE APPROACH FOR INCOMPLETE BINARY DATA

Jansen *et al.* (2003) developed the local influence approach for the BRD family of models (Section 15.5). They considered perturbations of a given BRD model in the direction of a model with one more parameter in which the original model is nested, implying that perturbations lie along the edges of Figure 15.4: for each of the nested pairs in Figure 15.4, the simpler of the two models equates two parameters from the more complex one. For example, BRD4 includes $\beta_{.k}$, ($k = 1, 2$), whereas in BRD1 only $\beta_{..}$ is included. For the influence analysis, ω_i is then included as a contrast between two such parameters; for the perturbation of BRD1 in the direction of BRD4, one considers $\beta_{..}$ and $\beta_{..} + \omega_i$. Such an ω_i is not a subject-specific parameter, but rather an infinitesimal perturbation. The vector of all ω_i defines the direction in which such a perturbation is considered. Clearly, other perturbation schemes are possible as well, or one could consider a different route of sensitivity analysis altogether. Ideally, several could be considered within an integrated sensitivity analysis. Note that our influence analysis focuses on the missingness model, rather than on the measurement model parameters. This may not at first sight be as expected, because usually scientific interest focuses on the measurement model parameters. However, it has been documented (discussion to Diggle and Kenward 1994; Kenward 1998; Verbeke *et al.* 2001b) that the missingness model parameters are often the most sensitive to misspecification and influential features. These may then, in turn, affect conclusions obtained from the measurement model parameters (e.g., time evolution) or combinations from both (e.g., covariate effects for certain groups of responders).

22.10   ANALYSIS OF THE FLUVOXAMINE DATA

We now apply the local influence ideas, outlined in the previous section, to the BRD models for comparison with the original conclusions of Section 15.5.1. Whereas all comparisons along the edges of Figure 15.4 are possible, we propose to focus principally on the comparison of BRD1 with BRD4 (Figure 22.29), as the first of these was found to be the most adequate model both in the absence of a duration effect and when duration is included in both parts of the model,

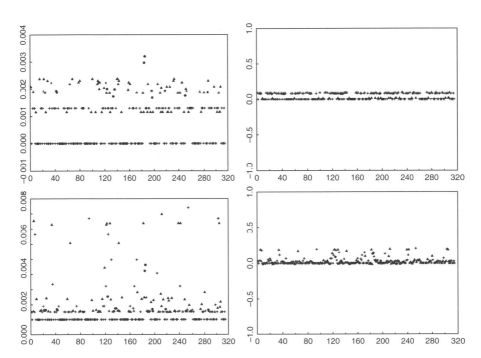

Figure 22.29   Fluvoxamine trial. Index plots of C_i (left panels) and of the components of the direction $\boldsymbol{h}_{\max}$ of maximal curvature (right panels) for comparison BRD1–4, without (top panels) and with (bottom panels) duration as a covariate in the missingness models.

whereas the second was the model of choice when duration is included in the measurement model only. In addition, we will consider the comparisons BRD4–7 (Figure 22.30) and BRD4–8 (plot not shown), the supermodels of BRD4. The symbols used in these figures are the following: +, both observations are available, (1,1) type; black triangle, only the first observation is available, (1,0) type; black square, only the second observation is available, (0,1) type; bullet, both measurements are missing, (0,0) type.

The overall C_i are considered, as well as the components of the direction of maximal curvature h_{max}. The top right-hand panel in Figure 22.29 shows essentially no structure, whereas on the top left there are two important observations. First, a clear layering effect is present, consistent with the analysis in Section 22.8. Again, this is not surprising, as there are quite a number of discrete features to the model: the responses and the missingness patterns. On the other hand, the continuous covariate duration is included in the measurement model. In this case, mainly the missingness patterns are noticeable, although the top layer shows a good deal of variability. These layers are reminiscent of a pattern-mixture structure (Little 1995), even though the model is of a selection nature.

Two views can be taken. One can focus can be on two observations, nos 184 and 185, that stand out. These subjects have no measurements at all for side effects. Alternatively, one can give further consideration to the entire pattern without follow-up measurements. We will return to this issue later in this section. This phenomenon is in contrast to the analyses by Verbeke *et al.* (2001b) and Molenberghs *et al.* (2001b) who found that the influential observations were invariably completers. In this case, the situation is different because the 'empty' observations are explicitly modelled in the BRD family. Therefore, assumptions about the perturbations in the direction of such observations have an impact on the values such an individual *would have had* had the measurements been made; hence a strong sensitivity. This is an illustration of the fact that studying influence by means of perturbations in the missingness model may lead to important conclusions regarding the measurement model parameters. Indeed, the measurement model conclusions depend not only on the observations actually made, but also on the expectation of the missing measurements. In an MNAR model, such expectations depend on the missingness model as well, since they are made *conditional on an observation being missing*. A high level of sensitivity means that the expectations of the missing outcomes and the resulting measurement model parameters strongly depend on the missingness model (Verbeke *et al.* 2001b). As stated earlier, the only continuous characteristics of the observations are the levels for duration. These are 38 and 41, respectively, the largest values within the group without observations and the 91st and 92nd percentile values within the entire sample. Thus, the conclusions are driven by a very high value of duration.

Consider now the bottom panels of Figure 22.29. The right-hand panel still shows little or no structure. On the left-hand side, the layering has been blurred due to the occurrence of duration as a continuous feature in the missingness model. The fact that no sets of observations stand out as such confirms the impression that a good fit has been obtained by including duration in both parts of the model.

We now turn to Figure 22.30. A qualitative difference with Figure 22.29 (top left) is that now the entire group with no follow-up measurements is more influential than all other subjects. In this case, h_{max} displays the same group of subjects with no follow-up. However, all of this disappears when one turns to the bottom panels, again underscoring the importance of duration in the missingness model.

The consequence of these findings is that, as soon as duration is included in the missingness model, a reasonable amount of confidence can be put in the conclusions so obtained. Nevertheless, based on the comparison BRD1–4, it seems wise to further study the effect of subjects 184 and 185, as well as from the group without follow-up measurements. To this end, three additional analyses are considered (Table 22.11). Two sets pertain to removal of subjects 184 and 185: without (I) and with (II) duration as a covariate in the measurement model. Note that we do not consider removal when duration is included

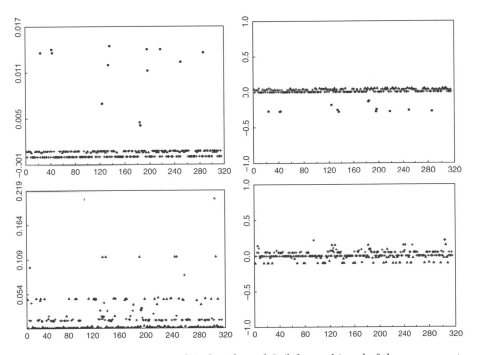

Figure 22.30 Fluvoxamine trial. Index plots of C_i (left panels) and of the components of the direction h_{max} of maximal curvature (right panels) for comparison BRD4–7, without (top panels) and with (bottom panels) duration as a covariate in the missingness models.

Table 22.11 Fluvoxamine trial. Negative log-likelihood values for three additional sets of analysis: I, observations 184 and 185 removed, no covariates; II, observations 184 and 185 removed, duration as covariate in the measurement model; III, all observations in the (0,0) group removed, duration as covariate in the measurement model.

Set	BRD1	BRD2	BRD3	BRD4	BRD5	BRD6	BRD7	BRD8	BRD9
I	559.59	558.18	558.70	558.18	558.97	557.59	557.32	557.59	557.32
II	543.65	541.87	542.16	540.35	542.43	540.61	538.53	538.81	540.34
III	496.19	494.33	495.26	492.53	495.53	493.71	491.67	491.95	493.43

in the missingness model because, in this case, these two subjects did not show up as locally influential. Finally, removing all subjects without follow-up measurements and using duration as a covariate in the measurement model is reported as family III.

In analysis I, BRD1 is still the preferred model; in II, evidence still points towards BRD4, although slightly less extreme than before: likelihood ratio test statistics for BRD1–4, BRD4–7, and BRD4–8 are 6.60, 3.64, and 3.08, respectively, compared to 7.10, 2.10, and 1.52 as obtained initially. However, while the two subjects deleted in I and II cannot explain the apparent non-random missingness, the same conclusions are reached when all subjects in pattern (0,0) are deleted (analysis III), as then a few likelihood ratios are above the significance threshold (7.17 attained for BRD3–7 and for BRD5–8; and 7.32 for BRD1–4). Thus, removing these subjects does not change the conclusions about the non-random nature of the data. This is useful supplemental information. Indeed, it is confirmed that the largest impact on the conclusion regarding the nature of the missingness mechanism is coming from the inclusion of the covariate duration, and neither from isolated individuals nor from a specific missingness pattern (those without measurements). A useful side effect of this conclusion is that the selected analysis encompasses all subjects and therefore avoids the need for subject deletion, which, if at all possible, should be avoided in statistical analysis.

These analyses can be seen as a useful component of a sensitivity analysis. Given the intrinsic problems with incomplete data models, one can never be completely sure the nature of the missingness mechanism is as posited in the model of choice and therefore several sensitivity assessments simultaneously and/or substantive knowledge have to be considered. When a number of possible causes for the observed non-randomness are found, one might ideally add substantive arguments as to their relative plausibility.

Subjects in an influence graph are displayed without a particular order. Several alternatives are possible, each with pros and cons. For example, one could order the subjects by covariate level, but this method cannot be considered when there are several covariates. Alternatively, the subjects could be ordered by C_i or h_i level, but then different orderings would exist on different plots.

22.11   CONCLUDING REMARKS

For many clinical trials, the assumption of an MAR missingness mechanism is a reasonable starting point. However, MNAR can never be completely ruled out. Understanding how the results depend on the specification of the missingness mechanism can be very helpful in understanding the relationship between the data and the conclusions drawn. Because the models for non-random dropout rest on strong and untestable assumptions, the optimal place for the MNAR analyses is within a sensitivity analysis framework. One such tool is local influence, which is used to depict anomalous subjects that lead to a seemingly MNAR mechanism. Although the original idea behind the use of local influence methods was to detect subjects that drop out non-randomly, several authors (Jansen *et al.* 2006b; Verbeke *et al.* 2001b) have shown that the influential subjects are commonly influential for other than missingness-related features. This is the subject of the next chapter. In this chapter, we applied local influence methods to the Diggle–Kenward selection model, the Dale model, and the BRD family, in a variety of application settings. Each analysis identifies specific features of one or a few subjects, many of which are completers. For example, a few cows in the mastitis study have unusually large increments, and some cows in the milk protein content trial have an uncommon serial correlation structure. In the depression trials, the most influential subject was patient 30. Belonging to the treatment group, this patient had the unusual profile of a very big improvement, but still dropped out after the first visit.

The Nature of Local Influence

23.1 INTRODUCTION

In the previous chapter, local influence was introduced as one mode of sensitivity analysis for MNAR models, such as the Diggle–Kenward model (Section 15.2), the Dale model (Section 15.4), and the BRD family of models (Section 15.5). The original idea behind the use of local influence methods was to detect observations that had a high impact on the conclusions *due to their aberrant missingness mechanism*. An example of such a scenario is where most missing measurements are MAR, while a few would be MNAR following one or a few deviation mechanisms. However, in most applications, such as the mastitis data (Section 22.3), the milk protein content trial (Section 22.5), the depression trials (Section 22.6), and the fluvoxamine trial (Sections 22.8 and 22.10), where a seemingly MNAR mechanism turned out to be MAR or even MCAR after removing the influential subjects identified upon the use of local influence, the situation turned out to be more complex than anticipated. For example, in the mastitis data set, the three influential cows had complete data but were identified by an extreme increase between the measurements at two subsequent years. Thus, the influential subjects often are influential for other than missingness-related reasons.

In this chapter, we study the method of local influence, not only to better understand its behaviour, but also to increase insight into the overall behaviour and impact of MNAR mechanisms. This is done using simulations and general modelling considerations, along the lines of Jansen *et al.* (2006b).

In Section 23.2, a testosterone inhibition study in rats is introduced, previously described and analysed by Verdonck *et al.* (1998), Verbeke and Molenberghs (2000, 2003), Verbeke *et al.* (2001b), and Jansen *et al.* (2006b).

Missing Data in Clinical Studies   G. Molenberghs and M.G. Kenward
© 2007 John Wiley & Sons, Ltd

The data are analysed and subjected to sensitivity analysis in Section 23.3. In Section 23.4, the behaviour of the local influence method is studied. In particular, the effect of sample size and anomalies in the measurement and missingness models is scrutinized. Also, confidence limits and confidence bands are constructed.

23.2   THE RATS DATA

These data come from a randomized experiment designed to study the effect of the inhibition of testosterone production in rats (Department of Orthodontics of the Catholic University of Leuven in Belgium (Verbeke and Lesaffre 1997; Verbeke and Molenberghs 2000). A total of 50 male Wistar rats were randomized to either the control or one of the two treatment groups (low or high dose of the drug Decapeptyl (triptorelin), a testosterone production inhibitor). Treatment started at the age of 45 days, and measurements were taken every 10 days, with the first observation taken at the age of 50 days. The response measurement is a characterization of the size of the skull, taken under anaesthesia. Many rats do not survive anaesthesia, implying that for only 22 (44%) rats could all seven designed measurements have been taken. The investigators' impression is that dropout is independent of the measurements.

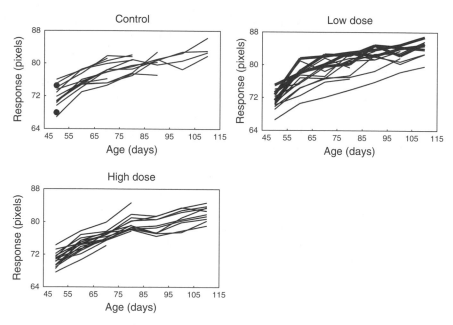

Figure 23.1   Rats data. Individual growth curves for the three treatment groups separately. Influential subjects are highlighted.

The individual profiles are shown in Figure 23.1. To linearize, we use the logarithmic transformation $t = \ln(1 + (\text{age} - 45)/10)$ for the time scale. Let y_{ij} denote the jth measurement for the ith rat, taken at $t = t_{ij}$, $j = 1, \ldots, n_i$, $i = 1, \ldots, N$. A simple statistical model, as considered by Verbeke *et al.* (2001b), then assumes that y_{ij} satisfies a model of the form (7.4) with common average intercept β_0 for all three groups, average slopes β_1, β_2 and β_3 for the three treatment groups respectively, and assuming a so-called compound symmetry covariance structure with common variance $\sigma^2 + \tau^2$ and common covariance τ^2.

23.3   ANALYSIS AND SENSITIVITY ANALYSIS OF THE RATS DATA

The rats data are analysed using model (7.4) with the following specific version of dropout model (15.2):

$$\text{logit}\,[P(D_i = j | D_i \geq j, \boldsymbol{y}_i)] = \psi_0 + \psi_1 y_{i,j-1} + \psi_2 y_{ij}. \qquad (23.1)$$

Parameter estimates are shown in Table 23.1. More details about these estimates and the performance of a local influence analysis can be found in Verbeke *et al.* (2001b). This section will focus on specific details of this local influence analysis.

Figure 23.2 displays overall C_i and influences for subvectors $\boldsymbol{\theta}$, $\boldsymbol{\beta}$, $\boldsymbol{\alpha}$, and $\boldsymbol{\psi}$. In addition, the direction $\boldsymbol{h}_{\max}$ corresponding to maximal local influence is given. Apart from the last of these graphs, the scales are not dimensionless and therefore it would be hard to use a common one for all of the panels. This implies that the main emphasis should be on *relative* magnitudes.

The largest C_i are observed for rats 10, 16, 35, and 41, and virtually the same picture holds for $C_i(\boldsymbol{\psi})$. They are highlighted in Figure 23.2. All four belong to the low-dose group. Arguably, their relatively large influence is caused by an interplay of three factors. First, the profiles are relatively high, and hence y_{ij} and h_{ij} in (22.12) are large. Second, since all four profiles are complete, the first factor in (22.12) contains a maximal number of large terms. Third, the computed v_{ij} are relatively large.

Examination of $C_i(\boldsymbol{\alpha})$ reveals peaks for rats 5 and 23. Both belong to the control group and drop out after a single measurement occasion. They are highlighted in the first panel of Figure 23.1. To explain this, observe that the relative magnitude of $C_i(\boldsymbol{\alpha})$, approximately given by (22.12), is determined by $1 - g(h_{id})$ and $h_{id} - \lambda(h_{id})$. The first term is large when the probability of dropout is small. Now, when dropout occurs early in the sequence, the measurements are still relatively low, implying that the dropout probability is rather small (see Table 23.1). This feature is built into the model by writing the dropout probability in terms of the raw measurements with time-independent

Table 23.1 Rats data. Maximum likelihood estimates (standard errors) of completely random, random and non-random dropout models, fitted to the rat data set, with and without modification.

Original data

Effect	Parameter	MCAR	MAR	MNAR
Measurement model				
Intercept	β_0	68.61 (0.33)	68.61 (0.33)	68.60 (0.33)
Slope control	β_1	7.51 (0.22)	7.51 (0.22)	7.53 (0.24)
Slope low dose	β_2	6.87 (0.23)	6.87 (0.23)	6.89 (0.23)
Slope high dose	β_3	7.31 (0.28)	7.31 (0.28)	7.35 (0.30)
Random intercept	τ^2	3.44 (0.77)	3.44 (0.77)	3.43 (0.77)
Measurement error	σ^2	1.43 (0.14)	1.43 (0.14)	1.43 (0.14)
Dropout model				
Intercept	ψ_0	−1.98 (0.20)	−8.48 (4.00)	−10.30 (6.88)
Previous measurement	ψ_1		0.08 (0.05)	0.03 (0.16)
Current measurement	ψ_2			0.07 (0.22)
−2 log-likelihood		1100.4	1097.6	1097.5

Modified data

Effect	Parameter	MCAR	MAR	MNAR
Measurement model				
Intercept	β_0	70.20 (0.92)	70.20 (0.92)	70.25 (0.92)
Slope control	β_1	7.52 (0.25)	7.52 (0.25)	7.42 (0.26)
Slope low dose	β_2	6.97 (0.25)	6.97 (0.25)	6.90 (0.25)
Slope high dose	β_3	7.21 (0.31)	7.21 (0.31)	7.04 (0.33)
Random intercept	τ^2	40.38 (0.18)	40.38 (0.18)	40.71 (8.25)
Measurement error	σ^2	1.42 (0.14)	1.42 (0.14)	1.44 (0.15)
Dropout model				
Intercept	ψ_0	−1.98 (0.20)	−0.79 (1.99)	2.08 (3.08)
Previous measurement	ψ_1		−0.015 (0.03)	0.23 (0.15)
Current measurement	ψ_2			−0.28 (0.17)
−2 log-likelihood		1218.0	1217.7	1214.8

coefficients rather than, for example, in terms of residuals. Furthermore, the residual $h_{id} - \lambda(h_{id})$ is large since these two rats are somewhat different from the corresponding mean. A practical implication of this is that the time-constant nature of the dropout model may be unlikely to hold. Therefore, a time-varying version was considered, where the logit of the dropout model takes form $\psi_0 + \psi_1 y_{i,j-1} + \nu_0 t_{ij} + \nu_1 t_{ij} y_{i,j-1}$. There is overwhelming evidence in favour of such a more elaborate MAR model (likelihood ratio statistic of 167.4 on 2 degrees of freedom). Thus, local influence can be used to call into question the posited

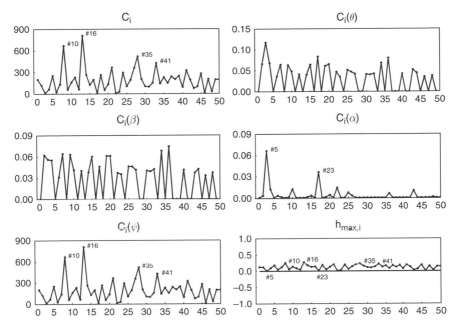

Figure 23.2 Rats data. Index plots of C_i, $C_i(\theta)$, $C_i(\beta)$, $C_i(\alpha)$, $C_i(\psi)$, and of the components of the direction $\boldsymbol{h}_{\max}$ of maximal curvature.

MAR (and MNAR) models, and to guide further selection of more elaborate, perhaps MAR, models.

As all deviations are rather moderate, we further explore our approach by considering a second analysis where all responses for rats 10, 16, 35, and 41 have been increased by 20 units. The effect of this distortion will primarily be seen in the variance structure. Such a change is likely to inflate the random-intercept variance, at the expense of the other variance components. In doing so, we show that (1) such a change is likely to show up in the assessment of the dropout model, underscoring the sensitivity, and (2) the local influence approach is able to detect such an effect. The parameter estimates for all three models are also shown in Table 23.1. Clearly, while the fixed-effects parameters remain virtually unchanged, the random-intercept parameter has, of course, drastically increased. Likewise, the dropout parameters are affected. In addition, the likelihood ratio statistic for MAR versus MCAR changes from 2.8 to 0.3 and for MNAR versus MAR changes from 0.1 to 2.9. Thus, the evidence has shifted from the first to the second test. While all of these statistics seem to be non-significant, there is an important qualitative effect. Moreover, as discussed in Section 19.6, the use of the classical χ^2 distribution is inappropriate for hypothesis tests involving MNAR assumptions

To check whether these findings are recovered by the local influence approach, we examine Figure 23.3. In line with the changes in parameter

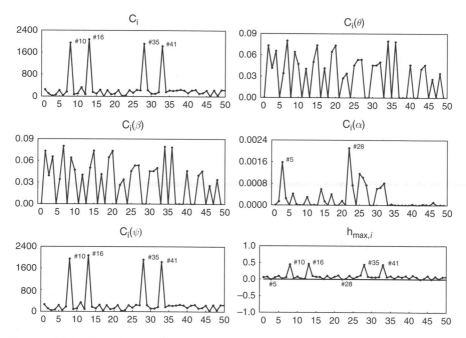

Figure 23.3 Rats data. Index plots of C_i, $C_i(\theta)$, $C_i(\beta)$, $C_i(\alpha)$, $C_i(\psi)$, and of the components of the direction h_{max} of maximal curvature, where four profiles have been shifted upward.

estimates, $C_i(\beta)$ shows no peaks in these observations, but peaks in $C_i(\alpha)$ and $C_i(\psi)$ indicate a relatively strong influence from the four extreme profiles.

It will be clear from the above that subjects may turn out to be influential, for reasons that are distinct from the nature of the dropout model. Indeed, increasing the profile by 20 units primarily changes the level of the random intercept and ultimately changes the form of the random-effects distribution. Nevertheless, this feature shows in our local influence analysis, where the perturbation is put in the dropout model and not, for example, in the measurement model. This feature requires careful study and will be addressed in the next section.

23.4 LOCAL INFLUENCE METHODS AND THEIR BEHAVIOUR

A number of concerns have been raised not only about sensitivity, but also about the tools used to assess sensitivity themselves. We have seen in the case studies in Chapter 22, as in the examples in Verbeke *et al.* (2001b), that the local influence tool, as defined and implemented in Section 22.2, is able to pick up anomalous features of study subjects that are not necessarily related to the missingness mechanism. Such characteristics include subjects with an unusually high profile, or a somewhat atypical serial correlation behaviour. At first sight, this is a little disconcerting, since the ω_i parameter in (22.1) is placed in the dropout model and not in the measurement model, necessitating further investigation regarding which effects are easy or difficult to detect with these local influence methods.

Jansen *et al.* (2006b) designed a simulation study to explore various sources of influence. First, interest lies in the relative magnitudes of the influence measures to assess how feasible it is to separate influence values that are in line with regular behaviour from those that are unduly large. This can be done by proposing a rule of thumb as well as by constructing sampling-based confidence limits and bounds. Second, the impact of one or a few subjects with an anomalous dropout mechanism is explored. Such anomalies are of the kind one would intuitively expect to be picked up by the proposed tool. Great care is needed. Third, the impact due to anomalies in the measurement model is explored. It follows that precisely such anomalies are picked up by the tool relatively easily, in spite of the fact that it is designed for anomalies in the missingness mechanism. An explanation is offered for why such behaviour is seen, which can be combined with explanations offered in Section 19.6.

23.4.1   Effect of sample size

Lesaffre and Verbeke (1998) applied local influence methods to the classical linear mixed-effects model. They introduced ω_i parameters as follows: $\ell = \sum_i \omega_i \ell_i$ where ℓ_i is the log-likelihood contribution for subject i. They were able to show that the sum of the influences is approximately equal to $2N$, where N is the sample size. Their result is based on the fact that, in their local influence contributions, Δ_i in (22.2) becomes

$$\Delta_i = \frac{\partial \ell_i}{\partial \boldsymbol{\theta}},$$

so that the entire expression has (approximately) the form of a contribution to the score test. In our case, as can be seen from (22.8) and (22.9), Δ_i is a second rather than a first derivative of the log-likelihood contributions, implying that a dependence on the sample size, perhaps linear, could be envisaged. Such a calibration would be beneficial since it would allow the determination of critical values, or at least rules of thumb, to assess how large a subject's influence needs to be to require further scrutiny.

To assess this, several data sets were generated, all under the assumption of MAR and with parameters equal to those from the rats example. The only difference between these simulations was the sample size. Selected quantiles for sample sizes 50, 500, and 1000 are shown in Table 23.2. Studying larger

Table 23.2 Simulation study. Selected quantiles of the local influence measures for data sets of different sample sizes, as obtained from simulations and after fitting a simple empirical model.

Sample size	Simulated results						Empirical model		
	50	50	50	500	500	1000	50	500	1000
Median	176.7	138.7	146.8	16.5	15.6	7.6	150.0	15.0	7.5
95th percentile	384.5	359.9	317.3	40.6	39.5	18.7	359.4	39.4	20.3
Maximum	683.7	674.1	950.7	138.0	137.8	53.6	—	—	—

sample sizes was prohibitive in terms of computation time. This is also the reason for considering a single run at size 1000. While the relationship is less clear, as is to be expected, for the maximum value, an obvious trend is seen in the median values and in the 95th percentile. It is seen that the influence for a subject decreases linearly with sample size, and hence the total influence for a data set is roughly constant. This is confirmed by a simple multiplicative regression model, which points to a constant product of the median and the sample size that is equal to 7500. In a similar way, the product of the 95th percentile and the sample size to the power 0.96 equals 15 367. To ensure calibration at the individual level, one could then multiply all influences by the sample size. This calibration result implies that the rescaled local influence can be used as a rough measure to determine whether large values are present. For example, one could investigate subjects for which the influence exceeds $1/N$ of the calibrated total with a certain amount. However, while this is useful in its own right, we still do not learn anything about the actual distribution of a local influence profile under the null hypothesis. To gain further insight into this problem, confidence limits and simultaneous confidence bounds will be derived next.

23.4.2   Pointwise confidence limits and simultaneous confidence bounds for the local influence measure

Because, for practical purposes, only high values of the influence measures are of interest, we will focus on one-sided (upper) limits and bounds. One thousand data sets of 50 rats were simulated, using the parameters of the MAR model. To produce a consistent ordering of the C_i values, rather than that based on the arbitrary order of the rats within the set of data, these were sorted from large to small.

Consider, say, 1000 repetitions of a bootstrap experiment with 50 grid points. At each grid point, the 95% pointwise upper confidence limit is the 95th percentile of the C_{ij} values at that particular grid point. Construction of the simultaneous confidence bounds is based on Besag *et al.* (1995). For each grid point j, the C_{ij} values are ordered to give the order statistics C_{ij} and their corresponding ranks $r_j^{(t)}, t = 1, \ldots, 1000$. Next, for fixed k, t_k is defined as the kth order statistic of the set

$$\left\{ \max\left(\max_{1 \leq j \leq 50} r_j^{(t)}; 1001 - \min_{1 \leq j \leq 50} r_j^{(t)} \right); t = 1, \ldots, 1000 \right\}.$$

Then, by construction, the intervals

$$\left\{ \left[C_{i,j}^{[1001-t_k]}; C_{i,j}^{[t_k]} \right]; j = 1, \ldots, 50 \right\}$$

have a global confidence level of at least $100(k/1000)\%$. To obtain the 95% simultaneous upper confidence bound, take $k = 900$, and restrict consideration to the upper bound $C_{i,j}^{[t_k]}$. A graphical representation of this result is given in Figure 23.4.

23.4.3 Anomalies in the missingness mechanism

To obtain an idea of the effect of anomalies in the dropout mechanism, the following procedure was used.

Generate an MNAR data set, fit these data assuming an MAR mechanism in model 15.2, and use the estimates of those model parameters to generate 1000 data sets, which are then used to construct the pointwise confidence limits and simultaneous confidence bounds as outlined in Section 23.4.2. Next, add the profile of ordered C_i values from the original MNAR data set on the

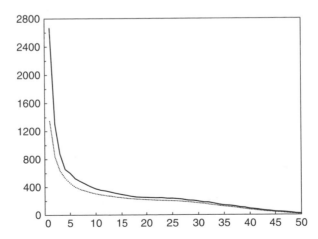

Figure 23.4 Simulation study. 95% pointwise upper confidence limit (dotted curve) and 95% simultaneous upper confidence bound (solid curve).

graph with the pointwise confidence limits and simultaneous confidence bounds. Several different settings to generate the MNAR data set were explored and will be discussed in the remainder of this section.

First, attention is paid to the creation of MNAR sets, based on the model parameters. This was done in the following ways: (1) a set of 50 rats was generated using the MNAR parameters from the original rats data, as presented in the upper part of Table 23.1; (2) the same parameters were used, except for ψ_2, which was increased to 0.5; (3) only 10% of the data (equivalent to 5 rats) were generated taking $\psi_2 = 0.2$, while for the remaining 90% of the data (45 rats) $\psi_2 = 0$; (4) using the incremental parameterization introduced in Thijs *et al.* (2001), 10% of the rats were generated with $\lambda_2 = 0.2$, and the other 90% with $\lambda_2 = 0$. The different settings of these simulations were repeated several times but, as they all gave similar results, a single result from each setting is discussed and presented in Figures 23.5 and 23.6.

A general trend is observed in settings 1–4. The C_i profile of the MNAR data set crosses neither the 95% pointwise upper confidence limit nor the simultaneous upper confidence bound for large values of C_i. On the other hand, in some settings they cross the 95% pointwise upper confidence limit for small values of C_i (near the end of the profile), but since we are only interested in highly

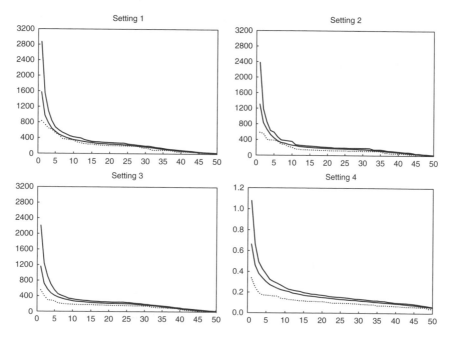

Figure 23.5 Simulation study. Graphical representation of the profiles of different parameter-based MNAR settings (dotted curves), compared with the 95% pointwise upper confidence limit and 95% simultaneous upper confidence bound (solid curves).

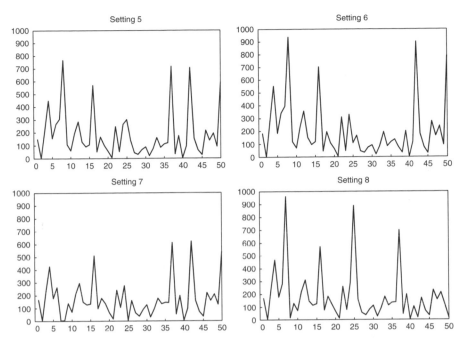

Figure 23.6 Simulation study. Graphical representation of the unordered C_i profiles of different settings with manually created anomalies in the missingness model.

influential subjects, this result is irrelevant for our purposes. Taking a closer look at the rats for whom $\psi_2 \neq 0$ (settings 3 and 4) we note that their C_i values are very small (all within the 10 lowest values). We can therefore conclude that this type of MNAR mechanism is undetectable using local influence. Note that the limit and bound for setting 2 is more ragged than for the others. The reason is that convergence is quite difficult to obtain for this setting, in line with general convergence problems for situations where ψ_2 is substantially different from zero. The scale for setting 4 in Figure 23.5 is completely different from the scale in the other settings, owing to the fact that setting 4 considers the effect of the difference between the current and the previous measurement on the dropout process, rather than the raw effect of the current measurement in the other three settings.

In a second round of settings, MNAR was created ministically. A data set was generated using the MAR parameters of the original rats data in Table 23.1 (the C_i profile of this data set is shown in Figure 23.7). Then the MNAR part was created by manually deleting values from some profiles as follows: (5) all values of skull height from the moment that one of them exceeded 86 mm; (6) all values of skull height from the moment that one of them exceeded 85 mm; (7) second to last values of skull height if the value at age 60 days (second value)

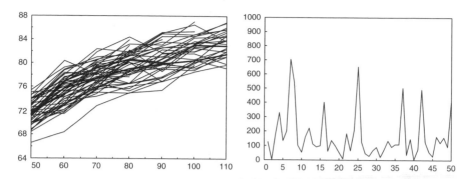

Figure 23.7 Simulation study. Individual growth curves (left-hand panel, subjects 3, 21, and 26 highlighted) and C_i profile (right) of the MAR data set which will be manipulated.

exceeded 78.83 mm (95th percentile); (8) third to last values of skull height if the value at age 70 days (third value) exceeded 80.82 mm (95th percentile).

Our interest is now in seeing how such sets of data give qualitatively different influence graphs than under the original rats data set. Therefore, we have to proceed somewhat differently from the simulation study done for settings 1–4. We now directly compare the influence graphs from the four settings 5–8 with the original one. Under setting 5, we see that the peak for rat 25, seen in the original analysis, is removed, while others appear, in the sense that some moderate peaks now become the largest ones. However, no rat really stands out to the extent that further investigation is needed. It is noteworthy, though, that those animals whose profiles have been shortened due to the action described under setting 5, have, as a consequence, a smaller influence value. A similar phenomenon is observed in Jansen *et al.* (2006b) for categorical responses. Settings 6–8 are similar in qualitative terms, even though the phenomena are slightly more extreme in setting 6 than in setting 5.

23.4.4 Anomalies in the measurement model

In this section, we shift attention to anomalies in the measurement model. For this purpose, four MAR data sets were generated, each with specific changes to the measurement model for three randomly selected rats: (1) mean profile increased by 20 units *after* the dropout probability was calculated, (2) mean profile increased by 20 units *before* the dropout probability was calculated, (3) variance component increased by 20 units, and (4) τ^2 (covariance for the compound symmetry) increased by 20 units. The starting data set, without any changes to the measurement model, is the same as was used in Figure 23.7.

In contrast to settings 3 and 4, which focus on the variance–covariance structure and show virtually no impact (Figure 23.8), settings 1 and 2 exhibit

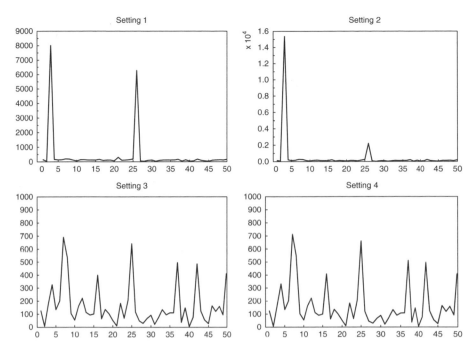

Figure 23.8 Simulation study. Graphical representation of the unordered C_i profiles of different settings with anomalies in the measurement model.

a dramatic effect. The impact is larger in setting 2 because there the dropout model is also affected. In both settings, rats 3 and 26 clearly stand out, although with differing relative magnitudes. The effect of rat 21 is negligible. These results can be explained by taking a closer look at the individual profiles of those rats.

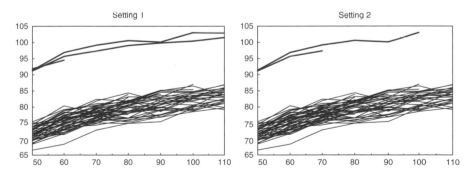

Figure 23.9 Simulation study. Individual growth curves for settings 1 and 2, where the mean profile is increased, before of after the dropout probability was calculated. Subjects 3, 21 and 26 are highlighted.

Figure 23.9 shows that in setting 1 rat 21 has only two observations, while rats 3 and 26 have complete profiles. In setting 2, the profile of rat 21 is reduced to only one observation, which explains the negligible influence, and the profiles of rats 3 and 26 are reduced to six and three measurements, respectively. This is consistent with earlier work that indicated that shortened profiles tend to give smaller influence values (Jansen *et al.* 2006b).

23.5   CONCLUDING REMARKS

The importance of sensitivity analysis in the missing data context has been repeatedly stressed in this book. One tool, among the wide range that have been proposed for such analyses, is local influence. At first sight this particular tool seems to behave in a counterintuitive way. The simulation results show that there can be little or no local influence stemming from a few subjects that drop out in a non-random way. On the other hand, there can be considerable influence in a number of settings where the measurement model is changed in the sense that a few profiles have outlying shapes. This indicates that the non-random parameter ψ_2, rather than capturing true MNAR missingness, has a strong tendency to pick up other deviations, primarily in the measurement model. Many authors have noted that there is very little information in many data sets for the parameter ψ_2, in addition to the information available for all other parameters. If this were to be true, it ought to show in the behaviour of the likelihood ratio test statistic for ψ_2, as well as in the structure of the information matrix for the vector of model parameters. We will explore this further in the next chapter.

A Latent-Class Mixture Model for Incomplete Longitudinal Gaussian Data

24.1 INTRODUCTION

In Section 3.3 the three main modelling frameworks – selection, pattern mixture, and shared parameter – were introduced. These were then explored in Chapters 15, 16, and 17, respectively. It is obviously possible, however, to formulate models that combine aspects of the three families; indeed Diggle (1998) places all three in one overall framework. One example of such a combination, as proposed by Beunckens *et al.* (2006), using latent classes, is the subject of the present chapter. This model provides a flexible modelling tool in its own right and can be used as a device for sensitivity analysis.

The so-called latent-class mixture model, proposed by Beunckens *et al.* (2006), is introduced in Section 24.2. The corresponding likelihood function and associated methods of estimation are discussed in Section 24.3. In Section 24.4 we explore how the method can be used as a device for classifying subjects into latent groups. Using simulations, some insight into its performance is provided in Section 24.5. In Section 24.6 we return to the depression trials data to illustrate the methodology.

24.2 LATENT-CLASS MIXTURE MODELS

As usual, let the random variable Y_{ij} denote the response of interest, for the ith individual, with measurements planned at times t_{ij}, $i = 1, \ldots, N$, $j = 1, \ldots, n_i$.

Missing Data in Clinical Studies   G. Molenberghs and M.G. Kenward
© 2007 John Wiley & Sons, Ltd

We group the outcomes into the vector $\boldsymbol{Y}_i = (Y_{i1}, \ldots, Y_{in_i})'$. We also define the dropout indicator D_i to have its usual meaning (Section 3.2).

Recall the shared-parameter model factorization (3.5), studied in Chapter 17. This can be expressed in dropout form as follows:

$$f(\boldsymbol{y}_i, d_i | \boldsymbol{b}_i, \boldsymbol{\theta}, \boldsymbol{\psi}) = f(\boldsymbol{y}_i | \boldsymbol{b}_i, \boldsymbol{\theta}) f(d_i | \boldsymbol{b}_i, \boldsymbol{\psi}).$$

We suppress explicit reference to the covariates in the notation. As stated in Chapter 17, the factorization above, in keeping with most shared-parameter models proposed in the literature, presumes the existence of a random-effects vector $\boldsymbol{b}_i$, conditional upon which the measurement and dropout processes are independent. This particular shared-parameter model can be represented as in Figure 24.1(a).

Beunckens *et al.* (2006) propose an extension to this model that captures unmeasured heterogeneity between the subjects through a latent variable. This extended model is called a *latent-class mixture model*, and a representation of it is shown in Figure 24.1(b). Thus, in addition to the shared parameters $\boldsymbol{b}_i$, the model contains a latent variable, $\boldsymbol{Q}_i$, that divides the population in g subgroups. This latent variable is a vector of group indicators $\boldsymbol{Q}_i = (Q_{i1}, \ldots, Q_{ig})$, defined as $Q_{ik} = 1$ if subject i belongs to group k, and 0 otherwise. Both the measurement and dropout processes depend on this latent variable, not only directly, but also through the subject-specific effects $\boldsymbol{b}_i$. The distribution of $\boldsymbol{Q}_i$ is multinomial and defined by $P(Q_{ik} = 1) = \pi_k$ ($k = 1, \ldots, g$). The component probabilities obey $\sum_{k=1}^{g} \pi_k = 1$. In what follows, π_k will also be called the prior probability of an observation belonging to the kth component of the mixture.

The measurement process is specified by means of a so-called heterogeneity linear mixed model, originally proposed by Verbeke and Lesaffre (1996) and also described by Verbeke and Molenberghs (2000, Chapter 12). The model is given by

$$\boldsymbol{Y}_i | q_{ik} = 1, \boldsymbol{b}_i \sim N(X_i \boldsymbol{\beta}_k + Z_i \boldsymbol{b}_i, \Sigma_i^{(k)}),$$

where, as usual, X_i and Z_i are design matrices, $\boldsymbol{\beta}_k$ are fixed effects, possibly depending on the group components, and $\boldsymbol{b}_i$ denotes the shared parameters,

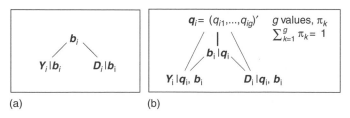

(a)   (b)

Figure 24.1 Representation of (a) shared-parameter models and (b) their extension to latent-class mixture models.

following a mixture of g normal distributions with mean vectors $\boldsymbol{\mu}_k$ and covariance matrices $\boldsymbol{D}_k$, that is,

$$(\boldsymbol{b}_i | q_{ik} = 1) \sim N(\boldsymbol{\mu}_k, D_k),$$

and therefore

$$\boldsymbol{b}_i \sim \sum_{k=1}^{g} \pi_k N(\boldsymbol{\mu}_k, D_k).$$

The measurement error terms $\boldsymbol{\varepsilon}_i$ follow a normal distribution with mean zero and covariance matrix $\Sigma_i^{(k)}$ and are assumed to be independent of the shared parameters. The mean and the variance of $\boldsymbol{Y}_i$ can be derived as

$$E(\boldsymbol{Y}_i) = X_i \sum_{k=1}^{g} \pi_k \boldsymbol{\beta}_k + Z_i \sum_{k=1}^{g} \pi_k \boldsymbol{\mu}_k, \tag{24.1}$$

$$\text{var}(\boldsymbol{Y}_i) = Z_i' \left[\sum_{k=1}^{g} \pi_k \boldsymbol{\mu}_k^2 - \left(\sum_{k=1}^{g} \pi_k \boldsymbol{\mu}_k \right)^2 + \sum_{k=1}^{g} \pi_k D_k \right] Z_i + \sum_{k=1}^{g} \pi_k \Sigma_i^{(k)}. \tag{24.2}$$

Furthermore, for identifiability reasons, we have to assume that the shared effects are 'calibrated', that is, that $\sum_{k=1}^{g} \pi_k \boldsymbol{\mu}_k = 0$. This leads to the following simplifications of (24.1) and (24.2):

$$E(\boldsymbol{Y}_i) = X_i \sum_{k=1}^{g} \pi_k \boldsymbol{\beta}_k,$$

$$\text{var}(\boldsymbol{Y}_i) = Z_i' \left[\sum_{k=1}^{g} \pi_k \boldsymbol{\mu}_k^2 + \sum_{k=1}^{g} \pi_k D_k \right] Z_i + \sum_{k=1}^{g} \pi_k \Sigma_i^{(k)}.$$

The dropout model is specified consistently with (15.2) and (15.3), but now the shared parameters $\boldsymbol{b}_i$ and the latent class membership indicators q_{ik} are part of the model:

$$g_{ij}(\mathbf{w}_{ij}, \boldsymbol{b}_i, q_{ik}) = P(D_i = j | D_i \geq j, \mathbf{w}_{ij}, \boldsymbol{b}_i, q_{ik} = 1),$$

where $\mathbf{w}_{ij}$ is a vector containing all relevant covariates. An obvious choice is to further assume that

$$\text{logit}[g_{ij}(\mathbf{w}_{ij}, \boldsymbol{b}_i, q_{ik})] = \mathbf{w}_{ij} \boldsymbol{\gamma}_k + \boldsymbol{\lambda} \boldsymbol{b}_i.$$

The joint likelihood of the measurement and dropout processes takes the form

$$f(\boldsymbol{y}_i, \boldsymbol{r}_i) = f(\boldsymbol{y}_i, d_i)$$

$$= \sum_{k=1}^{g} P(q_{ik} = 1) f(\boldsymbol{y}_i, d_i | q_{ik=1})$$

$$= \sum_{k=1}^{g} \pi_k \int f(\boldsymbol{y}_i, d_i | q_{ik=1}, \boldsymbol{b}_i) f_k(\boldsymbol{b}_i) d\boldsymbol{b}_i$$

$$= \sum_{k=1}^{g} \pi_k \int f(\boldsymbol{y}_i | q_{ik} = 1, \boldsymbol{b}_i, X_i, Z_i)$$

$$\times f(d_i | q_{ik} = 1, \boldsymbol{b}_i, \boldsymbol{w}_i) f_k(\boldsymbol{b}_i) d\boldsymbol{b}_i, \qquad (24.3)$$

where $f(\boldsymbol{y}_i | q_{ik} = 1, \boldsymbol{b}_i, X_i, Z_i)$ is the density function of the normal distribution $N(X_i\boldsymbol{\beta}_k + Z_i\boldsymbol{b}_i, \Sigma_i^{(k)})$, $f_k(\boldsymbol{b}_i)$ is the density function of $N(\boldsymbol{\mu}_k, D_k)$, and

$$f(d_i | q_{ik} = 1, \boldsymbol{b}_i, \boldsymbol{w}_i) = \begin{cases} g_{id_i}(\boldsymbol{w}_{id_i}, \boldsymbol{b}_i, q_{ik}) \times \prod_{j=2}^{d_i-1} [1 - g_{ij}(\boldsymbol{w}_{ij}, \boldsymbol{b}_i, q_{ik})] & \text{if incomplete,} \\ \prod_{j=2}^{n_i} [1 - g_{ij}(\boldsymbol{w}_{ij}, \boldsymbol{b}_i, q_{ik})] & \text{if complete.} \end{cases}$$

The latter equation is the latent-class mixture analogue of (15.2).

Whereas selection models and pattern-mixture models derive from two different factorizations of the joint density of the measurement and dropout processes, the latent-class mixture model is based on assuming an additional latent structure. In the pattern-mixture model, the observed dropout patterns are taken into account when modelling the measurement process. In the latent-class mixture models this idea is modified to allow grouping of the subjects through a latent variable, thereby accounting for inter-group differences in terms of both their dropout pattern and their measurement profiles.

24.3   THE LIKELIHOOD FUNCTION AND ESTIMATION

Estimation of the unknown parameters in the latent-class mixture model can be based on the maximum likelihood principle. The likelihood function of the latent-class mixture model is formulated in Section 24.3.1. Then, in Section 24.3.2, an outline is provided of how the likelihood can be maximized using the EM algorithm (see also Chapter 8) which follows the ideas in Redner and Walker (1984).

24.3.1   Likelihood function

Let $\boldsymbol{\pi}$ be the vector of component probabilities $\boldsymbol{\pi}' = (\pi_1, \ldots, \pi_g)$, and group all other unknown parameters of the measurement process in the vector $\boldsymbol{\theta}$, of the dropout process in $\boldsymbol{\psi}$, and of the mixture distribution in $\boldsymbol{\alpha}$. If $\boldsymbol{\sigma}$ denotes the vector of covariance parameters of all $\Sigma_i^{(k)}$, $\boldsymbol{\delta}$ the covariance parameters of all D_k, $\boldsymbol{\mu}' = (\boldsymbol{\mu}_1, \ldots, \boldsymbol{\mu}_g)$, and $\boldsymbol{\gamma}' = (\boldsymbol{\gamma}_1, \ldots, \boldsymbol{\gamma}_g)$, then $\boldsymbol{\theta} = (\boldsymbol{\beta}, \boldsymbol{\sigma})$, $\boldsymbol{\psi} = (\boldsymbol{\gamma}, \boldsymbol{\lambda})$ and $\boldsymbol{\alpha} = (\boldsymbol{\mu}, \boldsymbol{\delta})$. Denote by $\boldsymbol{\Omega}$ the vector containing all unknown parameters in the model, that is $\boldsymbol{\Omega}' = (\boldsymbol{\pi}', \boldsymbol{\theta}', \boldsymbol{\psi}', \boldsymbol{\alpha}')$. Estimation and inference for $\boldsymbol{\Omega}$ will now be based on the observed data likelihood, $L(\boldsymbol{\Omega}|\boldsymbol{y}^o, \boldsymbol{d})$, obtained by integrating out the unobserved data from the joint distribution of the measurement and dropout processes:

$$
\begin{aligned}
L(\boldsymbol{\Omega}|\boldsymbol{y}^o, \boldsymbol{d}) &= \prod_{i=1}^{N} f(\boldsymbol{y}_i^o, d_i|\boldsymbol{\Omega}) \\
&= \prod_{i=1}^{N} \int f(\boldsymbol{y}_i, d_i|\boldsymbol{\Omega}) \, d\boldsymbol{y}_i^m \\
&= \prod_{i=1}^{N} \int \left\{ \sum_{k=1}^{g} \pi_k \int f(\boldsymbol{y}_i|\boldsymbol{\theta}, \boldsymbol{b}_i, q_{ik} = 1) \right. \\
&\qquad \left. \times f(d_i|\boldsymbol{\psi}, \boldsymbol{b}_i, q_{ik} = 1) f_k(\boldsymbol{b}_i|\boldsymbol{\alpha}) d\boldsymbol{b}_i \right\} d\boldsymbol{y}_i^m \\
&= \prod_{i=1}^{N} \sum_{k=1}^{g} \pi_k \int \left\{ \int f(\boldsymbol{y}_i|\boldsymbol{\theta}, \boldsymbol{b}_i, q_{ik} = 1) \, d\boldsymbol{y}_i^m \right\} \\
&\qquad \times f(d_i|\boldsymbol{\psi}, \boldsymbol{b}_i, q_{ik} = 1) f_k(\boldsymbol{b}_i|\boldsymbol{\alpha}) d\boldsymbol{b}_i \\
&= \prod_{i=1}^{N} \sum_{k=1}^{g} \pi_k \int f(\boldsymbol{y}_i^o|\boldsymbol{\theta}, \boldsymbol{b}_i, q_{ik} = 1) f(d_i|\boldsymbol{\psi}, \boldsymbol{b}_i, q_{ik} = 1) \\
&\qquad \times f_k(\boldsymbol{b}_i|\boldsymbol{\alpha}) d\boldsymbol{b}_i,
\end{aligned}
\tag{24.4}
$$

where $\boldsymbol{y}^o = (\boldsymbol{y}_1^o, \ldots, \boldsymbol{y}_N^o)'$ is the vector containing all observed response values and $\boldsymbol{d} = (d_1, \ldots, d_N)$ is the vector of all values of the dropout indicator.

Note that this likelihood function is invariant under the $g!$ possible permutations of the parameters corresponding to each of the g mixture components. However, we can place constraints on the parameters to remove this lack of identifiability. We will use the constraint suggested by Aitkin and Rubin (1985): $\pi_1 \geq \pi_2 \geq \ldots \geq \pi_g$. The log-likelihood function corresponding to (24.4) is

$$
\begin{aligned}
\ell(\boldsymbol{\Omega}|\boldsymbol{y}^o, \boldsymbol{d}) &= \sum_{i=1}^{N} \ln \left\{ \sum_{k=1}^{g} \pi_k \int f(\boldsymbol{y}_i^o|\boldsymbol{\theta}, \boldsymbol{b}_i, q_{ik} = 1) \right. \\
&\qquad \left. \times f(d_i|\boldsymbol{\psi}, \boldsymbol{b}_i, q_{ik} = 1) f_k(\boldsymbol{b}_i|\boldsymbol{\alpha}) d\boldsymbol{b}_i \right\}.
\end{aligned}
\tag{24.5}
$$

To maximize (24.5) with respect to Ω, the EM algorithm (Dempster *et al.* 1977; see Chapter 8 above) will be employed. Here, the underlying latent variable Q_i, representing component membership, will be considered missing. Thus, the response vector Y_i^o and the dropout indicator D_i, together with the (unobserved) population indicators Q_i, can be seen as the so-called *augmented data*, whereas vectors Y_i^o and D_i constitute the observed data.

Clearly, the likelihood function $L(\Omega|y^o, d)$ still corresponds to the incomplete data. Since the joint density of Y_i^o, D_i and Q_i equals

$$f_i(\boldsymbol{y}_i^o, d_i, Q_{i1} = q_{i1}, \ldots, Q_{ig} = q_{ig})$$

$$= f_i(\boldsymbol{y}_i^o, d_i | Q_{i1} = q_{i1}, \ldots, Q_{ig} = q_{ig}) \cdot P(Q_{i1} = q_{i1}, \ldots, Q_{ig} = q_{ig})$$

$$= \left\{ \prod_{k=1}^{g} [f_{ik}(\boldsymbol{y}_i^o, d_i | \boldsymbol{\theta}, \boldsymbol{\psi}, \boldsymbol{\alpha})]^{q_{ik}} \right\} \cdot \left\{ \prod_{k=1}^{g} \pi_k^{q_{ik}} \right\}$$

$$= \prod_{k=1}^{g} [\pi_k f_{ik}(\boldsymbol{y}_i^o, d_i | \boldsymbol{\theta}, \boldsymbol{\psi}, \boldsymbol{\alpha})]^{q_{ik}},$$

the joint likelihood $L(\Omega|y^o, d, q)$ of the augmented data, that is, the likelihood function that would have been obtained if the values $\boldsymbol{q}_i = (q_{i1}, \ldots, q_{ig})'$ of the population indicators Q_i had been observed, would be

$$L(\Omega|\boldsymbol{y}^o, \boldsymbol{d}, \boldsymbol{b}) = \prod_{i=1}^{N} \prod_{k=1}^{g} [\pi_k f_{ik}(\boldsymbol{y}_i^o, d_i | \boldsymbol{\theta}, \boldsymbol{\psi}, \boldsymbol{\alpha})]^{q_{ik}}, \qquad (24.6)$$

with $\boldsymbol{q} = (\boldsymbol{q}_1, \ldots, \boldsymbol{q}_n)'$ the vector of all hypothetically observed population indicators. The log-likelihood function corresponding to the likelihood function (24.6) takes the form

$$\ell(\Omega|\boldsymbol{y}, \boldsymbol{d}, \boldsymbol{b}) = \sum_{i=1}^{N} \sum_{k=1}^{g} q_{ik} \{\ln \pi_k + \ln f_{ik}(\boldsymbol{y}_i^o, d_i | \boldsymbol{\theta}, \boldsymbol{\psi}, \boldsymbol{\alpha})\}. \qquad (24.7)$$

24.3.2   Estimation using the EM algorithm

Maximizing $\ell(\Omega|y^o, d, q)$ would be analytically and computationally easier than maximizing the log-likelihood $\ell(\Omega|y^o, d)$. However, the estimates obtained from maximizing $\ell(\Omega|y^o, d, q)$ with respect to Ω will depend on the unobserved indicators $\boldsymbol{q}$. Therefore, the EM algorithm is advisable, since then we will maximize the expected value of $\ell(\Omega|y^o, d, q)$ with respect to Ω, where the expectation is taken over all unobserved $\boldsymbol{q}$, that is, $E[\ell(\Omega|y^o, d, Q)|y, d]$. This conditional expectation of $\ell(\Omega|y^o, d, q)$ given y^o and d, is calculated within the E step of each iteration of the EM algorithm. In the M step the resulting expected log-likelihood function is then maximized. Denote by $\mathcal{O}$ the expected log-likelihood function and call this the objective function. The EM algorithm is an iterative procedure, that is, it starts from an initial value $\Omega^{(0)}$ for Ω, and then constructs a series of estimates $\Omega^{(t)}$ which converges to the maximum likelihood estimator $\widehat{\Omega}$ of Ω. Initial values can be obtained, for example, from considering separate models for the measurement and dropout processes. Given $\Omega^{(t)}$, the current estimate for Ω, the updated estimate $\Omega^{(t+1)}$ is obtained through one iteration of the EM algorithm. Iteration then continues until convergence, that is, until

$$\left| \ell(\Omega^{(t+1)}|\boldsymbol{y}^o, \boldsymbol{d}) - \ell(\Omega^{(t)}|\boldsymbol{y}^o, \boldsymbol{d}) \right| < \varepsilon^*,$$

for some small, prespecified $\varepsilon^* > 0$. More details are provided in the following.

24.3.3 The E step

We describe here the iteration step $t+1$, in which the estimate is updated to $\Omega^{(t+1)}$, using the estimate that results from iteration step t, $\Omega^{(t)}$. The E step consists of the calculation of the conditional expectation of $\ell(\Omega|\boldsymbol{y}^o, \boldsymbol{d}, \boldsymbol{q})$, given $\boldsymbol{y}^o$ and $\boldsymbol{d}$, which is given by

$$
\begin{aligned}
\mathcal{O}(\Omega|\Omega^{(t)}) &= E\left[\ell(\Omega|\boldsymbol{y}^o, \boldsymbol{d}, \boldsymbol{Q}) \,\middle|\, \boldsymbol{y}^o, \boldsymbol{d}, \Omega^{(t)} \right] \\
&= E\left[\sum_{i=1}^{N} \sum_{k=1}^{g} Q_{ik} \{\ln \pi_k + \ln f_{ik}(\boldsymbol{y}_i^o, d_i | \boldsymbol{\theta}, \boldsymbol{\psi}, \boldsymbol{\alpha})\} \,\middle|\, \boldsymbol{y}^o, \boldsymbol{d}, \Omega^{(t)} \right] \\
&= \sum_{i=1}^{N} \sum_{k=1}^{g} E\left[Q_{ik} \,\middle|\, \boldsymbol{y}^o, \boldsymbol{d}, \Omega^{(t)} \right] \{\ln \pi_k + \ln f_{ik}(\boldsymbol{y}_i^o, d_i | \boldsymbol{\theta}, \boldsymbol{\psi}, \boldsymbol{\alpha})\} .
\end{aligned}
$$

Therefore, we need to calculate:

$$
\begin{aligned}
E\left[Q_{ik} \,\middle|\, \boldsymbol{y}^o, \boldsymbol{d}, \Omega^{(t)} \right] &= P\left(Q_{ik} = 1 | \boldsymbol{y}^o, \boldsymbol{d}, \Omega^{(t)} \right) \\
&= \left. \frac{f_i\left(\boldsymbol{y}_i^o, d_i | Q_{ik} = 1\right) P(Q_{ik} = 1)}{f_i(\boldsymbol{y}_i^o, d_i)} \right|_{\Omega^{(t)}} \\
&= \left. \frac{\pi_k f_{ik}(\boldsymbol{y}_i^o, d_i | \boldsymbol{\theta}, \boldsymbol{\psi}, \boldsymbol{\alpha})}{\sum_{k=1}^{g} \pi_k f_{ik}(\boldsymbol{y}_i^o, d_i | \boldsymbol{\theta}, \boldsymbol{\psi}, \boldsymbol{\alpha})} \right|_{\Omega^{(t)}} = \pi_{ik}(\Omega^{(t)}),
\end{aligned}
$$

where $\pi_{ik}(\Omega^{(t)})$ is the posterior probability of the ith subject belonging to the kth component of the mixture. This means that the E step reduces to the calculation of posterior probabilities $\pi_{ik}(\Omega^{(t)})$, for $i = 1, \ldots, N$ and $k = 1, \ldots, g$.

24.3.4　The M step

The updated estimate $\mathbf{\Omega}^{(t+1)}$ is now obtained from maximizing $\mathcal{O}(\mathbf{\Omega}|\mathbf{\Omega}^{(t)})$ with respect to $\mathbf{\Omega}$. From the E step we know that

$$
\begin{aligned}
\mathcal{O}(\mathbf{\Omega}|\mathbf{\Omega}^{(t)}) &= \sum_{i=1}^{N}\sum_{k=1}^{g} \pi_{ik}(\mathbf{\Omega}^{(t)})\left\{\ln \pi_k + \ln f_{ik}(\boldsymbol{y}_i^o, d_i|\boldsymbol{\theta}, \boldsymbol{\psi}, \boldsymbol{\alpha})\right\} \\
&= \underbrace{\sum_{i=1}^{N}\sum_{k=1}^{g} \pi_{ik}(\mathbf{\Omega}^{(t)})\ln \pi_k}_{=\mathcal{O}_1(\boldsymbol{\pi}|\mathbf{\Omega}^{(t)})} + \underbrace{\sum_{i=1}^{N}\sum_{k=1}^{g} \pi_{ik}(\mathbf{\Omega}^{(t)})\ln f_{ik}(\boldsymbol{y}_i^o, d_i|\boldsymbol{\theta}, \boldsymbol{\psi}, \boldsymbol{\alpha})}_{=\mathcal{O}_2(\boldsymbol{\theta}, \boldsymbol{\psi}, \boldsymbol{\alpha}|\mathbf{\Omega}^{(t)})} \\
&= \mathcal{O}_1(\boldsymbol{\pi}|\mathbf{\Omega}^{(t)}) + \mathcal{O}_2(\boldsymbol{\theta}, \boldsymbol{\psi}, \boldsymbol{\alpha}|\mathbf{\Omega}^{(t)}).
\end{aligned}
\tag{24.8}
$$

The first term in (24.8) depends only on $\boldsymbol{\pi}$, whereas the second depends only on $\boldsymbol{\theta}$, $\boldsymbol{\psi}$, and $\boldsymbol{\alpha}$. So, to find the maximum of the $\mathcal{O}$ function with respect to $\mathbf{\Omega}' = (\boldsymbol{\pi}', \boldsymbol{\theta}', \boldsymbol{\psi}', \boldsymbol{\alpha}')$, we can maximize both terms separately.

We first maximize the $\mathcal{O}$ function with respect to $\boldsymbol{\pi}$. This requires the maximization of $\mathcal{O}_1$, since $\mathcal{O}_2$ is independent of $\boldsymbol{\pi}$. Under the restriction $\sum_{k=1}^{g} \pi_k = 1$, we can rewrite $\mathcal{O}_1$ as follows:

$$
\mathcal{O}_1(\boldsymbol{\pi}|\mathbf{\Omega}^{(t)}) = \sum_{i=1}^{N}\sum_{k=1}^{g-1} \pi_{ik}(\mathbf{\Omega}^{(t)})\ln \pi_k + \sum_{i=1}^{N} \pi_{ig}(\mathbf{\Omega}^{(t)})\ln\left(1 - \sum_{k=1}^{g-1}\pi_k\right).
$$

If we now set all first-order derivatives with respect to $\pi_1, \ldots, \pi_{g-1}$ equal to zero, the updated estimate satisfies

$$
\begin{aligned}
\frac{\partial \mathcal{O}_1}{\partial \pi_k} = 0 &\Leftrightarrow \sum_{i=1}^{N}\frac{\pi_{ik}(\mathbf{\Omega}^{(t)})}{\pi_k^{(t+1)}} - \sum_{i=1}^{N}\frac{\pi_{ig}(\mathbf{\Omega}^{(t)})}{1 - \sum_{k=1}^{g-1}\pi_k^{(t+1)}} = 0 \\
&\Leftrightarrow \sum_{i=1}^{N}\frac{\pi_{ik}(\mathbf{\Omega}^{(t)})}{\pi_k^{(t+1)}} = \sum_{i=1}^{N}\frac{\pi_{ig}(\mathbf{\Omega}^{(t)})}{\pi_g^{(t+1)}} \\
&\Leftrightarrow \frac{\pi_k^{(t+1)}}{\pi_g^{(t+1)}} = \frac{\sum_{i=1}^{N}\pi_{ik}(\mathbf{\Omega}^{(t)})}{\sum_{i=1}^{N}\pi_{ig}(\mathbf{\Omega}^{(t)})}.
\end{aligned}
\tag{24.9}
$$

This, in turn, implies that

$$
\begin{aligned}
1 = \sum_{k=1}^{g}\pi_k^{(t+1)} &= \sum_{k=1}^{g}\frac{\pi_g^{(t+1)}\sum_{i=1}^{N}\pi_{ik}(\mathbf{\Omega}^{(t)})}{\sum_{i=1}^{N}\pi_{ig}(\mathbf{\Omega}^{(t)})} \\
&= \frac{\pi_g^{(t+1)}\sum_{i=1}^{N}\overbrace{\sum_{k=1}^{g}\pi_{ik}(\mathbf{\Omega}^{(t)})}^{=1}}{\sum_{i=1}^{N}\pi_{ig}(\mathbf{\Omega}^{(t)})} = \frac{N\,\pi_g^{(t+1)}}{\sum_{i=1}^{N}\pi_{ig}(\mathbf{\Omega}^{(t)})},
\end{aligned}
$$

and hence

$$\pi_g^{(t+1)} = \frac{1}{N} \sum_{i=1}^{N} \pi_{ig}(\boldsymbol{\Omega}^{(t)}). \tag{24.10}$$

From (24.9) and (24.10) it follows that the updated estimates $\pi_k^{(t+1)}$, $k = 1, \ldots, g$, are given by

$$\pi_k^{(t+1)} = \frac{1}{N} \sum_{i=1}^{N} \pi_{ik}(\boldsymbol{\Omega}^{(t)}),$$

that is, the updated mixture component probabilities are equal to the average posterior probabilities.

Next, to maximize the $\mathcal{O}$ function with respect to $\boldsymbol{\theta}$, $\boldsymbol{\psi}$, and $\boldsymbol{\alpha}$, it suffices to maximize

$$\mathcal{O}_2(\boldsymbol{\theta}, \boldsymbol{\psi}, \boldsymbol{\alpha} | \boldsymbol{\Omega}^{(t)}) = \sum_{i=1}^{N} \sum_{k=1}^{g} \pi_{ik}(\boldsymbol{\Omega}^{(t)}) \ln f_{ik}(\boldsymbol{y}_i^o, d_i | \boldsymbol{\theta}, \boldsymbol{\psi}, \boldsymbol{\alpha})$$

with respect to these parameters. However, in general, this cannot be done analytically. Therefore, a classical numerical maximization procedure such as Newton–Raphson is needed. Note that in such cases, the EM algorithm is doubly iterative, which can have a non-negligible impact on the computation time.

24.3.5 Some remarks regarding the EM algorithm

It has been shown (Rubin 1987) that an iteration within the EM algorithm always increases the value of the likelihood function $\ell(\boldsymbol{\Omega} | \boldsymbol{y}^o, \boldsymbol{d})$, under mild regularity conditions, that is,

$$\ell(\boldsymbol{\Omega}^{(t+1)} | \boldsymbol{y}^o, \boldsymbol{d}) > \ell(\boldsymbol{\Omega}^{(t)} | \boldsymbol{y}^o, \boldsymbol{d}) \quad \text{for all } t.$$

This is called the monotonicity property of the EM algorithm, which guarantees convergence of the iterative procedure, provided a finite maximum exists. However, this convergence can be painfully slow, particularly with poorly selected starting values. Apart from the local maxima resulting from the non-identifiability problem, there may be local maxima yielding different likelihood values (Böhning 1999). This suggests the use of multiple sets of starting values. If regions exist where the likelihood is flat, it is said have a *ridge*. The EM algorithm is capable of converging to some particular point on such a ridge, which is not the case for many other, more classical, maximization algorithms.

24.4 CLASSIFICATION

Upon fitting the latent-class mixture model to an incomplete set of repeated measurements, one is in a position to classify the study subjects into the various mixture components, that is, into the population's latent subgroups. Through the structure of the latent-class mixture model, the subdivision of the population into latent groups depends on the number of observed measurements: on the dropout indicator or pattern, as well as on the values of the observed response measurements. Therefore, the classification of subjects into different latent groups can be useful to assess the level of coherence between the dropout process and the measurement process. In certain cases, such latent groups can have a biological or otherwise substantive meaning. For instance, subjects of one group could have higher response values and drop out earlier in the study, whereas subjects of another group might have lower values but remain longer in the study.

The decision as to which component of the mixture, or equivalently to which subgroup of the population, a specific subject is most likely to belong is based on the *posterior probabilities*. Recall that $P(Q_{ik} = 1) = \pi_k$, thus the component probabilities π_k, $k = 1, \dots, g$, express how likely it is that the ith subject belongs to group k, without taking into account either the observed response values $\boldsymbol{y}_i^o$ or the dropout indicator d_i for that subject. For this reason, the component probabilities are often called *prior* probabilities.

The *posterior* probability for subject i belonging to the kth group is given by

$$\widehat{\pi}_{ik} = \widehat{P}(Q_{ik} = 1 | \boldsymbol{y}_i^o, d_i) = \left. \frac{f_i(\boldsymbol{y}_i^o, d_i | Q_{ik} = 1)\, P(Q_{ik} = 1)}{f_i(\boldsymbol{y}_i^o, d_i)} \right|_{\widehat{\boldsymbol{\Omega}}}$$

$$= \left. \frac{\pi_k f_{ik}(\boldsymbol{y}_i^o, d_i | \boldsymbol{\theta}, \boldsymbol{\psi}, \boldsymbol{\alpha})}{\sum_{k=1}^{g} \pi_k f_{ik}(\boldsymbol{y}_i^o, d_i | \boldsymbol{\theta}, \boldsymbol{\psi}, \boldsymbol{\alpha})} \right|_{\widehat{\boldsymbol{\Omega}}},$$

where $\widehat{\boldsymbol{\Omega}}$ is the vector of parameter estimates resulting from the EM algorithm. This expresses how likely it is that the ith subject belongs to group k, taking into account the observed response $\boldsymbol{y}_i^o$ as well as the dropout indicator d_i of that subject. Using these posterior probabilities, we can apply the following classification rule

$$\text{Classify subject } i \text{ into component } k \quad \Longleftrightarrow \quad \widehat{\pi}_{ik} = \max_j \{\widehat{\pi}_{ij}\},$$

assigning subject i to the component to which it is most likely to belong.

However, we do need to be cautious with the resulting classification into latent subgroups because, for a particular subject i, the vector of posterior probabilities is given by $\widehat{\boldsymbol{\pi}}_i = (\widehat{\pi}_{i1}, \dots, \widehat{\pi}_{ig})$ with $\sum_{k=1}^{g} \widehat{\pi}_{ik} = 1$. Ideally, one of these posterior probabilities for subject i would be close to 1. However, another scenario is that two or more posterior probabilities are almost equal, of which one is the maximum of all posterior probabilities for that particular subject. For example, suppose we have $g = 2$ latent subgroups and subject i has posterior probabilities $(\pi_{i1}, \pi_{i2}) = (0.55, 0.45)$. In this case subject i would be allocated to group 1, but this should be done with low confidence. Perhaps it is safer to assert that this subject lies between both groups, in this sense being an outlier, or rather an 'inlier'. Therefore, rather than merely considering the classification of subjects into the latent subgroups using the posterior probabilities, it important to inspect the posterior probabilities in full.

A separate issue is the (prespecified) number g of latent groups. It is hard to choose g with great confidence purely on a priori grounds and therefore it is advisable to explore the stability of the conclusions, by way of additional sensitivity analysis, by varying g across a range.

24.5 SIMULATION STUDY

An advantage of the latent-class mixture model is its flexible structure, which potentially makes the model a helpful analysis tool for incomplete longitudinal data. However, as already seen in Section 24.3.2, the estimation of the model parameters is based on a doubly iterative method, which we might expect to be computationally intensive. To check whether this disadvantage counterbalances the advantage of model flexibility, Beunckens *et al.* (2006) performed a simulation study. We first describe in Section 24.5.1 a simplification of the latent-class mixture model which is used in the following simulation study as well as later in the application in Section 24.6. Following this, the design and results of the simulation study are outlined in Sections 24.5.2 and 24.5.3, respectively.

24.5.1 A simplification of the latent-class mixture model

In their simulation study, Beunckens *et al.* (2006) assumed equal covariance matrices for the different mixture components, $D_1 = \ldots = D_g = D$, as well as equal residual covariance matrices, $\Sigma_i^{(1)} = \ldots = \Sigma_i^{(g)} = \Sigma_i$, which leads to

$$Y_i | q_{ik} = 1, b_i \sim N(X_i\beta + Z_ib_i, \Sigma_i),$$

with

$$b_i \sim \sum_{k=1}^{g} \pi_k N(\mu_k, D).$$

Furthermore, they simplified the general latent-class mixture model in two steps. In the first step, it is assumed that there is only one subject-specific effect b_i,

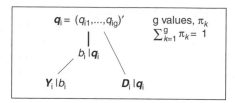

Figure 24.2   A simplification of the latent-class mixture model.

a shared intercept, which influences only the measurement process, not the dropout process. In the second step, the measurement process is assumed to depend on the latent variable only through the shared intercept. The model is depicted in Figure 24.2.

24.5.2   Design

The simulation study is structured as follows. Two-hundred and fifty data sets are simulated, each containing measurements and covariate information for 100 subjects. The latent variable in the model is assumed to split the subjects into two latent subgroups with component probabilities $\pi_1 = 0.6$ and $\pi_2 = 1 - \pi_1 = 0.4$, respectively. Measurements of a continuous outcome are simulated at five time points. Furthermore, these longitudinal data are assumed to follow a linear trend over time with intercept $\beta_0 = 9.4$ and slope $\beta_1 = 2.25$. The shared intercept follows a mixture of two normal distributions with different means for both latent groups: $\mu_1 = -4.4$ and $\mu_2 = -\pi_1\mu_1/\pi_2 = 6.6$. In line with Section 24.5.1, the variances of these two normal distributions are set equal and denoted by d. The measurement error variance is σ^2.

Three different settings are considered, based on varying these two variance parameters as shown in Table 24.1. In the first setting, both variance parameters are chosen to be relatively small. While only the measurement error variance is increased in the second setting, both variance parameters are increased in the third setting.

Finally, in the dropout model, the logistic regression is based on an intercept only, which differs for both groups, namely, $\gamma_1 = -2.5$ and $\gamma_2 = -1.25$,

Table   24.1 Simulation   study.   Variance parameters in three different simulation settings.

Setting	d	σ^2
1	2.0	0.25
2	2.0	0.75
3	3.5	1.00

respectively, with corresponding probabilities 0.73 and 0.45 of completing the study.

The latent-class mixture model can now be formulated as follows. For subject $i = 1, \ldots, 100$ belonging to latent group $k = 1, 2$, the measurement at time $j = 1, \ldots, 5$ is modelled by

$$Y_{ij} = \beta_0 + \beta_1 \, \text{time}_j + b_i + \varepsilon_{ij}^{(k)}, \qquad (24.11)$$

with

$$b_i \sim \pi_1 N\left(\mu_1, d^2\right) + \pi_2 N\left(\mu_2, d^2\right) \quad \text{and} \quad \varepsilon_i^{(k)} \sim N\left(\mathbf{0}, \sigma^2 I_5\right). \qquad (24.12)$$

Furthermore, the dropout model is expressed as

$$\text{logit}[g_{ij}(\mathbf{w}_{ij}, b_i, q_{ik})] = \gamma_k. \qquad (24.13)$$

24.5.3 Results

To get a better feel for the three simulation settings, a data set was selected randomly from the 250 simulated data sets for each setting. Figure 24.3 shows the individual profiles of these data set. Table 24.2 contains the results of the simulation study. As well as comparing the mean estimates and true values of the parameters through the bias, we also consider the mean squared error, simultaneously involving bias and precision.

We consider the three simulation settings in turn. For the first, Figure 24.3(a) shows a clear distinction between both groups, which is due to the small variance, d, of the mixture distribution, relative to the systematic difference between the group means, $\mu_1 - \mu_2$. Furthermore, the small measurement error variance, σ^2, ensures that the within-subject variability is small, resulting in almost straight individual profiles. From Table 24.2, the mean estimates of the parameters are close to the true values, with biases of the order 10^{-2} or less. Together with small MSE values, the magnitude of which does not exceed 10^{-4}, this indicates that the fit is excellent.

Increasing the measurement error variance in the second simulation setting leads to increased within-subject variability. The discrepancy between the two latent groups is still very obvious (Figure 24.3(b)). The bias increases slightly, but remains of the same order. For the MSE values, we observe a small increase, but its magnitude does not exceed 10^{-3}. We can therefore conclude the model fits the data well, even with a larger within-subject variability.

In the final simulation setting, both the measurement error variance and the variance in the mixture components are increased. In Figure 24.3(c) we

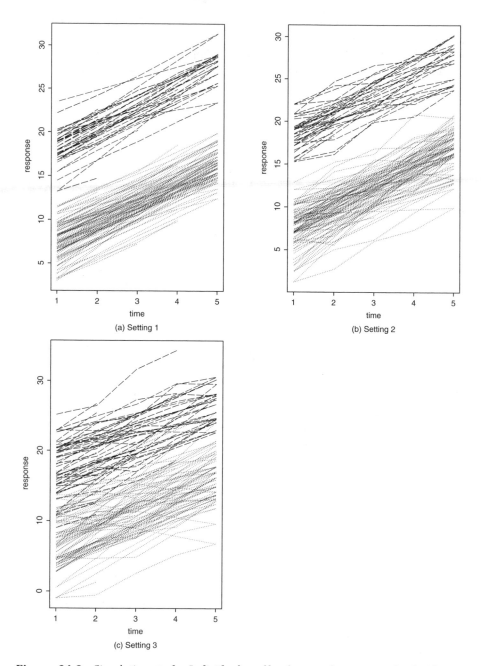

Figure 24.3 Simulation study. Individual profiles for one data set randomly chosen out of 250 simulated data sets, for each of the three simulation settings. Dotted lines correspond to subjects from the first latent group, dashed lines to subjects from the second.

Table 24.2 Simulation study. Mean and true value, bias, and mean squared error (MSE) of the parameters, under the three simulations settings.

Effect	Mean	True	Bias	MSE
Setting 1: *Measurement model*				
β_0	9.37	9.40	-2.84×10^{-2}	8.07×10^{-4}
β_1	2.25	2.25	1.30×10^{-4}	1.68×10^{-8}
σ	0.25	0.25	-2.49×10^{-4}	6.18×10^{-8}
μ_1	-4.39	-4.40	1.31×10^{-2}	1.73×10^{-8}
d	1.98	2.00	-1.70×10^{-2}	2.89×10^{-4}
π_1	0.60	0.60	4.60×10^{-4}	2.12×10^{-7}
Setting 1: *Dropout model*				
γ_1	-2.52	-2.50	-2.28×10^{-2}	5.19×10^{-4}
γ_2	-1.26	-1.25	-1.23×10^{-2}	1.53×10^{-4}
Setting 2: *Measurement model*				
β_0	9.34	9.40	-5.75×10^{-2}	3.31×10^{-3}
β_1	2.25	2.25	7.56×10^{-4}	5.72×10^{-7}
σ	0.75	0.75	6.27×10^{-4}	3.93×10^{-7}
μ_1	-4.36	-4.40	4.48×10^{-2}	2.00×10^{-3}
d	1.97	2.00	-2.53×10^{-2}	6.38×10^{-4}
π_1	0.60	0.60	4.22×10^{-3}	1.79×10^{-5}
Setting 2: *Dropout model*				
γ_1	-2.51	-2.50	-1.26×10^{-2}	1.58×10^{-4}
γ_2	-1.27	-1.25	-2.30×10^{-2}	5.27×10^{-4}
Setting 3: *Measurement model*				
β_0	9.44	9.40	3.83×10^{-2}	1.46×10^{-3}
β_1	2.25	2.25	1.91×10^{-4}	3.66×10^{-8}
σ	0.99	1.00	-5.45×10^{-3}	2.06×10^{-5}
μ_1	-4.69	-4.40	-2.86×10^{-1}	8.18×10^{-2}
d	3.43	3.50	-7.00×10^{-2}	4.90×10^{-3}
π_1	0.57	0.60	3.36×10^{-2}	1.13×10^{-3}
Setting 3: *Dropout model*				
γ_1	-2.61	-2.50	-1.07×10^{-1}	1.14×10^{-2}
γ_2	-1.27	-1.25	-2.04×10^{-2}	4.17×10^{-4}

observe that on top of the larger within-subject variability, the gap between the latent groups now vanishes. The discrepancy between the groups seems to have vanished, and the profiles appear to be homogeneous. We consider the results in Table 24.2 to examine influences on the model fit. For some of the parameters, the mean estimates deviates a little from the true value. Comfortingly, bias and MSE values remain small, the order of magnitude not exceeding 10^{-1} and 10^{-3}, respectively. Thus, here too, the latent-class mixture model fits the simulated data well.

From the three simulation settings we conclude that, whenever the model is correctly specified, it fits very well, as expected. The equivalent statement for a real application is that the fit allegedly will be good in most cases where the researcher has good insight into the true mean structure. Moreover, since computation time for each simulation run was of the order of one week, fitting the latent-class mixture model is not too time-consuming, perhaps somewhat against initial expectations.

24.6 ANALYSIS OF THE DEPRESSION TRIALS

We now apply the latent-class mixture model to the depression trials, introduced in Section 2.5, and then analysed in Chapter 6 and Sections 7.6, 10.5, and 22.6. First a latent-class mixture model is fitted to the depression trials and then a sensitivity analysis performed. The latter establishes the latent-class mixture model as a viable sensitivity tool.

24.6.1 Formulating a latent-class mixture model

A latent-class mixture model is fitted to the data from the depression trials, assuming the patients can be split into two latent subgroups. The mean structure is deliberately kept reasonably simple, and is based on a linear time trend. The heterogeneity linear mixed model for the change in $HAMD_{17}$ score includes as fixed effects an intercept, the treatment and time variables, and the interaction between treatment and time. The measurement error terms are assumed to be independent and to follow a normal distribution with mean 0 and variance σ^2. A shared intercept is included, which follows a mixture of two normal distributions with different means, μ_1 and μ_2 respectively, but with equal variance d. The dropout process is modelled through a logistic regression, including only an intercept, which can differ between both latent subgroups (γ_1 and γ_2). This latent-class mixture model has essentially the same structure as the one used in the simulation study in Section 24.5, based on (24.11)–(24.13), with the addition of terms to assess treatment. Parameter estimates with corresponding standard errors and p-values are shown in Table 24.3.

Once this latent-class mixture model has been fitted, the posterior probabilities can be used to classify the patients into two subgroups as shown in Section 24.4. In this way the 170 patients divide into 77 and 93 classified into the first and second groups, respectively. In Figure 24.4 solid lines represent the individual profiles of patients classified into the first latent group, and dashed lines represent the individual profiles of patients classified into the second group. Clearly, the first group corresponds to patients with lower $HAMD_{17}$ scores, which continue to decrease over time. This implies that these patients are the ones whose condition is improving. On the other hand, the second group contains patients

Table 24.3 Depression trials. Parameter estimates, standard errors, and p-values for the latent-class mixture model.

Effect	Estimate	s.e.	p-value
Measurement model			
Intercept : β_0	2.39	1.82	0.1903
Treatment : β_1	2.12	1.56	0.1743
Time : β_2	-1.36	0.17	<0.0001
Time $\times$ treatment : β_3	-0.49	0.24	0.0413
Measurement error : σ	4.31	0.13	<0.0001
Mean shared intercept group 1 : μ_1	-3.26	0.89	0.0003
Variance shared intercept : d	3.62	0.78	<0.0001
Prior probability group 1 : $\pi_1 = \pi$	0.49	0.22	0.0285
Dropout model			
Intercept group 1 : γ_1	-2.78	0.53	<0.0001
Intercept group 2 : γ_2	-1.71	0.26	<0.0001
Log-likelihood		-2358.84	

with a higher change with respect to baseline compared to the patients from the first group. Their changes in $HAMD_{17}$ score are around 0 – more specifically, somewhere in the interval between -10 and 10. In addition, without taking into account the within-subject variability, their profiles seem to be approximately constant over time.

A clear difference is evident in the incompleteness of the data in both latent groups. The first latent group mainly contains patients who complete the study, 67 in total. Of the 10 patients who drop out, only two do so at visit 6, two more at visit 7, and six patients miss the last visit only. The dropout percentage in the second latent group is larger, 54.8% (51 out of 93 patients) compared to 13.0% in the first group. Of these incompleters, 17 drop out after the first visit, 13 more at visit 6, and 12 at each of the penultimate and last visits.

Because the observed treatment groups are included in the mean structure of the measurement model, it is expected that the classification of subjects into latent subgroups is independent of their treatment classification. To verify this independence, the corresponding two-way table is shown in Table 24.4. From this table, we estimate the odds ratio between the latent variable and the treatment allocation to be 0.9955. The χ^2 test statistic for independence produces $p = 0.9884$. Clearly, this confirms the expectation of no association between the covariate treatment and the classified latent subgroups. Moreover, if the treatment variable were included in the dropout model, this independence would be even clearer.

However, as mentioned in Section 24.4, using this classification rule does not provide insight into how strongly patients are allocated to one group rather than the other. This depends on the magnitude of the maximal posterior probability.

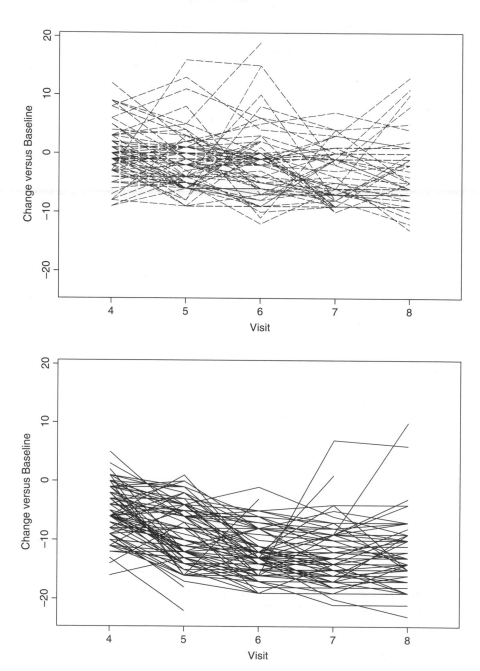

Figure 24.4   Depression trials. Classification of subjects based on a latent-class mixture model. Solid lines correspond to patients classified into first group (top), dashed lines to patients classified into second one (bottom).

Table 24.4 Depression trials. Two-way table with classification into latent subgroup and the treatment covariate.

	Experimental drug	Standard drug
Latent class 1	39	38
Latent class 2	47	46

Table 24.5 Depression trials. Classification of subjects based on the magnitude of posterior probabilities π_{i1}.

π_{i1}	Classification	No. of patients
0.80–1.00	Clearly group 1	49
0.60–0.80	Group 1	13
0.55–0.60	Doubtful, more likely group 1	5
0.45–0.55	Uncertain	21
0.40–0.45	Doubtful, more likely group 2	4
0.20–0.40	Group 2	32
0.00–0.20	Clearly Group 2	46

Since the latent-class mixture model considered here only contains two latent groups, we merely need to consider one of the posterior probabilities, for example the posterior probability that the subject belongs to group 1, π_{i1}. Based on this π_{i1}, the subjects can be classified following the guidelines of Table 24.5. If the posterior probability π_{i1} lies between 0.45 and 0.55, it is uncertain which group the subject can be classified into. Only 21 out of 170 patients in the depression trials are in this situation. For most patients, 140 or 82%, it is clear which group they can be classified into, since their maximal posterior probability is above 0.60.

24.6.2 A sensitivity analysis

We now illustrate the use of the latent-class mixture model as a sensitivity analysis tool. In addition to the latent-class mixture model introduced above, two selection models will be fitted to the depression trials, based on the selection models introduced by Diggle and Kenward (1994); see also Section 15.2 above. For the measurement model, a linear mixed model is considered, including the same fixed effects as were included in the latent-class mixture model: intercept, treatment and time variables, treatment-by-time interaction, and an unstructured covariance matrix. The dropout model takes the conventional form (15.3). We consider an MAR version as well as the full MNAR version of the model.

As the main focus of the depression trials was on the treatment effect at the last visit, Table 24.6 gives the estimates, standard errors, and p-values for this effect under the three fitted models. Clearly, the p-values resulting from all three

Table 24.6 Depression trials. Estimates (standard errors) and *p*-values for the treatment effect at visit 8, as well as the treatment-by-time interaction, for the latent-class mixture model and both selection models, assuming either MAR or MNAR.

Model	Treatment at endpoint		Treatment × time	
	Estimate (s.e.)	*p*-value	Estimate (s.e.)	*p*-value
Latent-class mixture	−1.801 (1.001)	0.072	−0.49 (0.24)	0.0413
MAR selection	−2.303 (1.293)	0.075	−0.56 (0.31)	0.0719
MNAR selection	−2.302 (1.294)	0.075	−0.56 (0.32)	0.0761

models are very similar and close to 0.07, yielding the same conclusion for the treatment effect at visit 8. Thus, the significance results are not sensitive to the model used, and hence more trust can be put in the conclusion, essentially, it seems, since a deflated estimate is combined with a reduced standard error. However, note that, using the latent-class mixture model, the standard error is reduced by 0.3 units, compared to either selection model, resulting in a more accurate confidence interval for the treatment effect at the last visit.

We continue by exploring the sensitivity of the treatment-by-time interaction by comparing the estimates, standard errors and *p*-values under the three fitted models in Tables 24.6. The *p*-values are close to the 0.05 boundary. The more significant result for the latent-class mixture model can perhaps be explained by increased precision, owing to the fact that otherwise unexplained variability is captured by the latent structure.

24.7 CONCLUDING REMARKS

Beunckens *et al.* (2006) proposed a latent-class mixture models for the analysis of longitudinal data subject to dropout. The model extends the shared-parameter model, in the sense that both the measurement and dropout processes are allowed to share a set of random effects, conditional upon which both processes are assumed to be independent. It can, at the same time, be seen as an extension of the pattern-mixture model, now with latent rather than explicitly observed groups. It uses ideas from random-effects and latent-class modelling. Therefore, it captures unobserved heterogeneity between latent subgroups of the population. The results from the simulation study underscore the fact that the flexibility of such latent-class mixture models outweighs the expected modelling complexity. Apart from a flexible modelling technique, the latent-class mixture model can be used for other purposes. First, clusters can be detected by classifying the subjects into the latent subgroups. Second, the latent-class mixture model can be used as a sensitivity analysis tool. Applying the tool to the depression trials increased the confidence level in the conclusions reached.

Part VI
Case Studies

25

The Age-Related Macular Degeneration Trial

The age-related macular degeneration trial was introduced in Section 2.8. In Chapter 13, simple methods (CC and LOCF) and direct likelihood methods were applied to both the continuous outcome, the difference in number of letters correctly read on a vision chart, as well as its dichotomized form (positive *versus* negative). For the binary outcome, GEE, weighted GEE, and GEE after multiple imputation (MI-GEE) were also used.

In this chapter, MNAR-based methods are applied to these data. In Section 25.1, the selection model of Diggle and Kenward (1994; see also Chapter 15 above) is fitted to the monotone response sequences. In Section 25.2, by way of sensitivity analysis, this is supplemented with local influence analysis (Chapter 22). In Section 25.3, the focus is on pattern-mixture models, as introduced in Chapter 16.

25.1 SELECTION MODELS AND LOCAL INFLUENCE

In this section, visual acuity in the age-related macular degeneration trial is first analysed using the full selection model proposed by Diggle and Kenward (1994), discussed in Section 15.2 above. Apart from explicitly modelling the three missing data mechanisms MCAR, MAR, and MNAR, an ignorable MAR analysis is also conducted in which the model for the response measurements only was fitted. For the measurement model, the linear mixed model was again used, assuming different intercepts and treatment effects for each of the four time points, with an unstructured covariance matrix, as in (13.2). In the full selection models, the dropout is modelled based on (15.3). Parameter estimates

Missing Data in Clinical Studies   G. Molenberghs and M.G. Kenward
© 2007 John Wiley & Sons, Ltd

Table 25.1 Age-related macular degeneration trial. Parameter estimates (standard errors) assuming ignorability, as well as explicitly modelling the missing data mechanism under MCAR, MAR, and MNAR assumptions, for all data.

Effect	Parameter	Ignorable	MCAR	MAR	MNAR
Measurement model					
Intercept 4	β_{11}	54.00 (1.47)	54.00 (1.46)	54.00 (1.47)	54.00 (1.47)
Intercept 12	β_{21}	53.01 (1.60)	53.01 (1.59)	53.01 (1.60)	52.98 (1.60)
Intercept 24	β_{31}	49.20 (1.74)	49.20 (1.73)	49.19 (1.74)	49.06 (1.74)
Intercept 52	β_{41}	43.99 (1.79)	43.99 (1.78)	43.99 (1.79)	43.52 (1.82)
Treatment 4	β_{12}	−3.11 (2.10)	−3.11 (2.07)	−3.11 (2.09)	−3.11 (2.10)
Treatment 12	β_{22}	−4.54 (2.29)	−4.54 (2.25)	−4.54 (2.29)	−4.67 (2.29)
Treatment 24	β_{32}	−3.60 (2.49)	−3.60 (2.46)	−3.60 (2.50)	−3.80 (2.50)
Treatment 52	β_{42}	−5.18 (2.59)	−5.18 (2.57)	−5.18 (2.62)	−5.71 (2.63)
Dropout model					
Intercept	ψ_0		−2.79 (0.17)	−1.86 (0.46)	−1.81 (0.47)
Previous	ψ_1			−0.020 (0.009)	0.016 (0.022)
Current	ψ_2				−0.042 (0.023)
−2 log-likelihood		6488.7	6782.7	6778.4	6775.9
Treatment effect at 1 year (*p*-value)		0.046	0.044	0.048	0.030

and corresponding standard errors of the fixed effects of the measurement model and of the dropout model parameters are given in Table 25.1.

As expected, the parameter estimates and standard errors coincide for the ignorable direct likelihood analysis and the selection models under MCAR and MAR, except for some negligible numerical noise.

Since our main interest lies in the treatment effect at 1 year, the corresponding *p*-values are displayed in Table 25.1. In all four cases, this treatment effect is significant.

Note that for the MNAR analysis, the estimates of the ψ_1 and ψ_2 parameter are more or less of the same magnitude, but with a different sign. This is in line with the argument of Molenberghs *et al.* (2001b), stating that the dropout often depends on the increment $y_{ij} - y_{i,j-1}$. This is because two subsequent measurements are usually positively correlated. By rewriting the fitted dropout model in terms of the increment,

$$\text{logit}\,[P(D_i = j|D_i \geq j, \boldsymbol{y}_i)] = -1.81 - 0.026 y_{i,j-1} - 0.042(y_{ij} - y_{i,j-1}),$$

we find that the probability of dropout increases with larger negative increments; that is, those patients who showed or would have shown a greater decrease in visual acuity from the previous visit are more likely to drop out.

25.2   LOCAL INFLUENCE ANALYSIS

Let us now turn to local influence. Figure 25.1 displays overall C_i and influences for subvectors $\boldsymbol{\theta}$, $\boldsymbol{\beta}$, $\boldsymbol{\alpha}$, and $\boldsymbol{\psi}$. In addition, the direction $\boldsymbol{h}_{\max}$, corresponding to maximal local influence, is given. What is of interest here are the relative

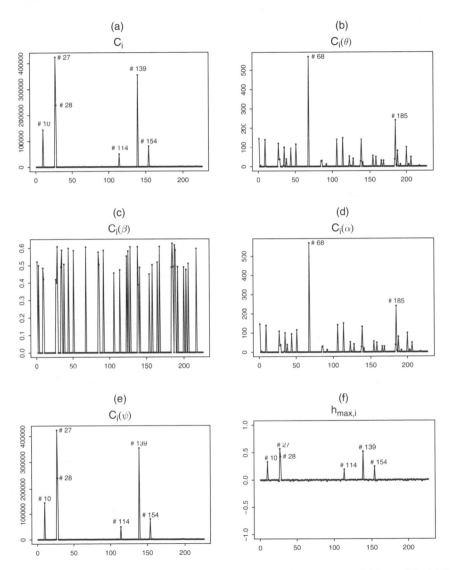

Figure 25.1   Age-related macular degeneration trial. Index plots of (a) C_i, (b) $C_i(\boldsymbol{\theta})$, (c) $C_i(\boldsymbol{\alpha})$, (d) $C_i(\boldsymbol{\beta})$, (e) $C_i(\boldsymbol{\psi})$, and (f) the components of the direction $\boldsymbol{h}_{\max,i}$ of maximal curvature.

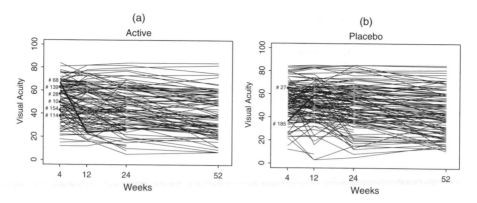

Figure 25.2 Age-related macular degeneration trial. Individual profiles for both treatment arms, with influential subjects highlighted.

magnitudes. We observe that patients 10, 27, 28, 114, 139, and 154 have larger C_i values compared to other patients, which means they can be considered influential. Virtually the same picture holds for $C_i(\psi)$.

Turning attention now to the influence on the measurement model, we see that for $C_i(\beta)$ there are no strikingly high peaks, whereas $C_i(\alpha)$ reveals noticeable peaks for patients 68 and 185. Note that both patients fail to have a high peak for the overall C_i, owing to the fact that the scale for $C_i(\alpha)$ is relatively small compared to the overall C_i. Nevertheless, these patients can still be considered influential. Finally, the direction of maximum curvature reveals the same six influential patients as the overall C_i.

In Figure 25.2 the individual profiles of the influential observations are highlighted. Let us take a closer look at these cases. The six patients strongly influencing the dropout model parameters are those dropping out after the first measurement is taken at week 4. All of these patients are in the active treatment arm, except for 27. On the other hand, the two patients with strong influence on the measurement model parameters stay in the study up to week 24 and then have no observation for the last measurement occasion at 1 year. Patient 68 received the active treatment, and his/her visual acuity decreases substantially after week 4, thereafter staying more or less level. Conversely, patient 185 is enrolled in the placebo treatment arm and his/her visual acuity increases after week 4, then sloping downward a little after week 12.

It is of interest to consider an analysis without these influential observations. Therefore, we applied the selection model to three subsets of the data. The first subset was obtained by removing all eight influential patients mentioned before. In the second subset of the data, patients 10, 27, 28, 114, 139, and 154 were removed, since these are overall the most influential ones. Finally, patients 68 and 185, who seemed to be influencing the measurement model the most, were removed, resulting in the third subset. Results of these analyses are shown in Table 25.2. We compare the results of the MAR and MNAR analyses.

Table 25.2 Age-related macular degeneration trial. Parameter estimates (standard errors) explicitly modelling the missing data mechanism under MAR and MNAR assumptions, after removing the following subsets of subjects: 10, 27, 28, 114, 139, 154, 68, 185 (Set 1); 10, 27, 28, 114, 139, 154 (Set 2); 68, 185 (Set 3).

Effect	Parameter	Set 1		Set 2		Set 3	
		MAR	MNAR	MAR	MNAR	MAR	MNAR
Measurement model							
Intercept 4	β_{11}	54.14 (1.51)	54.15 (1.49)	54.30 (1.47)	54.30 (1.46)	53.84 (1.48)	53.84 (1.47)
Intercept 12	β_{21}	53.09 (1.64)	53.06 (1.62)	53.16 (1.59)	53.13 (1.59)	52.94 (1.60)	52.91 (1.59)
Intercept 24	β_{31}	49.56 (1.77)	49.46 (1.75)	49.31 (1.74)	49.20 (1.72)	49.44 (1.73)	49.31 (1.72)
Intercept 52	β_{41}	44.40 (1.82)	43.97 (1.84)	44.00 (1.79)	43.58 (1.82)	44.38 (1.78)	43.90 (1.82)
Treatment 4	β_{12}	−3.13 (2.17)	−3.13 (2.11)	−3.28 (2.08)	−3.28 (2.06)	−2.95 (2.07)	−2.95 (2.05)
Treatment 12	β_{22}	−4.48 (2.36)	−4.63 (2.29)	−4.55 (2.26)	−4.69 (2.24)	−4.47 (2.26)	−4.60 (2.23)
Treatment 24	β_{32}	−3.80 (2.56)	−4.04 (2.49)	−3.55 (2.48)	−3.79 (2.44)	−3.85 (2.44)	−4.04 (2.42)
Treatment 52	β_{42}	−5.45 (2.66)	−6.12 (2.66)	−5.06 (2.59)	−5.72 (2.61)	−5.56 (2.55)	−6.09 (2.58)
Dropout model							
Intercept	ψ_0	−1.90 (0.47)	−1.85 (0.49)	−1.90 (0.47)	−1.85 (0.49)	−1.85 (0.46)	−1.81 (0.47)
Previous	ψ_1	−0.019 (0.010)	0.018 (0.022)	−0.019 (0.010)	0.017 (0.022)	−0.020 (0.009)	0.017 (0.022)
Current	ψ_2		−0.044 (0.024)		−0.043 (0.024)		−0.043 (0.024)
−2 log-likelihood		6535.3	6532.7	6606.9	6604.4	6706.4	6703.8
Treatment effect at 1 year (p-value)		0.040	0.021	0.051	0.028	0.029	0.018

After removing the patients who have large overall C_i and $C(\psi)$ values, the estimates of the dropout model parameters ψ_1 and ψ_2 are approximately the same, whereas the estimate of ψ_0 decreases from -1.86 to -1.90 under MAR, and from -1.81 to -1.85 under MNAR. The same can be seen after removing all influential patients. Considering the treatment effect at 1 year, its estimate under the MAR analysis increases from -5.18 to -5.06, yielding a slightly increased borderline p-value, whereas under the MNAR analysis it decreases with 0.01, and together with a decreased standard error this yields a small decrease in the p-value.

There is no impact on the likelihood ratio test for MAR against MNAR after removing either patients 10, 27, 28, 114, 139, and 154, or all influential patients, G^2 remains 2.5. If this likelihood ratio test followed a standard χ_1^2 distribution, we would fail to reject the null hypothesis, which leads us to the MAR assumption. However, the test of MAR against MNAR is non-standard and the conventional chi-squared approximation cannot be used for its null distribution (Rotnitzky *et al.* 2000; Jansen *et al.* 2006b).

Finally, we perform the same analyses on the third subset, with patients 68 and 185 removed. Both for the MAR and MNAR analysis, the estimate of the treatment effect at 1 year decreases quite a lot, from -5.18 to -5.56 and from -5.71 to -6.09, respectively. Consequently, the p-value also falls from 0.048 to 0.029 under MAR and from 0.030 to 0.018 under the MNAR analysis. The deviance for the likelihood ratio test for MAR against MNAR changes only slightly, from 2.5 to 2.6.

25.3   PATTERN-MIXTURE MODELS

We now consider the use of pattern-mixture models for these data. Here, we will apply strategy 1 from Section 16.4, making use of CCMV, NCMV, and ACMV identifying restrictions. The results for the three types of restrictions are shown in Table 25.3. After applying each of the three restrictions, as outlined in Section 16.4, the same selection model as before is fitted. It can be seen from the estimates and associated standard errors that there is little difference in conclusions between the strategies.

In the pattern-mixture approach, we use information from different patterns to multiply impute new values whenever the observations are missing. Borrowing information from more distant patterns, such as the complete cases, may introduce extra variability, depending on the nature of the conditional distributions sampled from. It is not unexpected, therefore, for the variability to be smallest when applying NCMV, as seen in the standard errors.

It can be seen from these analyses that the treatment effect at week 52 is not statistically significant, in contrast to the conclusions drawn in Chapter 13 and Section 25.1. The p-value is closest to significance with NCMV restrictions.

Table 25.3 Age-related macular degeneration trial. Parameter estimates (standard errors) and *p*-values resulting from the pattern-mixture model using identifying restrictions ACMV, CCMV, and NCMV.

Effect	Parameter	ACMV	CCMV	NCMV
Parameter estimate (standard error)				
Intercept 4	β_{11}	54.00 (1.47)	54.00 (1.47)	54.00 (1.47)
Intercept 12	β_{21}	52.87 (1.68)	52.92 (1.61)	52.86 (1.63)
Intercept 24	β_{31}	48.65 (2.00)	49.16 (1.87)	48.77 (1.78)
Intercept 52	β_{41}	44.19 (2.14)	44.69 (2.54)	44.00 (1.80)
Treatment 4	β_{12}	−3.11 (2.10)	−3.11 (2.10)	−3.11 (2.10)
Treatment 12	β_{22}	−4.18 (2.48)	−4.07 (2.30)	−4.40 (2.42)
Treatment 24	β_{32}	−4.36 (3.83)	−5.14 (3.61)	−4.19 (2.62)
Treatment 52	β_{42}	−5.04 (3.86)	−2.33 (4.93)	−4.89 (2.70)
p-values				
Intercept 4	β_{11}	—	—	—
Intercept 12	β_{21}	<0.0001	<0.0001	<0.0001
Intercept 24	β_{31}	<0.0001	<0.0001	<0.0001
Intercept 52	β_{41}	<0.0001	<0.0001	<0.0001
Treatment 4	β_{12}	—	—	—
Treatment 12	β_{22}	0.092	0.077	0.069
Treatment 24	β_{32}	0.271	0.173	0.110
Treatment 52	β_{42}	0.211	0.647	0.071

The fact that no significant treatment effect is found here suggests caution concerning the conclusions obtained under the selection model formulation. This implies that a significant treatment effect is conditional upon the MAR assumption holding. One would feel more comfortable about a significant treatment effect if it held across MAR and a number of MNAR scenarios. Thus, at best, it is fair to say there is a weak evidence only for a treatment effect.

25.4 CONCLUDING REMARKS

The age-related macular degeneration trial has been reanalysed using (1) MCAR, MAR, and NMAR selection models, (2) a sensitivity analysis tool in the form of local and global influence, and (3) pattern-mixture models. The selection model results, together with the global influence analysis, corroborate the evidence of a mild treatment effect at the end of the study (52 weeks), obtained using MAR analyses in Chapter 13. However, pattern-mixture model analyses, based on identifying restrictions, do not confirm this result. The main difference in the selection and pattern-mixture based analyses is in the assumptions made about the unseen missing data, specifically their conditional distribution given the given the observed measurements. A cautious conclusion therefore is that there is some (albeit far from overwhelming) evidence for a treatment effect at the end of the study.

26

The Vorozole Study

26.1 INTRODUCTION

The vorozole study was introduced and explored in Section 2.2. An extensive analysis within the pattern-mixture framework was reported on in Section 16.6. This analysis was restricted to the three initial measurements, enabling us to make a number of points about fitting and interpreting pattern-mixture models. In this chapter we will revisit the vorozole trial, now analysing the measurement sequence in full. A comprehensive data exploration exercise is described in Section 26.2, based on the ideas set out in Verbeke and Molenberghs (2000). Section 26.3 is devoted to selection modelling, while in Section 26.4 pattern-mixture analyses are presented. The vorozole study was also the subject of analysis in Thijs *et al.* (2002).

26.2 EXPLORING THE VOROZOLE DATA

The vorozole data will be explored in terms of their average evolution (Section 26.2.1), variance structure (Section 26.2.2), and covariance structure (Section 26.2.3), using general longitudinal data principles as in Verbeke and Molenberghs (2000). An exploration focusing on the incompleteness of the data is the subject of Section 26.2.4.

26.2.1 Average evolution

The average evolution describes how the profile for a number of relevant subpopulations (or the population as a whole) evolves over time. The results of

---

Missing Data in Clinical Studies G. Molenberghs and M.G. Kenward
© 2007 John Wiley & Sons, Ltd

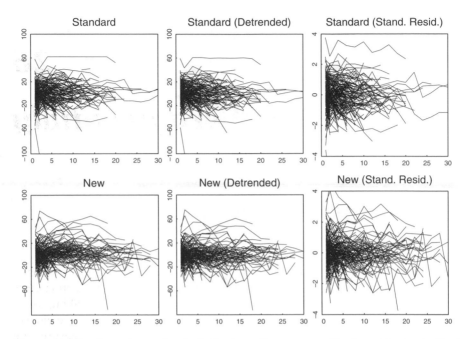

Figure 26.1 Vorozole study. Individual profiles, raw residuals, and standardized residuals.

this exploration will be useful in order to choose a fixed-effects structure for the linear mixed model.

The individual profiles are displayed in Figure 26.1, and the mean profiles, by treatment arm, are plotted in Figure 26.2. The average profiles indicate an increase over time which is slightly stronger for the vorozole group. In addition, the vorozole group is, with the exception of month 16, consistently higher than the megestrol acetate group. Of course, at this point it is not yet possible to decide on the statistical significance of this difference. It is useful to explore the treatment difference separately because this is usually of primary interest and can follow a simple model even when both individual treatment profiles are complicated, or vice versa. The treatment difference is plotted in Figure 26.3.

The individual profiles augment the averaged plot and provide a suggestion of the variability seen within the data. The thinning of the data towards the later study times suggests that trends at later times should be treated with caution. Although these plots also give some indication of the variability at given times and even of the correlation between measurements of the same individual, it is easier to base such considerations on residual profiles and standardized residual profiles.

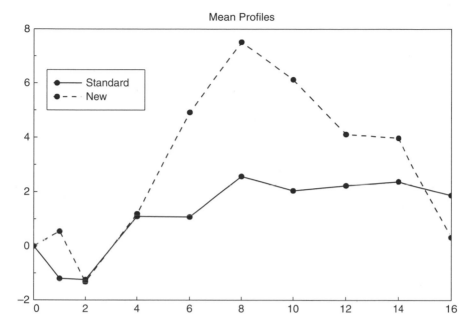

Figure 26.2   Vorozole study. Mean profiles.

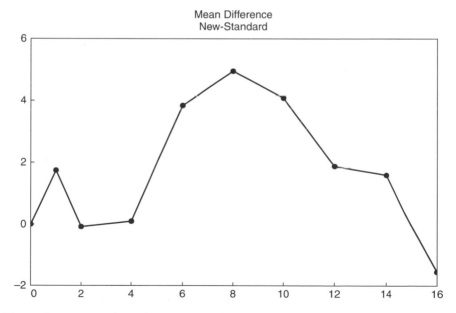

Figure 26.3   Vorozole study. Treatment difference.

26.2.2   Variance structure

To build an appropriate longitudinal model it is necessary to consider the evolution over time of both the mean and covariance structures. For the latter it is necessary to correct the measurements for the fixed-effects structure so raw residuals are used. Again, two plots are of interest. The first shows the average evolution of the variance as a function of time; the second shows the individual residual plots. The detrended profiles are displayed in Figure 26.1, and the corresponding variance function is plotted in Figure 26.4.

The variance function appears relatively stable and hence a constant variance model could be a plausible starting point. The individual detrended profiles show the tendency for this to decrease for subjects just before leaving the study, and this is most apparent in the vorozole group. In addition, the detrended profiles suggest that the variance decreases over time. This contradicts the variance function and is entirely due to the considerable attrition. This observation suggests that caution should exercised with such descriptive plots when used with incomplete data, a point to which we return in Section 26.2.4.

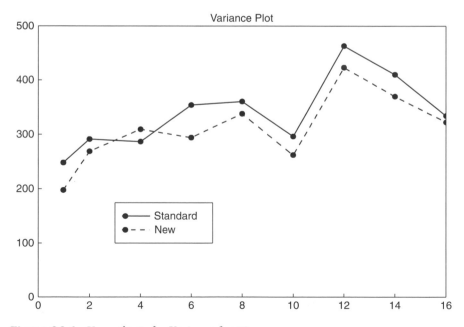

Figure 26.4   Vorozole study. Variance function.

26.2.3   Correlation structure

The correlation structure describes how measurements within a subject are mutually correlated. The correlation function depends on a pair of measurement occasions, and only under the assumption of stationarity does this pair simplify to the time lag only. This is important because many exploratory and modelling tools are based on the assumption of stationarity. A plot of standardized residuals is useful in this respect (Figure 26.1). The picture is not greatly different from the previous individual plots, and this can be explained by the relative flatness of both mean profile and variance functions. If one or both structures is varying with time, the standardized residuals will contribute useful additional information.

An alternative way of displaying the correlation structure is to use a scatter plot matrix, such as the one presented in Figure 26.5. The off-diagonal elements feature scatter plots of standardized residuals obtained from pairs of measurement occasions. The decay of correlation with time is studied by considering the evolution of the scatter plots with increasing distance from the main diagonal. Stationarity, on the other hand, implies that the scatter plots remain similar within diagonal bands *if measurement occasions are approximately*

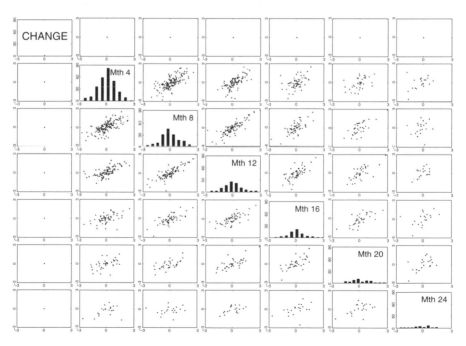

Figure 26.5 Vorozole study. Scatter plot matrix for selected time points. The same vertical scale is used along the diagonal to display the attrition rate as well.

equally spaced. In addition to the scatter plots, we place histograms on the diagonal, capturing the variance structure, including such features as skewness. If the axes are given the same scales, it is very easy to capture the attrition rate as well.

26.2.4 Missing data aspects

So far we have applied several descriptive methods in the context of the vorozole study to explore the longitudinal data graphically, both from the individual-level standpoint (Figures 26.1 and 26.5) and from the population-averaged or group-averaged perspective (Figures 26.2, 26.3, and 26.4). Such plots are designed to focus on various structural aspects, such as the mean structure, the variance function, and the association structure.

The incompleteness of the data, however, adds an additional dimension to the complexity of this exploration. The first issue to consider is the simple depletion of the study subjects. A decreasing sample size reduces the precision of estimators. In this respect, the vorozole study provides a dramatic example, as can be seen from Figure 26.6 and Table 26.1, showing both graphically and numerically the attrition in both treatment arms. Clearly, the dropout rate

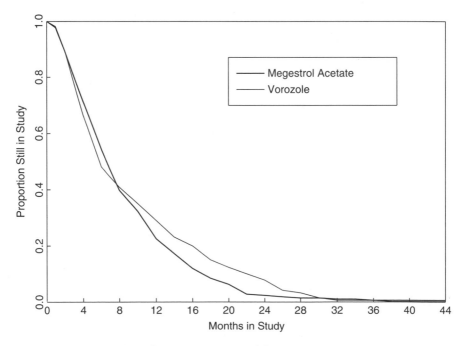

Figure 26.6 Vorozole study. Representation of dropout.

Table 26.1 Vorozole study. Evolution of dropout.

	Standard		Vorozole	
Week	No. of subjects	%	No. of subjects	%
0	226	100	220	100
1	221	98	216	98
2	203	90	198	90
4	161	71	146	66
6	123	54	106	48
8	90	40	90	41
10	73	32	77	35
12	51	23	64	29
14	39	17	51	23
16	27	12	44	20
18	19	8	33	15
20	14	6	27	12
22	6	3	22	10
24	5	2	17	8
26	4	2	9	4
28	3	1	7	3
30	3	1	3	1
32	2	1	1	0
34	2	1	1	0
36	1	0	1	0
38	1	0	0	0
40	1	0	0	0
42	1	0	0	0
44	1	0	0	0

is high *and* there is a hint of a differential rate between the two arms. This means we have identified one potential factor that could influence a patient's probability of dropping out. Although a large part of the trialist's interest focuses on the treatment effect, we should be aware that it is still a covariate and hence a design factor. Another question that will arise is whether dropout depends on observed or unobserved responses. An equivalent representation is given in Figure 26.7.

A consequence of dropout is seen if we consider the average profile in each treatment arm, with pointwise confidence limits added (Figure 26.8). Near the end of the study, these intervals become extremely wide, as opposed to the relatively narrow intervals at the start of the experiment. Thus, it is clear that dropout leads to efficiency loss. Of course, this effect can be due in part to increasing variability over time. Modelling is required to obtain more insight into this effect.

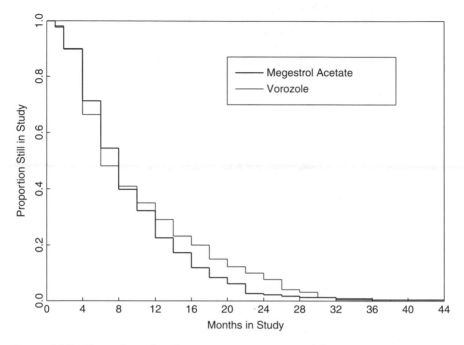

Figure 26.7   Vorozole study. Alternative representation of dropout.

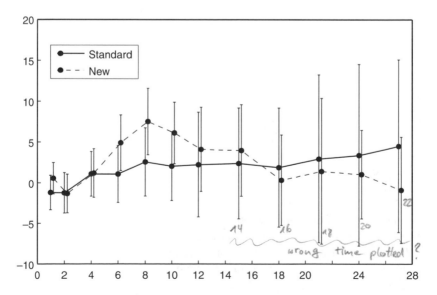

Figure 26.8   Vorozole study. Mean profiles, with 95% confidence intervals added.

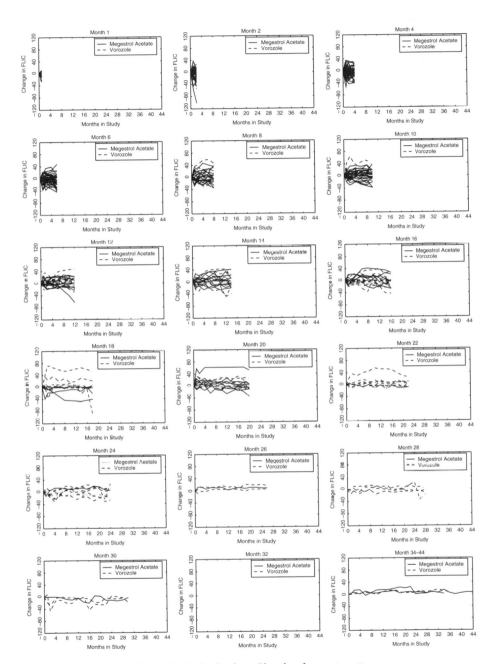

Figure 26.9 Vorozole study. Individual profiles, by dropout pattern.

To gain further insight into the impact of dropout, it is useful to construct dropout-pattern-specific plots. Figures 26.9 and 26.10 display the individual and averaged profiles for each pattern.

The individual profiles plot (Figure 26.9), by definition, displays all available data, but does have some intrinsic limitations. As is the case with any individual data plot, it tends to be fairly busy. As there is considerable early dropout, there are many short sequences, and since we have decided to use the same time axis for all profiles, including early dropouts, very little information can be extracted; the evolution over the first few sequences is not clear at all. Furthermore, the eye assigns more weight to the longer profiles, even though they are considerably less frequent.

Some of these limitations are removed in Figure 26.10, where the pattern-specific average profiles are displayed by treatment arm. Still, care has to be taken not to overinterpret the longer profiles and neglect the shorter profiles, bearing in mind that the shorter profiles represent more subjects than the longer profiles.

Several observations can be made at this point. Most profiles clearly show a quadratic trend, which seems to contrast with the relatively flat nature of the average profiles in Figure 26.8. This implies that the impression given when combining over patterns may differ greatly from a pattern-specific examination. These conclusions appear consistent across treatment arms. Another important observation is that those who drop out rather early seem to decrease from the start, whereas those who remain a relatively long time in the study exhibit, on average and in turn, a rise, a plateau, and then a decrease. This suggests that there are at least two important characteristics that make dropout increase:

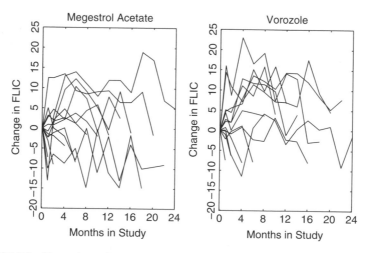

Figure 26.10 Vorozole study. Mean profiles, by dropout pattern, grouped by treatment arm.

(1) a low value of change versus baseline and (2) an unfavourable (downward) evolution.

When modelling these data, irrespective of the framework chosen, these features must be reflected. Sections 26.3 and 26.4 will consider the selection and pattern-mixture model frameworks, respectively.

26.3 A SELECTION MODEL FOR THE VOROZOLE STUDY

First, a linear mixed model will be considered, later supplemented with a dropout model of Diggle–Kenward (Section 15.2) type. Because we are modelling change with respect to baseline, all models are forced to pass through the origin. The following covariates were considered for the measurement model: baseline value, treatment, dominant site, stage, and time in months. Second-order interactions were considered as well. For design reasons, treatment was kept in the model in spite of its non-significance; an F test for treatment effect produces $p = 0.5822$. Apart from baseline, no other time-stationary covariates were kept. A quadratic time effect provided an adequate description of the time trend. We confined the random-effects structure to random intercepts and supplemented this with a Gaussian serial correlation component and measurement error. The final model is presented in Table 26.2.

The fitted profiles are displayed in Figures 26.11 and 26.12. In Figure 26.12, empirical Bayes estimates of the random effects are included, whereas in Figure 26.11 the pure marginal mean is used. For each treatment group, we obtain three sets of profiles. The fitted complete profile is the average curve that would be obtained had all individuals been observed completely. If we use only those predicted values that correspond to occasions at which an observation was

Table 26.2 Vorozole study. Selection model parameter estimates (standard errors).

Effect	Parameter	Estimate (s.e.)
Fixed-effects parameters		
Time	β_0	7.78 (1.05)
Time $\times$ baseline	β_1	-0.065 (0.009)
Time $\times$ treatment	β_2	0.086 (0.157)
Time^2	β_3	-0.30 (0.06)
Time $^2 \times$ baseline	β_4	0.0024 (0.0005)
Variance parameters		
Random intercept	d	105.42
Serial variance	τ^2	77.96
Serial association	λ	7.22
Measurement error	σ^2	77.83

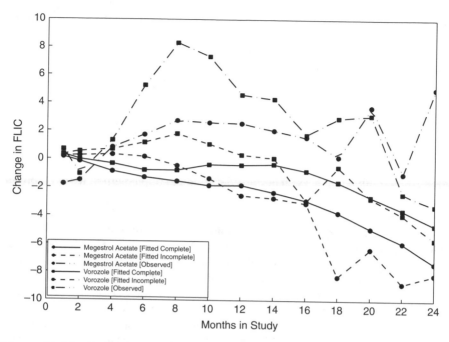

Figure 26.11 Vorozole study. Fitted profiles, averaging the predicted means for the incomplete and complete measurement sequences, without the random effects.

made, then the fitted incomplete profiles are obtained. The latter are somewhat higher that the former when the random effects are included, and somewhat lower when they are not, suggesting that individuals with lower measurements are more likely to disappear from the study. In addition, although the fitted complete curves are very close (the treatment effect was not significant), the fitted incomplete curves are not, suggesting that there is more dropout in the megestrol acetate arm than in the vorozole arm. This is in agreement with the dropout rate, displayed in Figure 26.6, and should not be seen as evidence of a bad fit. Finally, the observed curves, based on the measurements available at each time point, are displayed. These are higher than the fitted ones, but this should be viewed with the standard errors of the observed means in mind (see Figure 26.2).

The fitted variance structure is represented by means of the fitted variogram in Figure 26.13. The total correlation between two measurements, 1 month apart, equals 0.696. The residual correlation, which remains after accounting for the random effects, is still equal to 0.491. The serial correlation, obtained by further ignoring the measurement error, equals $\rho = \exp(-1/7.22^2) = 0.981$.

Next, we study factors that influence dropout. A logistic regression model, described by 15.2 and 15.3, is used. To begin with, we restrict attention to MAR processes, so that $\omega = 0$. The first model includes treatment, dominant

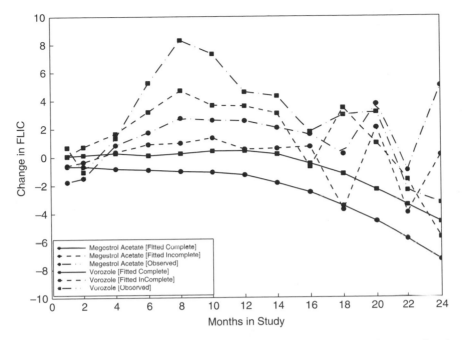

Figure 26.12 Vorozole study. Fitted profiles, averaging the predicted means for the incomplete and complete measurement sequences, including the random effects.

site, stage group, baseline, and the previous measurement, but only the last two are significant, giving

$$\text{logit}[g(\mathbf{h}_{ij})] = 0.080(0.341) - 0.014(0.003)\text{base}_i - 0.033(0.004)y_{i,j-1}. \quad (26.1)$$

We discussed earlier the important relationship between apparent MNAR relationships and the observed dependence of dropout on the measurement *increments* (Section 22.3.2) – that is, the difference between the current and previous measurements, $y_{ij} - y_{i,j-1}$. Clearly, a very similar quantity is found in $y_{i,j-1} - y_{i,j-2}$, but a major advantage of a model based on this particular compound measure is that it fits within the MAR framework. In our case, we obtain

$$\text{logit}[g(\mathbf{h}_{ij})] = 0.033(0.401) - 0.013(0.003)\text{base}_i$$

$$+ 0.012(0.006)y_{i,j-2} - 0.035(0.005)y_{i,j-1}$$

$$= 0.033(0.401) - 0.013(0.003)\text{base}_i$$

$$- 0.023(0.005)\frac{y_{i,j-2} + y_{i,j-1}}{2}$$

$$- 0.047(0.010)\frac{y_{i,j-1} - y_{i,j-2}}{2}, \quad (26.2)$$

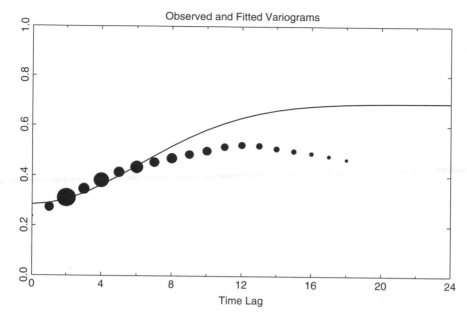

Figure 26.13 Vorozole study. Observed variogram (bullets with size proportional to the number of pairs on which they are based) and fitted variogram (solid line).

indicating that both size and increment are significant predictors for dropout. We conclude that dropout increases with a decrease in baseline, in overall level of the outcome variable, as well as with a decreasing evolution in the outcome. Recall that fitting the dropout model could be done using a logistic regression of the type (26.2) and based upon 15.2.

Both dropout models (26.1) and (26.2) can be compared with their MNAR counterparts, where y_{ij} is added to the linear predictor. The first one becomes

$$\text{logit}[g(\mathbf{h}_{ij}, y_{ij})] = 0.53 - 0.015\text{base}_i - 0.076y_{i,j-1} + 0.057y_{ij}, \qquad (26.3)$$

and the second one changes to

$$\text{logit}[g(\mathbf{h}_{ij}, y_{ij})] = 1.38 - 0.021\text{base}_i - 0.0027y_{i,j-2} - 0.064y_{i,j-1} + 0.035y_{ij}. \qquad (26.4)$$

It turns out that model (26.4) is not significantly better than (26.2) and, hence, we retain (26.2) as the most plausible description of the dropout process we have so far obtained.

26.4   A PATTERN-MIXTURE MODEL FOR THE VOROZOLE STUDY

In Section 26.2 the individual and average profiles for the vorozole study were plotted in a pattern-specific way (Figures 26.9 and 26.10). Figure 26.10 suggests that pattern-specific profiles are of a quadratic nature, with a sharp decline prior to dropout in most cases. This is in line with the fitted dropout mechanism (26.2). Therefore, it seems reasonable to expect this to be reflected in the pattern-mixture model. By analogy with the selection model, the profiles are forced to pass through the origin. This is done by allowing only time main effects and interactions of other covariables with time in the model.

The most complex pattern-mixture model we consider includes a separate parameter vector for each of the observed patterns. This is achieved by making all effects in the model interact with *pattern*, a factor variable. We then proceed by backward selection in order to simplify the model. First, it was found that the covariance structure is common to all patterns, encompassing random intercept, a serial exponential process, and measurement error.

For the fixed effects, we proceeded as follows. A backward selection procedure was conducted, starting from a model that included a main effect of time and

Table 26.3   Vorozole study. Parameter estimates and standard errors for the first pattern-mixture model.

Effect	Estimate (s.e.)	Effect	Estimate (s.e.)
Fixed-effects parameters			
Time	4.671 (0.844)	$Time^2$	-0.034 (0.029)
Time × pattern 1	-8.856 (2.739)	$Time^2$ × pattern 1	
Time × pattern 2	-0.796 (2.958)	$Time^2$ × pattern 2	-1.918 (1.269)
Time × pattern 3	-1.959 (1.794)	$Time^2$ × pattern 3	-0.145 (0.365)
Time × pattern 4	1.600 (1.441)	$Time^2$ × pattern 4	-0.541 (0.197)
Time × pattern 5	0.292 (1.295)	$Time^2$ × pattern 5	-0.107 (0.133)
Time × pattern 6	1.366 (1.035)	$Time^2$ × pattern 6	-0.181 (0.080)
Time × pattern 7	1.430 (1.045)	$Time^2$ × pattern 7	-0.132 (0.071)
Time × pattern 8	1.176 (1.025)	$Time^2$ × pattern 8	-0.118 (0.061)
Time × pattern 9	0.735 (0.934)	$Time^2$ × pattern 9	-0.083 (0.049)
Time × pattern 10	0.797 (1.078)	$Time^2$ × pattern 10	-0.078 (0.055)
Time × pattern 11	0.274 (0.989)	$Time^2$ × pattern 11	-0.023 (0.046)
Time × pattern 12	0.544 (1.087)	$Time^2$ × pattern 12	-0.026 (0.049)
Time × baseline	-0.031 (0.004)	Time × treatment	-0.067 (0.166)
Variance parameters			
Random intercept	78.45		
Serial variance	95.38		
Serial association	8.85		
Measurement error	73.77		

time², as well as interactions of time with baseline value, treatment effect, dominant site and pattern, and the interaction of pattern with time². This procedure revealed main effects of time and time², as well as interactions of time with baseline value, treatment effect, and pattern, and the interaction of pattern with time². This reduced model can be found in Table 26.3. As was the case with the selection model in Table 26.2, the treatment effect is non-significant. Indeed, a single-degree-of-freedom F test yields a p-value of 0.687. Note that such a single-degree-of-freedom test is possible because treatment effect does not interact with pattern, in contrast to the model which we will describe next. The fitted profiles are displayed in Figure 26.14. We observe that the profiles for both arms are very similar. This is due to the fact that treatment effect is not significant but perhaps also because we did not allow a more complex treatment effect. For example, we might consider an interaction of treatment with the square of time and, more importantly, a treatment effect which is pattern-specific. Some evidence for such an interaction is seen in Figure 26.10.

Our second, expanded model allowed for up to cubic time effects, the interaction of time with dropout pattern, dominant site, baseline value and treatment, as well as their two- and three-way interactions. After a backward selection procedure, the effects included are time and time², the two-way interaction of time and dropout pattern, as well as three-factor interactions

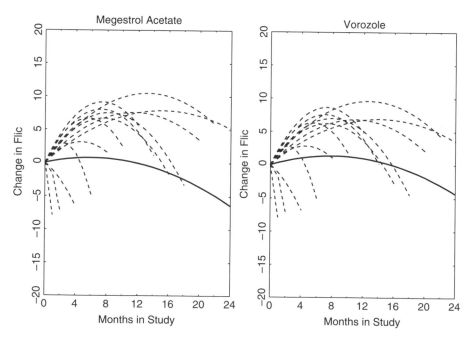

Figure 26.14 Vorozole study. Fitted selection (solid line) and first pattern-mixture models (dashed lines).

of time and dropout pattern with (1) baseline, (2) group, and (3) dominant site. Finally, time^2 interacts with dropout pattern and with the interaction of baseline and dropout pattern. No cubic time effects were necessary, which is in agreement with the observed profiles in Figure 26.10. The parameter estimates of this model are displayed in Table 26.4. The model is graphically represented in Figure 26.15.

Table 26.4 Vorozole study. Parameter estimates and standard errors for the second pattern-mixture model. Each column represents an effect, for which a main effect is given, as well as interactions with the dropout patterns.

Fixed-effects parameters

Effect	Time	Time × baseline	Time^2	Time^2 × baseline	Time × treatment	Time × domsite (1)	Time × domsite (2)	Time × domsite (3)
Main	5.468	−0.034	−0.271	0.002		−0.873	0.941	0.023
	(5.089)	(0.040)	(0.206)	(0.002)		(1.073)	(0.845)	(0.576)
Pattern 1	7.616	−0.119			0.445	−5.822	−9.320	1.431
	(21.908)	(0.175)			(5.095)	(17.401)	(9.429)	(9.878)
Pattern 2	44.097	−0.440	−18.632	0.1458	0.867	2.024	4.393	5.681
	(17.489)	(0.148)	(7.491)	(0.0644)	(1.552)	(3.847)	(2.690)	(2.642)
Pattern 3	22.471	−0.218	−5.871	0.0484	−1.312	2.937	0.940	1.414
	(10.907)	(0.089)	(2.143)	(0.0178)	(0.808)	(2.596)	(1.697)	(1.633)
Pattern 4	10.578	−0.055	−1.429	0.0080	−0.249	−1.378	−4.366	−3.237
	(9.833)	(0.079)	(1.276)	(0.0107)	(0.686)	(2.699)	(2.367)	(2.289)
Pattern 5	14.691	−0.123	−1.571	0.0127	−0.184	−0.547	−1.099	−1.015
	(8.424)	(0.069)	(0.814)	(0.0069)	(0.678)	(1.917)	(1.456)	(1.344)
Pattern 6	7.527	−0.061	−0.827	0.0058	0.527	1.302	−0.914	
	(6.401)	(0.052)	(0.431)	(0.0036)	(0.448)	(1.130)	(0.811)	
Pattern 7	−12.631	0.086	0.653	−0.0065	0.782	3.881	1.733	4.548
	(7.367)	(0.058)	(0.454)	(0.0038)	(0.502)	(1.485)	(1.226)	(1.218)
Pattern 8	14.827	−0.126	−0.697	0.0052	−0.809	2.359	−0.436	
	(6.467)	(0.053)	(0.343)	(0.0029)	(0.464)	(1.241)	(0.843)	
Pattern 9	5.667	−0.049	−0.315	0.0021	−0.080	1.138	−0.326	
	(6.050)	(0.049)	(0.288)	(0.0023)	(0.443)	(1.128)	(0.753)	
Pattern 10	12.418	−0.093	−0.273	0.0016	0.331		−3.595	
	(6.473)	(0.051)	(0.296)	(0.0024)	(0.579)		(0.996)	
Pattern 11	1.934	−0.022	−0.049	0.0003	−0.679	0.317	0.182	
	(6.551)	(0.053)	(0.289)	(00024)	(0.492)	(1.152)	(0.825)	
Pattern 12	6.303	−0.052	−0.182	0.0015	0.433		−1.694	
	(6.426)	(0.050)	(0.259)	(0.0021)	(0.688)		(0.972)	
Pattern 13					−1.323			
					(0.706)			

Variance parameters								
Random intercept							98.93	
Serial variance							38.86	
Serial association							6.10	
Measurement error							73.65	

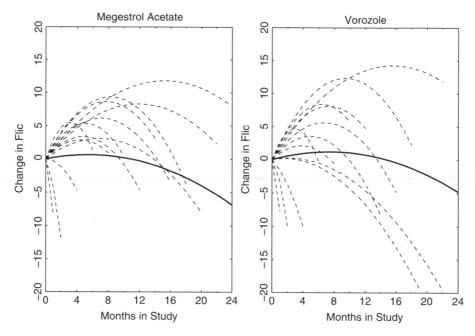

Figure 26.15 Vorozole study. Fitted selection (solid line) and second pattern-mixture models (dashed lines).

Because a pattern-specific parameter has been included, we have several options for the assessment of treatment. Since there are 13 patterns (recall that we cut off the patterns at 2 years), one can test the global hypothesis, based on 13 degrees of freedom, of no treatment effect. For this test we obtain $F = 1.25$, corresponding to $p = 0.240$, indicating that there is no overall treatment effect. Each of the treatment effects separately is at a non-significant level. Alternatively, the *marginal* effect of treatment can be calculated, which is the weighted average of the pattern-specific treatment effects, with weights given by the probability of occurrence of the various patterns. Its standard error is calculated using a straightforward application of the delta method, as in Section 16.6. This effect is equal to -0.286 (s.e. 0.288), producing $p = 0.321$, which is still non-significant.

The various assessments of treatment effect, based on the results obtained in this section and in Section 26.3, are summarized in Table 26.5. Thus, we obtain a non-significant treatment effect from all our different models, which gives more weight to the conclusion.

However, as has been made clear in Section 16.5, the apparently simpler Strategies 2a and 2b should be avoided where possible. We therefore shift attention to Strategy 1.

Table 26.5 Vorozole study. Summary of treatment effect assessment

Method	d.f.	p-value
Selection model	1	0.582
First pattern-mixture model	1	0.687
Second pattern-mixture model	13	0.240
Second pattern-mixture model	1	0.321

Table 26.6 Vorozole study. Distribution over patterns.

Pattern	Number of measurements	Number of subjects	Percentage
3	1	35	8.73
4	2	86	21.45
5	3	69	17.21
6	4	45	11.22
7	5	29	7.23
8	6	33	8.23
9	7	22	5.49
10	8	17	4.24
11	9	19	4.74
12	10	9	2.24
13	11	10	2.49
14	12	6	1.50
15	13	8	2.00
16	14	3	0.75
17	15	4	1.00
18	16	3	0.75
20	18	1	0.25
21	19	1	0.25
25	23	1	0.25

The distribution of subjects over patterns is described in Table 26.6. The largest portion of the subjects remains on study for less than 1 year, with very few in the subsequent 6-month period and only three subjects on trial after 18 months. Based on this information, we chose to remove the three subjects in the last patterns.

The selection of covariates was done by analogy with the earlier analyses. Covariates retained in the models were time, time interactions with baseline and treatment group, time^2 and the interaction between time^2 and baseline. We opted for NCMV, CCMV, and ACMV identifying restrictions (see Section 16.5).

Assessment of the marginal treatment effect leads to $p = 0.9407$ for NCMV, $p = 0.7570$ for CCMV, and $p = 0.0487$ for ACMV. This result is interesting and calls for careful discussion. First, there is a considerable difference with the assessment based on just three measurements (Section 16.6), where all three strategies yielded highly non-significant results. Second, the strategies lead to conclusions that differ dramatically from each other, which contrasts with the results from the earlier analysis. The MAR-based ACMV restrictions leads to a significant effect, albeit borderline, whereas the others do not lead to evidence in favour of a treatment difference. This suggests that the treatment effect found is conditional on the ACMV (MAR) assumption.

A graphical representation is given in Figure 26.16. It is, of course, rather difficult to get a clear message from the multitude of patterns, except that for ACMV, as opposed to the other two, the extrapolated profiles lie closer to the observed profiles.

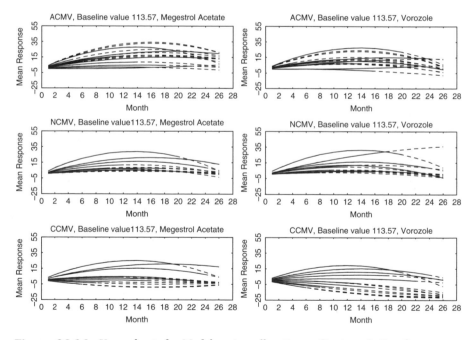

Figure 26.16 Vorozole study. Models using all patterns; Strategy 1. For the average level of baseline value and for both treatment arms, plots of mean profiles over time are presented. The (Solid lines from baseline until the last obtained measurement, while lines refer to extrapolations.)

26.5   CONCLUDING REMARKS

In a certain sense pattern-mixture modelling does not require modelling of the unobserved outcomes. Indeed, in its simplest form, a chosen measurement model (e.g., a linear mixed-effects model) can be fitted to the *observed* data in each of the dropout patterns separately. Together with estimating the (possibly covariate-dependent) probabilities of membership of each of the dropout patterns, the model is completed.

However, there are several reasons why more complex manipulations may be needed. First, there will often be interest in the marginal distribution of the responses, for which a mixture of an effect over the different dropout patterns is needed.

Second, there may be interest in the prediction of pattern-specific quantities, such as average profiles, *beyond* the time of dropout. This is where the underidentification of pattern-mixture models manifests itself. Several solutions have been proposed. Little (1993) suggested identifying restrictions (see Section 3.6). Alternatively, relatively simple models can be constructed such as linear or quadratic time evolutions, which allow for easy extrapolation – but for polynomials this is well known to have the potential for very unrealistic behaviour. Finally, dropout time can be incorporated as a covariate into the model, and information can be borrowed across patterns (Section 26.4). An advantage is that the assumptions are always very explicit, in contrast to selection modelling. This simplifies performing sensitivity analyses by investigating the effect of various assumptions on the final results.

Finally, as illustrated in our analyses, pattern-mixture models often comprise large numbers of parameters, some of which may be estimated very inefficiently, thereby possibly undermining results based on asymptotic considerations.

References

Aerts, M., Claeskens, G., Hens, N. and Molenberghs, G. (2002) Local multiple imputation. *Biometrika*, **89**, 375–388.

Afifi, A. and Elashoff, R. (1966) Missing observations in multivariate statistics I: Review of the literature. *Journal of the American Statistical Association*, **61**, 595–604.

Agresti, A. (1990) *Categorical Data Analysis*. New York: John Wiley & Sons, Inc.

Agresti, A. (2002) *Categorical Data Analysis* (2nd edn). New York: John Wiley & Sons, Inc.

Aitkin, M. and Rubin, D.B. (1985) Estimation and hypothesis testing in finite mixture models. *Journal of the Royal Statistical Society, Series B*, **47**, 67–75.

Albert, A. and Lesaffre, E. (1986) Multiple group logistic discrimination. *Computers and Mathematics with Applications*, **12**, 209–224.

Allison, P.D. (1987) Estimation of linear models with incomplete data. *Sociological Methodology*, **17**, 71–103.

Arnold, B.C. and Strauss, D. (1988) Pseudolikelihood estimation. Technical Report 164, University of California, Riverside, Dept. of Statistics.

Arnold, B.C. and Strauss, D. (1991) Pseudolikelihood estimation: some examples, *Sankhya, Series B*, **53**, 233–243.

Bahadur, R.R. (1961) A representation of the joint distribution of responses to *n* dichotomous items. In H. Solomon (ed.), *Studies in Item Analysis and Prediction*, Stanford Mathematical Studies in the Social Sciences VI. Stanford, CA: Stanford University Press.

Baker, S.G. (1992) A simple method for computing the observed information matrix when using the EM algorithm with categorical data. *Journal of Computational and Graphical Statistics*, **1**, 63–76.

Baker, S.G. (1994) Regression analysis of grouped survival data with incomplete covariates: non-ignorable missing-data and censoring mechanisms. *Biometrics*, **50**, 821–826.

Baker, S.G. (1995a) Marginal regression for repeated binary data with outcome subject to non-ignorable non-response. *Biometrics*, **51**, 1042–1052.

Baker, S.G. (1995b) Evaluating multiple diagnostic tests with partial verification. *Biometrics*, **51**, 330–337.

Baker, S.G. (2000) Analyzing a randomized cancer prevention trial with a missing binary outcome, an auxiliary variable, and all-or-none compliance. *Journal of the American Statistical Association*, **95**, 43–50.

Missing Data in Clinical Studies   G. Molenberghs and M.G. Kenward
© 2007 John Wiley & Sons, Ltd

Baker, S.G. and Laird, N.M. (1988) Regression analysis for categorical variables with outcome subject to non-ignorable non-response. *Journal of the American Statistical Association*, **83**, 62–69.

Baker, S.G., Rosenberger, W.F., and DerSimonian, R. (1992) Closed-form estimates for missing counts in two-way contingency tables. *Statistics in Medicine*, **11**, 643–657.

Beran, R. (1988) Prepivoting test statistics: a bootstrap view of asymptotic refinements. *Journal of the American Statistical Association*, **83**, 687–697.

Besag, J., Green, P.J., Higdon, D., and Mengersen, K. (1995) Bayesian computation and stochastic systems, *Statistical Science*, **10**, 3–66.

Best, N.G., Spiegelhalter, D.J., Thomas, A., and Brayne, C.E.G. (1996) Bayesian analysis of realistically complex models. *Journal of the Royal Statistical Society, Series A*, **159**, 323–342.

Beunkens, C., Molenberghs, G., and Kenward, M.G. (2005) Tutorial: Direct likelihood analysis versus simple forms of imputation for missing data in randomized clinical trials. *Clinical Trials*, **2**, 379–386.

Beunckens, C., Molenberghs, G., Verbeke, G., and Mallinckrodt, C. (2006) A latent-class mixture model for incomplete longitudinal Gaussian data. Submitted for publication.

Bickel, P.J. and Kwon, J. (2001) Inference for semiparametric models: some questions and an answer. *Statistica Sinica*, **11**, 920–936.

Birch, M.W. (1963) Maximum likelihood in three-way contingency tables. *Journal of the Royal Statistical Society, Series B*, **25**, 220–233.

Böhning D. (1999) *Computer-Assisted Analysis of Mixtures and Applications: Meta-analysis, Disease Mapping, and Others*. Boca Raton, FL: Chapman & Hall/CRC.

Breslow, N.E. and Clayton, D.G. (1993) Approximate inference in generalized linear mixed models. *Journal of the American Statistical Association*, **88**, 9–25.

Brown, C.H. (1990) Protecting against nonrandomly missing data in longitudinal studies. *Biometrics*, **46**, 143–155.

Buck, S.F. (1960) A method of estimation of missing values in multivariate data suitable for use with an electronic computer. *Journal of the Royal Statistical Society, Series B*, **22**, 302–306.

Burton, S.W. (1991) A review of fluvoxamine and its uses in depression. *International Clinical Psychopharmacology*, **6** (Suppl. 3), 1–17.

Buyse, M. and Molenberghs, G. (1998) The validation of surrogate endpoints in randomized experiments. *Biometrics*, **54**, 1014–1029.

Carpenter, J., Pocock, S., and Lamm, C.J. (2002) Coping with missing data in clinical trials: a model based approach applied to asthma trials. *Statistics in Medicine*, **21**, 1043–1066.

Carpenter, J., Kenward, M.G., Evans, S., and White, I. (2004) Last observation carry-forward and last observation analysis. Letter to the Editor. *Statistics in Medicine*, **23**, 3241–3244.

Carpenter, J.R., Kenward, M.G., and Vansteelandt, S. (2006) A comparison of multiple imputation and doubly robust estimation for analyses with missing data. *Journal of the Royal Statistical Society, Series A*, **169**, 571–584.

Catchpole, E.A. and Morgan, B.J.T. (1997) Detecting parameter redundancy. *Biometrika*, **84**, 187–196.

Catchpole, E.A., Morgan, B.J.T., and Freeman, S.N. (1998) Estimation in parameter-redundant models. *Biometrika*, **85**, 462–468.

Chatterjee, S. and Hadi, A.S. (1988) *Sensitivity Analysis in Linear Regression*. New York: John Wiley & Sons, Inc.

Chen, T. and Fienberg, S.E. (1974) Two-dimensional contingency tables with both completely and partially cross-classified data. *Biometrics*, **30**, 629–642.

Clayton, D. and Hills, M. (1993) *Statistical Methods in Epidemiology*. Oxford: Oxford University Press.

Clayton, D., Spiegelhalter, D., Dunn., D., and Pickles, A. (1998) Analysis of longitudinal binary data from multiphase sampling (with discussion). *Journal of the Royal Statistical Society, Series B*, **60**, 71–87.

Cochran, W.G. (1977). *Sampling Techniques*. New York: John Wiley & Sons, Inc.

Cohen, J. and Cohen, P. (1983) *Applied Multiple Regression/Correlation Analysis for the Behavioral Sciences* (2nd edn). Hillsdale, NJ: Erlbaum.

Conaway, M.R. (1992) The analysis of repeated categorical measurements subject to nonignorable nonresponse. *Journal of the American Statistical Association*, **87**, 817–824.

Conaway, M.R. (1993) Non-ignorable non-response models for time-ordered categorical variables. *Applied Statistics*, **42**, 105–115.

Cook, R.D. (1977) Detection of influential observations in linear regression. *Technometrics*, **19**, 15–18.

Cook, R.D. (1979) Influential observations in linear regression. *Journal of the American Statistical Association*, **74**, 169–174.

Cook, R.D. (1986) Assessment of local influence. *Journal of the Royal Statistical Society, Series B*, **48**, 133–169.

Cook, R.D. and Weisberg, S. (1982) *Residuals and Influence in Regression*. London: Chapman & Hall.

Copas, J.B. and Li, H.G. (1997) Inference from non-random samples (with discussion). *Journal of the Royal Statistical Society, Series B*, **59**, 55–96.

Cowles, M.K., Carlin, B.P., and Connett, J.E. (1996) Bayesian tobit modeling of longitudinal ordinal clinical trial compliance data with nonignorable missingness. *Journal of the American Statistical Association*, **91**, 86–98.

Cox, D.R. (1972) The analysis of multivariate binary data. *Applied Statistics*, **21**, 113–120.

Cox, D.R. and Hinkley, D.V. (1974) *Theoretical Statistics*. London: Chapman & Hall.

Crépeau, H., Koziol, J., Reid, N., and Yuh, Y.S. (1985) Analysis of incomplete multivariate data from repeated measurements experiments. *Biometrics*, **41**, 505–514.

Cressie, N.A.C. (1991) *Statistics for Spatial Data*. New York: John Wiley & Sons, Inc.

Cullis, B.R. (1994) Discussion of Diggle, P.J. and Kenward, M.G.: Informative dropout in longitudinal data analysis. *Applied Statistics*, **43**, 79–80.

Dale, J.R. (1986) Global cross-ratio models for bivariate, discrete, ordered responses. *Biometrics*, **42**, 909–917.

Davison, A.C. and Hinkley, D.V. (1997) *Bootstrap Methods and Their Application*. Cambridge: Cambridge University Press.

De Backer, M., van Lierde, M.A., De Keyser, P., De Vroey C., and Lesaffre E. (1995) A 12 weeks treatment for dermatophyte toe-onychomycosis: terbinafine 250 mg/d or itraconazole 200 mg/d? A double blind comparative trial. *Journal of the European Academy of Dermatology and Venereology*, **5** (Suppl. 1), 95.

DeGruttola, V. and Tu, X.M. (1994) Modelling progression of CD4 lymphocyte count and its relationship to survival time. *Biometrics*, **50**, 1003–1014.

Dempster, A.P. and Rubin, D.B. (1983) Overview. In W.G. Madow, I. Olkin, and D.B. Rubin (eds), *Incomplete Data in Sample Surveys, Vol. II: Theory and Annotated Bibliography*, pp. 3–10. New York: Academic Press.

Dempster, A.P., Laird, N.M., and Rubin, D. B. (1977) Maximum likelihood from incomplete data via the EM algorithm (with discussion). *Journal of the Royal Statistical Society, Series B*, **39**, 1–38.

Diggle, P.J. (1988) An approach to the analysis of repeated measures. *Biometrics*, **44**, 959–971.

Diggle, P.J. (1989) Testing for random dropouts in repeated measurement data. *Biometrics*, **45**, 1255–1258.

Diggle, P.J. (1990) *Time Series: A Biostatistical Introduction*. Oxford: Oxford University Press.

Diggle, P.J. and Kenward, M.G. (1994) Informative drop-out in longitudinal data analysis (with discussion). *Applied Statistics*, **43**, 49–93.

Diggle, P.J., Liang, K.-Y., and Zeger, S.L. (1994) *Analysis of Longitudinal Data*. Oxford: Clarendon Press.

Diggle, P.J., Heagerty, P.J., Liang, K.-Y., and Zeger, S.L. (2002) *Analysis of Longitudinal Data* (2nd edn). Oxford: Clarendon Press.

Dmitrienko, A., Offen, W.W., Faries, D., Chuang-Stein, C., and Molenberghs, G. (2005). *Analysis of Clinical Trial Data Using the SAS System*. Cary, NC: SAS Publishing.

Draper, D. (1995) Assessment and propagation of model uncertainty (with discussion). *Journal of the Royal Statistical Society, Series B*, **57**, 45–97.

Edwards, A.W.F. (1972) *Likelihood*. Cambridge: Cambridge University Press.

Efron, B. (1979) Bootstrap methods: another look at the jackknife. *Annals of Statistics*, **7**, 1–26.

Efron, B. and Hinkley, D.V. (1978) Assessing the accuracy of the maximum likelihood estimator: observed versus expected Fisher information. *Biometrika*, **65**, 457–487.

Efron, B. and Tibshirani, R.J. (1998) The problem of regions. *Annals of Statistics*, **26**, 1687–1718.

Ekholm, A. and Skinner, C. (1998) The Muscatine children's obesity data reanalysed using pattern mixture models. *Applied Statistics*, **47**, 251–263.

Faucett, C.L. and Thomas, D.C. (1996) Simultaneously modelling censored survival data and repeatedly measured covariates: a Gibbs sampling approach. *Statistics in Medicine*, **15**, 1663–1685.

Fay, R.E. (1986) Causal models for patterns of nonresponse. *Journal of the American Statistical Association*, **81**, 354–365.

Fay, R.E. (1992) When are inferences from multiple imputations valid? *Proceedings of the Survey Research Methods Section of the American Statistical Association*, 227–232.

Fitzmaurice, G.M., Laird, N.M., and Lipsitz, S.R. (1994) Analysing incomplete longitudinal binary responses: a likelihood-based approach. *Biometrics*, **50**, 601–612.

Fitzmaurice, G.M., Molenberghs, G., and Lipsitz, S.R. (1995) Regression models for longitudinal binary responses with informative dropouts. *Journal of the Royal Statistical Society, Series B*, **57**, 691–704.

Fitzmaurice, G.M., Laird, N.M., and Ware, J.H. (2004) *Applied Longitudinal Analysis*. Hoboken, NJ: John Wiley & Sons, Inc.

Follmann, D. and Wu, M. (1995) An approximate generalized linear model with random effects for informative missing data. *Biometrics* **51**, 151–168.

Foster, J.J. and Smith, P.W.F. (1998) Model-based inference for categorical survey data subject to non-ignorable non-response. *Journal of the Royal Statistical Society, Series B,* **60**, 57–70.

Fowler, Jr., F.J. (1988) *Survey Research Methods.* Newbury Park, CA: Sage.

Friedman, L.M., Furberg, C.D., and DeMets, D.L. (1998) *Fundamentals of Clinical Trials.* New York: Springer.

Gelman, A., Van Mechelen, I., Verbeke, G., Heitjan, D.F., and Meulders, M. (2005) Multiple imputation for model checking: completed-data plots with missing and latent data. *Biometrics,* **61**, 74–85.

Geys, H., Molenberghs, G., and Ryan, L. (1999) Pseudolikelihood modeling of multivariate outcomes in developmental toxicology. *Journal of the American Statistical Association,* **94**, 734–745.

Gibbons, R.D., Hedeker, D., Waternaux, D., Kraemer, H.C., Greenhouse, J.B., Shea, M.T., Imber, S.D., Sotsky, S.M., and Watkins, J.T. (1993) Some conceptual and statistical issues in analysis of longitudinal psychiatric data. *Archives of General Psychiatry,* **50**, 739–750.

Glynn, R.J., Laird, N.M., and Rubin, D.B. (1986) Selection modelling versus mixture modelling with non-ignorable nonresponse. In H. Wainer (ed.), *Drawing Inferences from Self Selected Samples,* pp. 115–142. New York: Springer.

Goss, P.E., Winer, E.P., Tannock, I.F., and Schwartz, L.H. (1999) Breast cancer: randomized phase III trial comparing the new potent and selective third-generation aromatase inhibitor vorozole with megestrol acetate in postmenopausal advanced breast cancer patients. *Journal of Clinical Oncology,* **17**, 52–63.

Gould, A.L. (1980) A new approach to the analysis of clinical drug trials with withdrawals. *Biometrics,* **36**, 721–727.

Green, S., Benedetti, J., and Crowley, J. (1997) *Clinical Trials in Oncology.* London: Chapman & Hall.

Greenlees, W.S., Reece, J.S., and Zieschang, K.D. (1982) Imputation of missing values when the probability of response depends on the variable being imputed. *Journal of the American Statistical Association,* **77**, 251–261.

Hartley, H.O. and Hocking, R. (1971) The analysis of incomplete data. *Biometrics,* **27**, 783–808.

Harville, D.A. (1974) Bayesian inference for variance components using only error contrasts. *Biometrika,* **61**, 383–385.

Heckman, J.J. (1976) The common structure of statistical models of truncation, sample selection and limited dependent variables and a simple estimator for such models. *Annals of Economic and Social Measurement,* **5**, 475–492.

Hedeker, D. and Gibbons, R.D. (1997) Application of random-effects pattern-mixture models for missing data in longitudinal studies. *Psychological Methods,* **2**, 64–78.

Heitjan, D.F. (1994) Ignorability in general incomplete-data models. *Biometrika,* **81**, 701–708.

Heitjan, D.F. and Rubin, D.B. (1991) Ignorability and coarse data. *Annals of Statistics,* **19**, 2244–2253.

Henderson, R., Diggle, P., and Dobson, A. (2000) Joint modelling of longitudinal measurements and event time data. *Biostatistics,* **1**, 465–480.

Henderson, R., Diggle, P., and Dobson, A. (2002). Identification and efficacy of longitudinal markers for survival. *Biostatistics,* **3**, 33–50.

Herzog, T.N. and Rubin, D.B. (1983) Using multiple imputations to handle nonresponse in sample surveys. In W.G. Madow, H. Nisselson, and I. Olkin (eds), *Incomplete Data in Sample Surveys, Volume 2: Theory and Bibliographies,* pp. 115–142. New York: Academic Press.

Heyting, A., Tolboom, J.T.B.M., and Essers, J.G.A. (1992) Statistical handling of drop-outs in longitudinal clinical trials. *Statistics in Medicine,* **11**, 2043–2061.

Hogan, J.W. and Laird, N.M. (1997) Mixture models for the joint distribution of repeated measures and event times. *Statistics in Medicine,* **16**, 239–258.

Hogan, J.W. and Laird, N.M. (1998) Increasing efficiency from censored survival data by using random effects to model longitudinal covariates. *Statistical Methods in Medical Research,* **7**, 28–48.

Horton, N.J. and Lipsitz, S.R. (2001) Multiple imputation in practice: comparison of software packages for regression models with missing variables. *American Statistician,* **55**, 244–254.

Horvitz, D.G. and Thompson D.J. (1952) A generalization of sampling without replacement from a finite universe. *Journal of the Americal Statistical Association,* **47**, 663–685.

Ibrahim, J.G. and Lipsitz, S. R. (1996) Parameter estimation from incomplete data in binomial regression when the missing data mechanism is nonignorable. *Biometrics,* **52**, 1071–1078.

Ibrahim, J., Lipsitz, S.R., and Chen, M. (1999) Missing covariates in generalized linear models when the missing data mechanism is nonignorable. *Journal of the Royal Statistical Society, Series B,* **61**, 173–190.

International Conference on Harmonisation E9 Expert Working Group (1999) Statistical principles for clinical trials: ICH Harmonised Tripartite Guideline. *Statistics in Medicine,* **18**, 1905–1942.

Jansen, I. and Molenberghs, G. (2005) A flexible marginal modeling strategy for non-monotone missing data. Submitted for publication.

Jansen, I., Molenberghs, G., Aerts, M., Thijs, H., and Van Steen, K. (2003) A local influence approach applied to binary data from a psychiatric study. *Biometrics,* **59**, 410–419.

Jansen, I., Beunckens, C., Molenberghs, G., Verbeke, G., and Mallinckrodt, C. (2006a) Analyzing incomplete discrete longitudinal clinical trial data. *Statistical Science,* **21**, 52–69.

Jansen, I., Hens, N., Molenberghs, G., Aerts, M., Verbeke, G., and Kenward, M.G. (2006b) The nature of sensitivity in missing not at random models. *Computational Statistics and Data Analysis,* **50**, 830–858.

Jennrich, R.I. and Schluchter, M.D. (1986) Unbalanced repeated measures models with structured covariance matrices. *Biometrics,* **42**, 805–820.

Kahn, H. and Sempos, C.T. (1989) *Statistical Methods in Epidemiology.* New York: Oxford University Press.

Kenward, M.G. (1998) Selection models for repeated measurements with nonrandom dropout: an illustration of sensitivity. *Statistics in Medicine,* **17**, 2723–2732.

Kenward, M.G. and Molenberghs, G. (1998) Likelihood based frequentist inference when data are missing at random. *Statistical Science,* **12**, 236–247.

Kenward, M.G. and Molenberghs, G. (1999) Parametric models for incomplete continuous and categorical longitudinal studies data. *Statistical Methods in Medical Research,* **8**, 51–83.

Kenward, M.G. and Roger, J.H. (1997) Small sample inference for fixed effects from restricted maximum likelihood. *Biometrics*, **53**, 983–997.

Kenward, M.G., Lesaffre, E., and Molenberghs, G. (1994) An application of maximum likelihood and generalized estimating equations to the analysis of ordinal data from a longitudinal study with cases missing at random. *Biometrics*, **50**, 945–953.

Kenward, M.G, Goetghebeur, E.J.T., and Molenberghs, G. (2001) Sensitivity analysis of incomplete categorical data. *Statistical Modelling*, **1**, 31–48.

Kenward, M.G., Molenberghs, G., and Thijs, H. (2003) Pattern-mixture models with proper time dependence. *Biometrika*, **90**, 53–71.

Koch, G., Singer, J., Stokes, M., Carr, G., Cohen, S. and Forthofer, R. (1992) Some aspects of weighted least-squares analysis for longitudinal categorical data. In J.H. Dwyer, M. Feinleib, P. Lipper, and H. Hoffmeister (eds), *Statistical Models for Longitudinal Studies of Health*, pp. 215–260. Oxford: Oxford University Press.

Laird, N.M. (1988) Missing data in longitudinal studies. *Statistics in Medicine*, **7**, 305–315.

Laird, N.M. (1994) Discussion of Diggle, P.J. and Kenward, M.G.: Informative dropout in longitudinal data analysis. *Applied Statistics*, **43**, 84.

Laird, N.M. and Ware, J.H. (1982) Random effects models for longitudinal data. *Biometrics*, **38**, 963–974.

Laird, N.M., Lange, N., and Stram, D. (1987) Maximum likelihood computations with repeated meausres: application of the EM algorithm. *Journal of the American Statistical Association*, **82**, 97–105.

Lapp, K., Molenberghs, G., and Lesaffre, E. (1998) Local and global cross ratios to model the association between ordinal variables. *Computational Statistics and Data Analysis*, **28**, 387–411.

Lavalley, M.P. and DeGruttola, V. (1996) Models for empirical Bayes estimators of longitudinal CD4 counts. *Statistics in Medicine*, **15**, 2289–2305.

Lavori, P.W., Dawson, R., and Shera, D. (1995) A multiple imputation strategy for clinical trials with truncation of patient data. *Statistics in Medicine*, **14**, 1913–1925.

Le Cessie, S. and Van Houwelingen, J.C. (1994) Logistic regression for correlated binary data. *Applied Statistics*, **43**, 95–108.

Lesaffre, E. and Verbeke, G. (1998) Local influence in linear mixed models. *Biometrics*, **54**, 570–582.

Li, K.H., Raghunathan, T.E., and Rubin, D.B. (1991) Large-sample significance levels from multiply imputed data using moment-based statistics and an *F* reference distribution. *Journal of the American Statistical Association*, **86**, 1065–1073.

Liang, K.-Y. and Zeger, S.L. (1986) Longitudinal data analysis using generalized linear models. *Biometrika*, **73**, 13–22.

Lilienfeld, D.E. and Stolley, P.D. (1994) *Foundations of Epidemiology*. New York: Oxford University Press.

Lipsitz, S.R., Zhao, L.P., and Molenberghs, G. (1998) A semi-parametric method of multiple imputation. *Journal of the Royal Statistical Society, Series B*, **60**, 127–144.

Lipsitz, S.R., Molenberghs, G., Fitzmaurice, G.M., and Ibrahim, J.G. (2004) A protective estimator for linear regression with nonignorably missing Gaussian outcomes. *Statistical Modelling*, **4**, 3–17.

Little, R.J.A. (1976) Inference about means for incomplete multivariate data. *Biometrika*, **63**, 593–604.

Little, R.J.A. (1993) Pattern-mixture models for multivariate incomplete data. *Journal of the American Statistical Association*, **88**, 125–134.

Little, R.J.A. (1994a) A class of pattern-mixture models for normal incomplete data. *Biometrika*, **81**, 471–483.

Little, R.J.A. (1994b) Discussion to Diggle, P.J. and Kenward, M.G.: Informative dropout in longitudinal data analysis. *Applied Statistics*, **43**, 78.

Ⴟ Little, R.J.A. (1995) Modeling the drop-out mechanism in repeated measures studies. *Journal of the American Statistical Association*, **90**, 1112–1121.

Little, R.J.A. and Rubin, D.B. (1987) *Statistical Analysis with Missing Data*. New York: John Wiley & Sons, Inc.

Little, R.J.A. and Rubin, D.B. (2002) *Statistical Analysis with Missing Data* (2nd edn). New York: John Wiley & Sons, Inc.

Little, R.J.A. and Wang, Y. (1996) Pattern-mixture models for multivariate incomplete data with covariates. *Biometrics*, **52**, 98–111.

Little, R.J.A. and Yau, L. (1996) Intent-to-treat analysis in longitudinal studies with dropouts. *Biometrics*, **52**, 1324–1333.

Louis, T.A. (1982) Finding the observed information matrix when using the EM algorithm. *Journal of the Royal Statistical Society, Series B*, **44**, 226–233.

Mallinckrodt, C.H., Clark, W.S., and Stacy R.D. (2001a) Type I error rates from mixed-effects model repeated measures versus fixed effects analysis of variance with missing values imputed via last observation carried forward. *Drug Information Journal*, **35**, 1215–1225.

Mallinckrodt, C.H., Clark, W.S., and Stacy R.D. (2001b) Accounting for dropout bias using mixed-effects models. *Journal of Biopharmaceutical Statistics*, **11**, 9–21.

Mallinckrodt, C.H., Carroll, R.J., Debrota, D.J., Dube, S., Molenberghs, G., Potter, W.Z., Sanger, T.D., and Tollefson, G.D. (2003a) Assessing and interpreting treatment effects in longitudinal clinical trials with subject dropout. *Biological Psychiatry*, **53**, 754–760.

Mallinckrodt, C.H., Scott Clark, W., Carroll, R.J., and Molenberghs, G. (2003b) Assessing response profiles from incomplete longitudinal clinical trial data with subject dropout under regulatory conditions. *Journal of Biopharmaceutical Statistics*, **13**, 179–190.

McArdle, J.J. and Hamagami, F. (1992) Modeling incomplete longitudinal and cross-sectional data using latent growth structural models. *Experimental Aging Research*, **18**, 145–166.

McCullagh, P. and Nelder, J.A. (1989) *Generalized Linear Models*. London: Chapman & Hall.

McLachlan, G.J. and Krishnan, T. (1997) *The EM Algorithm and Extensions*. New York: John Wiley & Sons, Inc.

Meilijson, I. (1989) A fast improvement to the EM algorithm on its own terms. *Journal of the Royal Statistical Society, Series B*, **51**, 127–138.

Meng, X.-L. (1994) Multiple-imputation inferences with uncongenial sources of input. *Statistical Science*, **9**, 538–558.

Meng, X.-L. and Rubin, D.B. (1991) Using EM to obtain asymptotic variance covariance matrices: the SEM algorithm. *Journal of the American Statistical Association*, **86**, 899–909.

Michiels, B. and Molenberghs, G. (1997) Protective estimation of longitudinal categorical data with nonrandom dropout. *Communications in Statistics*, **26**, 65–94.

Michiels, B., Molenberghs, G., Bijnens, L., and Vangeneugden, T. (2002) Selection models and pattern-mixture models to analyze longitudinal quality of life data subject to dropout. *Statistics in Medicine*, **21**, 1023–1041.

Michiels, B., Molenberghs, G., and Lipsitz, S.R. (1999). Selection models and pattern-mixture models for incomplete categorical data with covariates. *Biometrics*, **55**, 978–983.

Minini, P. and Chavence, M. (2004a) Sensitivity analysis of longitudinal normal data with drop-outs. *Statistics in Medicine*, **23**, 1039–1054.

Minini, P. and Chavance, M. (2004b) Sensitivity analysis of longitudinal binary data with non-monotone missing values. *Biostatistics*, **5**, 531–544.

Molenberghs, G. and Goetghebeur, E. (1997) Simple fitting algorithms for incomplete categorical data. *Journal of the Royal Statistical Society, Series B*, **59**, 401–414.

Molenberghs, G. and Lesaffre, E. (1994) Marginal modelling of correlated ordinal data using a multivariate Plackett distribution. *Journal of the American Statistical Association*, **89**, 633–644.

Molenberghs, G. and Lesaffre, E. (1999) Marginal modelling of multivariate categorical data. *Statistics in Medicine*, **18**, 2237–2255.

Molenberghs, G. and Verbeke, G. (2005) *Models for Discrete Longitudinal Data*. New York: Springer.

Molenberghs, G. and Verbeke, G. (2006) Likelihood ratio, score, and Wald tests in a constrained parameter space. *American Statistician*, **61**, 1–6.

Molenberghs, G., Kenward, M. G., and Lesaffre, E. (1997) The analysis of longitudinal ordinal data with non-random dropout. *Biometrika*, **84**, 33–44.

Molenberghs, G., Michiels, B., and Kenward, M.G. (1998a) Pseudo-likelihood for combined selection and pattern-mixture models for missing data problems. *Biometrical Journal*, **40**, 557–572.

Molenberghs, G., Michiels, B., Kenward, M.G., and Diggle, P.J. (1998b) Missing data mechanisms and pattern-mixture models. *Statistica Neerlandica*, **52**, 153–161.

Molenberghs, G., Goetghebeur, E.J.T., Lipsitz, S.R., Kenward, M.G. (1999a) Non-random missingness in categorical data: strengths and limitations. *American Statistician*, **53**, 110–118.

Molenberghs, G., Michiels, B., and Lipsitz, S.R. (1999b) A pattern-mixture odds ratio model for incomplete categorical data. *Communications in Statistics: Theory and Methods*, **28**, 2843–2869.

Molenberghs, G., Kenward, M.G., and Goetghebeur, E. (2001a) Sensitivity analysis for incomplete contingency tables: the Slovenian plebiscite case. *Applied Statistics*, **50**, 15–29.

Molenberghs, G., Verbeke, G., Thijs, H., Lesaffre, E., and Kenward, M.G. (2001b) Mastitis in dairy cattle: influence analysis to assess sensitivity of the dropout process. *Computational Statistics and Data Analysis*, **37**, 93–113.

Molenberghs, G., Thijs, H., Jansen, I., Beunckens, C., Kenward, M.G., Mallinckrodt, C., and Carroll, R.J. (2004) Analyzing incomplete longitudinal clinical trial data. *Biostatistics*, **5**, 445–464.

Molenberghs, G., Beunckens, C., Jansen, I., Thijs, H., Van Steen, K., Verbeke, G., and Kenward, M.G. (2005) The analysis of incomplete data. In C. Chuang-Stein and R. D'Agostino (eds), *Pharmaceutical Statistics with SAS*. Cary, NC: SAS Publishing.

Murray, G.D. and Findlay, J.G. (1988) Correcting for the bias caused by drop-outs in hypertension trials. *Statistics in Medicine*, **7**, 941–946.

Muthén, B., Kaplan, D., and Hollis, M. (1987) On structural equation modeling with data that are not missing completely at random. *Psychometrika*, **52**, 431–462.

Nelder, J.A. and Mead, R. (1965) A simplex method for function minimisation. *Computer Journal*, **7**, 303–313.

Nelder, J.A. and Wedderburn, R.W.M. (1972) Generalized linear models. *Journal of the Royal Statistical Society, Series B*, **135**, 370–384.

Newey, W.K. (1990) Semiparametric efficiency bounds. *Journal of Applied Econometrics*, **5**, 99–135.

Nordheim, E.V. (1984) Inference from nonrandomly missing categorical data: an example from a genetic study on Turner's syndrome. *Journal of the American Statistical Association*, **79**, 772–780.

Park, T. and Brown, M.B. (1994) Models for categorical data with nonignorable nonresponse. *Journal of the American Statistical Association*, **89**, 44–52.

Patel, H.I. (1991) Analysis of incomplete data from clinical trials with repeated measurements. *Biometrika*, **78**, 609–619.

Pawitan, Y. and Self, S. (1993) Modeling disease marker processes in AIDS. *Journal of the American Statistical Association*, **88**, 719–726.

Philips, M.J. (1993) Contingency tables with missing data. *The Statistician*, **42**, 9–18.

Pharmacological Therapy for Macular Degeneration Study Group (1997) Interferon α-IIA is ineffective for patients with choroidal neovascularization secondary to age-related macular degeneration. Results of a prospective randomized placebo-controlled clinical trial. *Archives of Ophthalmology*, **115**, 865–872.

Piantadosi, S. (1997) *Clinical Trials: A Methodologic Perspective*. New York: John Wiley & Sons, Inc.

Pinheiro, J.C. and Bates, D.M. (1995). Approximations to the log-likelihood function in the nonlinear mixed-effects model. *Journal of Computational and Graphical Statistics*, **4**, 12–35.

Pinheiro, J.C. and Bates, D.M. (2000) *Mixed Effects Models in S and S-Plus*. New York: Springer.

Potthoff, R.F. and Roy, S.N. (1964) A generalized multivariate analysis of variance model useful especially for growth curve problems. *Biometrika*, **51**, 313–326.

Prasad, N.G.N. and Rao, J.N.K. (1990) The estimation of mean squared error of small-area estimators. *Journal of the American Statistical Association*, **85**, 163–171.

Press, W.H., Teukolsky, S.A., Vetterling, W.T., and Flannery, B.P. (1992) *Numerical Recipes in FORTRAN* (2nd edn). Cambridge: Cambridge University Press.

Quenouille, M.H. (1956) Notes on bias in estimation. *Biometrika*, **43**, 353–360.

Redner, R.A. and Walker, H.F. (1984) Mixture densities, maximum likelihood, and the EM algorithm. *SIAM Review*, **26**, 195–239.

Reisberg, B., Borenstein, J., Salob, S.P., Ferris, S.H., Franssen, E., and Georgotas, A. (1987) Behavioral symptoms in Alzheimer's disease: phenomenology and treatment. *Journal of Clinical Psychiatry*, **48**, 9–13.

Renard, D., Geys, H., Molenberghs, G., Burzykowski, T., and Buyse, M. (2002) Validation of surrogate endpoints in multiple randomized clinical trials with discrete outcomes. *Biometrical Journal*, **44**, 921–935.

Rizopoulos, D., Verbeke, G., and Molenberghs, G. (2006) Shared parameter models under random-effects misspecifications. Submitted for publication.

Roberts, D.T. (1992) Prevalence of dermatophyte onychomycosis in the United Kingdom: results of an omnibus survey, *British Journal of Dermatology*, **126** (Suppl. 39), 23–27.

Robins, J.M. and Gill, R. (1997) Non-respone models for the analysis of non-monotone ignorable missing data. *Statistics in Medicine*, **16**, 39–56.

Robins, J.M. and Rotnitzky, A. (1995) Semiparametric efficiency in multivariate regression models with missing data. *Journal of the Americal Statistical Association*, **90**, 122–129.

Robins, J.M., Rotnitzky, A., and Zhao, L.P. (1994) Estimation of regression coeficients when some regressors are not always observed. *Journal of the Americal Statistical Association*, **89**, 846–866.

Robins, J.M., Rotnitzky, A., and Zhao, L.P. (1995) Analysis of semiparametric regression models for repeated outcomes in the presence of missing data. *Journal of the American Statistical Association*, **90**, 106–121.

Robins, J.M., Rotnitzky, A., and Scharfstein, D.O. (1998) Semiparametric regression for repeated outcomes with non-ignorable non-response. *Journal of the American Statistical Association*, **93**, 1321–1339.

Rosenbaum, P.R. and Rubin, D.B. (1983) The central role of the propensity score method in observational studies for causal effects. *Biometrika*, **70**, 41–55.

Rotnitzky, A. and Robins, J.M. (1995) Semi-parametric estimation of models for means and covariances in the presence of missing data. *Scandinavian Journal of Statistics*, **22**, 323–334.

Rotnitzky, A. and Robins, J.M. (1997) Analysis of semi-parametric regression models for repeated outcomes in the presence of missing data. *Statistics in Medicine*, **16**, 81–102.

Rotnitzky, A. and Wypij, D. (1994). A note on the bias of estimators with missing data. *Biometrics*, **50**, 1163–1170.

Rotnitzky, A., Cox, D.R., Bottai, M., and Robins, J. (2000) Likelihood-based inference with singular information matrix. *Bernouilli*, **6**, 243–284.

X Rubin, D.B. (1976) Inference and missing data. *Biometrika*, **63**, 581–592.

Rubin, D.B. (1977) Formalizing subjective notions about the effect of nonrespondents in sample surveys. *Journal of the American Statistical Association*, **72**, 538–543.

Rubin, D.B. (1978) Multiple imputations in sample surveys – a phenomenological Bayesian approach to nonresponse. In *Imputation and Editing of Faulty or Missing Survey Data*, pp. 1–23. Washington, DC: US Department of Commerce.

Rubin, D.B. (1987) *Multiple Imputation for Nonresponse in Surveys*. New York: John Wiley & Sons, Inc.

Rubin, D.B. (1994) Discussion of Diggle, P.J. and Kenward, M.G.: Informative dropout in longitudinal data analysis. *Applied Statistics*, **43**, 80–82.

Rubin, D.B. (1996) Multiple imputation after 18+ years. *Journal of the American Statistical Association*, **91**, 473–489.

Rubin, D.B. and Schenker, N. (1986) Multiple imputation for interval estimation from simple random samples with ignorable nonresponse. *Journal of the American Statistical Association*, **81**, 366–374.

Rubin, D.B., Stern H.S., and Vehovar V. (1995) Handling 'don't know' survey responses: the case of the Slovenian plebiscite. *Journal of the American Statistical Association*, **90**, 822–828.

Satterthwaite, F.E. (1941) Synthesis of variance. *Psychometrika*, **6**, 309–316.

Schafer J.L. (1997) *Analysis of Incomplete Multivariate Data*. London: Chapman & Hall.

Schafer, J.L. (1999) Multiple imputation: a primer. *Statistical Methods in Medical Research*, **8**, 3–15.

Schafer, J.L. and Schenker, N. (2000) Inference with imputed conditional means. *Journal of the American Statistical Association*, **95**, 144–154.

Schafer J.L., Khare M., and Ezatti-Rice T.M. (1993) Multiple imputation of missing data in NHANES III. In *Proceedings of the Annual Research Conference*, pp. 459–487. Washington, DC: Bureau of the Census.

Scharfstein, D.O., Rotnitzky, A., and Robins, J.M. (1999) Adjusting for nonignorable drop-out using semiparametric nonresponse models (with discussion). *Journal of the Americal Statistical Association*, **94**, 1096–1146.

Schipper, H., Clinch, J., McMurray, A., and Levitt, M. (1984) Measuring the quality of life of cancer patients: the Functional Living Index-Cancer: development and validation. *Journal of Clinical Oncology*, **2**, 472–483.

Schluchter, M.D. (1992) Methods for the analysis of informatively censored longitudinal data. *Statistics in Medicine*, **11**, 1861–1870.

Seber, G.A.F. (1984) *Multivariate Observations*. New York: John Wiley & Sons, Inc.

Selvin, S. (1996) *Statistical Analysis of Epidemiologic Data*. New York: Oxford University Press.

Sheiner, L.B., Beal, S.L., and Dunne, A. (1997) Analysis of nonrandomly censored ordered categorical longitudinal data from analgesic trials. *Journal of the American Statistical Association*, **92**, 1235–1244.

Shih, W.J. and Quan, H. (1997) Testing for treatment differences with dropouts in clinical trials – a composite approach. *Statistics in Medicine*, **16**, 1225–1239.

Siddiqui, O. and Ali, M.W. (1998) A comparison of the random-effects pattern-mixture model with last-observation-carried-forward (LOCF) analysis in longitudinal clinical trials with dropouts. *Journal of Biopharmaceutical Statistics*, **8**, 545–563.

Skrondal, A. and Rabe-Hesketh, S. (2004) *Generalized Latent Variable Modeling*. Boca Raton, FL: Chapman & Hall/CRC.

Stasny, E.A. (1986) Estimating gross flows using panel data with nonresponse: an example from the Canadian Labour Force Survey. *Journal of the American Statistical Association*, **81**, 42–47.

Stram, D.O. and Lee, J.W. (1994) Variance components testing in the longitudinal mixed effects model. *Biometrics*, **50**, 1171–1177.

Stram, D.A. and Lee, J.W. (1995) Correction to: Variance components testing in the longitudinal mixed effects model. *Biometrics*, **51**, 1196.

Tanner, M.A. and Wong, W.H. (1987) The calculation of posterior distributions by data augmentation. *Journal of the American Statistical Association*, **82**, 528–550.

Taylor, J.M.G., Cumberland, W.G., and Sy, J.P. (1994) A stochastic model for analysis of longitudinal AIDS data. *Journal of the American Statistical Association*, **89**, 727–736.

Taylor, M.G., Cooper, K.L., Wei, J.T., Sarma, A.V., Raghunathan. T.E., and Heeringa, S.G. (2002) Use of multiple imputation to correct for nonresponse bias in a survey of urologic symptoms among African-American men. *American Journal of Epidemiology*, **156**, 774–782.

Thijs, H., Molenberghs, G., and Verbeke, G. (2000) The milk protein trial: influence analysis of the dropout process. *Biometrical Journal*, **42**, 617–646.

Thijs, H., Molenberghs, G., Michiels, B., Verbeke, G., and Curran, D. (2002) Strategies to fit pattern-mixture models. *Biostatistics*, **3**, 245–265.

Tierny, L. and Kadane, J.B. (1986) Accurate approximations for posterior moments and marginal densities. *Journal of the American Statistical Association*, **81**, 82–86.

Troxel, A.B., Harrington, D.P., and Lipsitz, S.R. (1998) Analysis of longitudinal data with non-ignorable non-monotone missing values. *Applied Statistics*, **47**, 425–438.

Tsiatis, A.A. (2006) *Semiparametric Theory and Missing Data*. New York: Springer.

Tsiatis, A.A., DeGruttola, V., and Wulfsohn, M.S. (1995) Modeling the relationship of survival to longitudinal data measured with error. Applications to survival and CD4 counts in patients with AIDS. *Journal of the American Statistical Association*, **90**, 27–37.

Tuerlinckx, F., Rijmen, F., Molenberghs, G., Verbeke, G., Briggs, D., Van den Noortgate, W., Meulders, M., and De Boeck, P. (2004) Estimation and software. In P. De Boeck and M. Wilson (eds), *Explanatory Item Response Models: A Generalized Linear and Nonlinear Approach*, pp. 343–373, New York: Springer.

Vach, W. and Blettner, M. (1995) Logistic regresion with incompletely observed categorical covariates – investigating the sensitivity against violation of the missing at random assumption. *Statistics in Medicine*, **12**, 1315–1330.

Van Buuren, S., Boshuizen, H.C., and Knook, D.L. (1999) Multiple imputation of missing blood pressure covariates in survival analysis. *Statistics in Medicine*, **18**, 681–694.

Van der Laan M.J. and Robins, J. (2003) *Unified Methods for Censored Longitudinal Data and Causality*. New York: Springer.

Van Steen, K., Molenberghs, G., Verbeke, G., and Thijs, H. (2001) A local influence approach to sensitivity analysis of incomplete longitudinal ordinal data. *Statistical Modelling*, **1**, 125–142.

Vansteelandt, S., Goetghebeur, E., Kenward, M.G., and Molenberghs, G. (2006) Ignorance and uncertainty regions as inferential tools in a sensitivity analysis. *Statistica Sinica*, **16**, 953–979.

Verbeke, G. and Lesaffre, E. (1996) A linear mixed-effects model with heterogeneity in the random-effects population. *Journal of the American Statistical Association*, **91**, 217–221.

Verbeke, G. and Lesaffre, E. (1997) The effect of misspecifying the random-effects distribution in linear mixed models for longitudinal data. *Computational Statistics and Data Analysis*, **23**, 541–556.

Verbeke, G. and Molenberghs, G. (1997) *Linear Mixed Models in Practice: A SAS-Oriented Approach*, Lecture Notes in Statistics 126. New York: Springer.

Verbeke, G. and Molenberghs, G. (2000) *Linear Mixed Models for Longitudinal Data*. New York: Springer.

Verbeke, G. and Molenberghs, G. (2003) The use of score tests for inference on variance components. *Biometrics*, **59**, 254–262.

Verbeke, G., Lesaffre, E., and Spiessens, B. (2001a) The practical use of different strategies to handle dropout in longitudinal studies. *Drug Information Journal*, **35**, 419–434.

Verbeke, G., Molenberghs, G., Thijs, H., Lesaffre, E., and Kenward, M.G. (2001b) Sensitivity analysis for non-random dropout: a local influence approach. *Biometrics*, **57**, 7–14.

Verbyla, A.P. and Cullis, B.R. (1990) Modelling in repeated measures experiments. *Applied Statistics*, **39**, 341–356.

Verdonck, A., De Ridder, L., Verbeke, G., Bourguignon, J.P., Carels, C., Kuhn, E.R., Darras, V., and de Zegher, F. (1998). Comparative effects of neonatal and prepubertal castration on craniofacial growth in rats. *Archives of Oral Biology*, **43**, 861–871.

Wang-Clow, F., Lange, N., Laird, N.M., and Ware, J.H. (1995) A simulation study of estimators for rate of change in longitudinal studies with attrition. *Statistics in Medicine*, **14**, 283–297.

Ware, J.H., Dockery, D.W., Spiro, A., III, Speizer, F.E., and Ferris, B.G., Jr. (1984) Passive smoking, gas cooking, and respiratory health of children living in six cities. *American Review of Respiratory Diseases*, **129**, 366–374.

White, I.R. and Goetghebeur, E.J.T. (1998) Clinical trials comparing two treatment policies: which aspects of the treatment policies make a difference? *Statistics in Medicine*, **17**, 319–339.

Wolfinger, R. and O'Connell, M. (1993) Generalized linear mixed models: a pseudo-likelihood approach. *Journal of Statistical Computation and Simulation*, **48**, 233–243.

Woolson, R.F. and Clarke, W.R. (1984) Analysis of categorical incomplete longitudinal data. *Journal of the Royal Statistical Society, Series A*, **147**, 87–99.

Wu, M.C. and Bailey, K.R. (1988) Analysing changes in the presence of informative right censoring caused by death and withdrawal. *Statistics in Medicine*, **7**, 337–346.

Wu, M.C. and Bailey, K.R. (1989) Estimation and comparison of changes in the presence of informative right censoring: conditional linear model. *Biometrics*, **45**, 939–955.

Wu, M.C. and Carroll, R.J. (1988) Estimation and comparison of changes in the presence of informative right censoring by modeling the censoring process. *Biometrics*, **44**, 175–188.

Wulfsohn, M.S. and Tsiatis, A.A. (1997) A joint model for survival and longitudinal data measured with error. *Biometrics*, **53**, 330–339.

Xu, J. and Zeger, S.L. (2001) Joint analysis of longitudinal data comprising repeated measures and times to events. *Applied Statistics*, **50**, 375–387.

Zeger, S.L. and Liang, K.-Y. (1986) Longitudinal data analysis for discrete and continuous outcomes. *Biometrics*, **42**, 121–130.

Index

Missing Data in Clinical Studies   G. Molenberghs and M.G. Kenward
© 2007 John Wiley & Sons, Ltd

Statistics in Practice

Human and Biological Sciences

Berger – Selection Bias and Covariate Imbalances in Randomized Clinical Trials
Brown and Prescott – Applied Mixed Models in Medicine, Second Edition
Chevret (Ed) – Statistical Methods for Dose Finding Experiments
Ellenberg, Fleming and DeMets – Data Monitoring Committees in Clinical Trials:
A Practical Perspective
Hauschke, Steinijans and Pigeot – Bioequivalence Studies in Drug Development:
Methods and Applications
Lawson, Browne and Vidal Rodeiro – Disease Mapping with WinBUGS and
MLwiN
Lui – Statistical Estimation of Epidemiological Risk
*Marubini and Valsecchi – Analysing Survival Data from Clinical Trials and
Observation Studies
O'Hagan – Uncertain Judgements: Eliciting Experts' Probabilities
Parmigiani – Modeling in Medical Decision Making: A Bayesian Approach
Senn – Cross-over Trials in Clinical Research, Second Edition
Senn – Statistical Issues in Drug Development
Spiegelhalter, Abrams and Myles – Bayesian Approaches to Clinical Trials and
Health-Care Evaluation
Whitehead – Design and Analysis of Sequential Clinical Trials, Revised Second
Edition
Whitehead – Meta-Analysis of Controlled Clinical Trials
Willan – Statistical Analysis of Cost-effectiveness Data

Earth and Environmental Sciences

Buck, Cavanagh and Litton – Bayesian Approach to Interpreting Archaeological
Data
Glasbey and Horgan – Image Analysis in the Biological Sciences
Helsel – Nondetects and Data Analysis: Statistics for Censored Environmental
Data
McBride – Using Statistical Methods for Water Quality Management
Webster and Oliver – Geostatistics for Environmental Scientists

Industry, Commerce and Finance

Aitken – Statistics and the Evaluation of Evidence for Forensic Scientists, Second Edition
Balding – Weight-of-evidence for Forensic DNA Profiles
Lehtonen and Pahkinen – Practical Methods for Design and Analysis of Complex Surveys, Second Edition
Ohser and Mücklich – Statistical Analysis of Microstructures in Materials Science
Taroni, Aitken, Garbolino and Biedermann – Bayesian Networks and Probabilistic Inference in Forensic Science

*Now available in paperback